# CRITICAL CARE NURSING SECRETS

# CRITICAL CARE NURSING SECRETS

## Hildy M. Schell, RN, MS, CCRN

Clinical Nurse Specialist, Adult Critical Care
Department of Nursing
University of California at San Francisco Medical Center
Assistant Clinical Professor
Department of Physiological Nursing
School of Nursing
University of California, San Francisco
San Francisco, California

## Kathleen A. Puntillo, RN, DNSc, FAAN

Associate Professor of Nursing
Director, Critical Care/Trauma Graduate Program
Department of Physiological Nursing
School of Nursing
University of California, San Francisco
San Francisco, California

HANLEY & BELFUS, INC./ Philadelphia

Publisher:     HANLEY & BELFUS, INC.
               Medical Publishers
               210 South 13th Street
               Philadelphia, PA 19107
               (215) 546-7293; 800-962-1892
               FAX (215) 790-9330
               Web site: http://www.hanleyandbelfus.com

Note *to the reader*: Although the information in this book has been carefully reviewed for correctness of dosage and indications, neither the authors nor the editors nor the publisher can accept any legal responsibility for any errors or omissions that may be made. Neither the publisher nor the editors make any warranty, expressed or implied, with respect to the material contained herein. Before prescribing any drug, the reader must review the manufacturer's current product information (package inserts) for accepted indications, absolute dosage recommendations, and other information pertinent to the safe and effective use of the product described.

Library of Congress Cataloging-in-Publication Data

Critical care nursing secrets / edited by Hildy M. Schell, Kathleen A. Puntillo.
        p. ; cm.—(The Secrets Series®)
    Includes bibliographical references and index.
    ISBN 1-56053-454-0 (alk. paper)
       1. Intensive care nursing—Examinations, questions, etc.  I. Schell, Hildy M, 1965-
II. Puntillo, Kathleen A.  III. Series.
    |DNLM: 1. Critical Care—methods—Examination Questions.  2. Critical
Illness—nursing—Examination Questions.  3. Nursing Care—methods—Examination
Questions.  WY 18.2 C9345 2001|
    RT120.15 C777 2001
    610.73'61—dc 21
                                                                        00-058132

**CRITICAL CARE NURSING SECRETS**                    ISBN 1-56053-454-0

Last digit is the print number:   9  8  7  6  5  4  3  2

## DEDICATION

To my dear husband, Mike Chaple, for his support and patience throughout this project, and to my son, Alex, for the love and joy he brings to this world.

Hildy

To my students in critical care nursing—past, present, and future—who make a difference in the lives of critically ill patients and families. And to my husband, Richard, who makes the biggest difference in my life.

Kathleen

# CONTENTS

## II. RESPIRATORY SYSTEM

## III. INFECTION CONTROL, HEMATOLOGY, ONCOLOGY, AND IMMUNOLOGY

# CONTRIBUTORS

**Gabull M. Abdullah, RN, MS, ACNP**
Acute Care Nurse Practitioner, Cardiac Services, Kaiser Permanente, San Francisco, California

**Mary G. Adams, RN, MS**
Critical Care Educator, University of California at San Francisco Medical Center, and Instructor, San Francisco State University School of Nursing, San Francisco, California

**Lisa M. Boulais, RN, MS, CCRN, CEN**
Clinical Nurse Specialist, Emergency Department, Stanford Hospital and Clinics, Stanford, California

**Suzanne M. Burns, RN, MSN, RRT, ACNP-CS, CCRN**
Associate Professor of Nursing and Clinician 5, Acute and Specialty Care (School of Nursing) and Medical Intensive Care, University of Virginia Health System, Charlottesville, Virginia

**Debra Busta-Moore, RN, MS**
Clinical Nurse Specialist, Lactation Specialist, University of California at San Francisco Medical Center, San Francisco, California

**Kristina J. Carson, RN, MS**
San Jose, California

**Vicki Casella-Gordon, RN, MS, CCRN**
Clinical Nurse Specialist, Critical Care, Kaiser Permanente, Walnut Creek, California

**Lisa J. Cianfichi, MS, RN, NP**
Nurse Practitioner, Interventional Cardiology, University of California at Los Angeles, Los Angeles, California

**Heidi D. Clay, RN, MS, CCRN, CCNS**
Clinical Nurse Specialist, Department of Neurosurgery, University of California at San Francisco Medical Center, San Francisco, California

**Christine M. Corcoran, RN, MS**
Nurse Coordinator, Division of Vascular Surgery, Stanford Hospital and Clinics, Stanford, California

**Linda M. Couts, RN, MS, ACNP-CS, CEN, MICN**
Acute Care Nurse Practitioner, Cardiovascular Unit, Porter Adventist Hospital, Denver, Colorado

**Ann Marie Daleiden, RN, BA**
Patient Care Manager, Interventional Cardiology, Hospital Department, University of California at San Francisco Medical Center Hospital, San Francisco, California

**Brian M. Daniel, RCP, RRT**
Clinical Coordinator, Respiratory Care Service and Cardiovascular Research; Assistant Clinical Professor, UCSF School of Nursing, University of California at San Francisco, San Francisco, California

**Lisa J. Day, RN, PhD**
Assistant Clinical Professor, Department of Physiological Nursing, School of Nursing, University of California, San Francisco, San Francisco, California

**Debbie L. Dempel, RN, BSN, CCRN**
Clinical Nurse, Intensive Cardiac Care, University of California at San Francisco Medical Center, San Francisco, California

**Margaret H. Doherty, RN, MSN, CCRN**
Assistant Professor, Department of Nursing, Sonoma State University, Rohnert Park; Staff Nurse, ICU, Petaluma Valley Hospital, Petaluma, California

**Siobhan M. Geary, RN, MS**
Clinical Nurse Specialist, Sutter Medical Center, Sacramento; Assistant Clinical Professor, Department
of Physiological Nursing, School of Nursing, University of California, San Francisco, California

**Sheila Kathleen Gleeson, RN, BSN**
Assistant Patient Care Manager, Department of Nursing, University of California at San Francisco
Medical Center, San Francisco, California

**Laura Greicus, RN, MSN, ACNP, CCRN**
Registered Nurse Practitioner, Medicine, Veterans Affairs Medical Center, Menlo Park, California

**Theresa Lynn Griffin, RN, MS, CCRN, TNCC**
Clinical Nurse Specialist, Medical/Surgical/Trauma ICU, Department of Nursing, Stanford Hospital
and Clinics, Palo Alto, California

**Stacey Anne Hallatt, RN, MS**
Clinical Nurse III, Intensive Care Unit, University of California at San Francisco Medical Center, San
Francisco, California

**KellyJane Harris, RN, MS, CEN, CCRN**
Staff Nurse, Emergency Department, Kaiser Permanente Medical Center, Vallejo, California

**Lynn Houweling, RN, MS, CCRN**
Clinical Nurse II, Intensive Cardiac Care Unit, University of California, San Francisco, San Francisco,
California

**Jill N. Howie, RN, CS, MS, ACNP**
Assistant Clinical Professor and Director, Acute Care Nurse Practitioner Program, Department of
Physiological Nursing, School of Nursing, University of California, San Francisco, San Francisco,
California

**Cheryl Hubner, RN, MS**
Associate Clinical Professor, Department of Physiological Nursing, School of Nursing, University of
California, San Francisco, and Veterans Affairs Medical Center, San Francisco, California

**Brigid Ide, MS, RN**
Clinical Nurse Specialist in Cardiology and Director of Clinical Resource Management, University of
California at San Francisco Medical Center; Assistant Clinical Professor, School of Nursing,
University of California, San Francisco, San Francisco, California

**Maribeth Inturrisi, RN, MS**
Clinical Nurse Specialist, High-Risk Obstetrics; University of California at San Francisco Medical
Center; Assistant Professor, Department of Family Health Care Nursing, University of California, San
Francisco, San Francisco, California

**Kris Ishii, MS, PT, CCS**
Assistant Clinical Professor, Department of Physical Therapy and Rehabilitative Science, UCSF/SFSU
Graduate Program in Physical Therapy; Cardiopulmonary Clinical Specialist, University of California
at San Francisco Medical Center, San Francisco, California

**Marilyn L. Jordan, RN, BS, MPH**
Infection Control Practitioner, University of California at San Francisco Medical Center, San
Francisco; Kaiser Foundation Hospital, San Rafael, California

**Roberta Kaplow, RN, PhD, CCNS, CCRN**
Critical Care Nurse Educator, Department of Nursing Education, Memorial Sloan-Kettering Cancer
Center, New York, New York

**Steven R. Kayser, PharmD**
Clinical Professor of Pharmacy, Department of Clinical Pharmacy, School of Pharmacy, University of
California at San Francisco, San Francisco, California

**S. Jill Ley, RN, MS, CCRN, CNS**
Clinical Nurse Specialist, Cardiac Revascularization, California Pacific Medical Center; Associate Clinical Professor, University of California, San Francisco, San Francisco, California

**Lori Kennedy Madden, RN, MS, ACNP**
Nurse Practitioner, Department of Neurological Surgery, University of California at Davis, Sacramento, California

**Robin D. Marci, RN, MS, CCRN**
Clinical Instructor, Department of Nursing, Sonoma State University, Rohnert Park; Clinical Nurse Specialist, Inpatient Nursing, Kaiser Medical Center, San Rafael, California

**Martie Mattson, RN, MSN, CCRN**
Clinical Education Specialist, Critical Care, Department of Nursing Education, California Pacific Medical Center, San Francisco, California

**Christine L. Nelson, BSN, RN, CCRN**
Staff Nurse, Surgical Intensive Care Unit, David Grant Medical Center, Travis Air Force Base, California

**Colleen O'Leary-Kelley, RN, MS, CNSN**
Doctoral student, Department of Physiological Nursing, University of California, San Francisco, San Francisco, California

**Anna Omery, RN, DNSc**
Nurse Scientist and Director of Nursing Research, Patient Care Services, California Division, Kaiser Permanente, Pasadena, California

**Kathleen A. Puntillo, RN, DNSc, FAAN**
Associate Professor of Nursing, Director, Critical Care/Trauma Graduate Program, University of California at San Francisco Medical Center; Department of Physiological Nursing, School of Nursing, University of California, San Francisco, San Francisco, California

**Mary Reid-Finlay, RN, MS, ACNP, CCRN, OCN**
Clinical Nurse, Department of Nursing, Memorial Sloan Kettering Cancer Center, New York, New York

**Celia Rifkin, RN, BSN**
Heart and Lung Transplant Coordinator, Department of Cardiothoracic Surgery, University of California, San Francisco, San Francisco, California

**Ted S. Rigney, RN, MS, ACNP**
The Permanente Medical Group, Cardiovascular Services, Kaiser Hospital, San Francisco, California

**Susan L. Robertson, RN, MS, CNN**
Research Coordinator, Department of Medicine, Division of Nephrology, University of California at San Francisco Medical Center, University of California, San Francisco, San Francisco, California

**Sandra C. Rowlee, MS, RN, CNS, ACNP-CS**
Trauma Nurse Practitioner, Trauma Program, Mercy San Juan Hospital, Carmichael, California

**Nancy Ann Rudisill, RN, MSN**
Research Coordinator, Department of Neurological Surgery, University of California at Davis, Sacramento, California

**Hildy M. Schell, RN, MS, CCRN**
Clinical Nurse Specialist, Adult Critical Care, Department of Nursing, University of California at San Francisco Medical Center; Assistant Clinical Professor, Department of Physiological Nursing, School of Nursing, University of California, San Francisco, San Francisco, California

**Dianne Marie Schultz, RN, BS, BSN**
Clinical Nurse III, Intensive Care Unit, Department of Nursing, University of California, San Francisco, San Francisco, California

**Dianne L. Sodt-Davitt, RN, BS**
Nursing Services, University of Michigan, Ann Arbor, Michigan

**Daphne Stannard, RN, PhD**
Assistant Professor, San Francisco State University School of Nursing, San Francisco, California;
Assistant Clinical Professor and Critical Care Educator, University of California at San Francisco
Medical Center, San Francisco, California

**James R. Stotts, RN, MS**
Clinical Nurse Specialist, Cardiology, Stanford Hospital and Clinics, Stanford; Adjunct Clinical
Faculty, University of California at San Francisco Medical Center; Department of Physiological
Nursing, School of Nursing, University of California, San Francisco, San Francisco, California

**Nancy A. Stotts, RN, EdD**
Professor, Department of Physiological Nursing, School of Nursing, University of California, San
Francisco, San Francisco, California

**Margaret M. Sullivan, RN**
Clinical Nurse III, Intensive Care Unit, Department of Nursing, University of California at San
Francisco Medical Center, San Francisco, California

**Jeffrey L. Tarnow, RRT**
Adult Clinical Coordinator, Department of Respiratory Care; Clinical Research Coordinator,
Department of Anesthesia, University of California, San Francisco, San Francisco, California

**Evelyn Taverna, RN, MS, CCRN**
Cardiology Clinical Nurse Specialist, California Pacific Medical Center, San Francisco, California;
Assistant Clinical Professor, Department of Physiological Nursing, School of Nursing, University of
California, San Francisco, San Francisco, California

**Carrie Ann Taylor, RN, MS, CCRN**
Auxiliary Clinical Faculty, Adult Health and Illness, Ohio State University, Columbus, Ohio

**Charlene Trouillot, RN, MS, ANP**
Oncology Nurse Practitioner, University of Colorado Cancer Center, Denver, Colorado

**Carol S. Viele, RN, MS**
Clinical Nurse Specialist, Hematology/Oncology, University of California at San Francisco Medical
Center; Assistant Clinical Professor, Department of Physiological Nursing, School of Nursing,
University of California, San Francisco, San Francisco, California

**Kathleen M. Vollman, MSN, RN, CCNS, CCRN**
Clinical Nurse Specialist, Medical Critical Care, Henry Ford Hospital, Detroit, Michigan

**Mariann M. Ward, RN, MS, ANP-CS**
Nurse Practitioner and Clinical Nurse Specialist, Department of Neurological Surgery, University of
California, San Francisco, San Francisco, California

**Charles L. Witherell, RN, CS, MSN**
Assistant Clinical Professor of Nursing, Department of Physiological Nursing, School of Nursing,
University of California, San Francisco; Clinical Nurse Specialist, Department of Electrophysiology,
University of California at San Francisco Medical Center, San Francisco, California

# PREFACE

The care of critically ill patients is becoming increasingly more complex. Critical care nurses, working in the rapid-paced ICU environment, need a quick reference to consult for answers to the many questions about a patient's disease process, key assessment criteria, therapies, and patient care issues. This book is designed to help both experienced and inexperienced nurses understand the important aspects of monitoring and managing their critically ill patients. For example, this book can help the new critical care nurse perform a basic interpretation of an ECG rhythm strip as well as provide the preceptor or experienced nurse the rationale for potassium replacement for the patient with diabetic ketoacidosis and normal potassium. This book focuses on essential "what," "why," and "how" questions of patient assessment, monitoring, and therapeutic interventions for critical care patients. It provides evidence-based information as well as clinical pearls of wisdom from many expert clinicians. We hope that this book provides nurses information that will enhance their clinical practice and positively impact their patients, from early detection or symptom management to interventions that affect survival.

We would like to acknowledge and thank our interdisciplinary team of nurses, care assistants, physicians, respiratory therapists, nutritionists, pharmacologists, social workers, and physical therapists for their contributions to this book and for their dedication to the highest quality of care for their critically ill patients. We would also like to thank the many patients and families that we have cared for in our clinical practices. They have been our best teachers.

Hildy M. Schell, RN, MS, CCRN
Kathleen A. Puntillo, RN, DNSc, FAAN

# I. Cardiovascular System

# 1. CARDIAC ASSESSMENT

*Lisa J. Cianfichi, RN, MS, NP*

**1. What are the key components in the cardiac history?**

History-taking is a vital component before the cardiac physical examination. It guides appropriate diagnosis and helps to determine whether the patient has a cardiac problem. The history assessment can prevent unnecessary diagnostic tests, thus decreasing pain, stress, and cost.

It is important to gather specific information about the problem by asking key questions about the onset, character, location, severity, frequency, and duration of pain; associated symptoms (e.g., fatigue, cough, dyspnea on exertion or at rest, claudication, peripheral edema, palpitations, cyanosis, dizziness, and syncope); precipitating factors; and alleviating factors. Other essential information includes a list of medications, family history, medical history, surgical history, allergies to medications, social history, and review of systems. Asking questions related to each system helps to formulate a diagnosis and rule out other active problems.

**2. How do I begin the cardiac physical examination?**

The clinician should stand on the patient's right side. Begin with general inspection, which includes assessment of skin, eyes, arteries, veins, and precordium. Proceed to palpation of the arteries and precordium, followed by percussion and auscultation of the precordium. This systematic approach helps to avoid oversight of key elements.

**3. How are the peripheral arterial pulses assessed?**

Peripheral arterial pulses should be inspected and palpated bilaterally. Examine the skin for cyanosis, pallor, warmth, and breakdown. Palpate bilateral peripheral pulses and grade them on a scale of 0–4:

| | |
|---|---|
| 0 | absent pulse |
| 1+ | diminished pulse |
| 2+ | normal pulse |
| 3+ | increased pulse |
| 4+ | hyperdynamic pulse |

Hyperdynamic pulsations with 4+ grade may suggest aortic regurgitation, thyrotoxicosis, anemia, anxiety, and possibly peripheral arteriovenous fistula.

**4. What is the difference between arterial insufficiency and venous congestion?**

With **arterial insufficiency**, peripheral pulses less than 2+ may suggest obstructive atherosclerotic disease of the aorta, iliac arteries, or femoral arteries. The following physical signs suggest chronic weak or absent arterial pulses, which usually occur distal to the artery:

1. Pallor, rubor, or cyanotic skin with atrophied muscles
2. Slow capillary refill time
3. Loss of hair, ulcerated areas, or nonhealing areas distal to the absent pulse
4. Complaints of pain with ambulation, which is relieved with rest

**Acute venous insufficiency** occurs with thrombophlebitis, which produces edema, erythema, or cyanosis in the affected area and superficial vein engorgement. Chronic venous occlusion or insufficiency may occur over time. The skin shows brown discoloration and/or edema. If possible, the patient should be examined in the supine as well as the standing position to assess for arterial and venous disorders.

### 5. What is pulsus alternans?

Pulsus alternans is the alternation between strong and weak pulsations. It can be identified when the peripheral arterial pulses are palpated. Pulsus alternans results when the damaged ventricle is unable to contract to a normal impulse. After a weak contraction, the ventricle has time to recover and produces a normal contraction. Pulsus alternans occurs in left ventricular failure due to multiple myocardial infarctions and/or dilated cardiomyopathy. Do not confuse pulsus alternans with bigeminal rhythms. Bigeminal rhythms occur with alternating sinus beats and premature ventricular contractions.

Pulsus alternans can be confirmed during auscultation of blood pressure or analysis of the arterial waveform, if an arterial line is present. When pulsus alternans and an S3 gallop are identified in patients with left ventricular failure, the prognosis is often poor.

### 6. What is a paradoxical pulse?

Paradoxical pulse is variation of the pulse with respirations. The pulse may be stronger with expiration and weaker with inspiration. Paradoxical pulse is noted with pericardial tamponade and constrictive pericarditis because inspiration decreases right and left ventricular filling and therefore left ventricular contractions. Expiration increases left ventricular filling, and the pulse is increased. Other causes of paradoxical pulse are obstructive lung disease, asthma, pulmonary embolism, hypovolemic shock, and morbid obesity. Pulsus paradoxus can be verified with invasive arterial pressure monitoring or indirect sphygmomanometry with a blood pressure cuff. During deflation, measure the difference of the first Korotkoff sound heard with expiration and the presence of Korotkoff sounds with every beat. A decrease of more than 20 mmHg in systolic pressure with inspiration is diagnostic for pulsus paradoxus.

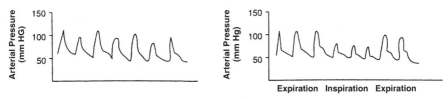

Pulsus alternans *(left)* and pulsus paradoxus *(right)*. (From Chatterjee K: Textbook of Cardiovascular Medicine. Philadelphia, Lippincott-Raven, 1998, p 297, with permission.)

### 7. How is the jugular venous pulse (JVP) measured?

First, it is important to differentiate between internal and external JVP. External jugular pulse reflects distention, whereas internal jugular pulse provides detailed information about measurement of visible pulsations in the patient's neck. Assist the patient to the supine position with the head of the bed elevated by 30–40°. Measure the pulsation from the patient's right side, which better reflects right atrial pressure. Have the patient turn his or her head toward the left, relaxing the neck muscles. The sternal angle of Louis is used as a reference point for measuring JVP because it reflects 5 cm above the right atrium. With a ruler perpendicular to the sternal angle, observe and measure the jugular pulsation with tangential light. Normal JVP is 6–7 cm.

If the JVP appears normal but the clinician is convinced that the patient is in right ventricular failure, the hepatojugular maneuver may be helpful. The clinician instructs the patient to breathe normally while applying pressure in the right upper quadrant of the abdomen for approximately 10 seconds. If right ventricular failure is present, blood volume is enhanced, causing an increase in the JVP. It may be difficult to obtain an accurate measurement of the JVP in patients with obstruction in the peripheral venous circulation.

8. **What is the difference between carotid pulsation and jugular venous pulsation?**
   • The carotid pulse rises and falls, whereas the JVP has three waves (a, c, v waves).
   • Application of pressure above the clavicle does not affect the carotid pulse but obliterates the JVP.
   • Raising the head of the bed increases the prominence of the carotid pulse but decreases JVP.
   • Application of abdominal compression does not affect the carotid pulse but may cause the JVP to increase.

9. **How are cardiac function and edema related?**
   Generalized edema is associated with congestive heart failure (CHF). The increase in central venous pressure leads to an increase in capillary pressure that increases transudation of fluid from the intravascular to the interstitial space, resulting in tissue edema. The decrease in cardiac output associated with CHF causes, in turn, a decrease in arterial blood pressure. The low pressure activates the renin-angiotensin-aldosterone system, which leads to retention of sodium and water. Edema results from gravitational factors and/or hydrostatic pressure, especially in the periphery or sacral areas. Sacral edema commonly occurs in patients with CHF during bed rest.

10. **How is edema assessed?**
    Edema causes a shiny appearance of the skin and can be depressed with palpation. Pitting edema can be quantitated by depressing the affected area and making a subjective assessment of the amount of edema:
    1+ Mild edema; 2-mm induration that quickly disappears
    2+ Moderate edema; 4-mm induration that disappears within 10–15 seconds
    3+ Moderately severe edema; 6-mm induration that takes minutes to disappear
    4+ Severe pitting edema; 8-mm induration that may take 2–5 minutes to disappear

11. **Distinguish between left ventricular and right ventricular failure.**
    Left-sided heart failure may manifest as exertional dyspnea, orthopnea, and paroxysmal dyspnea with pulmonary congestion and edema because of increased pressure in the left atrium and pulmonary veins. In contrast, right ventricular failure causes accumulation of fluid in the viscera of the abdomen and extremities secondary to increased pressure in the systemic veins and capillaries.

12. **What is the difference between a bruit and a thrill?**
    A **bruit** reflects turbulent flow in an artery and sounds like a murmur. When auscultating the carotid arteries, note whether bruits are present. They warrant further evaluation with noninvasive testing because they suggest partial obstruction of cerebral blood flow. Bruits may be present in patients with carotid atheromatous plaque, anemia, and thyrotoxicosis. In some patients with aortic stenosis, a transmitted murmur is heard over the carotid arteries. Thus, it may be difficult to differentiate between a transmitted cardiac murmur and carotid atherosclerotic plaque. Other noninvasive tests may help. The clinician should auscultate the abdominal aorta and renal arteries. A bruit may suggest obstructive renal artery lesions caused by atherosclerosis.
    A **thrill** is a palpable murmur over the base of the heart (second intercostal space at the right or left sternal border). Palpation with the palm of the nondominant hand is recommended because it is typically more sensitive with less callus. A palpable thrill may suggest disruption of blood flow in a semilunar valve (e.g., aortic stenosis or pulmonary stenosis with or without pulmonary hypertension). If the thrill is palpable, it should be accompanied by a murmur. Systolic thrills can be palpated before the apical impulse, diastolic thrills after the apical impulse.

13. **What hemodynamic parameters are important in cardiac assessment?**
    Basic vital signs include temperature, pulse, respirations, and blood pressure. Blood pressure should be obtained in bilateral upper extremities. Large discrepancies between pressures may suggest other problems, such as atherosclerotic vascular disease, dissecting aortic aneurysm, coarctation of the aorta, and supravalvular aortic stenosis.

Other important hemodynamic parameters are obtained with a pulmonary artery catheter. Although not necessary in all patients, the placement of a pulmonary artery catheter may be essential in unstable patients with an unclear diagnosis. It may help to differentiate among septic shock, cardiogenic shock, and hypovolemic shock. It also may aid in the management of patients with CHF. Right atrial pressure, pulmonary arterial pressure, pulmonary capillary wedge pressure, cardiac output, cardiac index, venous oxygen saturation, systemic vascular resistance, and pulmonary vascular resistance may help the clinician to make treatment decisions.

**14. What areas of the heart should the clinician inspect and palpate?**

1. **Pulmonic area:** located at the second intercostal space at the sternal border. Pulmonic stenosis and pulmonary hypertension may manifest as a palpable systolic thrill radiating to the left side of the neck.

2. **Aortic area:** a systolic thrill by the second intercostal space, which radiates to the right side of the neck, may suggest aortic stenosis or aortic regurgitation. An abnormal pulsation in the aortic area may suggest a dilated ascending aorta due to aneurysm or chronic regurgitation.

3. **Left parasternal area:** located in the third, fourth, and fifth intercostal parasternal spaces. A thrill in this area may suggest ventricular septal defect or tricuspid regurgitation. Abnormal pulsations may suggest right ventricular hypertrophy or dilation. A pericardial lift may indicate moderate-to-severe mitral regurgitation.

4. **Apical area:** located at the fifth intercostal space at the left midclavicular line (also known as the point of maximal impulse). A hyperdynamic apex may suggest moderate left ventricular failure or mitral or aortic regurgitation. A sustained impulse may suggest left ventricular hypertrophy.

5. **Ectopic area:** located between the pulmonary and apical areas. The clinician may observe ectopic pulsation, which is suggestive of cardiomyopathy.

6. **Epigastric area:** hepatic movements in the epigastric area are associated with tricuspid regurgitation, tricuspid stenosis, right ventricular dilatation or hypertrophy, or pulmonary hypertension due to chronic lung disease.

**15. Is percussion always used in the cardiac exam?**

No. However, if one is concerned about cardiomegaly and pericardial effusion, it may be helpful to percuss the precordial area to obtain a gross measurement. Start with the left axillary line and percuss horizontally to the sternal borders. Listen to the difference between dullness and resonance. Percussion may be of limited value in making important diagnostic decisions.

**16. What is the difference between the diaphragm and bell of the stethoscope?**

The stethoscope tubing should not be longer than 12 inches to avoid diminishing high-frequency transmission. The diaphragm of the stethoscope is used to auscultate high-pitched sounds, which include murmurs, S1, and S2. The bell of the stethoscope is used to auscultate low-pitched sounds such as S3 and S4.

**17. Describe a systematic approach to auscultating the heart.**

A systematic approach to auscultation helps to avoid missing key assessments. The heart is auscultated in the following order:

1. **Aortic area:** the second heart sound is louder than the first heart sound at the right sternal border. The first component of the S2 is the louder than the second component in this area.

2. **Pulmonic area:** the second heart sound is louder than the first heart sound. The splitting of the S2 sounds is best heard in this area.

3. **Erb's point** (also known as the second pulmonic area) is located at the third intercostal space at the left sternal border.

4. **Tricuspid area:** located at the fourth intercostal space at the left lower sternal border.

5. **Apex:** the sound of the mitral valve as it closes precedes closure of the tricuspid valve. The S1 component is louder than the S2 component.

When auscultating the heart, the clinician should palpate either the apical or carotid pulse simultaneously to help delineate systolic and diastolic cycles.

**18. Can certain patient positions help to elucidate different heart sounds?**

Yes. Different positions may help to identify murmurs not heard in the supine position.

• The supine position helps to elucidate pulmonic and tricuspid murmurs.

• The left lateral position helps to identify low-pitched diastolic rumble (e.g., mitral stenosis) or low-pitched diastolic sounds (e.g., gallops) because the heart is against the chest.

• Sitting may help to differentiate diastolic blowing murmurs with aortic regurgitation or pulmonary regurgitation at Erb's point. Have the patient sit, lean forward, and hold the breath during exhalation. This maneuver helps to identify splitting of S2 sounds and friction rubs.

ª The upright position is helpful for patients with pulmonary emphysema or distant heart sounds. Auscultate below the xiphoid area.

• If possible, position the patient on knees and elbows to hear faint friction rubs.

**19. What are split S2 heart sounds?**

Split S2 heart sounds reflect closure of the aortic and pulmonic valves. They normally occur at the end of systole. The first component of the S2 sound is the closure of the aortic valve (A2); the second component is the closure of the pulmonic valve (P2).

**20. Describe the various types of S2 splits.**

A **physiologic split** can be heard in many people. The best place to auscultate split S2 sounds is at the left or right sternal border at the second intercostal space. Have the patient take a big inspiration and hold it; the S2 split becomes wider. However, when the patient exhales and holds, the S2 split becomes closer. This finding indicates a physiologic split S2.

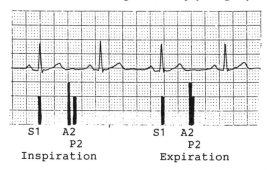

Physiologic split S2.

A **wide split** may suggest right bundle-branch block, Wolff-Parkinson-White syndrome, or pulmonary stenosis. The split S2 is prolonged during expiration and becomes even longer during inspiration .

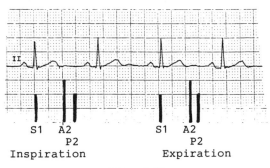

Wide split S2.

A **fixed split** is not affected by the respiratory cycle. It occurs with large atrial septal defects, ventricular septal defects with left-to-right shunt, and right ventricular failure.

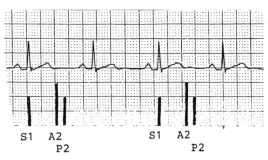

Fixed split S2.

A **paradoxical split** occurs when the pulmonic valve (P2) closes before the aortic valve (A2). The split is prolonged during expiration and shortened during inspiration. This finding may suggest left bundle-branch block or Wolff-Parkinson-White syndrome.

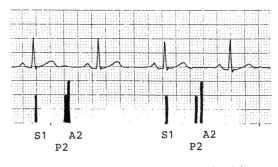

Paradoxical split S2.

### 21. What is the difference between S3 and S4?

S3 is a third heart sound. It may be heard after closure of the aortic and pulmonic valves. An S3 is also known as a gallop and can be heard in patients with CHF. Repeating either "Tenn-es-see" or "I believe" provides a rhythmic feel for how the S3 may sound on auscultation. An S3 can be heard in children, adolescents, athletes, and young adults. It is rarely heard in healthy adults older than 40 years. The best position for auscultation is the left lateral decubitus position with the bell of the stethoscope placed on the apex.

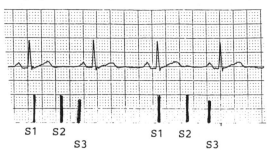

S3 gallop.

**S4** represents ejection of blood in the ventricles following atrial contraction. An S4 occurs before S1, which is the closure of the mitral and tricuspid valves. An S4 is heard in many patients after a myocardial infarction. Repeating either "Ken-tuc-ky" or "Believe me" may help the clinician identify an S4. It is commonly heard in people older than 50 years.

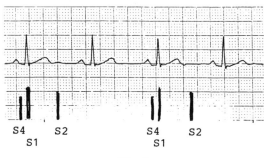

S4 gallop.

## 22. What is a murmur?

A murmur is the sound that represents turbulence or disruption of blood flow. The sound of a murmur is affected by the function of the valve, blood flow, and myocardial intensity or thickness. Cardiac murmurs can be auscultated with the diaphragm of the stethoscope and suggest an increase in the turbulence of blood flow through a narrow area, irregular area, or both. For example, stenosis is the inability of the valve to open completely, whereas regurgitation is the inability of the valve to close completely. There are three kinds of murmurs: systolic, diastolic, and continuous.

## 23. Are all systolic murmurs pathologic?

No. Some systolic murmurs are physiologic (benign). A continuous murmur (known as venous hum) may be heard in children. It usually is located in the neck and chest and can be heard when the patient is sitting upright. Other systolic physiologic murmurs can be heard during the last few months of pregnancy at the second intercostal space at the left sternal border. A mammary bruit may accompany this murmur. A systolic murmur, called a hemic murmur, can be heard in anemic patients.

## 24. What causes an abnormal systolic murmur?

Abnormal systolic murmurs are related to narrow or irregular valves. They are heard during systole, when the mitral and tricuspid valves are closed and the aortic and pulmonic valves are open. Any disruption in the closure of the mitral or tricuspid valve (e.g., regurgitation) may present as a systolic murmur. Systolic murmurs also may be heard when the aortic or pulmonic valve is narrowed or stenotic. Aortic valve stenosis, pulmonary valve stenosis, idiopathic hypertrophic subaortic stenosis, mitral regurgitation, rupture of the mitral valve chordae tendineae, papillary muscle rupture or dysfunction, and tricuspid regurgitation may present with a systolic murmur.

A mnemonic useful in remembering systolic murmurs is **MR. PASS** and **MVP:**

**M** = **M**itral
**R** = **R**egurgitation

**P** = **P**hysiologic
**A** = **A**ortic
**S** = **S**tenosis
**S** = **S**ystolic murmurs

**MVP** = mitral valve prolapse

From Fitzgerald MA: Cardiac Exam: NP Review–1988. North Andover, MA, Fitzgerald Health Education Associates, 1998, p 39, with permission.

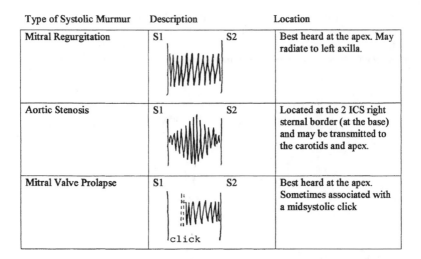

| Type of Systolic Murmur | Description | Location |
| --- | --- | --- |
| Mitral Regurgitation | S1          S2 | Best heard at the apex. May radiate to left axilla. |
| Aortic Stenosis | S1          S2 | Located at the 2 ICS right sternal border (at the base) and may be transmitted to the carotids and apex. |
| Mitral Valve Prolapse | S1          S2    click | Best heard at the apex. Sometimes associated with a midsystolic click |

## 25. What is an innocent murmur?

Innocent murmurs occasionally occur with an intense myocardial contraction that forces blood through a small chamber and/or blood vessel. They are heard primarily in children, adolescents, and young athletes. An innocent murmur is usually described as a soft midsystolic murmur located at the second intercostal space at the left sternal border without radiation. It is associated with a split S2 and is best heard when the patient is supine. Remember that innocent murmurs are different from benign murmurs.

## 26. Are diastolic murmurs benign or pathologic?

During diastole the aortic and pulmonic valves are closed while the mitral and tricuspid valves are open, allowing the ventricles to fill. Any disturbances in the opening of the mitral or tricuspid valve can cause a diastolic murmur and suggests a pathologic origin. With an incompetent aortic or pulmonic valve, the clinician may hear a diastolic murmur. Aortic regurgitation, mitral stenosis, and pulmonary regurgitation can present with diastolic murmurs.

A mnemonic useful for remembering diastolic murmurs is **MS. ARD**:

**M** = **M**itral
**S** = **S**tenosis
**A** = **A**ortic
**R** = **R**egurgitation
**D** = Both are **D**iastolic murmurs

From Fitzgerald MA: Cardiac Exam: NP Review–1988. North Andover, MA, Fitzgerald Health Education Associates, 1998, p 39, with permission.

| Type of Diastolic Murmur | Description | Location |
| --- | --- | --- |
| Mitral Stenosis | S1          S2 | Best heard at the apex with the patient in the left lateral decubitus position |
| Aortic Regurgitation | S1          S2 | Aortic area and perhaps radiate to the apex |

### 27. How are murmurs characterized?
Murmurs are described by the following characteristics:
- Timing (during systole or diastole)
- Location
- Pitch (low, medium, or high)
- Quality (harsh, musical, raspy, blowing, or rumbling)
- Radiation (present or absent)
- Intensity (loudness)

### 28. What is the grading system for systolic and diastolic murmur intensity?
| | |
|---|---|
| Grade 1 | Very faint murmur |
| Grade 2 | Faint murmur |
| Grade 3 | Moderately loud murmur |
| Grade 4 | Very loud murmur with a thrill |
| Grade 5 | Extra-loud murmur with the stethoscope placed lightly on the chest and a palpable thrill |
| Grade 6 | Murmur that is audible without a stethoscope and accompanied by a visible and palpable thrill |

### 29. What laboratory tests can provide additional data for cardiac assessment?
The serum laboratory tests to obtain when myocardial ischemia or necrosis is suspected are **creatine kinase** (CK) and its **MB isoenzyme** (CK-MB). CK increases 4–6 hours after onset of symptoms, peaks within 24 hours, and returns to baseline 3–4 days later. CK cannot diagnose acute myocardial infarction or differentiate between rhabdomyolysis and musculoskeletal injury.

Another laboratory test that may be useful for diagnosing cardiac ischemia is **lactate dehydrogenase** (LDH). LDH increases within 12 hours of onset of symptoms and peaks within 24–48 hours. LDH levels can remain elevated as long as 10–14 days. This test may not be sensitive because of coexisting conditions such as megaloblastic anemia, hemolysis, and renal insufficiency, all of which affect LDH.

Currently, the more specific serum tests for myocardial injury are **troponin I** and **troponin T**. Like CK and CK-MB, these serial markers increase 4–6 hours after the beginning of infarction and peak at 24 hours. Unlike CK and CK-MB, however, troponin I and troponin T last as long as 6 days, which may aid in the diagnosis of late myocardial infarctions. They also help to rule out false-positive CK and CK-MB findings. In the emergency setting, point-of-care devices are available to test for troponin.

#### BIBLIOGRAPHY
1. Adams JE, Bodor GS, Davila-Roman VG, et al: Cardiac troponin I. A marker with high specificity for cardiac injury. Circulation 88:101–106, 1993.
2. Braunwald E: The clinical examination. In Goldman L, Braunwald E (eds): Primary Cardiology. Philadelphia, W.B. Saunders, 1998, pp 27–43.
3. Chatterjee K: Physical examination. In Topol EJ (ed): Textbook of Cardiovascular Medicine. Philadelphia, Lippincott-Raven, 1998, pp 293–331.
4. Fitzgerald MA: Cardiac Exam: NP Review–1998. North Andover, MA, Fitzgerald Health Education Associates,1998, pp 39–44.
5. Froelicher VF, Quaglietti S: Handbook of Ambulatory Cardiology. Philadelphia, Lippincott-Raven, 1997.
6. Guzzetta CE, Seifert PC: Cardiovascular assessment. In Kinney MR, Packa DR, Andreoli KG (eds): Comprehensive Cardiac Care, 7th ed. St. Louis, Mosby, 1991, pp 10–48.
7. Hamm CW, Goldman BU, Heeschen C, et al: Emergency room triage of patients with acute chest pain by means of rapid testing for cardiac troponin T or troponin I. N Engl J Med 337:1648–1653, 1997.
8. Hurst JW: Cardiovascular Diagnosis: The Initial Examination. St. Louis, Mosby, 1993.
9. Hurst JW: The examination of the heart: The importance of initial screening masters in medicine. Dis-Month 36(5):254–313, 1990.
10. Kusumoto F: Cardiovascular disorders: Heart disease. In McPhee SJ (ed): Pathophysiology of Disease: An Introduction to Clinical Medicine, 2nd ed. Stamford, CT, Appleton & Lange, 1997, pp 219–254.

11. Mair J, Wagner I, Puschendorf B, et al: Cardiac troponin I to diagnose myocardial injury. Lancet 341:838–839, 1993.
12. Marriott HJ: Bedside Cardiac Diagnosis. Philadelphia, Lippincott, 1993.
13. O'Rourke RA, Shaver JA, Saleuni R, et al: The history, physical examination, and cardiac auscultation. In Alexander RW (ed): Hurst's The Heart, Arteries and Veins, vol. 1, 9th ed. New York, McGraw-Hill, 1998, pp 229–342.
14. Perloff JK: Physical Examination of the Heart and Circulation, 2nd ed. Philadelphia, W.B. Saunders, 1990.
15. Seidel HM, Ball JW, Dains JE, Benedict GW: Mosby's Guide to Physical Examination, 4th ed. St. Louis, Mosby, 1999, pp 409–482.
16. Willerson JT: Cardiac signs and symptoms. In Willerson JT (ed): Cardiovascular Medicine. New York, Churchhill Livingstone, 1995, pp 1–30.
17. Winters KJ Eisenber, PR: Ischemic heart disease. In Carey CF (ed): The Washington Manual of Medical Therapeutics, 29th ed. Philadelphia, Lippincott-Raven, 1998, pp 81–108.

# 2. BASIC CARDIAC MONITORING

*Martie Mattson*, RN, MSN, CCRN

**1 Describe the heart's normal conduction system.**

The heart contracts in response to an electrical stimulus arising spontaneously from specialized pacemaker cells. This impulse then spreads across the myocardium via the electrical conduction system, which consists of the following structures:

- Sinoatrial (SA) node
- Atrioventricular (AV) node
- Bundle of His
- AV junction
- Bundle branches
- Purkinje fibers

The names of the different rhythms are derived from their site of origin. For example, the normal rhythm of the heart originates in the sinus node and is called **sinus rhythm**; a rhythm that originates in the AV junction is called a **junctional rhythm**; and a rhythm that originates in the ventricle is called a **ventricular rhythm**.

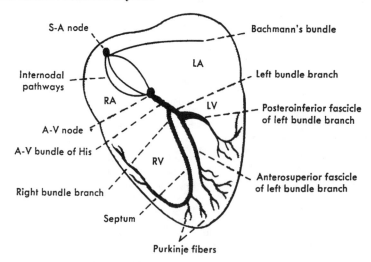

Cardiac conduction system. (From Kinney MR, Packa DR, Andreoli KG, Zipes DP: Comprehensive Cardiac Care, 7th ed. St. Louis, Mosby Year Book, 1991, with permission.)

## 2. Describe the location and function of the SA node.

The SA node, more commonly called the sinus node, lies in the right atrium near the entrance of the superior vena cava. Normally the sinus node is the primary pacemaker, fires first, and controls the heart rate. Other areas in the conduction system can initiate an impulse, but usually only if the higher, faster pacer fails to fire. If a lower pacemaker site for some reason fires faster than SA node, it may take over the pacing function. The impulse travels across Bachmann's bundle to the left atrium and rapidly down the internodal tracts to the AV node. The electrical stimulation also travels through the muscle of both atria, resulting in contraction. The intrinsic rate for the sinus node is 60–100 beats per minute, and autonomic nervous system influence may slow or increase the rate.

## 3. Describe the location and function of the AV node.

The AV node lies low in the right atrium near the tricuspid valve and septum. It is composed of many intricate pathways that slow down the electrical impulse. This delay allows atrial contraction to occur just before ventricular contraction, thus adding "atrial kick" to the stroke volume.

## 4. What is the bundle of His?

The Bundle of His is the short segment of conduction tissue between the AV node and the bundle branches. Here the electrical signal speeds up just before entering the ventricular septum.

## 5. What is the AV junction?

The AV junction is made up of the AV node and the bundle of His. Areas in the AV junction can take over as the pacemaker of the heart and have an intrinsic rate of 40–60 beats per minute.

## 6. Describe the location and function of the bundle branches.

The right and left bundle branches are located in the ventricular septum and conduct the electrical impulse rapidly to the right and left ventricles. Because the left ventricle has a large muscle mass, shortly after entering the septum the left bundle divides into the left anterior and posterior fascicles.

## 7. What are Purkinje fibers?

Bundle branches terminate in the Purkinje fibers, which are a network of fine fibers spread throughout the ventricular endocardium. The Purkinje fibers have the ability to fire spontaneously if the higher pacemakers fail. The intrinsic rate of this ventricular pacemaker is 20–40 beats per minute.

## 8. Describe the waves, complexes, intervals, and segments in a rhythm strip. What do they represent?

In interpreting a rhythm strip, it is necessary to identify the presence or absence and sometimes the amplitude of particular waves, the duration of intervals and complexes, and the relative position of certain segments to the baseline.

*ECG Pattern*

| | REPRESENTS | NORMAL | WHERE TO MEASURE |
|---|---|---|---|
| P wave | Atrial depolarization | < 0.10 sec, ≤ 2.5 mm high | From beginning to end of P-wave length and height |
| QRS complex | Ventricular depolarization | 0.06–0.10 sec | From point where complex leaves baseline to where it returns to baseline |
| T wave | Ventricular repolarization | Rounded and asymmetric, < 5 mm high in lead II and < 10 mm in $V_{1-6}$ | From beginning of rise from baseline to peak |
| U wave | Possibly Purkinje cell repolarization | If present, small, rounded wave after T wave; same polarity as T wave | Do not measure |

*Table continued on following page.*

*ECG Pattern (Continued)*

|              | REPRESENTS                                                                                  | NORMAL                                                                                                                                      | WHERE TO MEASURE                                                     |
| ------------ | ------------------------------------------------------------------------------------------- | ------------------------------------------------------------------------------------------------------------------------------------------- | ------------------------------------------------------------------- |
| PR interval  | Time for impulse to travel through atrium and AV node and initiate ventricular contraction | 0.12–0.20 sec                                                                                                                               | From beginning of P wave to beginning of QRS complex               |
| QT interval  | Duration of ventricular depolarization and repolarization                                   | Varies with heart rate and gender, but generally, if corrected for heart rate, it should be < 0.44 in men and < 0.45 in women | From beginning of QRS complex to end of T wave                      |
| ST segment   | Initial ventricular repolarization                                                          | Isoelectric and < 0.12 sec in duration                                                                                                      | From end of QRS complex to beginning of T wave                      |

### 9. How do you measure the waves, complexes, intervals, and segments?

ECG recording paper is standardized for all cardiac monitoring systems. It is composed of 1-mm squares. Time is represented along the horizontal axis and voltage and amplitude on the vertical axis. Each small square is 0.04 seconds in duration, 0.1 mV in voltage, and 1 mm in amplitude. Every fifth vertical and horizontal line is darkened and makes a large square. Each large square is 0.20 seconds in duration, 0.5 mV in voltage, and 5 mm in amplitude. By placing calipers at the beginning and end or peak of a particular wave, complex, interval, or segment and counting how many small or large squares lie between, the duration of the event or the voltage or amplitude of the event can be measured. In addition to the squares, ECG recording paper has a short, usually vertical, line at the top of the paper every 3 seconds. These slash marks are helpful in measuring the heart rate.

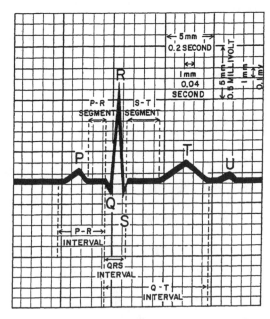

ECG recording of waves, complexes, intervals, and segments. (From Lessig ML, Lessig PM: The cardiovascular system: Nursing assessment data base. In Alspach JG (ed): AACN Core Curriculum for Critical Care Nursing, 5th ed. Philadelphia, W.B. Saunders, 1998, p 173, with permission.)

**10. When is cardiac monitoring indicated?**

The American College of Cardiology and the American Association of Critical Care Nurses recommend cardiac monitoring for any condition in which life-threatening arrhythmias are likely to be a symptom or complication. Examples of such conditions include acute myocardial infarction (MI), suspected MI (until ruled out), recent resuscitation from cardiac arrest, heart failure, shock from any cause, acute drug or chemical poisoning with agents known or suspected to cause cardiac arrhythmias, acute myocarditis, unstable angina, and high-risk coronary lesions. In addition, monitoring is recommended during and after certain procedures. Examples include cardiac surgery, percutaneous coronary interventions, catheter ablation for arrhythmias, and initiation and loading of type I or III antiarrhythmics.

**11. Where are the electrodes placed on the patient?**

Placement of electrodes on the chest depends on the number of lead wires that the cable has and which cardiac lead is to be monitored. Three-lead cables have a positive, negative, and ground lead wire. In older monitoring systems, the polarity is fixed and usually is indicated on the cable where the lead wires attach. With a three-lead system, cardiac leads I, II, III, $MCL_1$, and $MCL_6$ can be monitored. The recommended lead to monitor is $MCL_1$ because cardiac rhythms with a wide QRS complex can be diagnosed more accurately. These rhythms include ventricular tachycardia, supraventricular tachycardia with aberrant conduction, pacemaker rhythms, and bundle-branch blocks. To monitor $MCL_1$ the positive electrode is placed in the fourth intercostal space at the right sternal border, the negative electrode is placed just below the left clavicle close to the juncture of the left arm and torso, and the ground electrode is placed at the fifth intercostal space at the left midaxillary line. The lead selection switch on the monitor should be placed at lead I. If, for some reason, the positive electrode cannot be placed in the exact position for $MCL_1$, $MCL_6$ is the next best choice of lead to monitor. The electrodes can stay in the same place, but the monitor lead selector is switched to lead II. This changes the left midaxillary line electrode to positive and the fourth intercostal space electrode to ground.

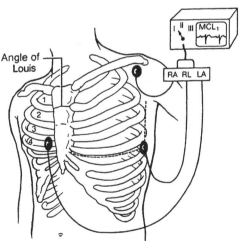

Placement of electrodes. (From Drew BJ: Bedside Electrocardiogram Monitoring. AACN Clin Issues 1:25-33, 1993, with permission.)

**12. What are the advantages of five-lead cables? Where are the electrodes placed?**

Five-lead cables are preferable to three-lead cables, because they allow monitoring of multiple limb leads (I, II, III aVR, aVL, aVF) and one precordial lead. The lead wires on five-lead cables are standardized among manufacturers and are labeled and color coded: RA (white), LA (black), RL (green), LL (red), and C (brown).

The RA and LA electrodes are placed just below the right and left clavicles close to the junctures of the arms and torso. The RL and LL electrodes are placed in the lower abdomen, close to the junctures of the legs and the torso. The C lead usually is placed in the fourth intercostal space at the right sternal border to monitor $V_1$, but it can be placed at any precordial lead position for continuous monitoring, if appropriate.

Electrodes must be placed in the correct position. Although it is desirable to see an arrhythmia on a 12-lead ECG, many arrhythmias are transient and can be captured only on a cardiac monitoring rhythm strip. Inaccurately placed electrodes can change the ECG complexes from those normally expected for a particular lead and invalidate the criteria that help to differentiate arrhythmias.

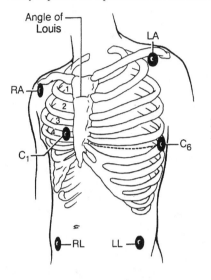

Placement of five-lead cables. (From Drew BJ: Bedside Electrocardiogram Monitoring. AACN Clin Issues 1:25-33, 1993, with permission.)

### 13. Which leads are the best to monitor with a five-lead cable?

The choice is a clinical decision based on the patient's arrhythmias or potential arrhythmias and cardiac disease. Monitoring systems allow two or sometimes three channels of the ECG to be monitored simultaneously, but only one can be a V lead. It is recommended that $V_1$ always be among the monitored leads, because criteria to differentiate cardiac rhythms with a wide QRS complex can be applied with increased accuracy. Rhythms with a wide QRS complex include ventricular tachycardia, supraventricular tachycardia with aberrant conduction, pacemaker rhythms, and bundle-branch blocks. If the chest lead for $V_1$ cannot be placed correctly, $V_6$ should be monitored, because it is the second best lead for recognition of ventricular arrhythmia.

The choice of the second lead to monitor is based on the location of the cardiac disease and ischemia. The lead that shows the most significant ST segment deviation with an ischemic episode or balloon occlusion during angioplasty should be monitored. If the lead with the most significant ST segment deviation cannot be determined, research indicates that ST segment ischemic changes are noted more frequently in aVF than in other limb leads, no matter which coronary artery is diseased. If a third ECG channel can be selected, lead I is the best choice because it can help to detect lateral wall ischemic changes and, in combination with aVF, can be used to determine the cardiac axis.

### 14. What is the best way to analyze an ECG rhythm strip?

The best way to analyze a rhythm strip is to use a consistent, systematic approach. Assess the following elements and ask the following questions to identify the rhythm:

**Heart rate.** Determine both the atrial rate (look at the P waves) and the ventricular rate (look at the QRS complexes). Are they the same? Are they greater than 100 or less than 60?

**Rhythm.** Are the intervals between the QRS complexes regular? If they are irregular, is there a pattern to the irregularity? Are early beats present? Groups of QRS complexes, then a space? Or is there no noticeable pattern?

**P waves.** Are P waves present? Does every QRS have a P wave? Are there P waves without a QRS? Do some T waves look different from other T waves? Could it be a P wave on top of them?

**PR interval.** Is the duration between 0.12 and 0.2 seconds? Is it the same for every QRS that is preceded by a P wave?

**QRS complex.** Is the duration between 0.06 and 0.10 seconds? Do all the QRS complexes look the same?

These questions allow you to match the answers to specific criteria for different rhythms. Several other elements should be assessed, depending on the patient's condition.

**QT interval.** For patients taking drugs that prolong cardiac repolarization, the QT interval must be measured. Examples include quinidine, procainamide, disopyramide, amiodarone, sotalol, ibutilide, haloperidol, and IV erythromycin. Prolonging the AV conduction time lengthens the QT interval and can be proarrhythmic.

**ST segment.** Observe for any sudden elevation or depression of the ST segment, and assess the patient immediately if it occurs. A sudden elevation or depression may indicate cardiac ischemia. Many monitoring systems have the capability to do continuous ST segment monitoring.

## 15. How is the heart rate determined from an ECG rhythm strip?

The easiest way to determine the heart rate from a rhythm strip is to count the number of QRS complexes that occur in 6 seconds, which is the distance between three slash marks at the top of the ECG paper, and to multiply the sum by 10. Although not exact, this method can be used with both regular and irregular rhythms and is accurate enough for making clinical decisions. Two other methods to determine heart rate are (1) to divide 300 by the number of large boxes between two QRS complexes and (2) to divide 1500 by the number of small boxes between two QRSs. Both methods require a regular rhythm and take more time.

## 16. What can be done to improve the quality of the ECG tracing?

The most important points in achieving and sustaining a high-quality rhythm strip are to place the electrodes in the correct position and to apply and maintain them properly. Prepare the skin by clipping excessive hair; washing the site with soap, rinsing, and drying thoroughly; cleaning with an alcohol wipe; and abrading the skin gently with a washcloth or gauze pad before applying the electrodes. Check that the electrode gel has not dried out, then apply it to the prepared skin areas by firmly pressing the entire adhesive perimeter, avoiding pressure on the gel pad. If the patient is diaphoretic, tincture of benzoin may be applied first under the adhesive area only. If the patient is unstable and electrodes must be applied quickly without adequate skin preparation, change the electrodes and apply properly as soon as the patient has stabilized. At a minimum, electrodes should be replaced every 48 hours to ensure that the gel is still moist. If for some reason a specific electrode needs to be changed at an earlier point, all electrodes should be changed at the same time to maintain equal transmission of the signal from each lead wire. Keep lead wires and cables away from electrical equipment, and be sure that lead wires are not frayed to prevent electrical interference.

## 17. What must be documented for patients with continuous cardiac monitoring? How often?

The American Association of Critical Care Nurses recommends documenting a rhythm strip in the patient's chart on admission, during every shift, and with any significant change in the rhythm. Individual hospitals may require more frequent documentation. The date, time, lead, heart rate, PR interval, QRS duration, and interpretation of the rhythm should be identified on every documented strip. Some of this information may be printed on the strip by the monitor recorder, but it should be verified. If the patient is taking a medication that can prolong the QT interval, the QT interval should be documented at least once during each shift and at least every 4 hours if the medication is administered intravenously.

### BIBLIOGRAPHY

1. American College of Cardiology Policy Statement: Recommended guidelines for in-hospital cardiac monitoring of adults for detection of arrhythmia. J Am Coll Cardiol 18:1431–1433, 1991.
2. Drew BJ: Bedside electrocardiogram monitoring. AACN Clin Issues 1:25– 33, 1993.

3. Drew BJ, Tisdale LA: ST segment monitoring for coronary artery reocclusion following thrombolytic therapy and coronary angioplasty: Identification of optimal bedside monitoring leads. Am J Crit Care 2:280–292, 1993.
4. Jacobson C: AACN: Bedside Cardiac Monitoring Protocol. Aliso Viejo, CA, American Association of Critical-Care Nurses, 1996.
5. Kinney MR, Packa DR, Andreoli KG, Zipes DP: Comprehensive Cardiac Care, 7th ed. St. Louis, Mosby, 1991.
6. Lessig ML, Lessig PM: The cardiovascular system: Nursing assessment data base. In Alspach JG (ed): AACN Core Curriculum for Critical Care Nursing, 5th ed. Philadelphia, W.B. Saunders, 1998, pp 160–199.
7. Mims BC, Toto KH, Luecke LE, Roberts MK: Critical Care Skills: A Clinical Handbook. Philadelphia, W.B. Saunders, 1996.
8. Paul S, Hebra JD: The Nurse's Guide to Cardiac Rhythm Interpretation: Implications for Patient Care. Philadelphia, W.B. Saunders, 1998.
9. Wagner GS. Marriott's Practical Electrocardiography, 9th ed. Baltimore, Williams & Wilkins, 1994.

# 3. ARRHYTHMIAS

*Mary G. Adams*, RN, MS

### 1. How do we assess the effects of an arrhythmia?

Whenever there is a change in the electrocardiogram (ECG), assess the patient, record a rhythm strip, and report significant findings. Heart rates below 50 or above 140 beats/min decrease cardiac output and may require prompt attention. Be prepared for emergency action. Careful observation of the patient determines the need and urgency of intervention. Evaluate the following parameters to assess whether the arrhythmia is compromising cardiovascular function.

**Radial pulse**
• Pulse deficits may occur with blocks or atrial arrhythmias.
• A weak or absent pulse suggests diminished cardiac output.

**Blood pressure** (BP): low BP may be a warning of congestive heart failure (CHF) or impending shock.

**Signs and symptoms**
• Chest pain, palpitations, labored or rapid breathing, or an inability to breathe when lying flat indicates inadequate cardiac oxygenation.
• Restlessness, confusion, lethargy, personality changes, or loss of consciousness may indicate inadequate cerebral oxygenation.
• Cool, moist skin and pallor indicate reduced blood flow to the periphery.

### 2. What are some arrhythmias that originate above the ventricles?

• Premature atrial contractions (PAC)
• Premature atrial tachycardia (PAT)
• Atrial flutter
• Atrial fibrillation
• Junctional rhythm
• Junctional tachycardia
• Wandering pacemaker

### 3. What is the effect of supraventricular arrhythmias on the QRS complex?

Unless aberrantly conducted, supraventricular arrhythmias conduct through the ventricular pathway in a normal manner. The QRS shape is not affected and should remain < 12 msec.

### 4. What are some arrhythmias that originate in the ventricles?

• Premature ventricular contractions (PVCs)
• Ventricular tachycardia (VT)
• Torsades de pointes
• Ventricular fibrillation (VF)
• Idioventricular rhythm
• Accelerated idioventricular rhythm
• Ventricular standstill

### 5. How are antiarrhythmic drugs classified?

Most cardiac drugs are classified by their action in blocking sodium, potassium, or calcium channels or blocking the effect of the sympathetic nervous system.

*Current Classification of Antiarrhythmic Drugs*

| CLASSIFICATION | PRIMARY ACTION | EXAMPLES |
|---|---|---|
| Class I | Sodium channel blockade | |
| IA | | Quinidine, procainamide |
| IB | | Lidocaine, tocainide |
| IC | | Propafenone, encainide |
| Class II | Beta blockade | Propranolol, esmolol, metoprolol |
| Class III | Potassium channel blockade | Amiodarone, bretylium, sotalol |
| Class IV | Calcium channel blockade | Verapamil, diltiazem |

### 6. How common is a proarrhythmic effect with antiarrhythmic drugs?

A proarrhythmic effect has been reported in all of the cardiac drug classifications. The incidence varies primarily because of the definition of proarrhythmia but ranges from 5–15%. Subsequently, the clinical use of antiarrhythmic agents focuses on treatment rather than prevention.

### 7. What are the causes and treatment options for sinus tachycardia (ST)?

Excessive sympathetic nerve stimulation causes ST when the QRS complexes are normal and exceed 90 beats/minute. A fast cardiac rate is relatively ineffectual and may lead to CHF. Since ST is almost always a secondary arrhythmia, the underlying cause should be determined and treated, if necessary.

*Causes of Sinus Tachycardia*

| NORMAL EVENTS | NONCARDIAC ABNORMALITIES | CARDIAC ABNORMALITIES |
|---|---|---|
| Exercise | Fever | Poor left ventricular function (CHF) |
| Anxiety | Hemorrhage | Sympathomimetics (dopamine, epinephrine) |
| Stimulants | Infection | Vagolytics (atropine) |
| | Pain | Vasodilators (nitroglycerin) |

### 8. What is the difference between premature atrial complexes (PACs) and atrial tachycardia?

**PACs** are beats initiated by an ectopic atrial focus that appears early in the cardiac cycle. Because the impulse arises from a site other than the sinus node, the shape of the P wave and the length of the PR interval usually are different. A characteristic pause follows the beat. PACs indicate atrial irritability and are associated with myocardial ischemia or infarction, low potassium or magnesium, and hypoxia. They often are an early sign of heart failure as the myocardium is stretched.

**Atrial tachycardia** is an abrupt episode of tachycardia with the heart rate between 140 and 250 beats/minute. Because, like PACs, the beats are initiated by an ectopic atrial focus, the P wave may be abnormally shaped or not seen because it is buried in the preceding T wave. Cardiac output decreases because of shortened ventricular filling time. Atrial tachycardia is seen in young adults, patients with cardiomyopathy, and patients who have had previous atrial surgery.

### 9. What is the difference between atrial fibrillation (afib) and atrial flutter?

Both are fast atrial rates that arise from many ectopic foci in the atrium. Because the impulses fire so rapidly, the atrioventricular (AV) node cannot accept and conduct each one; therefore, some degree of blockage occurs at the AV node.

**Atrial flutter** has a regular ventricular response rate and is due to a reentrant mechanism, presumably a single stable reentrant circuit located in the right atrium. For example, if the atrial rate is 300 impulses/minute, the ventricle rate (same as the pulse rate) may be 150. Thus, the block is said to be 2:1; in other words, there are two atrial impulses for each ventricular response.

**Afib** has an irregular ventricular response in which it is difficult to discern the P waves because they resemble a wavy line on the ECG. However, the atrial rate is certainly much faster than the ventricular rate.

### 10. What risk factors are associated with atrial flutter?
Transient atrial flutter is a typical complication after open-heart surgery and may be seen in the acute phase of myocardial infarction (MI) . Chronic atrial flutter often is seen in patients over the age of 40 and is associated with organic heart disease; thus termination and prevention of the arrhythmia are important. Patients with accessory pathways who have atrial flutter are particularly at risk because of the high ratio of ventricular response (sometimes 1:1).

### 11. How is atrial flutter treated?
- Cardioversion (<50 joules)
- Rapid atrial pacing
- Slowing of ventricular response (beta blockers or calcium channel blockers)
- Radiofrequency ablation of the accessory pathway
- Maintenance of sinus rhythm (class IA, IC, or III drugs)

### 12. What risk factors are associated with afib?
Afib is one of the most common symptomatic sustained arrhythmias. It often is seen in acute MI or hypertension or after open-heart surgery. The most serious risk of afib is thrombi formed by the stasis of blood in the left atrium. When the thrombus embolizes, it may lodge in the brain, causing a stroke, which often leaves the patient severely disabled. In addition, cardiac output may drop by as much as 30% because of the loss of atrial contraction (atrial kick).

### 13. How is afib treated?
- Anticoagulation for prophylaxis of systemic thromboembolism
- Control of ventricular response (digoxin, beta blockers, and calcium channel blockers)
- Return of atria to sinus rhythm (antiarrhythmic drugs, including quinidine or amiodarone)

### 14. Why do we no longer treat asymptomatic premature ventricular complexes (PVCs)?
The unexpected results of the Cardiac Arrhythmia Suppression Trial in 1989 (CAST I), which studied patients with a prior MI, showed that class IC antiarrhythmic drugs produced an increased mortality rate in most patient populations. Thus, prophylactic use of lidocaine is no longer indicated for patients with acute MI and rarely is indicated for patients without symptomatic arrhythmias or sustained VT or VF.

### 15. How do we distinguish among the types of AV block?
An AV block is the delayed conduction or nonconduction of an atrial impulse. The three types are first-, second-, and third-degree block.

*Types of Atrioventricular Block*

| TYPE | PR INTERVAL | QRS COMPLEX | AV CONDUCTION | TREATMENT |
|---|---|---|---|---|
| First-degree | > 0.20 sec | Normal | All sinus beats are conducted to ventricles | None |
| Second-degree | | | | |
| Type I | Becomes progressively longer until one P is dropped | Normal | More Ps than QRS | Close observation |
| Type II | Same from beat to beat | Broad (> 0.12 sec) | More Ps than QRS | Pacemaker |
| Third-degree | Does not apply; no relationship with QRS | Usually normal | Independent of atrium because atrium and ventricles are disassociated | Pacemaker |

**16. Why is it important to differentiate torsades de pointes from polymorphic ventricular tachycardia?**

The correct identification of torsades de pointes is critical because it is not treated like other VTs and can be exacerbated by the administration of some antiarrhythmics. Torsades de pointes is associated with a prolonged QT interval and initiated by a pause; it has a typical undulating pattern in which the QRS peaks appear to be first up and then down. Most patients with polymorphic VT have coronary artery disease or ischemic conditions, whereas torsades de pointes is either congenital or iatrogenically acquired by QT-lengthening medications. Polymorphic VT has a similar morphologic appearance but does not have a prolonged QT, nor is it preceded by a pause.

**17. What is the treatment for torsades de pointes?**
- Immediate discontinuation of any agent that may lengthen the QT interval
- Intravenous potassium to correct any abnormality
- Intravenous magnesium (Mg) suppresses torsades de pointes and has the advantage of safety because it does not aggravate other forms of VT. Although easily administered, Mg is contraindicated in patients with renal failure, loss of deep tendon reflexes, serum Mg > 5 mEq/L, drop in systolic pressure < 80 mmHg, or drop in heart rate < 60 beats/min.
- Overdrive ventricular pacing
- Cardioversion

**18. What are bundle-branch blocks?**

A bundle-branch block is an obstruction in the right or left ventricular conduction pathway. The impulse travels first through the unobstructed branch and then is conducted to the opposite ventricle. The resulting QRS is > 0.12 seconds because the aberrant pathway requires a longer time for activation of the ventricles. However, the P wave is normal because the impulse originates in the normal pacer (SA node).

**19. How do you differentiate between right bundle-branch block (RBBB) and left bundle-branch block (LBBB)?**

To determine which bundle branch is blocked, look at the precordial lead $V_1$ or modified chest lead 1 ($MCL_1$). **RBBB patterns** show an upward deflection, representing delayed right ventricular activation and resulting in the typical rSR' complex. **LBBB patterns** show that the right ventricle and septum are activated simultaneously and immediately followed by left ventricular activation, producing a wide, deep V-shaped complex. RBBB is more common because the branch is long, narrow, more superficial, and hence more vulnerable to injury.

## BIBLIOGRAPHY

1. Cardiac Arrhythmia Suppression Trial (CAST) Investigators: Preliminary report: Effect of encainide and flecainide on mortality in a randomized trial of arrhythmia suppression after myocardial infarction. N Engl J Med 321:406–412, 1989.
2. Conover MB: Understanding Electrocardiography, 7th ed. St Louis, Mosby, 1996.
3. Marriott HJL, Conover MB: Advanced Concepts in Arrhythmias, 3rd ed. St. Louis, Mosby, 1998
4. Podrid PJ, Kowey PR: Cardiac Arrhythmia: Mechanisms, Diagnosis and Management. Baltimore, Williams & Wilkins, 1995.
5. Staton MS, Prystowsky, EN, Fineberg, et al: Arrhythmogenic effects of antiarrhythmic drugs: A study of 506 patients treated for ventricular tachycardia or fibrillation. J Am Coll Cardiol 14: 209–215, 1989.
6. Van Gelder IC, Brugemann J, Crijns HJGM: Current treatment recommendations in antiarrhythmic therapy. Drugs 55:331–343, 1998.
7. Wagner GS: Marriott's Practical Electrocardiography, 9th ed. Baltimore, Williams & Wilkins, 1994.
8. Working Group on Arrhythmias: The silicon gambit: A new approach to the clarification of antiarrhythmic drugs based on their actions on arrhythmogenic mechanisms. Circulation 81:1831–1851, 1991.

# 4. TEMPORARY PACING

*Charles L. Witherell, RN, CS, MSN*

### 1. What are temporary pacemakers?

Temporary pacemakers provide electrical stimulation to the heart to promote a normal heart rate and synchronous contraction of the atria and ventricles, just as "permanent" (implanted) pacemakers do. These battery-powered devices work external to the body.

### 2. What are the indications for temporary pacing?

Temporary pacing may be useful in patients with postsurgical or infarct-related heart block, patients who are symptomatically bradycardic, patients who require overdrive dysrhythmia control, and patients whose native rates may be depressed by medications. When the expected duration of a state of block or bradycardia is in doubt, some clinicians do not wish to commit immediately to a permanent pacemaker and elect temporary pacing for some days in hope of a natural resolution.

### 3. What types of temporary pacemakers are available?

Transcutaneous, transvenous, and epicardial.

### 4. Which type is preferable? Why?

Transvenous and epicardial temporary pacemakers are preferable to transcutaneous pacing in all but emergent situations for two reasons:

1. If both atrial and ventricular wires are installed, transvenous and epicardial pacing allow sequential atrioventricular contractions, providing atrial kick to maximize cardiac output. They also can be used to deliver high rate atrial pacing. Transcutaneous pacing causes ventricular contraction only.

2. Transvenous and epicardial pacing use relatively little energy to provoke contraction, because their electrodes are in direct contact with the myocardium. Transcutaneous pacing relies on its large energy output to cross the chest wall, and therefore can be intensely uncomfortable for a patient who is conscious to any degree.

### 5. When is transcutaneous pacing used?

When rate support is urgently needed, transcutaneous pacing may be invaluable; it is noninvasive and can be instituted in moments to buy time for more definitive treatment.

### 6. What do the letters of the pacemaker code mean?

The NASPE/BPEG (NBG) Generic Pacemaker Code, devised in 1987 by the North American Society for Pacing and Electrophysiology and the British Pacing and Electrophysiology Group, provides three- to five-letter designations to describe the operation of pacemakers.

The first letter refers to the chamber paced. The second indicates the chamber sensed, that is, the chamber whose intrinsic electrical activity, if any, is detected. The third letter stands for the pacemaker's response to sensed events. The fourth and fifth letters in the code pertain primarily to functions of permanent pacemakers.

### 7. What do the letters VVI and AAI mean?

**VVI:** The paced chamber is the ventricle (V); the sensed chamber is the ventricle (V); and the pacemaker's response is inhibited (I). The inhibited response means that the pacer will be inhibited from pacing if the ventricle is depolarizing unaided.

**AAI:** The paced chamber is the atrium (A); the sensed chamber is the atrium (A); and the pacemaker's response is inhibited (I). If the pacemaker senses native P waves, it is inhibited from pacing.

**8. What is the DDD mode?**

The DDD provides atrioventricular (AV) synchrony, preserving or restoring atrial kick and thereby boosting cardiac output. It is useful in patients with second-degree (either classic or Wenckebach type) and third-degree block. The Ds stand for "dual": either the atrium or the ventricle or both may be paced; either native P waves or native R waves may be sensed; and the pacemaker may be inhibited or triggered to pace, depending on the combination of events it detects.

**9. Define AV delay in the DDD mode.**

AV delay is the pacemaker's own PR interval, i.e., the time that the pacemaker allows between atrial and ventricular events. This value can be controlled by the clinician.

**10. The pacemaker is set in the DDD mode to a rate of 60 beats/min and to an AV delay of 180 msec. What will the pacemaker do if the patient's native rhythm is sinus, with a rate of 70 and a PR interval of 0.16 (i.e., 160 msec)? Why?**

It will not pace at all, because the native rate exceeds 60 beats/min and because native R waves follow native P waves before the pacemaker's 180-msec deadline has passed. These events inhibit the pacer from firing for either chamber.

**11. What if the same patient has sinus bradycardia at a rate of 50 beats/min and a PR interval of 0.2?**

The pacemaker will pace both atrium and ventricle. It is triggered to do so because the patient's rate is less than its lower rate limit and the pacer's AV delay of 180 msec elapses before the native P waves can conduct to the ventricle.

**12. In the same patient, when would the DDD mode pace only the atrium or only the ventricle?**

The DDD mode paces only the atrium if it conducts quickly to the ventricle but at a slower rate than 60 beats/min. It may pace only the ventricle if the atrial rate is greater than 60, but conduction is delayed beyond 180 msec.

**13. What do the letters AOO, VOO, and DOO mean?**

The first letters of these modes indicate pacing in the atrium (AOO), the ventricle (VOO), or both chambers (DOO). In OO modes, the pacemaker does not detect native events (as indicated by the O in second position). And, because the pacer is not sensing, it naturally can have no response to sensed events (as indicated by the O in third position).

**14. What are the advantages and disadvantages of the VVI and AAI modes?**

**VVI** is good for simple rate support in bradycardias or heart block, but it is less useful if the patient requires atrial kick. Some patients tolerate VVI quite poorly if their paced ventricular depolarizations conduct retrogradely to the atria, producing pacemaker syndrome.

Pacing in **AAI** gives excellent support because it maintains atrial kick, provided that the patient has intact AV conduction. If second- or third-degree heart block develops or is likely to develop, however, AAI will be inadequate because it produces only atrial contractions.

**15. What are the advantages and disadvantages of the DDD mode?**

In DDD mode, the pacer uses the patient's native atrial rate as its cue, pacing the ventricle at exactly the same rate, if needed. In patients with heart block and a normal atrial rhythm, DDD is the most physiologic mode and generally gives the best cardiac output. Patients with atrial dysrhythmias (e.g., atrial tachycardia, flutter, or fibrillation) do not fare as well with temporary pacers in DDD mode, because the pacer will attempt to synchronize the ventricle to the arrhythmic atrium; VVI may give better support.

**16. When are the AOO, VOO, and DOO modes used?**

AOO, VOO, and DOO are called asynchronous pacing modes. A pacer set to the DOO mode will simply pace in the atrium and the ventricle at the selected rate, regardless of the presence of any native P or R waves. This mode may work well enough if the patient is profoundly bradycardic and the pacer is set at a rate of 60 or 70 beats/min. However, if the patient's native rate occasionally exceeds the set pacing rate, the pacer will compete. Moreover, if the patient is easily stimulated into dysrhythmias, the VOO or DOO mode may produce ventricular tachycardia or fibrillation by pacing in the relative refractory period of the T wave. If a patient arrives in your unit with one of these modes selected, determine the reason and ask if AAI, VVI, or DDD may be used instead.

### 17. What should you assess in patients with a temporary pacemaker?

1. Observe the patient's response to pacing at the current settings. If blood pressure and cardiac output are inadequate, ask whether a different mode or rate might improve hemodynamics.

2. Determine and document the capture and sensing thresholds, and set the pacemaker appropriately (see questions 18 and 19).

3. Determine when the battery was last changed. If indicated according to the manufacturer's instructions, replace the battery and document the change.

4. Examine the insertion sites of the temporary pacing leads to ensure that they are properly dressed, according to institutional protocol.

5. Because microshocks can be transmitted via a pacing wire to the myocardium and provoke serious dysrhythmia, carefully wrap uninsulated portions of the wire with a nonconductive material, such as a portion of a latex glove.

6. Be alert for the possibility of postpericardiotomy syndrome, which is characterized by blood in the pericardium, fever, leukocytosis, elevated erythrocyte sedimentation rate, pericardial or pleural pain and dyspnea, arthralgias, and pericardial friction rubs.

### 18. How is the proper rate setting determined?

The proper rate is the rate that provides the patient with the optimal cardiac output for his or her needs. Commonly some rate within the normal adult range of 60–100 beats/min is selected—and usually works well. Occasionally, it may be necessary to test a more fragile patient's cardiac output at a variety of rates to determine the best one.

### 19. What is the pacing or capture threshold?

The pacing or capture threshold is the smallest amount of energy from the pacemaker that consistently provokes contraction of the target chamber. The energy output of most temporary pacemakers is measured in milliamperes (mA). It is important to know this "absolute minimum" value so that you can provide a safety margin for the patient by setting an output at least two or three times as large.

### 20. How is the capture threshold assessed?

1. Gradually slow the pacing rate, observing carefully for patient tolerance, until the patient is in his or her own native rhythm.

2. Check the threshold one chamber at a time, beginning with the ventricle, which is the more important chamber because it is the supplier of systemic circulation.

3. Set the output to a low value (e.g., 1 mA), then raise the pacing rate to a level slightly higher than the patient's own rate.

4. If you see only pacing artifacts (spikes) with no corresponding depolarizations at the same rate or with only intermittent response from the heart, you have not yet reached the capture threshold. Increase the output by another milliampere and test again.

5. Repeat until every spike is followed immediately by depolarization of the target chamber. Then dial in at least twice as much output for the chamber you are evaluating.

6. Document the threshold.

### 21. What is an acceptable capture threshold?

A good capture threshold is one that you can exceed by at least a factor of two. That is, if the capture threshold in the patient's ventricle is 12 mA and the maximal output of the temporary pacer is 20 mA, the threshold is too high. It may be time for a decision about placing new temporary pacing wires (which probably will have a lower threshold), discontinuing the temporary pacer (if patient tolerance allows), or implanting a permanent pacemaker. Check capture thresholds once daily, because with temporary pacing wires they can change quickly.

**22. What is the sensing threshold?**

The pacer must be able to detect native cardiac signals—P and R waves—reliably, because when they appear, they should inhibit the device from pacing. These signals are often small; therefore the pacer's sensitivity threshold must be set so that they are reliably detected, preventing competition by the pacer with the native rhythm. The sensing threshold, measured in millivolts (mV), is the minimal amount of sensitivity that achieves this goal.

**23. How is the sensing threshold assessed?**

1. As with pacing thresholds, check one chamber at a time, again starting with the ventricle.

2. Gradually reduce the pacing rate until the patient's underlying rhythm has fully emerged.

3. Purposely make the pacer as insensitive to the ventricle as you can by setting ventricular sensitivity to the highest numeric value, perhaps 15 mV.

4. Set the pacing rate a bit higher than the patient's native rate.

5. If the pacer's sensitivity is insufficient, it will not be able to detect the patient's R waves and will begin to pace at the set rate. Therefore, increase the sensitivity a bit by setting it to a smaller number (e.g., 13 mV), and repeat the procedure.

6. Continue testing at smaller and smaller numeric values until at last no more pacing occurs; at this point the pacer is sensitive enough to detect every native R wave. The value now dialed into the pacer is the ventricular sensing threshold.

7. Document the sensing threshold, and set the sensitivity at least twice as high by decreasing the value to half its numeric size. For example, if the ventricular sensing threshold is 6 mV, you may choose a final setting of 3 mV for the ventricle.

8. Move on to the atrial channel, and repeat the procedure.

9. Check sensing thresholds once daily.

**24. What is oversensing?**

Oversensing is the pacemaker's detection of noncardiac electrical signals and results in failure to pace the patient when pacing in fact is required. The pacer is designed to receive the very small electrical impulses that the heart produces. If other, more powerful signals in the pacer's vicinity "drown out" the P or R waves and are of a particular character, the pacer may interpret these stray impulses as adequate heart rate, the pacer is inhibited from pacing, and cardiac output may suffer.

**25. How is oversensing remedied?**

Oversensing betrays itself as failure to pace where pacing is needed. If the pacer is set for 60 beats/min and the displayed rate is 40 beats/min with no visible pacer spikes, oversensing is the most likely culprit. Your first response should be to decrease the sensitivity in the chamber that requires pacing by dialing in higher and higher numeric values until at last you see consistent pacing at the desired rate. Try to find and eliminate possible sources of electromagnetic interference in the patient's environment. Ungrounded or short-circuited electrical equipment may be responsible; report any suspect items for testing by biomedical engineers. Only hospital-tested equipment should be in the patient's room, and the use of walkie-talkies or cellular phones in the critical care area should be strictly prohibited. Avoid passing lines with electric power near the pacemaker or its leads.

**26. What is undersensing?**

Undersensing is the opposite of oversensing: the pacer fails to detect native cardiac events that actually occur. In other words, the pacer is not sensitive enough. This problem manifests as unnecessary pacing.

**27. How is undersensing remedied?**

Your first response should be to increase the sensitivity in the problem chamber. To do so, dial in a smaller numeric value (2 mV is more sensitive than 4 mV), and continue in steps until the unnecessary pacing ceases. Then set the sensitivity still higher to provide a safety margin.

**28. What is failure to capture? How is it remedied?**

Failure to capture is the inability of the pacer to depolarize the target chamber with the output as set. This problem manifests as pacer spikes that are not followed immediately by depolarizations.

**29. How is failure to capture remedied?**

A number of difficulties can result in failure to capture. If the pacer's battery is very low, if the leads have shifted position in the heart, or if the myocardium is damaged or ischemic at the point of lead contact, failure to capture is the likely result. Often, however, simply increasing the output is the solution. Maintain the pacing rate, and in steps of 1 mA increase the output to the problem chamber until depolarization follows every pacer spike. Then double the output from that threshold value. Sudden failure to capture after satisfactory pacing thresholds in previous days is always cause for close evaluation of the adequacy of the temporary pacing leads.

BIBLIOGRAPHY

1. Baas LS, Beery TA, Hickey CS: Care and safety of pacemaker electrodes in intensive care and telemetry nursing units. Am J Crit Care 6:302–311, 1997
2. Bajaj BP, Evans KE, Thomas P: Postpericardiotomy syndrome following temporary and permanent transvenous pacing. Postgrad Med J 75:357–358, 1999.
3. Beery TA, Baas LS, Hickey CS: Infection precautions with temporary pacing leads: A descriptive study. Heart Lung 25(3):182–189, 1996.
4. Cooper JP, Swanton RH: Complications of transvenous temporary pacemaker insertion. Br J Hosp Med 53(4):155–161, 1995.
5. Cottle S: Temporary transvenous cardiac pacing. Nurs Times 93(48):48–51, 1997.
6. Davis GK, Roberts DH: Experience and training in temporary transvenous pacing [see comments]. J R Coll Physicians [London] 30:432–434, 1996.
7. Ettin D, Cook T: Using ultrasound to determine external pacer capture. J Emerg Med 17:1007–1009, 1999.
8. Gal Th J, Chaet MS, Novitzky D: Laceration of a saphenous vein graft by an epicardial pacemaker wire. J Cardiovasc Surg 39:221–222, 1998.
9. Gerstenfeld EP, Hill MR, French SN, et al: Evaluation of right atrial and biatrial temporary pacing for the prevention of atrial fibrillation after coronary artery bypass surgery. J Am Coll Cardiol 33:1981–1988, 1999.
10. Halldorsson AO, Vigneswaran WT, Podbielski FJ, Evans DM: Electrophysiological and clinical comparison of two temporary pacing leads following cardiac surgery. Pacing Clin Electrophysiol 22:1221–1225, 1999.
11. Keenan J: Cardiology update: Temporary cardiac pacing. Nurs Standard 9(20):50–51, 1995.
12. Kosmas CE, Ryder RG, Poon MJ, et al: Time-limited efficacy of pacing electrodes following open heart surgery. Ind Heart J 48:681–684, 1996.
13. Liebold A, Reodig G, Birnbaum DE: Performance of temporary epicardial stainless steel wire electrodes used to treat atrial fibrillation: A study in patients following open heart surgery. Pacing Clin Electrophysiol 22:315–319, 1999.
14. Macedo W Jr, Sturmann K, Kim JM, Kang J: Ultrasonographic guidance of transvenous pacemaker insertion in the emergency department: A report of three cases. J Emerg Med 17:491–496, 1999.
15. Murphy JJ: Current practice and complications of temporary transvenous cardiac pacing. BMJ 312:1134, 1996.
16. Pacifico AD: Management of temporary epicardial ventricular pacing wires [letter]. J Card Surg 13:228, 1998.
17. Preisman S, Cheng DC: Life-threatening ventricular dysrhythmias with inadvertent asynchronous temporary pacing after cardiac surgery. Anesthesiology 91:880–883, 1999.
18. Samuels LE, Samuels FL, Kaufman MS, et al: Temporary epicardial atrial pacing electrodes: Duration of effectiveness based on position. Am J Med Sci 315(4):248–250, 1998.
19. Sheldon R. Role of pacing in the treatment of vasovagal syncope. Am J Cardiol 84(8A):26Q–32Q, 1999.
20. Trigano AJ, Azoulay A, Rochdi M, Campillo A: Electromagnetic interference of external pacemakers by walkie-talkies and digital cellular phones: Experimental study. Pacing Clin Electrophysiol 22(4 Pt 1):588–593, 1999.
21. Wollan DL: Removal of epicardial pacing wires: An expanded role for nurses. Prog Cardiovasc Nurs 10(4):21–26, 1995.

# 5. BLOOD PRESSURE MONITORING: INVASIVE AND NONINVASIVE

*Carrie A. Taylor, RN, MS, CCRN*

### 1. What are the physiologic determinants of blood pressure?

Cardiac output and total peripheral resistance are the two major determinants of blood pressure. The volume of blood ejected from the heart per minute reflects **cardiac output**, which is influenced directly by stroke volume and heart rate. **Total peripheral resistance** (vascular resistance) is determined by the diameter and elasticity of blood vessels and blood viscosity. The arterioles demonstrate most of the resistance in the circulation. Arterial blood pressure varies with each cardiac cycle.

Various **chemical mediators**, either circulating or released, affect arteriolar diameter and blood pressure. Angiotensin II, vasopressin, and certain prostaglandins cause vasoconstriction and blood pressure elevation. Histamine, nitric oxide, and other prostaglandins reduce blood pressure.

### 2. Describe the role of baroreceptors in regulating blood pressure.

Baroreceptors in the carotid sinus and aortic arch regulate arterial blood pressure by sensing changes in mean arterial pressure and sending impulses to the medulla of the brainstem. An increase in the baroreceptor firing rate leads to a decrease in sympathetic response and an increase in parasympathetic response. Parasympathetic outflow causes a slowing of the heart rate and vasodilation, with subsequent reduction in arterial blood pressure. The opposite occurs with a sensed decrease in arterial mean pressure. (See figure on following page.)

### 3. How is blood pressure most commonly measured?

Blood pressure is measured most commonly with an inflatable cuff, sphygmomanometer, and stethoscope. The brachial artery is occluded by inflation of the cuff, and heart tones are auscultated during the deflation of the cuff. The auscultated heart tones are called Korotkoff sounds and signify the return of blood flow through the arterial vessels. The description and phases of the Korotkoff heart sounds are described in the table below.

*Korotkoff Phases and Heart Sounds*

| PHASE | SOUND | INDICATION |
|-------|-------|------------|
| I | First appearance of faint, clear heart sounds | Systolic blood pressure |
| II | Sounds developing a murmur or muffled quality | No indication |
| III | Sounds become clearer and increase | No indication |
| IV | Abrupt muffling of sounds | Diastolic blood pressure (in children) |
| V | Sounds disappear | Diastolic blood pressure (in adults) |

### 4. Define systolic blood pressure (SBP) and diastolic blood pressure (DBP).

SBP reflects the maximal pressure in the arterial vessels following ventricular ejection or systole. During ventricular ejection, pressure in the aorta and major arteries averages 120 mmHg in the healthy adult.

DBP represents the minimal pressure in the arterial vessels following the ventricular resting state or diastole. The average DBP in the healthy adult is 80 mmHg. DBP is often used to estimate systemic vascular resistance because both are influenced by the diameter of the arterial vessel. Both SBP and DBP are directly influenced by changes in volume (cardiac output) and pressure (total peripheral resistance).

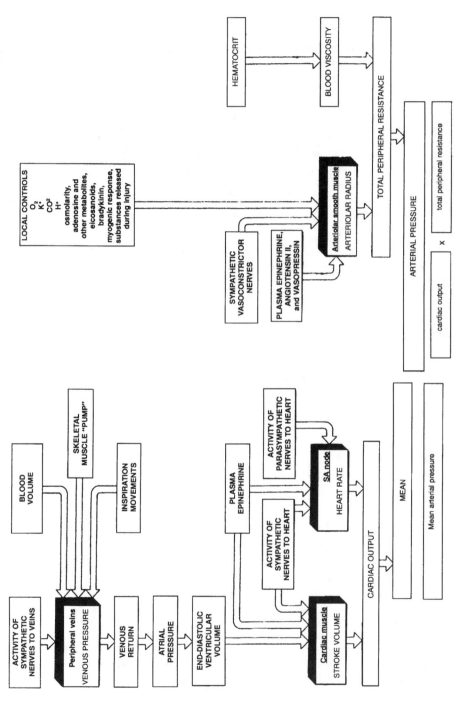

Determination of arterial blood pressure. (From Vander AJ, Sherman JH, Luciano DS: Human Patho-physiology: The Mechanisms of Body Function, 5th ed. New York, McGraw-Hill, 1990, pp 404–405, with permission.)

**5. Why is the mean arterial pressure (MAP) often monitored instead of SBP/DBP?**

The MAP is the product of cardiac output multiplied by total peripheral resistance, the two main determinants of blood pressure. MAP is estimated by adding the diastolic pressure to one-third of the pulse pressure. Pulse pressure is the difference between SBP and DBP. Because more time is spent in the diastolic phase, it is weighted more heavily:

$$MAP = \frac{SBP - DBP}{3} + DBP \quad or \quad \frac{DBP \times 2 + SBP}{3}$$

Because close monitoring of blood pressure is essential in critically ill patients, the MAP may be a more sensitive indicator for acute changes in the arterial system. Systolic pressure differs in the central and peripheral circulations, but diastolic and mean pressures do not. In clinical conditions associated with alterations in peripheral vascular resistance, the MAP is the more stable choice for blood pressure monitoring. In patients with vasoconstrictive shock, hypothermia, arterial occlusive lesions or stenosis, or vasodilator therapy and in patients who have undergone cardiopulmonary bypass, the MAP is a more accurate clinical indicator of the dynamic response of the arterial system than SBP/DBP measurement.

**6. What are the methods of indirect blood pressure measurement?**

| METHOD | DESCRIPTION | INDICATIONS |
|---|---|---|
| Palpation | The brachial artery is palpated while cuff is inflated until the pulse disappears. Cuff inflation continues for an additional 30 mmHg, then cuff is gradually deflated until the pulse reappears. This number is recorded as SDP/P. No DBP is recorded with. this method. | For quick measurement of SBP in emergency situations or when auscultation is not possible. Also for patients with peripheral vascular disease or hypotension. |
| Doppler | Doppler is used over the brachial or radial artery to determine SBP/D (D for Doppler), using the same procedure described above. | Patients with severe hypotension or peripheral vascular disease when Doppler is needed to enhance SBP sounds. |
| Auscultation | Stethoscope is used over the brachial artery during deflation of cuff; listen and record first heart tones (SBP) and disappearance of heart tones (DBP). | Most common method of blood pressure measurement. Used in all patients, excluding situations mentioned above. |
| Oscillometric (automatic blood pressure devices) | This method requires use of an automatic blood pressure cuff. Pulsatile blood flow creates turbulence or oscillations in blood vessel, which is transmitted to blood pressure cuff and recorded electronically on monitor. | When patient requires frequent blood pressure measurements, automatic devices help to free the nurse to perform other important patient management functions. |

**7. Why should the SBP be palpated before the auscultation method is used?**

The presence of an auscultatory gap can provide an erroneously low SBP reading if the palpation method is not used before auscultation of the blood pressure. The auscultatory gap most often occurs in patients with hypertension. After the SBP is auscultated, the heart tones disappear or become muffled briefly, reappear, then disappear again, and are recorded as the DBP. If the SBP is not palpated before auscultation, the cuff may not be inflated high enough, and the auscultatory gap will be misinterpreted as SBP (lower than actual). Once the presence or absence of a gap is determined, palpation is not needed on subsequent readings.

## 8. What factors influence noninvasive blood pressure measurement?

The importance of the **correct cuff size** cannot be stressed enough. The cuff size or bladder width must be 40% of the arm circumference. All cuffs and bladders have a sizing range on the outside of the cuff that can be used to identify the appropriate size for each patient. The standard cuff size for the average adult is 12–14 cm. Cuffs for clients with obese arms or for use on thighs should be 18–22 cm. If the cuff bladder width is < 40% of arm circumference, blood pressure recordings are higher than normal. If the cuff bladder width is > 40% of arm circumference, readings will be falsely low.

The **ideal location of the arm** for blood pressure measurement is at the level of the heart (phlebostatic axis). The bell of the stethoscope is placed at the position of the brachial artery, which should be at the level of the phlebostatic axis. Blood pressure readings increase as the arm is lowered from the level of the heart. When manual blood pressure readings are taken from different positions, such as standing and sitting, the placement of the stethoscope head must remain at the level of the heart. Thus, the arm must be supported and placed on a bedside table so that the measurement is taken at the level of the heart. The position of the manometer for the auscultatory method has no direct bearing on blood pressure measurement, but it should be placed at eye level so that mistakes are not made during the actual reading of mmHg.

## 9. What physiologic variables decrease the accuracy of noninvasive blood pressure measurement?

**Cardiac dysrhythmias.** Blood pressure can fluctuate from one cycle to the next in patients with frequent or regular premature ventricular contractions or atrial fibrillation because blood volumes change with each stroke. For patients with dysrhythmias, an estimation of the blood pressure is recorded along with the apical pulse and actual dysrhythmia.

**Shock.** The blood pressure of patients who are in shock with hypotension (septic or cardiogenic), elevated systemic vascular resistance, and decreased cardiac output (congestive heart failure, cardiomyopathy) is difficult to measure accurately with noninvasive methods. During auscultation Korotkoff sounds often are diminished or absent, resulting in lower recorded readings than by direct arterial measurement. For patients in this state, Doppler is the more reliable noninvasive method. The ideal method is direct arterial pressure readings.

**Obesity.** In morbidly obese patients, noninvasive blood pressure readings are often taken with the wrong size cuff and bladders (< 40% of arm circumference). The frequent results are falsely elevated blood pressure recordings and higher reporting of hypertension. This problem is found with both auscultatory and oscillatory methods.

**Peripheral vascular disease.** Patients with peripheral vascular disease require extremely high cuff inflations because of the resistance of the blood vessel to pressure. Measurements often are recorded at a higher level than in fact is present.

## 10. Discuss the reliability and recommendations for blood pressure measurement in the thigh and forearm.

At times it may be clinically necessary to avoid the use of the upper arm for blood pressure measurement. The thigh and forearm can provide accurate blood pressure readings if the appropriate techniques are applied. If the thigh is used, select a cuff and bladder that is specific for the thigh or 18–22 cm wide. Have the patient lie face down and apply the cuff around the upper thigh so that the inflation bladder is over the posterior aspect of the mid thigh. Place the stethoscope bell over the popliteal fossa and auscultate. SBP measured in the thigh can be 20–30 mmHg higher than in the upper arm. DBP is usually the same as the arm measurement.

When the patient is morbidly obese and a large cuff cannot be found, the forearm can be used with the regular adult cuff. The radial artery is palpated and auscultated. Forearm pressure measurements usually are avoided because they provide falsely elevated diastolic readings.

## 11. Is there a more direct way to measure systemic blood pressure?

True systemic pressure can be measured with a centrally placed aortic pressure monitoring device such as an intraaortic balloon pump (IABP) catheter. However, placement of an IABP catheter strictly for blood pressure monitoring is not recommended. The use of intraarterial pressure monitoring with a catheter directly inserted into the radial, brachial, or femoral artery is the most common direct method for arterial pressure monitoring. Pressure from the artery is transmitted through a transducer that converts it into a measurable waveform.

**12. When should invasive methods of blood pressure monitoring be used?**
 • For patients in whom cardiac output or peripheral vascular resistance may be compromised, such as shock or low flow states
 • For titration of vasoactive medications (e.g., Nipride for treatment of severe hypertension)
 • For clinical conditions in which frequent blood gas analyses are necessary (avoids painful needle sticks).

**13. What is the proper position for the transducer of an intraarterial line during blood pressure monitoring?**
Regardless of where the catheter is located (brachial, radial, or femoral artery), the goal of intraarterial monitoring is the same: to obtain readings that reflect central aortic pressure. The reference point for leveling the transducer should be as close to the right atrium as possible. The reference stopcock of the transducer must be leveled at the phlebostatic axis (heart level). The phlebostatic axis is located at the junction of the fourth intercostal space and the lower left sternal border. The level must be reevaluated after a change in the patient's position. Moving from sitting to supine position without releveling the transducer leads to false readings. If the transducer is placed too high, abnormally low readings result; if the transducer is placed too low (or, as commonly occurs, falls to the floor), abnormally high readings result.

**14. What factors influence the accuracy of intraarterial blood pressure monitoring?**
**Technical factors** include problems with the transducer, tubing, and catheter. Transducers must be placed consistently at the level of the phlebostatic axis to prevent effects from hydrostatic and atmospheric pressure. The system must be zeroed before insertion, after all disconnections from the cable, whenever clinical conditions question the accuracy of the pressure, and routinely during every shift. Tubing used for pressure monitoring should be of appropriate length and compliance (rigid). Tubing with air in line, inappropriate extensions, additional stopcocks, or increased compliance (flexible) can reduce the accuracy of the pressure reading by as much as 30 mmHg.
**Clinical factors** may influence the arterial waveform during respirations. Examples include asthma, chronic obstructive pulmonary disease, cardiac tamponade, constrictive pericarditis, and pulsus paradoxus. In such situations, readings should be taken consistently at the end of expiration.

**15. Which is more accurate—intraarterial line pressure or cuff pressure?**
This question continues to plague critical care clinicians. It is interesting that clinicians continue to compare cuff and arterial line pressure readings when clearly they do not measure the same thing. Cuff measurements by oscillometry (automatic blood pressures) record flow in the arterial system. The direct measurement using the arterial line records pressure in the arterial system. Pressure does not equal flow. However, a positive relationship does exist as long as peripheral resistance remains the same. As discussed above, because many clinical conditions alter peripheral resistance, it often does not remain constant. The current suggestion for the continuing dilemma of cuff vs. arterial line is to select the best method of blood pressure measurement for the clinical situation, optimize that method, and stop comparing the two.

## BIBLIOGRAPHY

1. Bridges ME, Middleton R: Direct arterial vs oscillometric monitoring of blood pressure: Stop comparing and pick one (a decision-making algorithm). Cardiovasc Med 17:58–72, 1997.
2. Dobbin KR: Protocols for practice: Applying research at the bedside: Noninvasive blood pressure monitoring. Crit Care Nurs 18: 101–102, 1998.
3. Frolich ED, Grim C, Labarthe DR, et al: Recommendations for human blood pressure determination by sphygmomanometers. Ann Intern Med 109:612, 1988.

4. Henshaw C: Alterations in blood pressure. In Copstead LC (ed): Perspectives on Pathophysiology. Philadelphia, W.B. Saunders, 1995, pp 325–335.
5. Imperial-Perez F, McRae M: Protocols for practice: Applying research at the bedside: Arterial pressure monitoring. Crit Care Nurs 19:105–107, 1999.
6. Larrivee C, Joseph DH: Strategies for teaching decision making: Discrepancies in cuff versus invasive blood pressures. Dimens Crit Care Nurs 11:278–285, 1992.
7. Smith SF, Duell DJ: Clinical Nursing Skills: Basic to advanced skills, 4th ed. Norwalk, CT, Appleton & Lange, 1996, pp 229–237.
8. Thelan LA, Davie JK, Urden LD: Critical Care Nursing: Diagnosis and Management, 3rd ed. St. Louis, Mosby, 1998.
9. Venus B, Mathru M, Smith R, Pham C: Direct versus indirect blood pressure measurements in critically ill patients. Heart Lung 14:228–231, 1985.

# 6. HEMODYNAMIC MONITORING

*Jim Stotts, RN, MS*

**1. What parameters are included in the hemodynamic profile?**

Various parameters are included in the hemodynamic profile. They are obtained by invasive direct measurement of pressure and/or volume or by physiologic calculations.

**Parameters measured directly**

- Right atrial pressure (RAP) or central venous pressure (CVP)
- Right ventricular pressure (RVP): systolic (RVS), diastolic (RVD), and mean (RVM) pressures
- Right ventricular end-diastolic pressure (RVEDP)
- Pulmonary artery pressure (PAP): systolic (PAS), diastolic (PAD), and mean (PAM) pressures
- Pulmonary artery wedge pressure (PAWP)
- Left ventricular end-diastolic pressure (LVEDP)
- Systemic systolic (SBP), diastolic (SDP), and mean arterial (MAP) blood pressures
- Pulse pressure (PP)
- Heart rate (HR)

**Indirect measurements**

- *Work indices:* cardiac output (CO), cardiac index (CI), stroke volume (SV), stroke volume index (SVI), stroke work (SW) or stroke work index (SWI) of the right ventricle (RVSW or RVSWI) and left ventricle (LVSW or LVSWI), ejection fraction (EF), and rate-pressure product (RPP)
- *Resistance states*: systemic vascular resistance (SVR), systemic vascular resistance index (SVRI), pulmonary vascular resistance (PVR), and pulmonary vascular resistance index (PVRI)
- Coronary artery perfusion pressure (CPP)

**2. What are the normal values for hemodynamic parameters?**

*Normal Values for Hemodynamic Parameters*

| PARAMETER | FORMULA | NORMAL RANGES | CLINICAL RELEVANCE |
|---|---|---|---|
| BP | CO × SVR | SBP ~ 120 mmHg<br>DBP~ 80 mmHg | Determinant of tissue perfusion<br>Affected by state of resistance in vessels, SV, and aortic elasticity |
| PP | SBP – DBP | 40–60 mmHg | Reflects increase or decrease in SV |

*Table continued on following page*

*Normal Values for Hemodynamic Parameters (Continued)*

| PARAMETER | FORMULA | NORMAL RANGES | CLINICAL RELEVANCE |
|---|---|---|---|
| MAP | $\dfrac{SBP + 2(DBP)}{3}$ (loses accuracy with HR > 120 bpm) | > 60 mmHg needed for adequate tissue perfusion | Average pressure in arterial system, determined by CO and SVR. Used to evaluate tissue perfusion |
| CVP | Direct measurement | 0–6 mmHg | Used to determine volume status and RV function; correlates with RVEDP |
| RVP | Direct measurement | RVS: 20–30 mmHg RVD: 0–6 mmHg | Used to determine RV function and volume |
| PAP | Direct measurement | PAS: 20–30 mmHg PAD: 6–10 mmHg | Used to determine state of resistance in pulmonary vasculature and RV function |
| PAM | $\dfrac{PAS + 2(PAD)}{3}$ | < 20 mmHg | Used in formulas to determine PVR and total pulmonary resistance |
| PAWP | Direct measurement | 4–12 mmHg | Used to determine LV function; correlates with LVEDP |
| Right-to-left pressure gradient | PAD – PAWP | 0–6 mmHg | Determines whether pulmonary disease is a cause of increased PAD. Value > 6 mmHg indicates pulmonary problem; normal gradient in presence of ↑ PAD indicates high PA pressures due to pump failure or fluid overload |
| CPP | MAP – PAWP Diastolic BP – PAWP | 60–80 mmHg | CPP < 40 mmHg is inadequate to maintain coronary artery flow. |
| RPP | HR × SBP | < 12000 mmHg/beats/ min | Used to evaluate oxygen consumption |
| CO | SV × HR | 4–8 L/min | Describes blood flow through tissues and reflects adequacy of cardiac function |
| CI | $\dfrac{CO}{BSA}$ | 2.5–4 L/min/m$^2$ | Indexes CO to body surface area (BSA)* |
| SV | $\dfrac{CO}{HR} \times 1000$ | 60–80 ml/beat | Amount of blood ejected during systole; decreased SV indicates ventricular dysfunction |
| SVI | $\dfrac{CI}{HR} \times 1000$ | 33–47 ml/beat/m$^2$ | SV referenced to BSA |
| PVR | $\dfrac{PAM - PAWP}{CO} \times 80$ $\dfrac{PAM - PAWP}{CO}$ | 20–120 dynes/sec/cm$^{-5}$ 0.25–1.7 Wood units | Describes state of resistance in pulmonary vasculature |
| PVRI | $\dfrac{PAM - PAWP}{CI} \times 80$ | 200–300 dynes/sec/ cm$^{-5}$/m$^2$ | PVR referenced to BSA |
| SVR | $\dfrac{MAP - CVP}{CO} \times 80$ $\dfrac{MAP - CVP}{CO}$ | 770–1500 dynes/sec/ cm$^{-5}$ 10–25 Wood units | Describes state of resistance in systemic vasculature |
| SVRI | $\dfrac{MAP - CVP}{CI} \times 80$ | 1900–2400 dynes/sec/ cm$^{-5}$/m$^2$ | SVR referenced to BSA |
| RVSW | $(PAM - CVP) \times SV$ $\times 0.0136$[†] | 10–15 g-m/beat | Defines how hard RV is working to pump blood; determined by average pressure generated by ventricular contraction multiplied by amount of blood ejected |

*Table continued on following page*

*Normal Values for Hemodynamic Parameters (Continued)*

| PARAMETER | FORMULA | NORMAL RANGES | CLINICAL RELEVANCE |
|---|---|---|---|
| RVSWI | (PAM − CVP × SVI × 0.0136[†] | 5–10 g-m/beat/m$^2$ | RSVW referenced to BSA |
| LVSW | (MAP − PAWP) × SV × 0.0136[†] | 60–80 g-m/beat | Defines how hard LV is working to pump blood |
| LVSWI | (MAP − PAWP) × SVI × 0.0136[†] | 45–75 g-m/beat/m$^2$ | LVSW referenced to BSA |

For key to abbreviations, see question 1.
* BSA is determined from the Dubois table using the patient's height and weight. It standardizes values to surface area.
[†] Conversion factor from mmHg/ml to gram-meters (g-m).

### 3. How are direct parameters measured?

Hemodynamic pressures are measured with a catheter situated in a vessel or in the heart and attached to a monitoring system. Typically a fluid-filled monitoring system is used, consisting of a catheter, pressure tubing, transducer, and electric cable attached to a monitor. Various catheter types are used to measure hemodynamic pressures, including sheaths and intraaortic, atrial, single- or multilumen central, and peripheral catheters. Pulsatile waves created by systolic and diastolic pressures are transmitted from the catheter tip via special low-compliance tubing to the pressure transducer. For accurate pressure and waveform conductance, the catheter and tubing must be filled only with fluid (free of air bubbles and blood), and all connections must be tightened. Use of other than low-compliance/noncompressible tubing, unnecessarily long tubing, and/or air or blood in the line produces distortions of waveform data. Pressure pulsations caused by the pressure changes between systole and diastole induce motion on the transducer diaphragm. These pulsations are converted to low-voltage electric signals, which are transmitted to the monitoring hardware, where they are amplified, filtered, and displayed as a pressure waveform and numerical data.

### 4. Describe the pulmonary artery (PA) catheter.

The signature characteristic of the PA catheter is that the catheter tip is situated in the pulmonary artery. A balloon located near the tip of the catheter, when inflated, assists in placement in the pulmonary artery and prevents trauma to cardiac structures as the tip travels through the heart chambers and valves. PA catheters may have a single lumen solely to monitor PA pressures or multilumens with ports exiting into the right ventricle, right atrium, and/or vena cava. Other features of various PA catheters include a thermistor to measure blood temperature, electrodes for cardiac pacing, a fiberoptic diode at the tip for measuring mixed venous oxygen saturation, and a warming coil to heat blood during thermodilution continuous measurements of cardiac output.

### 5. What other types of central lines are used?

The many other types of central lines, such as introducers and single-lumen and multilumen catheters, are used to administer fluids and measure right atrial pressure. Intraaortic lines are placed percutaneously, either through the femoral artery into the aorta or directly into the aortic arch, to measure aortic pressure. Intraatrial catheters are used to measure left atrial pressure in cardiac surgical patients with prosthetic tricuspid or pulmonic valves or high pulmonary artery pressures.

### 6. Describe the proper maintenance of a monitoring system.

1. Tubing is attached to a flush bag after the air has been removed from the bag. The flush bag is pressurized to 300 mm Hg. This counterpressure prevents back flow of blood into the catheter and tubing, assists in rapidly purging the system during manual flush, and allows delivery of a continuous 3–5-ml flush per hour while the monitoring system is in use.

2. Either 5% dextrose in water ($D_5W$) or 0.9 normal saline is used as the flush solution. Clinicians working with heart failure patients prefer $D_5W$ to avoid the added sodium burden of a saline flush; however, $D_5W$ may support growth of gram-negative bacteria.

3. Monitoring tubing is packaged with vented caps over each open stopcock port. These caps are necessary for gas sterilization but must be exchanged for female or dead-ended caps to maintain a closed system and preserve sterility.

4. Some institutions still require that flush solutions be heparinized at various concentrations. A large, randomized clinical trial conducted by the American Association of Critical Care Nurses (AACN) found no difference in patency rates for heparinized and nonheparinized arterial lines discontinued before 4 days. In general, however, patency is maintained for a longer period with heparinized line set-ups. No large randomized study has evaluated the use of heparin versus no heparin in central line monitoring, although at some institutions no heparin is used.

5. Institutional standards vary with regard to when tubings, flush bags, and dressings should be changed, which type of dressings should be used over arterial and central lines, and when central and arterial catheters should be replaced.

6. Other routine activities associated with hemodynamic monitoring include leveling and zeroing the transducer, assessing the system's dynamic response, and, in some instances, instrument and transducer calibration. These procedures are discussed as aspects of quality assurance.

### 7. How is right atrial (RA) pressure measured? What do normal RA pressure waveforms look like?

RA (CVP) pressures are measured using any port of a triple- or dual-lumen central line, single-lumen central line, or venous introducer catheter. The RA pressure waveform has three characteristic waves during the cardiac cycle: *a* wave, *c* wave, and *v* wave.

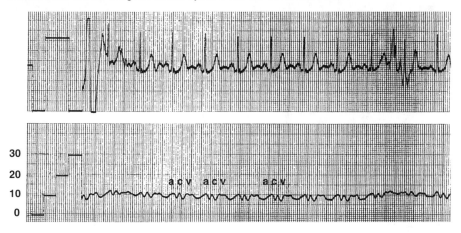

Normal right atrial pressure waveform.

### 8. What is the significance of the *a* wave?

The *a* wave denotes atrial systolic contraction and represents atrial kick. As the walls contract, blood volume is moved under pressure from the atrium to the ventricles. The increased intraatrial pressure creates an elevated pressure wave on the CVP/PAWP waveform. Atrial pressure falls as blood empties into the ventricle. At the beginning of ventricular systole, rising intraventricular pressure closes the AV valves.

### 9. What is the significance of the *c* wave?

During isovolumetric ventricular systolic contraction, the AV valves billow upward into the atria, creating the *c* wave. The *c* wave descent correlates with the opening of the pulmonic and aortic valves and ventricular systolic ejection.

**10. When does the *v* wave occur?**

With the AV valves closed, blood fills the atria, causing a rise in atrial pressure represented as the *v* wave. The *v* wave occurs during ventricular systole and soon after the descent of the *c* wave. When the ventricles relax during diastole, the AV valves once again open, allowing blood to flow from the atrium into the ventricle.

**11. How is left atrial (LA) pressure measured? What do normal LA pressure waveforms look like?**

LA pressure (PAWP) waveforms are obtained either from a left atrial catheter or from the tip of a PA catheter during balloon inflation. Typically they have the same *a*, *c*, and *v* waves as RA waveforms. The *c* wave, however, may be absent in the PAWP waveform for two reasons: (1) the PA/PAWP waveform typically is monitored in a 0–60-mmHg scale, which may be too large to show the subtle transition from *a* to *v* wave, and (2) as the PAWP readings travel from the left atrium through lung vessels back to the PA tip, there is loss of subtle waveform definition.

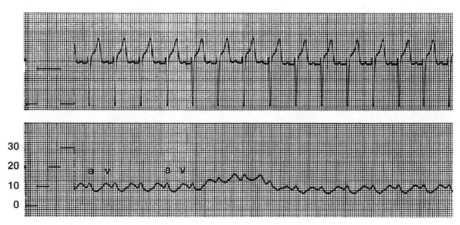

Normal left atrial pressure waveform.

**12. What is the advantage of simultaneous ECG and pressure recording of RA waveforms?**

Simultaneous ECG and pressure recording of either RA or PAWP waveforms is helpful in recognizing abnormal pressure waveforms. In the CVP waveform, the *a* wave comes closely after the P wave of an ECG; the *c* wave is at end of the QRS complex; and the *v* wave occurs near the end of the T wave. PAWP waveform propagation is delayed so that the *a* wave occurs at the end of the QRS complex, the *c* wave within the ST segment, and the *v* wave later into the T-P segment.

**13. What do normal right ventricular (RV) pressure waveforms look like?**

The RV pressure waveform is not routinely monitored on a continuous basis, but it is important for clinicians to recognize. The RV waveform is characterized by a steep upstroke at the beginning of systole. The peak pressure is 2–3 times higher than the mean CVP reading. RV pressure drops from the peak with a sharp downstroke to the lowest nadir; then sharply rises, signifying rapid ventricular filling; and finally tapers as pressure slowly rises during slower RV filling to the next sharp systolic rise. The point at which RV systolic ejection begins marks the end of RV diastole and, in patients without tricuspid valve disease, is equal to RA mean pressure readings. RV systolic pressure is equal to PA systolic pressure. These two similarities help the clinician assess PA catheter tip position so that inadvertent RV location can be avoided.

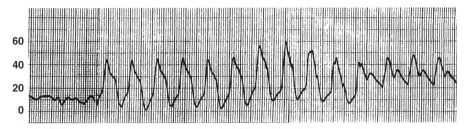

CVP to RV to PA pressure waveform.

### 14. What do normal PA and systemic arterial pressure waveforms look like?

PA and systemic arterial pressure waveforms are characterized by a sharp upstroke coming to a peak and a sharp downstroke interrupted by another short upstroke or plateau, followed by a tapered pressure drop to the nadir immediately before the next systolic beat. The dicrotic notch, the wave that interrupts the sharp pressure fall, represents closure of the pulmonic valve (PA waveform) or aortic valve (systemic arterial waveform) and the beginning of pulmonary or systemic arterial diastole. The dicrotic notch may or may not be observed on systemic arterial pressure waveforms. The PA diastolic pressure is read at the end of diastole and is higher than RV diastolic pressure.

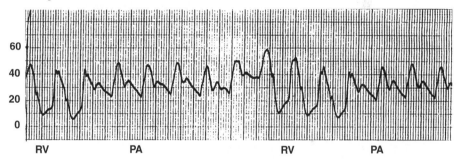

RV to PA pressure waveform.

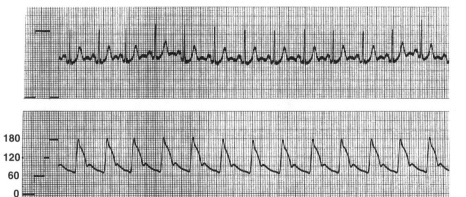

Systemic arterial pressure waveform.

### 15. Why should PA and systemic arterial pressure waveforms be correlated with ECG?

As with RA and PAWP readings, PA and systemic arterial pressures should be correlated with the ECG rhythm superimposed above the pressure waveform. The end of PA diastole is read immediately at the end of the QRS complex, whereas the end of systemic arterial diastolic pressure is at the end of the T wave. If a presystolic pressure wave is present in a PAP waveform, diastolic pressure should be read at the end of the QRS complex. If this reading falls within the middle of the presystolic wave, plot a continuation of the diastolic run-off through the extra wave.

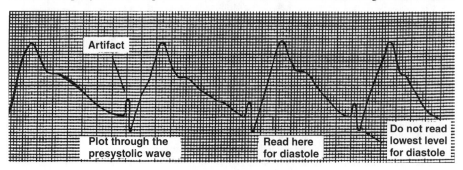

Presystolic pulmonary diastolic determination. (From Ahrens AS, Taylor LA: Hemodynamic Waveform Analysis. Philadelphia, W.B. Saunders, 1992, p 148, with permission.)

### 16. Discuss the relationships among preload pressure readings.

In the absence of abnormal valves, RA pressure represents RVEDP, whereas PAWP represents LVEDP. End-diastolic pressure reflects ventricular function. Rises or falls in RVEDP or LVEDP denote changes in ventricular function and/or fluid/blood volume. In the absence of cardiopulmonary dysfunction, PAWP pressure can be estimated at 2 times the CVP reading plus 2. For example if the CVP is 5 mmHg pressure, the PAWP is 12 or $(5 \times 2) + 2$. The PAD correlates within 1–4 mmHg of the PAWP in the absence of pulmonary hypertension or mitral stenosis; PAD is higher as a result of greater resistance to blood flow in the pulmonary circulation. When the PAD correlates with the PAWP, many clinicians trend PAD pressures as an indication of ventricular performance.

### 17. What conditions cause PAWP to overestimate LVEDP?

- Pulmonary hypertension
- Reduced LV compliance (due to LV hypertrophy, septal displacement, acute myocardial infarction, myocardial fibrosis, and amyloidosis)
- Elevations in pressure around the heart (e.g., cardiac tamponade, ascites, use of military antishock trousers, increased intrathoracic pressure).

### 18. How can I ensure accurate and reliable data?

Checking the dynamic response of the tubing/catheter system and zeroing, calibration, and leveling of the monitoring system should be done routinely to ensure accurate and reliable data.

### 19. Define dynamic response.

Dynamic response is the ability of the fluid-filled catheter and tubing system to reproduce accurately the patient's pulse without distortion on the amplifier/monitor. The square-wave or fast-flush test is used to assess dynamic response. When a fast flush is performed, an optimally damped system creates a sharp upstroke that peaks and plateaus. This should be followed by a rapid downstroke extending below the baseline with 1 or 2 oscillations and then a return to a normal pressure waveform. An overdamped system produces a waveform with a somewhat slurred upstroke, peak plateau, a rapid downstroke that does not extend below the baseline, and no oscillations after the flush. Overdamping underestimates systolic pressure and overestimates diastolic pressure. An underdamped system shows numerous oscillations above and below the baseline at the end of a fast flush. With underdamping systole is artificially elevated, and diastole is falsely low.

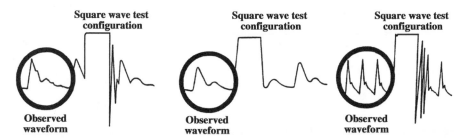

*Left,* Optimally damped waveform. *Center,* Overdamped waveform. *Right,* Underdamped waveform. (From Darovic GO, Vanriper S, Vanriper J: Fluid-filled monitoring systems. In Darovic GO (ed): Hemodynamic Monitoring: Invasive and Noninvasive Clinical Application. Philadelphia, W.B. Saunders, 1995, pp 161–162, with permission.)

### 20. How do I minimize problems with dynamic response?

1. Use a system with as few stopcocks and manifolds as necessary.
2. Use catheters no smaller than 18 gauge or 7 French.
3. Use low-compliance tubing no longer than 3–4 feet.
4. Ensure that nothing other than fluid (i.e., air or blood) fills the tubing and that all connections are tight.
5. Use a continuous-flush device maintained at 300 mmHg.
6. Ensure that tubing is protected from sources of extraneous movement.
7. Zero balancing, leveling, and calibration are also important.

Over- and underdamping are concerns for arterial pressures only. If either is present and uncorrectable, mean pressures are the most reliable values to report and document.

### 21. Why is zero balancing important? How is it done?

Zero balancing the monitoring system to a standard or reference pressure (i.e., atmospheric pressure) eliminates interference from other pressure sources and ensures that recorded pressures reflect intravascular pressure changes only.

The stopcock closest to the tranducer is turned to the off position in the direction of the patient. The dead-end cap is removed, creating an air-to-fluid interface. The zeroing process is initiated when the zero function on the monitor is engaged. Re-zeroing on a consistent basis eliminates the possibility that the monitoring system has drifted from the zero pressure mark. Zeroing should be performed according to hospital protocol (usually once a shift, when the clinician questions the validity of data, and when the displayed values or waveforms do not correlate with the clinical picture).

### 22. Why is leveling important? How is it done?

The stopcock used for zeroing should be leveled to the point where the catheter tip is located. Fluoroscopic examinations have shown that for central and aortic catheters this point is at the intersection of the midaxillary line and fourth intercostal space, also called the phlebostatic axis. If the stopcock is below this axis, hydrostatic pressure from the fluid within the tubing exerts additional pressure on the tranducer diaphragm, artificially elevating pressure readings. If the stopcock is above the phlebostatic axis, less hydrostatic pressure is applied to the transducer because of gravity, and the pressure reading is falsely low. Leveling is done whenever the transducer stopcock is not level with the phlebostatic axis (e.g., when the patient changes position).

### 23. Why is calibration important? When is it done?

A calibration is done to check the reliability of the monitor's electronic performance. By pressing the calibration button, a known signal is presented to the monitor and causes a square wave up to a standard pressure height, then back to zero. Calibration of disposable transducers is done simultaneously with zero balancing.

### 24. How are RA and PAWP pressure readings determined?

Several different methods are used to determine RA and PAWP pressure readings. Clinicians should not simply record pressure values from the monitor screen or draw a line bisecting all of the waves to determine mean pressure. They should analyze the waveform for abnormalities associated with fling, valve pathology, respiratory cycle, and dampening. The *a* wave analysis provides the most accurate method of determining RA and PAWP pressure, except in patients with mitral stenosis.

### 25. How is waveform analysis performed?

Three methods have been proposed: (1) calculate the mean between the peak of the *a* wave and the end of the *x* descent; (2) read the mean at the plateau immediately before the beginning of the *a* wave (the *h* wave); and (3) read the mean at the onset of the *c* wave (the *z* point). When determining PAWP, keep the balloon inflated for at least 2–3 respiratory cycles so that end-expiration can be accurately identified. In patients with mitral stenosis, pressure is higher on the atrial side than on the ventricular side, resulting in an artifical elevation of *a* wave pressures. In this case the *v* wave may correlate more closely with LVEDP.

### 26. Where should the PA catheter tip be located? How is its location assessed?

For accurate PAWP readings, the PA catheter tip should be located in zone III of the lung vascular tree. In zone III both arterial and venous pressures exceed alveolar pressure. If alveolar pressure exceeds arterial pressure (zone I), the PA pressure reflects alveolar pressure. If alveolar pressure does not exceed arterial pressure but does exceed venous pressure (zone II), the PA catheter may not provide accurate left atrial waveforms and pressures. The tip is located in a zone III position if it is located below the left atrium on radiographs.

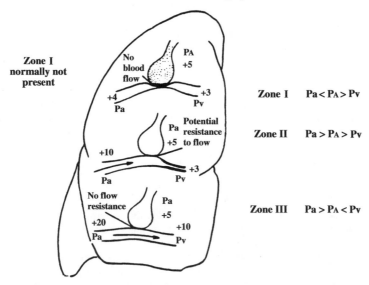

Catheter tip location in lung zones. (From Ahrens AS, Taylor LA: Hemodynamic Waveform Analysis. Philadelphia, W.B. Saunders, 1992, p 37, with permission.)

### 27. How should the patient be positioned for pressure readings?

All pressure readings should be done while the patient is in the supine position. The head of the bed can be elevated as much as 45°, provided that the transducer system is leveled to the phlebostatic axis. Studies with patients in the supine position at head elevations greater than 45° and in the lateral lying position are not conclusive in terms of correct transducer placement and accuracy of values. All pressures should be read at the end-expiratory phase of the respiratory cycle.

### 28. What is the nurse's role in PA catheter insertion?

Nursing responsibility with PA catheter insertion is changing with the advent of advanced nursing practice roles. Specific tasks include patient/family teaching, acquiring consent, assembling equipment, assisting the physician, premedicating the patient, preparing the monitor and tubing, and, in some settings, actually inserting the catheter.

### 29. Describe the procedure for PA catheter insertion.

Because PA catheter insertion is a sterile procedure, caps and masks are necessary for everyone involved. The patient is heavily draped and may require sedation and coaching to tolerate the procedure. The nurse assists with the following tasks:
- Flushing the tubing with fluid to purge it of air
- Checking the balloon by dipping it in sterile saline or water while it is inflated to ensure that the balloon is competent
- Leveling and zeroing the transducer before line insertion
- Setting the PA channel to a 60-mmHg scale so that changes in waveforms are easily seen
- Recording and watching the waveform progression from RA to RV to PA to PAWP to help determine optimal placement of the catheter tip.

### 30. What does hemodynamic monitoring reveal about tricuspid and mitral valve pathology?

The presence of large *a* waves on the CVP and PAWP tracing represents tricuspid and mitral valve stenosis, respectively. Large *v* waves signify tricuspid and mitral valve regurgitation. An ECG graphic should be run concurrently with the CVP or PAWP tracing to distinguish *a* waves from *v* waves. Elevated *a* and *v* waves artificially elevate the CVP and PAWP mean digital readings on the monitor, justifying measurement of these parameters from the graphic tracing instead.

### 31. What does hemodynamic monitoring reveal about aortic valve stenosis?

Advanced aortic valve stenosis and insufficiency can alter the normal appearance of the arterial waveform. In aortic stenosis, the upstroke of systole is slurred, prolonged, and gradual. Overall pulse pressure is reduced because of a decrease in systolic peak pressure while diastolic peak pressure remains the same. Often the dicrotic notch is blurred or appears as a bend in the waveform because of slower closure of the stiff valve leaflet.

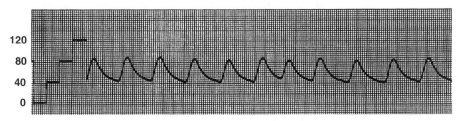

Aortic stenosis waveform. Note that the dicrotic notch is blurred between descending systolic and diastolic pressures.

### 32. What does hemodynamic monitoring reveal about aortic regurgitation?

The arterial waveform of aortic regurgitation has a sharp upstroke and wide pulse pressure due to elevated systolic and reduced end-diastolic pressure. In some cases, two systolic peaks are present, producing two palpable pulses. The two peaks may be equal, or one may be larger than the other. The dicrotic notch may be absent, and end-diastole pressure may be elevated higher than the diastolic nadir. Aortic diastolic pressure continues to decline because of an insufficient valve, while at the same time filling of the ventricle from the aorta and left atrium occurs. End-diastolic aortic pressure is elevated by reflections of an elevated LVEDP.

### 33. What are the complications of hemodynamic monitoring?

The many complications of hemodynamic monitoring have fueled a long-standing debate over its risk/benefit ratio. Most complications are unrelated to monitoring per se; they result instead from the insertion and presence of a catheter in the heart. The list of complications includes hemorrhage, vascular erosions, arrhythmias, infection, fluid overload, thromboemoblic events, electrical microshock, venous air embolism, perforation of cardiac chambers, pneumothorax, prolonged hospital stay, and death.

### 34. What are the major arguments against hemodynamic monitoring?

Opponents of PA monitoring cite not only unacceptable risks but also studies showing that many clinicians are not experienced with line insertion and cannot interpret the data correctly. In addition, clinical presentation does not correlate well with hemodynamic findings.

### 35. What are the benefits of hemodynamic monitoring?

The benefits of hemodynamic monitoring remain unproved. A few small studies suggest that benefits of monitoring tissue oxygenation, especially in patients at high risk or with multisystem failure, may outweigh the risks. Many clinicians use hemodynamic monitoring when LV function is in question.

### 36. What is the nurse's role in discontinuance of hemodynamic monitoring?

With the advent of reduced Medicare funding for medical training and with more advanced practice nurses in intensive care units, nurses are asked with increasing frequency to remove PA catheters. Although nurses can perform this procedure safely, complications such as valve disruption and emboli sheer when the PA catheter is pulled into the introducer may occur. Hypothetically, the nurse performing the procedure alone may find him- or herself in an emergency situation without immediate back-up from a physician. Still, with adequate training and competency testing and a two-nurse team, the procedure can be done as safely by a nurse as by a physician.

### BIBLIOGRAPHY

1. Amercian Association of Critical Care Nurses Thunder Project: Evaluation of the effects of heparinized and non-heparinzed flush solutions on the patency of arterial pressure monitoring lines. Am J Crit Care 2:3, 1993.
2. Ahrens AS, Taylor LA: Hemodynamic Waveform Analysis. Philadelphia, W.B. Saunders, 1992.
3. Bond EF, Halpenny CJ: Physiology of the heart. In Woods SL, Sivarajan Froelicher ES, Halpenny CJ, Motzer SU (eds): Cardiac Nursing, 3rd ed. Philadelphia, Lippincott, 1995, pp 46–47.
4. Daily EK, Schroeder JS: Techniques in Bedside Hemodynamic Monitoring, 4th ed. St. Louis, Mosby, 1989, pp 179–199.
5. Freeman GL, Klein LW, Darovic GO: Valvular heart disease. In Darovic GO (ed): Hemodynamic Monitoring: Invasive and Noninvasive Clinical Application. Philadelphia, W.B. Saunders, 1995.
6. Gardner PE, Bridges EJ: Hemodynamic monitoring. In Woods SL, Sivarajan Froelicher ES, Halpenny, CJ, Underhill Motzer, S (eds): Cardiac Nursing, 3rd ed. Philadelphia, Lipponcott, 1995.
7. Kern L: Hemodynamic monitoring. In Boggs RL, Wooldridge-King M (eds): American Association of Critical Care Nursing Procedure Manual for Critical Care, 3rd ed. St. Louis, Mosby, 1993, pp 281–367.

# 7. CARDIAC OUTPUT MONITORING

*Jim Stotts*, RN, MS

### 1. Define cardiac output (CO). What is its normal range?

CO is the volume of blood, measured in liters, ejected each minute during ventricular contraction. CO measurement represents flow through any part of the circulatory system, assuming the absence of intracardiac shunts and regurgitant valves. For most adults, normal resting CO is 4–8 L/minute, an average of 5 quarts/minute or 75 gallons/hour.

### 2 What variables affect "normal" CO values?

In coordination with blood pressure, CO fluctuates in response to changing **tissue metabolic demands**. An increase in metabolic or oxygen demand is met with a rise in CO and vice versa. Because of their greater metabolic needs, children have a higher resting CO than adults.

**Body composition and size** also affect CO. People with less skeletal muscle mass and more body fat have lower COs than people with more muscle mass and less fat. Adipose tissue is less vascular and requires less metabolic energy than skeletal muscle tissue. Larger body mass, in general, requires a higher CO than smaller body frames to achieve adequate tissue perfusion.

**Changes in body position**—for example, from lying to standing—lead to a decrease in resting CO. Disparity among CO values with position changes supports the standard of determining CO with the patient in the supine position, with the head of the bed raised no more than 20°.

### 3. What is cardiac index (CI)? What is its normal range?

CI is a means of adjusting CO for body size. Blood flow is represented relative to 1 square meter ($m^2$) of body surface area (BSA). The normal range for CI is 2.5–4.5 $L/min/m^2$.

### 4. How is CI calculated?

By dividing CO by BSA. BSA can be determined by plotting the patient's weight and height onto the Dubois nomogram. CI does not accommodate for differences in metabolic rate, as in patients with diseases such as hyper- or hypothyroidism, or body mass (i.e., an obese person vs. a well-muscled person of equal weight and height).

### 5. What are the determinants of CO?

CO is the product of heart rate (HR) and stroke volume (SV). HR is controlled principally by the autonomic nervous system. SV is the volume of blood ejected during ventricular systole and ranges between 60 and 130 ml. SV is affected by preload, afterload, and contractility. A change in heart rate, preload, afterload, or contractility causes a corresponding change in CO.

### 6. How does HR affect CO?

The continuous fluctuations in HR are due to various degrees of sympathetic and vagal nerve stimulation and blockade in response to alterations in tissue oxygenation, blood volume, blood pressure, emotional reactions, and other factors. Stimulation of beta$_1$ receptors in the heart produces an increase in HR, which is associated with increased influx of calcium into the cell's sarcoplasmic reticulum and thus an increase in contractile force and CO. The beneficial effect of an increase in contractility is offset by reductions in diastolic filling or preload and underlying myocardial disease. Faster heart rates limit ventricular filling time and in turn decrease CO. A slower heart rate, with its prolonged diastolic filling time, augments CO. Profound bradycardia, however, induces reduced contractile force and myofibril overstretch, causing CO to decline.

### 7. Define preload. How does it affect CO?

Preload refers to the amount of myofibril stretch caused by blood volume at the end of diastole. The greater the volume, the greater the stretch. Myofibril extension is beneficial to CO. At the beginning of diastole, actin and myosin filaments overlap. With the addition of volume, the myofibrils are stretched; actin and myosin filaments become disassociated or pulled apart. During a contractile stimulus, the actin and myosin filaments interact, in the presence of calcium, to pull closer, producing a forceful contraction. Greater myofibril stretch produces a greater contraction and increased CO; less stretch results in reduced CO.

### 8. Why are we interested in the volume of blood at the end of diastole?

The end of diastole is the point of maximal myofibril stretch. If we could stop the heart at this point in the cardiac cycle, insert a catheter, and withdraw the contents, we would be able to measure the actual volume in the heart. Because volume quantification is impractical, we evaluate preload by measuring end-diastolic pressure. A basic principle of physics states that pressure within a closed chamber increases as volume increases. Direct application of this principle to cardiac physiology is confounded by the elasticity of heart tissue. Starling noted that increases in left ventricular volume at the end of diastole were associated with an increase in active pressure and CO—within limits. Beyond a certain point, a greater volume results in greater pressure but a drop in CO.

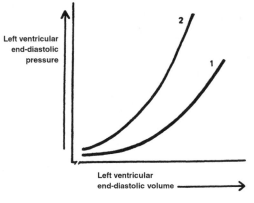

Pressure/volume relationship. Both curves demonstrate that as left ventricular end-diastolic pressure increases, so does left ventricular volume. Curve 1 represents conditions of normal ventricular muscle stiffness. Curve 2 represents increasing stiffness. (From Bond EF, Halpenny CJ: Physiology of the heart. In Woods SL, Sivarajan Froelicher ES, Halpenny CJ, Motzer SU (eds): Cardiac Nursing, 3rd ed. Philadelphia, J.B. Lippincott, 1995, p 47, with permission.)

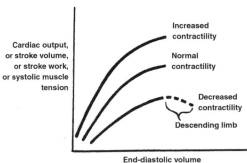

Volume/CO relationship. As left ventricular volume increases, there is a corresponding increase in CO. With increases in contractility at the same volume, there is an increase in CO. With decreased contractility, as with heart failure, a limit exists, so that with higher preloads there is a corresponding decline in CO. (From Bond EF, Halpenny CJ: Physiology of the heart. In Woods SL, Sivarajan Froelicher ES, Halpenny CJ, Motzer SU (eds): Cardiac Nursing, 3rd ed. Philadelphia, J.B. Lippincott, 1995, p 46, with permission.)

### 9. How is end-diastolic pressure evaluated?

Central venous pressure (CVP) is used to evaluate right ventricular end-diastolic pressure. The normal range of CVP is 0–6 mmHg. Pulmonary artery wedge pressure (PAWP) is used to evaluate left ventricular end-diastolic pressure. The normal range of PAWP is 4–12 mmHg. PAWP above 20–25 mmHg, seen in patients with left ventricular failure, causes pulmonary congestion, pulmonary edema, and adventitious lung sounds.

### 10. Define afterload. How does it affect CO?

Afterload is the force or pressure that opposes ventricular systolic ejection and emptying during contraction. The variables that contribute to afterload are the condition of the aortic valve, elastic compliance of the aorta, blood volume, blood viscosity, and the state of meta-arteriole vasoactivity. Of these five factors, afterload is most affected by meta-arteriole vasoactivity. The greater the afterload, the greater the resistance against ventricular emptying, the slower the ventricular contraction, and the less volume ejected. The overall result is a decrease in CO. Coronary artery perfusion is also adversely affected as a consequence of elevated preload at greater afterloads.

### 11. How is afterload measured?

Afterload cannot be measured directly. Indirect measurements of afterload at the bedside include pulmonary artery mean (PAM) and pulmonary artery diastolic (PAD) pressures, mean systemic arterial pressure (MAP), diastolic arterial pressure (DBP), systemic vascular resistance (SVR), and pulmonary vascular resistance (PVR).

### 12. How is SVR calculated?

Calculation of SVR is based on the principle that resistance is equal to pressure divided by flow. Either of two equations may be used:

$$SVR = \frac{MAP - CVP}{CO} \times 80 \qquad or \qquad SVR = \frac{MAP - CVP}{CO}$$

If the *first equation* is used, normal values range from 770–1500 dynes/sec/cm$^{-5}$. Pressure in mmHg is changed to dynes/cm$^{-2}$, and flow in L/min is changed to cm$^{-3}$, the unit most often used in clinical practice.

If the *second equation* is used, normal values range from 9.9–18.9 mmHg/L/min or Wood or R units. Values for flow are expressed in volume (L/min) vs. velocity flow, and values for pressure are expressed in mmHg, the unit most commonly used in laboratories.

### 13. How is PVR calculated?

Calculation of PVR is based on the same principle as calculation of SVR. Either of two equations may be used:

$$PVR = \frac{PAM - PAWP}{CO} \times 80 \qquad or \qquad PVR = \frac{PAM - PAWP}{CO}$$

If the *first equation* is used, normal values range from 20–120 dynes/sec/cm$^{-5}$.

If the *second equation* is used, normal values range from 0.25–1.7 mmHg/L/min or Wood or R units.

### 14. Define contractility. How does it affect CO?

Contractility refers to the inherent ability of the myocardium to shorten muscle fiber length and develop tension, regardless of preload and afterload. Contractility cannot be measured directly. Clinical decision-making is based on the patient's ventricular curves and perfusion status. Inotropy describes the force of contraction. Factors such as sympathomimetic agents and exercise increase contractility and produce a steeper function curve that shifts upward and to the left, demonstrating an increase in CO at a given preload pressure. Negative inotropic agents lower CO. (See figure at top of following page.)

### 15. How do I use this information clinically?

The integration of hemodynamic data with clinical presentation allows the clinician to evaluate the patient's response to therapy. Given any abnormal CO value, the clinician should be able to analyze the hemodynamic profile consisting of HR, preload, and SVR and to suggest treatments that will shift CO toward normal. Analysis depends on comparing measured values with norms, determining abnormal values, and deciding which abnormal values contribute to altered CO. Treatment depends on which values are abnormal.

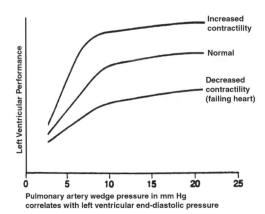

Ventricular function curve. Note that with increased contractility left ventricular performance improves. With states of relatively depressed contractility, ventricular performance deteriorates. (From Darovic GO: Pulmonary artery pressure monitoring. In Darovic GO (ed): Hemodynamic Monitoring: Invasive and Noninvasive Clinical Application. Philadelphia, W.B. Saunders, 1995, p 290, with permission.)

### 16. Specify the cause and treatment of major hemodynamic abnormalities.

*Hemodynamic Abnormalities Leading to Decreased CO and Recommended Treatments*

| PARAMETER | CAUSE | TREATMENT |
|---|---|---|
| ↓ Preload | ↓ Fluid/blood volume | Fluid replacement |
| ↑ Preload | Overhydration ↓ Ventricular performance | Diuresis, inotropic or sympathomimetic agent to increase contractility |
| ↓ HR | Pacemaker failure, conduction failure, or vagal stimulation | Atropine, pacemaker, treatments to remove source of vagal stimulation |
| ↑ HR | Physiologic stress—i.e., fever, pain, anxiety, hypoxemia, ventricular dysfunction; may be side effect of sympathomimetic or vaso-active agent | Correct causative condition; if warranted, slow HR with beta blockers, calcium channel blockers |
| ↓ Afterload | Vasodilation | Determine cause. If endotoxins, treat with antibiotics; if vasodilating drugs, reduce dose or discontinue. Treat with vasopressors such as dopamine, epinephrine, neosynephrine. |
| ↑ Afterload | Vasoconstriction | Vasodilators; titrate to keep MAP at desired level. |

Other parameters that give an indication of CO adequacy include venous oxygen saturation, heart rhythm, color, and level of consciousness.

### 17. Describe the procedure for measuring CO by the thermodilution method.
Measurement of CO by thermodilution involves instilling a known quantity of fluid, either dextrose or saline, at a known temperature into the right atrium, which cools the surrounding blood. A thermistor located 4 cm from the tip of the PA detects the change in blood temperature. This information is fed back to either the bedside monitor or a stand-alone CO computer, which creates a thermodilution curve and a digital display of CO. The area under the curve is used to calculate CO mathematically and is inversely proportional to the flow rate of blood. If a high CO is measured, the area under the curve is small; for low CO, the area is large. The procedure is repeated until two determinations are within 10% of the median value.

### 18. What are the limitations of measuring CO by thermodilution?
Limitations include inaccuracy in patients with tricuspid regurgitation (TR), ventricular septal defect (VSD), and the potential for volume overload associated with volume restrictions.

Measurement of change in blood temperature over time with the thermodilution method depends on blood flowing forward with no contamination of blood from another source. Both TR and VSD allow mixing of blood either because of backflow between the right atrium and ventricle (TR) or blood from the right and left ventricle (VSD).

**19. What potential sources of error are inherent in the thermodilution method?**
- Using the wrong computation factor for the catheter, volume, or temperature of injectate
- Overhandling of injectate syringe, which warms the injectate fluid
- Infusing injectate for more than 4 seconds, which causes slower mixing of cool injectate with warm blood
- Infusing injectate during inspiration, which is associated with a lower PA temperature
- Determining CO during concomitant drug or fluid administration
- Determining CO during arrhythmias
- Infusing injectate through a proximal port that exits within the introducer sheath instead of the right atrium
- Determining CO using a catheter with a dampened waveform.

**20. How does a continuous CO PA catheter determine CO?**
PA catheters with a heating filament can determine CO continuously. This method uses the same theoretical principle as thermodilution with a cold injectate, but the wire warms the blood in cycles to a known temperature. No ill effects have been reported from heating blood elements to a temperature of 43°C. Continuous CO measurements are not affected by technician errors but are invalid in the presence of TR and VSD.

**21. How can we be sure that our data are reliable and accurate?**
Careful attention to detail while performing a thermodilution CO is paramount:

1. Position the patient in a supine position at a backrest elevation of less than 20°. Studies evaluating the correlation between supine and side-lying positions are not conclusive. CO readings done at backrest elevations greater than 20° are artificially low.

2. Make sure that the thermistor is working properly. If measurements of blood temperature are inaccurate, CO measurement will be inaccurate.

3. Use the manufacturer's recommendation to determine the correct computation factor. The wrong index can give either a low CO (index set too low) or high CO (index set too high).

4. Infuse exact amounts of injectate.

5. Avoid overhandling the injectate, and draw and infuse injectate within 30 seconds. Overhandling and exposing iced injectate to room temperature for longer than 30 seconds can increase the injectate temperature, giving higher than expected CO.

6. Injectate infusion bags should be kept out of direct sunlight.

7. Infuse injectate smoothly within 4 seconds. Infusing longer than 4 seconds produces a lower than expected CO. Uneven infusions produce an irregular upslope of the CO curve. Use of an automatic injector does not improve reproducibility or accuracy of CO determinations.

8. Because PA blood temperature is lower with inspiration (an effect that may be exaggerated with mechanical ventilation), most texts recommend infusing the injectate close to the end of expiration. Mechanical ventilation may decrease CO overall, especially with higher inspiratory pressures and higher levels of peak end-expiratory pressure (PEEP).

9. Make sure that the RA and PA waveforms are not dampened.

10. If possible, concomitant infusions should be turned off, although research validating this practice is inconclusive. Infusions of more than 150 ml/hr cause an artificially low CO.

11. It takes 60–90 seconds for blood temperature to equalize to baseline. Do not repeat CO determinations until at least 90 seconds have elapsed.

12. Perform a series of CO determinations until two readings are within 10% of the median value. Dysrhythmias during injectate infusion may cause a wide variation in serial CO measurements.

### 22. How does injectate affect CO?

Too much injectate produces a low CO; too little, a higher than expected CO. Saline injectates produce a 2% lower CO reading than dextrose. Studies have shown that iced and room-temperature injectates and 10-, 5-, and 3-ml injectate volumes produce comparable data. (For recommended injectate volume and temperature in select patient populations, see question 24). The use of iced injectate increases the signal-to-noise ratio (the greater the difference in temperature, the greater the signal-to-noise ratio) between injectate and blood temperature.

### 23. What is the significance of a dampened RA or PA waveform?

A **dampened RA waveform** may suggest that the proximal infusion port is within the introducer sheath or that a fibrin sheath or clot has formed over the exit port. In the case of catheter misplacement, the catheter can be inserted further into the heart as long as the PA distal port does not demonstrate wedging. If a clot is suspected and cannot be removed with aspiration, the venous infusion port or side port of the introducer can be used to infuse the injectate without an appreciable threat to validity.

A **dampened PA waveform** may indicate that the catheter is too distal, resulting in an artificially high CO.

### 24. Outline injectate volume and temperature recommendations for the following patient populations.

| | |
|---|---|
| Normothermic patients | 5–10 ml iced or 10 ml at room-temperature |
| Hypothermic patients | 10 ml iced or at room temperature |
| Hyperthermic patients | 10 ml iced |
| Hyperdynamic patients | 10 ml iced or at room temperature |
| Patients with low CO | 10 ml iced |

### 25. Describe the Fick method for measurement of CO.

The Fick principle describes flow in terms of changes in oxygen tension and oxygen consumption. The premise of the Fick equation is that the amount of oxygen picked up by blood as it passes through the lungs must be equal to the amount of oxygen taken up by the patient's lungs during breathing. The amount of oxygen uptake, or oxygen consumption, is measured noninvasively by sampling exhaled gases at the mouth. The amount of oxygen picked up by the blood is measured by drawing arterial and mixed venous blood samples. Normal oxygen consumption in the resting state is 220–229 ml/min. Measurement of oxygen consumption at the bedside is time-consuming and labor-intensive and requires a resting oxygen consumption state. An estimated Fick CO uses an average oxygen consumption value of 125 ml/min/m$^2$, multiplied by the patient's BSA. The difference in oxygen concentration, depicted as the difference between arterial and mixed venous oxygen concentration in volume % saturation (ml/dl), reflects oxygen uptake per unit of blood as it flows through the lungs. Volume % saturation is the amount of oxygen saturation per 100 ml of blood.

### 26. What formula is used to calculate CO by the Fick method?

$$CO\ (L/min) = \frac{\text{Oxyen consumption (125 ml/min/m}^2) \times BSA}{(\text{Arterial} - \text{venous saturation}) \times \text{hemoglobin} \times 1.34 \times 10}$$

where 1.34 ml represents the amount of blood that each gram of hemoglobin can carry and 10 is the factor used to convert arteriovenous oxygen saturation difference from ml/dl to L/min.

### 27. How accurate is the Fick method compared with thermodilution?

Both the thermodilution and Fick methods apply the law of conservation of mass. The accuracy of the Fick method is not affected by TR, but VSD invalidates the formula because shunting of blood contaminates the validity of venous oxygen saturation measurement. The Fick method is more valid for low CO states and patients with TR, whereas the thermodilution method is more valid for higher CO states. Thermodilution tends to overestimate CO in low-flow states, a problem frequently compensated for by using iced injectate. Like thermodilution, the Fick method evaluates CO at only one point in time.

**28. What simpler method may be used to gain a rough estimate of CO?**

Look at the difference between arterial and venous oxygen content ($AVDO_2$). The normal range for $AVDO_2$ is 3–5.5 ml/dl. An $AVDO_2$ less than 3 indicates that blood flows quickly past the tissues so that less oxygen dissociates from hemoglobin, producing a smaller difference between arterial and venous oxygen content. An $AVDO_2$ greater than 5.5 indicates that flow is slow through the tissues, giving more time for a greater amount of oxygen to dissociate from the hemoglobin and producing a greater difference between arterial and venous oxygen content.

**29. How often should CO be measured?**

There is no standard answer to this question, although some critical care units have guidelines to facilitate decision-making. CO should be measured as often as needed to evaluate patient response to therapy. In general, if vasoactive agents, inotropes, or fluids are added or weaned, CO should be determined at least every 1–2 hours, depending on how quickly the treatments are added or removed. Between CO determinations the clinician should monitor preload (CVP, PAWP), blood pressure, HR, and cardiac rhythm closely to observe for acute changes that suggest a change in CO or the patient's condition. If the patient becomes hemodynamically stable, CO should be measured once during each shift until the central line is discontinued.

**30. List three noninvasive methods used to measure CO.**
1. Doppler ultrasound
2. Bioimpedance
3. Expired carbon dioxide

**31. How is Doppler ultrasound used to measure CO? How accurate is it?**

Doppler ultrasound, in conjunction with echocardiography, can plot blood flow velocity and points within the ventricle and aortic root to determine diameter. Flow velocity and left ventricular outflow diameter are used to compute CO. The reliability and sensitivity of this method is highly observer-dependent and tends to underestimate CO.

**32. How is bioimpedance used to measure CO? How accurate is it?**

Transthoracic electrical bioimpedance (TEB) measures stroke volume using a low-energy current that is discharged through the thorax. The impulse course of travel through the body is either impeded or conducted. Tissues that impede conduction include fat, cardiac and skeletal muscle, lung, vascular tissue, bone, and the ratio of air to liquids in the thorax. Overall thoracic impedance to voltage conduction, called baseline impedance, remains relatively unchanged. Blood, on the other hand, is highly conductive. Because blood volume is greater during systole, electrical conduction is enhanced, whereas the smaller blood volume during diastole decreases conduction. Sensors placed on either side of the chest and neck detect changes in voltage conduction through the body and heart rate. Blood volume changes in the aorta, the vessel with the largest blood volume, and subsequent phasic changes in bioimpedance are used to determine SV. CO is then calculated by multiplying SV by HR. CO determinations by TEB correlate well with CO measurements via Doppler ultrasound, indirect Fick, and thermodilution methods. (See figures at top of following page.)

**33. How is expired carbon dioxide ($CO_2$) used to measure CO? How accurate is it?**

The Fick $CO_2$ rebreathing measurement is based on the principle that $CO_2$ output is a product of CO multiplied by the difference in arterial and venous $CO_2$ concentration. Arterial $CO_2$ is inferred from the end-tidal expired $CO_2$. A mixed venous $CO_2$ is measured by having the patient rebreathe from a bag or circuit that contains a precise concentration of oxygen and $CO_2$. Measurement of mixed venous $CO_2$ and oxygen/$CO_2$ gas concentration is controlled by a separate machine. $CO_2$ output is measured as a routine part of an exercise test or is calculated by a machine that measures flow and $CO_2$ from the circuit of a ventilated patient. The partial $CO_2$ rebreathing method for determining CO correlates well with thermodilution techniques.

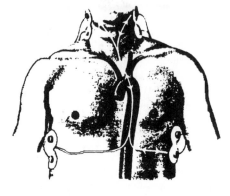

Surface electrode placement for thoracic electrical bioimpedance monitoring. The outer electrodes (upper electrodes on the neck, bottom electrodes on the chest) introduce the current, whereas the inner electrodes sense corresponding voltage changes through the cardiac cycle. (Reprinted with permission from CardioDynamic International Corporation.)

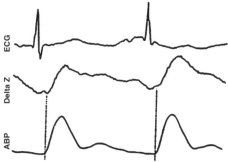

Comparision of ECG, arterial waveform, and voltage conduction wave (delta Z). Voltage conduction increases (bioimpedance decreases) milliseconds after QRS and arterial systole, then decreases during diastole to the lowest point of conduction at the end of diastole, the point of baseline thoracic impedance. (Reprinted with permission from CardioDynamic International Corporation.)

## BIBLIOGRAPHY

1. Bond EF, Halpenny CJ: Physiology of the heart. In Woods SL, Sivarajan Froelicher ES, Halpenny CJ, Underhill Motzer S (eds): Cardiac Nursing, 3rd ed. Philadelphia, Lippincott, 1995, pp 46–47.
2. Daily EK, Schroeder JS: Techniques in Bedside Hemodynamic Monitoring, 4th ed. St. Louis, Mosby, 1989, pp 179–199.
3. Darovic GO: Pulmonary artery pressure monitoring. In Darovic GO (ed): Hemodynamic Monitoring: Invasive and Noninvasive Clinical Application. Philadelphia, W.B. Saunders, 1995, p 290.
4. Darovic GO, Yacone-Morton LA: Monitoring CO. In Darovic GO (ed): Hemodynamic Monitoring: Invasive and Noninvasive Clinical Application. Philadelphia, W.B. Saunders, 1995, pp 323–346.
5. Gardner PE, Bridges EJ: Hemodynamic monitoring. In Woods SL, Sivarajan Froelicher, ES, Halpenny CJ, Underhill Motzer S (eds): Cardiac Nursing, 3rd ed. Philadelphia, Lippincott, 1995, p 447.
6. Kadota LT: Hemodynamic monitoring. In Clochesy JM, Breu C, Cardin S, et al (eds): Critical Care Nursing. Philadelphia, W.B. Saunders, 1993, pp 155–182.
7. Kern L: Hemodynamic monitoring. In Boggs RL, Wooldridge-King M (eds): AACN Procedure Manual for Critical Care, 3rd ed. St. Louis, Mosby, 1993, pp 281–367.
8. Moran CM, McDicken WN, Hoskins PR, Fish PJ: Developments in cardiovascular ultrasound. Part 3: Cardiac applications. Med Biol Eng Comput 36:529–543, 1998.
9. Osypka MJ, Bernstein DP: Electrophysiologic principles and theory of stroke volume determination by thoracic electrical bioimpedance. AACN Clin Issues10:388–399, 1999.
10. Watt RC, Loeb RG, Orr J: Comparison of a new non-invasive CO technique with invasive bolus and continuous thermodilution. Anesthesia 89:A536, 1998.

# 8. SvO₂ and AVDO₂ MONITORING

*Christine Corcoran, RN, MS*

### 1. What is SvO₂?

Mixed venous oxygen saturation ($SvO_2$) is the measurement of oxygen saturation of the pooled venous blood that returns to the heart from systemic tissues after the tissues have extracted the oxygen necessary for energy production. $SvO_2$ is an indirect measure of oxygen delivery and consumption. Therefore, it can be used to assess the balance between oxygen supply and demand in critically ill patients. To understand how clinicians use $SvO_2$, one must understand the primary function and normal circulation of the cardiopulmonary system and the principles of oxygen delivery and consumption.

### 2. What is the primary function of the cardiopulmonary system?

The primary function of the cardipulmonary system is the oxygenation and delivery of blood to systemic tissues to prevent hypoxia and to support aerobic metabolism. The viability of the human cell depends on a continuous source of oxygen and its adequate delivery to the tissues for the production of adenosine triphosphate (ATP). ATP is the major source of energy used to support aerobic metabolism at the cellular level. Without adequate oxygen and mechanisms of delivery, the tissues become hypoxic, anaerobic metabolism replaces aerobic metabolism, and lactic acidosis develops. This sequence of events leads to cellular dysfunction that can precipitate major organ dysfunction and failure if treatment is not initiated.

### 3. Describe the normal circulatory process.

Pooled venous blood returns to the right heart via the superior and inferior vena cava and is pumped into the pulmonary artery, at which point it is considered to be true, mixed venous blood. It then circulates through the pulmonary bed to be oxygenated and returns to the left side of the heart via the pulmonary vein. Normal red blood cells in a healthy person are approximately 100% saturated with oxygen on their return to the left heart. This blood is then pumped through the arterial system to the systemic tissues for utilization in cellular metabolism.

### 4. Define oxygen delivery. How is it calculated?

Oxygen delivery ($DO_2$) is the volume of oxygen delivered to the systemic tissues every minute. $DO_2$ is measured in ml/min or ml/min/m² (when CO is replaced with cardiac index [CI]). Using CI to calculate $DO_2$ takes into consideration body surface area (BSA) and is, therefore, a more accurate measurement for the individual patient. $DO_2$ can be calculated with one of the following equations, in which the constant 10 allows conversion of hemoglobin (Hgb) from gm/dl to gm/1000 ml of blood:

$$DO_2 = CO \times CaO_2 \times 10$$
$$DO_2 = CI \times CaO_2 \times 10$$

### 5. What are the main determinants of DO₂?

**Cardiac output** (CO), the volume of blood that the heart pumps out every minute, is the most important determinant of $DO_2$. Metabolic demands of the tissues cannot be met if blood flow to the tissues is inadequate. Normal CO for the average adult is 4–8 L/min.

**Arterial oxygen content** ($CaO_2$), the amount of oxygen in each 100 ml of arterial blood, is the second major determinant of $DO_2$. Defining components of $CaO_2$ are the partial pressure of oxygen in arterial blood ($PaO_2$), arterial oxygen saturation ($SaO_2$), and Hgb level.

### 6. How is CaO₂ calculated?

$$CaO_2 = (Hgb \times 1.38 \times SaO_2) + (0.003 \times PaO_2)$$

$SaO_2$ equals the amount of oxygen bound to Hgb divided by the total Hgb available. It is the actual amount of oxygen carried by Hgb vs. the total amount that the Hgb could carry. Each gram of Hgb is capable of carrying 1.38 ml of oxygen. Therefore, Hgb × 1.38 = oxygen-carrying capacity of arterial blood.

### 7. How do you determine the actual amount of oxygen bound to the Hgb?

Simply take the equation in question 6 one step further:

$$Oxygen\ bound\ to\ Hgb = Hgb \times 1.38 \times SaO_2$$

The majority of the oxygen is transported in the bloodstream bound to Hgb; however, a small quantity is dissolved in the plasma. This amount of oxygen is represented in the $CaO_2$ equation as $0.003 \times PaO_2$, where 0.003 is the solubility coefficient for oxygen and $PaO_2$ is the partial pressure of oxygen. If the normal $PaO_2$ of 100 mmHg is multiplied by 0.003, the result is 0.3 ml of oxygen dissolved in the plasma. Because this number is such a small portion of the total arterial oxygen content, it is considered acceptable to delete this part of the equation in clinical practice and to calculate $CaO_2$ with the following equation:

$$CaO_2 = Hgb \times 1.38 \times SaO_2$$

With $PaO_2$ greater than 60 mmHg, $SaO_2$ is > 90%, resulting in an inconsequential effect on oxygen content. When the $PaO_2$ drops below 60 mmHg, the impact on $SaO_2$ and oxygen content is significant.

### 8. What is the oxygen supply-demand ratio?

Under normal physiologic conditions, the amount of oxygen delivered generously exceeds tissue requirements to support aerobic metabolism. Normal $DO_2$ for resting adults is 1000 ml/min. The tissues use approximately 25% (250 ml) of the oxygen delivered. The remaining 75% (750 ml) is returned to the heart, yielding an oxygen supply-demand ratio of approximately 4:1. The oxygen that returns to the heart and pulmonary artery, bound to the Hgb, is referred to as the venous reserve and is measured as $SvO_2$.

### 9. Why monitor $SvO_2$ when you can monitor variables such as CO, $SaO_2$, and $PaO_2$?

$SvO_2$ measurement allows you to monitor oxygen utilization at the tissue level. Other parameters such as CO, $PaO_2$, and $SaO_2$ monitor the volume of blood flow and its oxygen content. They do not necessarily indicate oxygen consumption ($VO_2$) and venous reserve. Despite adequate oxygen delivery, critically ill patients may present with an imbalance between oxygen supply and demand.

### 10. What is the clinical significance of $SvO_2$?

The $SvO_2$ reading may be an earlier indicator than other hemodynamic measurements that the clinical picture is changing at the cellular level. Frequently, substantial changes in blood pressure (BP) and heart rate (HR) are late indicators of a significant physiologic event because the body attempts to compensate in the early stages of hemodynamic compromise. $SvO_2$ usually changes at the time that the balance between oxygen supply and demand is offset and may be a valuable indicator of events to come. For example, in the early stages of bleeding when intravascular volume is compromised, the systemic vascular resistance (SVR) and HR may increase to compensate for the low BP. Eventually, if unrecognized, the CO and BP will drop as the HR rises. With continuous monitoring of $SvO_2$, the nurse may see a more immediate change as the patient reacts to a compromise in oxygen delivery at the tissue level. In this case, one would expect to see a drop in $SvO_2$ as the tissues attempt to extract more oxygen from a limited supply (e.g., inadequate $DO_2$).

### 11. Can you monitor $SvO_2$ without monitoring other variables?

$SvO_2$ monitoring should not replace the monitoring of other hemodynamic parameters but rather should be used as an adjunctive technique that provides the nurse with critical information. For example, CO and stroke volume (SV) are indicators of myocardial function, and $SaO_2$ measures available circulating oxygen. A change in $SvO_2$ does not differentiate whether the problem is related to cardiac dysfunction, hemorrhage, or oxygen delivery. However, it does indicate a change associated with oxygen supply and demand that warrants reassessment of one or more parameters that are indicative of specific physiologic functions.

## 12. How is SvO$_2$ monitored?

SvO$_2$ can be monitored by intermittent sampling of blood from a pulmonary artery (PA) catheter, or it can be monitored continuously using a fiberoptic PA catheter. Intermittent sampling requires that the mixed venous blood sample be analyzed in a central blood gas laboratory. Continuous monitoring techniques allow continuous SvO$_2$ readings at the bedside. Through contact with the red blood cells, the fiberoptic PA catheter transmits information about mixed venous blood to a computer module. Light emitted from the catheter tip is reflected off the red blood cells. Oxygenated blood reflects light back to the fiberoptic catheter more readily than deoxygenated blood. The computer interprets the wavelength of the light and then converts this information to a numeric value that is displayed continuously, as a percentage, on the computer screen. This percentage is the average of SvO$_2$ values from the previous 5 seconds.

## 13. What is the acceptable range of SvO$_2$ values?

Normal SvO$_2$ is 75%, with an acceptable range of 60–80%. A value less than 60% implies an increase in oxygen demand or a decrease in oxygen supply to the tissues. A value > 80% indicates an increased oxygen supply, decreased oxygen extraction by the tissues, or inability of the tissues to utilize available oxygen. Whenever the SvO$_2$ drops below 60%, rises above 80%, or changes by 10% from the baseline for more than 3 minutes or for more than 10 minutes after a position change, the patient's condition should be reevaluated.

## 14. How does SvO$_2$ monitoring assist in the assessment of DO$_2$?

Evaluation of SvO$_2$ alerts the clinician to potential problems associated with DO$_2$. During times of increased oxygen demand, the body attempts to augment DO$_2$. The primary compensatory mechanism to increase DO$_2$ is to increase CO, thereby increasing blood flow to the tissues. Another mechanism may be an increase in minute ventilation, which potentially increases CaO$_2$. A severe disease state can alter these mechanisms so that DO$_2$ remains inadequate, oxygenation of circulating blood in the pulmonary bed is compromised, or the tissues are unable to extract the oxygen. If DO$_2$ remains inadequate to support aerobic metabolism, the tissues will extract more oxygen. An increase in oxygen extraction is indicated by a fall in the SvO$_2$ reading (a depletion of venous reserve). If the DO$_2$ is adequate but the tissues are unable to extract the oxygen, a rise in SvO$_2$ is noted. A change in the SvO$_2$ reading should alert the nurse that assessment of the components of DO$_2$ (CaO$_2$, CO) is warranted to determine the origin of the oxygen deficit. Energy expenditures should also be evaluated in the presence of a falling SvO$_2$, because physiologic factors and medical or nursing interventions may contribute to an imbalance between oxygen supply and demand.

## 15. Define oxygen consumption.

Oxygen consumption (VO$_2$) is the volume of oxygen extracted by the tissues every minute. VO$_2$ depends on the availability of oxygen and the ability of tissues to extract the oxygen from the capillaries. Because it is a measurement of how much oxygen is consumed by the tissues, VO$_2$ is used as an indirect measurement of tissue oxygen demand. Tissues extract only the amount of oxygen that is needed to support aerobic metabolism.

## 16. How is VO$_2$ calculated?

VO$_2$ can be calculated with one of the following equations. Note that the VO$_2$ can be indexed to account for the patient's size by substituting the cardiac index (CI) for CO in the equation. CI is the CO divided by BSA.

$$VO_2 = (SaO_2 - SvO_2) \times Hgb \times 1.38 \times CO \times 10$$
$$VO_2 \text{ index} = (SaO_2 - SvO_2) \times Hgb \times 1.38 \times CI \times 10$$

## 17. What is AVDO$_2$?

AVDO$_2$ is the difference between arterial oxygen content (CaO$_2$) and mixed venous oxygen content (CvO$_2$). It represents the amount of oxygen uptake by body tissues for aerobic metabolism. Assessment of AVDO$_2$ helps in decision making about treatment strategies to maximize DO$_2$ and meet the patient's oxygen demands. It is another method used to assess the oxygen supply-demand balance of critically ill patients.

## 18. What is the normal value of AVDO$_2$?

Normal arterial and venous oxygen contents are measured in ml/dl of blood or vol %. Normal CaO$_2$ is 20 mg/dl, and normal CvO$_2$ is 15 mg/dl. Plugging these numbers into the following equation defines normal AVDO$_2$:

$$CaO_2 - CvO_2 = AVDO_2$$
$$20 \text{ mg/dl} - 15 \text{ mg/dl} = 5 \text{ mg/dl}$$

## 19. What is the significance of changes in AVDO$_2$ values?

As oxygen demands increase in the presence of inadequate oxygen supply, the AVDO$_2$ increases. Similarly, as oxygen utilization decreases (e.g., in patients with sepsis), so does AVDO$_2$.

## 20. What factors affect the accuracy of AVDO$_2$ assessment?

The bedside nurse can calculate AVDO$_2$ when using SvO$_2$ monitoring techniques. Nursing technique for obtaining the necessary blood samples can affect accuracy of the calculated AVDO$_2$:

1. Arterial and mixed venous (MV) blood samples must be drawn simultaneously.
2. The distal port of the PA catheter is used to draw the MV sample.
3. The MV sample is drawn slowly (over 1 minute) to prevent collection of arterial/oxygenated blood.
4. Intravenous infusions into the PA line should be withheld while the MV sample is drawn to prevent dilution of the Hgb value.

## 21. How does SvO$_2$ monitoring aid in assessing overall tissue oxygen consumption?

Monitoring of SvO$_2$ offers a mechanism to assess overall tissue oxygen consumption. From the VO$_2$ equations above, one sees that a change in VO$_2$ is reflected in the SvO$_2$ reading. If VO$_2$ increases and DO$_2$ does not increase accordingly, SvO$_2$ decreases because the tissues extract more oxygen from the circulating supply and the venous oxygen content returning to the heart is lower. If VO$_2$ decreases, the inverse occurs.

## 22. Is oxygen supply and demand equal for all organs?

Neither DO$_2$ nor VO$_2$ is uniform for individual organs. For example, the kidneys require a high volume of blood flow for normal function, yet VO$_2$ is approximately 10% of the volume perfused. In contrast, the myocardium requires a relatively small volume of blood flow but extracts nearly 70% of the delivered oxygen. Because of this disparity in oxygen utilization, the measurement of SvO$_2$ is indicative of an overall trend in oxygen supply and demand rather than an indicator of specific tissue or organ VO$_2$. Technology has been unable to develop a mechanism by which clinicians can directly measure the oxygen consumption of individual organs.

## 23. What physiologic events can cause a decrease in SvO$_2$?

A decrease in SvO$_2$ indicates that oxygen demands exceed oxygen supply. This deficit may be related to a decrease in DO$_2$ or an increase in VO$_2$.

| Decrease in DO$_2$ | Increased VO$_2$ |
|---|---|
| 1. Decreased CO | 1. Fever |
| • Congestive heart failure | 2. Pain |
| • Hypovolemia | 3. Shivering |
| • Arrhythmias | 4. Increased work of breathing |
| • Increased peak end-expiratory pressure | 5. Interventions/procedures |
|    (positive-pressure ventilation) | 6. Infection |

2. Decreased SaO$_2$
   - Respiratory failure (altered gas exchange)
   - Interventions such as suctioning
3. Low hematocrit/Hgb
   - Hemorrhage
   - Hemodilution
   - Anemia

### 24. Describe the likely clinical scenario in a ventilated patient who has recently undergone major abdominal surgery and experiences significant physiologic stress. How should the nurse respond?

Two compromising conditions exist in this clinical situation. First, VO$_2$ is increased by stressors such as the surgical procedure, pain, work of breathing, catecholamine release, and wound healing. More oxygen is extracted by the tissues to provide energy during hypermetabolism. Secondly, DO$_2$ is compromised (low CO and low SaO$_2$) and most likely unable to support the increased tissue demand. The result is increased oxygen extraction from the capillary bed and lower venous oxygen content as blood returns to the heart. An imbalance in the oxygen supply-demand ratio can be recognized using SvO$_2$ monitoring techniques. A fall in the SvO$_2$ reading should prompt reassessment of the components of DO$_2$ and the reasons for increased VO$_2$. Interventions may include volume resuscitation with blood products and vasoactive medications to augment DO$_2$. Sedation and pain medication may be necessary to alleviate stress and discomfort, thereby decreasing metabolic demands.

### 25. What physiologic events cause an increase in SvO$_2$?

An increase in oxygen supply (improved or augmented DO$_2$), a decrease in oxygen demand, and decreased oxygen utilization due to inability of the tissues to extract oxygen may cause an increase in the SvO$_2$ value.

**Increase in oxygen supply**
1. Increased CO
   - Volume replacement
   - Inotropic agents
   - Intraaortic balloon pump
2. Increase in SaO$_2$
   - Supplemental oxygen
   - Mechanical ventilation
   - Improved respiratory status
3. Improved hematocrit/Hgb
   - Blood transfusions

**Decrease in oxygen demand**
1. Treatment of pain, infection, anxiety
2. Anesthesia
3. Hypothermia

**Decreased oxygen utilization**
1. Left shift of oxyhemoglobin dissociation curve
2. Cellular dysfunction (e.g., sepsis)
3. Cyanide toxicity

### 26. How does sepsis increase SvO$_2$?

The cellular dysfunction and impaired oxygen transport associated with sepsis are related to a systemic inflammatory response, maldistribution of blood flow, vasodilation and regional vasoconstriction, increased capillary permeability, and hypermetabolism. Blood is shunted to organs that normally consume lower amounts of oxygen rather than organs that consume higher amounts of oxygen. Increased capillary permeability at the microcirculatory level causes interstitial edema that interferes with blood flow as well as oxygen transport into the cells. The hyperdynamic state of sepsis increases metabolic needs, but compromised oxygen transport results in either shunting of blood flow or decreased oxygen extraction by tissues. Ultimately, vasoconstriction occurs, interfering with CO and DO$_2$. In late sepsis, cardiac failure ensues, compromising CO and DO$_2$. At this point the patient suffers from multisystem organ dysfunction, and outcomes are often poor.

### 27. How does cyanide toxicity increase SvO$_2$?

Cyanide toxicity is a rare occurrence associated with the administration of sodium nitroprusside. Toxic levels of this medication can interfere with the utilization of oxygen by the mitochondria, resulting in an increased SvO$_2$ secondary to a reduction in VO$_2$.

**28. How does SvO$_2$ monitoring help to diagnose an intracardiac shunt?**

In the presence of an intracardiac shunt (either atrial septal or ventricular septal), arterial blood is shunted from the right side of the heart to the left, causing a mixing of venous blood with arterial blood. The physician may be able to identify the development of a septal defect in a patient who experiences a myocardial infarction (involving the septum) with SvO$_2$ monitoring techniques. A sudden increase in the SvO$_2$ may indicate the presence of a left-to-right shunt. As arterial blood mixes with venous blood in the right heart, it circulates into the pulmonary artery, where SvO$_2$ is measured and, in this situation, becomes elevated. The patient needs further evaluation to verify the existence of a new cardiac defect.

**29. Now that I know what SvO$_2$ is all about, how do I apply it at the bedside?**

The important message is that changes in the SvO$_2$ reading indicate changes in the patient's overall clinical status; they do not reflect specific organ function or dysfunction. A drop in SvO$_2$ should prompt reassessment of the patient for changes in DO$_2$ and VO$_2$ and their underlying cause. If a current therapy is adjusted, a new therapy is added, or the patient undergoes an intervention based on a change in the SvO$_2$ reading, the patient's condition should improve. Pharmacologic, medical, and surgical interventions should increase DO$_2$ and possibly decrease VO$_2$, leading to normalization or stabilization of the oxygen supply and demand balance, as reflected in an increase in SvO$_2$. For example, a patient with congestive heart failure who is unable to maintain an adequate CO may demonstrate an SvO$_2$ in the 50% range. In this case, DO$_2$ is inadequate to meet the demands. After initiation of therapies such as intravenous medications and insertion of an intraaortic balloon pump, SvO$_2$ should rise, indicating improved CO, adequate arterial oxygenation, and normalization of cellular function.

Monitoring SvO$_2$ can also assist evaluation of patient response to bedside interventions and activities. For example, suctioning is an invasive procedure that can temporarily decrease oxygenation and increase patient anxiety. Ambulation or getting the patient out of bed to a chair increases the work of breathing and may elicit pain. Both scenarios increase metabolic demands and can disrupt the oxygen supply-demand balance. Knowledge of how a patient reacts physically and how long it takes for the patient to recover help to plan the patient's daily schedule. Recovery periods between activities may be necessary so that efforts to provide adequate and safe care do not result in periods of physiologic decompensation.

**30. What do I really need to know about the technology and equipment?**

1. The technology is only as good as the person who is monitoring the equipment. If you do not understand why it is being used or how to evaluate the numbers, SvO$_2$ monitoring does the clinician no good.

2. Probably the most important point is that the insertion of a PA catheter is an invasive procedure not without risk to the patient. Consider the necessity of invasive monitoring in each case, and weigh the risks against the benefits. If information provided by the PA catheter is not used to guide therapies, it may not be worth the risk.

3. For continuous SvO$_2$ monitoring, the computer module must be calibrated upon PA catheter insertion and then on a daily basis. Consult the user manual for instructions, troubleshooting techniques, and regular maintenance issues. In addition, enlist the assistance of a colleague who is familiar with the equipment before initial use or troubleshooting.

4. If SvO$_2$ is monitored intermittently, calibration is usually done daily in conjunction with the central laboratory.

5. Equipment can and will fail. Always look at the patient and assess each situation clinically.

6. If you get an unexpectedly high reading, make sure that the PA catheter is not wedged farther out in the pulmonary artery. The fiberoptic piece may be "looking" at arterial blood instead of mixed venous blood.

7. If the intermittent sampling technique is used, be sure to draw the blood back slowly to get a good mixed venous sample.

**31. What questions should you ask before beginning continuous SVO$_2$ monitoring?**

Continuous SvO$_2$ monitoring must be cost-effective. The fiberoptic source is more expensive than a standard PA catheter. The following are important questions to ask:

1. Does knowledge of the SvO$_2$ value provide clinical information that cannot be derived through other means?

2. Are nurses and physicians using this information to its full potential?

3. Does monitoring SvO$_2$ save time and make patient care more efficient, or is it just another number to write on the flowsheet?

4. In what clinical situations does SvO$_2$ correlate or not correlate with other hemodynamic parameters?

5. How will this information guide therapies?

The answers to these questions and many others may depend on the nurse or physician assessing the patient or implementing therapies during a particular shift. Institutions should look at clinical indicators for development of guidelines that define the most appropriate use of SvO$_2$ monitoring techniques.

### BIBLIOGRAPHY

1. Aherns T: Continuous mixed venous SvO$_2$ monitoring: Too expensive or indispensable? Crit Care Nurs Clin North Am 11: 33–48, 1999.
2. Ahrens T: Technology utilization in the cardiac surgical patient: SvO$_2$ and capnography monitoring. Crit Care Nurs Q 21:24–40, 1998.
3. Cathelyn JL, Samples DA: SvO$_2$ monitoring: Tool for evaluating patient outcomes. Dimens Crit Care Nurs 17(2):58–63, 1998.
4. Epstein CD: Oxygen transport variable in the identification and treatment of tissue hypoxia. Heart Lung 22:328–345, 1993.
5. Headley JM: Strategies to optimize the cardiorespiratory status of the critically ill. AACN Clin Issues 6:121–134, 1995.
6. Hayden RA: Trend spotting with SvO$_2$ monitor. Am J Nurs Jan:26–33, 1993.
7. Hennemann EA, Gawlinski A: Evaluating cardiopulmonary instability with continuous monitoring of mixed venous oxygen saturation. Crit Care Nurs Clin North Am 6:855–862, 1994.
8. Mims, BC: Physiologic rationale of SvO$_2$ monitoring. Crit Care Nurs Clin North Am 1:619–628, 1989.
9. White KM: Using continuous SvO$_2$ to assess oxygen supply/demand balance in the critically ill patient. AACN Clin Issues 4:134–147, 1993.

---

# 9. POSTOPERATIVE MANAGEMENT OF THE CARDIAC SURGERY PATIENT

S. Jill Ley, RN, MS, CCRN, CNS

---

**1. What are distinguishing features of traditional vs. minimally invasive cardiac surgery procedures?**

**Traditional cardiac surgery** is performed via a median sternotomy incision on a quiet, bloodless heart with the use of a cardiopulmonary bypass (CPB) machine, which maintains total body oxygenation and perfusion despite cardiac arrest. Injection of cardioplegia solution directly into the coronary circulation stops the heart while providing necessary nutrients for myocardial preservation despite the absence of cardiac blood flow. Traditional approaches are associated with varying degrees of hypothermia, coagulopathy, hemodilution (resulting in anemia and tissue edema), and postoperative mechanical ventilation.

**Minimally invasive surgery** (MIS) modifies one or more of the above techniques to accomplish similar surgical outcomes through use of small incisions with or without CPB (e.g., "off pump"). If MIS can be performed with similar surgical precision and durability as a traditional approach, it ultimately may offer the benefits of reduced complications, length of stay, and resource use.

## 2. What concerns are important in admitting the postoperative cardiac surgery patient?

The basic ABCs of airway, breathing, and circulation are paramount on admission. First ensure a patent airway (with or without an endotracheal tube), adequate respirations, and appropriate tissue perfusion. Prompt establishment of continuous monitoring of the electrocardiogram (ECG), arterial pressure, central venous or pulmonary artery (PA) pressures, and pulse oximetry readings is essential. Restoration of cardiac output may be accomplished by manipulation of preload (volume loading), afterload (vasodilators), contractility (inotropes), and/or heart rate (temporary pacing). Bleeding abnormalities from surgical sites or coagulopathies are manifest as increased chest tube output and a falling hematocrit, which warrant prompt correction to maintain hemodynamic stability. Although dysrhythmias may occur in response to electrolyte abnormalities, atrial fibrillation (the most common complication of cardiac surgery) typically does not appear until the second or third postoperative day. Extubation and mobilization proceed promptly once hemodynamic stability is established.

## 3. What assessment findings can be expected?

Traditional signs of hypoperfusion, including hypotension and oliguria, can be masked in the immediate postoperative period by hypothermia, the catecholamine response to surgery, and mannitol-induced diuresis. Vasoconstriction, evidenced by elevated systemic vascular resistance (SVR), often leads to hypertension regardless of fluid status. In patients with impaired ventricular function, afterload reduction is essential to overcome resistance to cardiac ejection and optimize cardiac output. Postoperative fluid status and filling pressure readings are quite variable, depending on preoperative conditions (e.g., valve disease, pulmonary edema, renal failure) as well as intraoperative fluid management. Typically, patients exhibit varying degrees of hypovolemia and require mild-to-moderate fluid resuscitation in the immediate postoperative period. Contractility may be mildly depressed from anesthesia and myocardial ischemia, warranting careful assessment of cardiac function and intervention with inotropic agents as necessary. Tachycardia is common (and generally self-limiting), although varying degrees of heart block may occur, more commonly after valve surgery.

## 4. How is the patient's respiratory status managed after cardiac surgery?

The intraoperative use of short-acting anesthetics and low-dose opioids promotes minimal intubation times; in some MIS cases, the patient is extubated intraoperatively. Criteria for extubation include recovery of neuromuscular function, hemodynamic stability, absence of bleeding or hypothermia, and adequate lung mechanics. Management of pain and sedation are geared toward early (4–6 hours postoperatively) extubation, using adjuncts such as short-acting anesthetics (propofol) and nonsteroidal agents (ketorolac) to minimize opioid-induced respiratory depression. Rigorous use of the incentive spirometer is encouraged after extubation to overcome the effects of intraoperative hypoinflation.

## 5. How is pain managed after cardiac surgery?

The pain response to cardiac surgery is affected by the type of incision (thoracotomy incisions reportedly are more painful than sternotomy incisions), painful rib manipulation with some MIS procedures, and individual pain tolerance. Intermittent intravenous opioids generally are required for the first 24 hours postoperatively, with occasional need for continuous patient-controlled analgesia (PCA). Additional adjuncts in the management of early postoperative pain include intrathecal or intrapleural opioid administration as well as nonsteroidal agents. Oral opioids are introduced on the first postoperative day; few patients require intravenous analgesia after this time. Removal of chest tubes, usually on the first or second postoperative day, is a painful procedure that requires additional, well-timed intravenous analgesia.

### 6. How is hypertension managed after cardiac surgery?

Hypertension is common in the immediate postoperative period, even in patients without a prior history, in part because of the stress response to surgery. Short-acting intravenous agents are used to control blood pressure (BP), which may be quite labile as a result of fluid depletion, recovery from anesthesia, and rewarming. When tachycardia also is present, short-acting beta blockers (e.g., esmolol) are effective in controlling both heart rate (HR) and BP responses to surgery. In patients with a contraindication to beta blockers, vasodilators such as nitroprusside are indicated. Oral antihypertensive agents are resumed as indicated after extubation.

### 7. Describe the general management of a low cardiac output.

Management of low cardiac output (CO) begins with a systematic assessment of the determinants of CO, represented by the following formula:

$$CO = HR \times SV$$

where stroke volume (SV) is a function of preload, afterload, and contractility. Although a PA catheter is not placed intraoperatively in many cardiac surgery patients, those exhibiting signs of significant cardiac impairment (hypotension, tachycardia, oliguria, cold extremities) require postoperative PA line insertion for adequate assessment and intervention in this potentially life-threatening disorder. Decreased HR is treated with temporary cardiac pacing. A compensatory tachycardia associated with low CO rarely requires direct intervention; any abrupt decrease in HR may worsen cardiac function. Instead, pay attention to other determinants of CO. Preload should be optimized with fluid resuscitation to individualized endpoints.

### 8. How is the Frank-Starling curve used?

Plotting a Frank-Starling curve using serial hemodynamic assessments of the relationship between fluid status (pulmonary wedge pressure [PWP]) and cardiac function (e.g., CO, cardiac

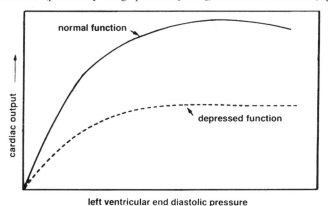

Frank-Starling ventricular function curves.

index, SV index), as illustrated below, reveals that CO can be improved with fluid therapy, up to a point. Once CO has plateaued, however, additional fluids contribute to cardiac overdistention and impair heart function. In the presence of an adequate hematocrit, failure to respond to initial resuscitation with 1–2 liters of crystalloid (e.g.. normal saline, lactated Ringer's solution) warrants a trial of colloid therapy (e.g., hetastarch or albumin).

If low output persists despite optimal volume status, agents that normalize afterload and contractility are indicated. In the presence of increased afterload (represented by a high SVR), vasodilator agents are useful in lowering resistance to cardiac ejection. In patients with a low CO, these agents are combined with inotropes to maintain BP and offer needed support of contractile function. Mechanical cardiac support with an intraaortic balloon pump or ventricular assist device is reserved for patients refractory to high-dose pharmacologic therapy.

**9. Describe the role of epicardial pacing wires in the postoperative patient.**

Temporary atrial and ventricular pacing wires are placed on the epicardial surface of the heart at the completion of surgery to aid in maintenance of electrical stability in the postoperative period. When attached to a temporary pacemaker generator, maintenance of adequate HR (80–100 beats/min) and atrioventricular synchrony provides optimal cardiac efficiency. Although atrial leads are not always inserted, they offer atrial pacing capabilities as well as dysrhythmia analysis via an atrial ECG. After connecting the atrial wire to the V1 pole of the ECG machine, a heightened atrial impulse is evident in the ECG recording of V1, helping to identify the atrial signal and differentiate the rhythm disorder. Atrial and ventricular pacing wires also can be used to terminate atrial flutter and ventricular tachycardia, respectively, via overdrive pacing. Pacing wires generally are discontinued 2–3 days postoperatively by gently pulling the wires out through the chest wall.

**10. Describe the role of inotropic agents in the postoperative period.**

Inotropic agents are widely used after cardiac surgery to support varying degrees of postoperative contractile dysfunction. Although all agents augment contractility via increased intracellular calcium levels, their actions and effects vary in a dose-dependent fashion, with differing effects by drug classification and receptor stimulation.

Sympathomimetic agents bind with end-organ adrenergic receptors, stimulating a combination of alpha ($\alpha$), beta$_1$ ($\beta_1$), beta$_2$ ($\beta_2$), and dopaminergic (DA) receptors. Alpha stimulation results in vasoconstriction. Beta$_1$ effects include increased inotropy and chronotropy, whereas $\beta_2$ stimulation leads to vasodilation and bronchodilation. DA receptor stimulation leads to vasodilation and increased perfusion in specific target organs, including the renal, mesenteric, and splanchnic vascular beds. Phosphodiesterase inhibitors (PDI) act via enzymatic pathways, producing increased contractility and systemic vasodilation without affecting receptor stimulation.

Pharmacologic therapy, either singly or in combination, is directed at increasing contractile force with inotropes, decreasing ventricular afterload with vasodilators, or, in cases of refractory hypotension or low SVR, increasing peripheral resistance with vasopressors.

*Hemodynamic Effects of Commonly Used Vasoactive Medications*

|  | RECEPTOR | HR | MAP | PWP | CI | SVR |
|---|---|---|---|---|---|---|
| Dobutamine | $\beta_1, \beta_2$ | =/↑ | ↑/↓ | =/↓ | ↑ | ↓ |
| Amrinone | None | = | =/↓ | ↓ | ↑ | ↓ |
| Dopamine | $\alpha, \beta_1, \beta_2$, DA | ↑ | ↑ | ↑ | ↑ | =/↑ |
| Epinephrine | $\alpha, \beta_1, \beta_2$ | ↑↑ | ↑ | ↑ | ↑ | ↑ |
| Norepinephrine | $\alpha, \beta_1$ | ↑ | ↑↑ | ↑ | ↑/↓ | ↑↑ |
| Isoproterenol | $\beta_1, \beta_2$ | ↑↑ | =/↓ | ↓ | ↑ | ↓ |
| Phenylephrine | $\alpha$ | = | ↑↑ | ↑ | =/↓ | ↑↑ |

HR = heart rate, MAP = mean arterial pressure, PWP = pulmonary wedge pressure, CI = cardiac index, SVR = systemic vascular resistance.

**11. Describe the role of mechanical cardiac support in the postoperative period.**

Perioperative mechanical cardiac support is indicated for low cardiac output states refractory to optimal fluid resuscitation and pharmacologic therapy. The **intraaortic balloon pump** (IABP) is placed percutaneously (or, rarely, surgically) in the descending thoracic aorta. Balloon mechanics are carefully timed via an ECG or arterial pressure signal to inflate when the heart is in diastole, thus raising coronary perfusion pressure, and to deflate just before systole, thus reducing afterload. Unlike pharmacologic therapy, CO is augmented without increased myocardial oxygen consumption. The IABP may be used preoperatively for patients with cardiogenic shock, preinfarction angina, or mechanical cardiac defects (e.g., mitral regurgitation or ventricular septal defect), before induction of anesthesia in high-risk patients, or at the conclusion of surgery if weaning from CPB proves difficult.

A **ventricular assist device** (VAD) is indicated for severe cardiac dysfunction unresponsive to IABP and pharmacologic therapy. A VAD is placed surgically to divert blood away from a failing heart via large-bore cannulas, similar to the CPB machine, and provides up to 100% of total CO. VADs provide myocardial rest while maintaining organ perfusion, allowing either recovery of the native heart or a bridge to cardiac transplantation. They can provide either continuous flow via a centrifugal-type pump or pulsatile flow via a pneumatic pump. Important complications, including hemorrhage, thromboembolism, stroke, and infection, limit their use to select candidates with an optimal chance for recovery.

### 12. Describe the management of mediastinal bleeding after cardiac surgery.

Intraoperative placement of **mediastinal chest tubes** (CT) promotes surgical drainage while allowing recognition of postoperative hemorrhage. CT output depends on procedure type, prior cardiac surgery, underlying coagulopathy, and use of intraoperative hemostatic agents (e.g., epsilon aminocaproic acid, aprotinin). CTs are assessed every 30–60 minutes initially. Outputs exceeding 150–200 ml/hr warrant physician notification and intervention.

Management of postoperative bleeding includes **reversal of heparin effect** with protamine and correction of coagulation deficits with factor specific therapy.

**Packed red cells** (PRCs) and **fresh frozen plasma** are administered to maintain the desired hematocrit and prothrombin time/partial thromboplastin time, respectively.

**Cryoprecipitate** is used if fibrinogen levels are low. If bleeding is excessive, platelets may be administered despite a relatively normal laboratory count to counteract platelet dysfunction after CPB.

**Leukodepleted PRCs** and **platelet transfusions** significantly reduce the morbidity and mortality associated with blood transfusions. In patients with active bleeding, efforts at blood conservation must be balanced against the hemodynamic consequences of "getting behind" in blood replacement therapies. Ongoing autotransfusion of CT drainage promotes maintenance of intravascular blood volume while avoiding exogenous blood transfusions.

**Surgical reexploration** should be considered if CT output exceeds 200 ml/hr for 2 consecutive hours after clotting factors have been restored. Patients receiving procoagulants should be monitored closely for the development of acute cardiac tamponade, particularly if abrupt cessation of CT output is noted. Hallmark clinical findings include hypotension, tachycardia, and elevation with equalization of filling pressures.

### 13. What causes acute coronary ischemia in the postoperative period.

Important postoperative coronary ischemia may be due to technical problems (e.g., inadequate cardioplegia, graft misalignment, inadvertent suture of a coronary artery) or incomplete revascularization due to poor target vessels. It also may occur during an MIS approach intended to be combined with subsequent angioplasty (called hybrid procedures). Acute coronary spasm, seen more commonly with arterial conduits (e.g., radial or gastroepiploic arteries), may cause profound ischemia or infarction.

### 14. Describe the recognition and management of acute coronary ischemia in the postoperative period.

Standard methods of detecting ischemia are used postoperatively, including ST-segment monitoring or 12-lead ECG analysis. Such events occur acutely in the immediate postoperative period and usually are associated with hemodynamic instability and/or dysrhythmias. Once the problem is detected, a rapid return to the operating room or cardiac catheterization lab is indicated in an attempt to salvage viable myocardium. Intravenous antianginal agents such as nitroglycerin, nicardipine, or diltiazem may be used for treatment or prophylaxis of coronary ischemia. Given the infrequency of such events, institutional practices regarding routine ECGs and antianginal use are quite variable. Many centers report a low utilization of ST-segment monitoring in cardiac surgery patients.

### 15. How is perioperative myocardial infarction (POMI) diagnosed?

Because of the trauma involved in cardiac surgery, diagnosis of POMI is more complex than in nonsurgical patients. Analysis of the 12-lead ECG is performed in standard fashion but may be misleading because of J-point elevation due to hypothermia or ST-T wave changes associated with pericardial inflammation. Lead-specific changes are useful in pinpointing the anatomic site of infarction. Careful interpretation of cardiac enzymes is required, including levels of creatine kinase isoenzymes (CPK) and troponin. Findings suggestive of a POMI include total CPK $> 2 \times$ normal, CPK-MB $> 5\%$ of total CPK, or CPK-MB $> 50$ IU. Cardiac troponin levels are reportedly more sensitive and specific for the diagnosis of POMI than CPK. Research to determine precisely the level associated with POMI in cardiac surgical patients is ongoing. Given the high incidence of false positives seen with enzyme analysis, echocardiography documenting a new wall motion abnormality is considered the gold standard for diagnosing MI after cardiac surgery. The incidence of POMI is approximately 6–10% after revascularization procedures.

### 16. What complications are common after cardiac surgery?

**Atrial dysrhythmias** are the most common complication after cardiac surgery (25–60% of patients). Advanced age is the most important risk factor for atrial fibrillation. Evidence indicates that prophylactic beta-blocker or amiodarone therapy is effective.

**Atelectasis** is a universal finding due to lung underinflation during CPB and may contribute to pneumonia if pulmonary hygiene efforts are inadequate.

**Pleural effusions** are also common because of the extensive dissection required in harvesting the internal mammary artery as a bypass conduit.

**Fluid overload** with anasarca is related to large-volume infusions and requires aggressive diuresis to achieve baseline weight.

**Significant neurologic deficits** occur in 5–6% of patients undergoing coronary artery bypass surgery, including strokes, transient ischemic attacks, and coma. Perioperative strokes can be attributed to microemboli of air or fat, mural thrombus, or disruption of atheromatous plaque by the aortic cross-clamp. A reduced incidence of neurologic impairment has been noted after MIS, attributed in part to avoidance of CPB. Although many patients recover from stroke within a few weeks, the postoperative mortality rate is doubled.

**Sternal wound infection** occurs in less than 2% of patients. Risk factors include obesity, immunosuppression, and diabetes. Strict control of blood glucose levels in the postoperative period has been shown to significantly reduce infection rates in diabetic patients. Early treatment of infected sternal wounds with debridement and pectoralis muscle flap has decreased the mortality rate from 60% to 20–30% in recent years.

### BIBLIOGRAPHY

1. Acuff TE, Landreneau RJ, Griffith BP, et al: Minimally invasive coronary artery bypass grafting. Ann Thorac Surg 61:135–137, 1996.
2. Benetti FJ, Naselli G, Wood M, Geffner L: Direct myocardial revascularization without extracorporeal circulation: Experience in 700 patients. Chest 100:312–316, 1991.
3. Cameron A, Davis KB, Green G, Schaff HV: Coronary bypass surgery with internal-thoracic-artery grafts: Effects on survival over a 15-year period. N Engl J Med 334:216–219, 1996.
4. Cheng DC, Karski J, Peniston C, et al: Morbidity outcome in early versus conventional tracheal extubation after coronary artery bypass grafting: A prospective randomized controlled trial. J Thorac Cardiovasc Surg 112:755–764, 1996.
5. Earp JK, Mallia G: Myocardial protection for cardiac surgery: The nursing perspective. AACN Clin Issues Crit Care Nurs 8:20–32, 1997.
6. Engleman RM, Rousou JA, Flack JE, et al: Fast-track recovery of the coronary bypass patient. Ann Thorac Surg 58:1742–1746, 1994.
7. Furnary AP, Zerr KJ, Grunkemeier, Starr A: Continuous intravenous insulin infusion reduces the incidence of deep sternal wound infection in diabetic patients after cardiac surgical procedures. Ann Thorac Surg 67:352–362, 1999.
8. Gensini GF, Fusi C, Conti AA, et al: Cardiac troponin I and Q-wave perioperative myocardial infarction after coronary artery bypass surgery. Crit Care Med 26:1986–1990, 1998.
9. Jones G, Jurkiewicz MJ, Bostwick J, et al: Management of the infected median sternotomy wound with muscle flaps. The Emory 20-year experience. Ann Surg 225:766–776, 1997.
10. Ley SJ: Myocardial depression following cardiac surgery: Pharmacologic and mechanical support. AACN Clin Issues Crit Care Nurs 4:293–308, 1993.

11. Ley SJ: Patient advocacy through outcomes management: A cardiac surgery example. Crit Care Nurs Clin 10:135–154, 1998.
12. Page PL, Pym J: Atrial fibrillation following cardiac surgery. Can J Cardiol 12(Suppl A):40A–44A, 1996.
13. Roach GW, Kanchuger M, Mangano CM, et al: Adverse cerebral outcomes after coronary bypass surgery. N Engl J Med 335:1857–1863, 1996.
14. Shaughnessy TE: Postoperative care of cardiothoracic surgery patients. In Parsons PE, Wiener-Kronish JP (eds): Critical Care Secrets, 2nd ed. Philadelphia, Hanley & Belfus, 1998.
15. Staples JR, Ramsay JG: Advances in anesthesia for cardiac surgery: An overview for the 1990s. AACN Clin Issues Crit Care Nurs 8:41, 1997.
16. van de Watering LMG, Hermand J, Houbiers JGA, et al: Beneficial effects of leukocyte depletion of transfused blood on postoperative complications in patients undergoing cardiac surgery: A randomized clinical trial. Circulation 97:562–568, 1998.

# 10. HEART AND LUNG TRANSPLANTATION

*Celia Rifkin, RN*

## HEART TRANSPLANTATION

### 1. What are the indications for heart transplant?

Patients who are selected for cardiac transplantation have end-stage heart disease for which there is no other effective medical or surgical therapy. End-stage cardiac disease usually is characterized by signs and symptoms of low cardiac output despite adequate ventricular preload. Other cardiovascular manifestations may include life-threatening arrhythmias, intractable angina, or thromboembolic events. End-stage cardiac disease is associated with a poor prognosis, an estimated survival period of 6–12 months, and severely impaired quality of life.

*Clinical Indications for Heart Transplant*

- Idiopathic dilated cardiomyopathy
- Coronary artery disease not amenable to direct attempts at revascularization (coronary artery bypass grafting [CABG] or percutaneous transluminal coronary angioplasty [PTCA]) or aneurysmectomy
- Valvular heart disease not amenable to attempts at repair or replacement
- Congenital heart disease not amenable to definitive repair or acceptable palliation
- Miscellaneous forms of cardiomyopathy, including familial, peripartum, viral, drug- or toxin-induced, and hypertrophic

### 2. What are the absolute contraindications to heart transplant?

- Irreversible pulmonary hypertension
- Concurrent carcinoma with metastases or a high likelihood of uncontrollable recurrence following immunosuppression
- HIV or other uncontrollable infection
- Irreversible and life-threatening or limiting disease in another organ system (renal, pulmonary, hepatic, neurologic, vascular)
- Active drug addiction, including alcohol
- Major affective disorder, maladaptive behavior, or suicidal ideation
- Severe mental retardation
- Severe cardiac cachexia. Malnutrition associated with significant loss of muscle mass increases the operative mortality rate and early risk of pulmonary complications, and infection. Cachectic patients who do not appear to have the capacity to withstand the transplant procedure and its attendant complications are excluded.

### 3. How are patients tested for irreversible pulmonary hypertension?

Pulmonary hypertension frequently accompanies chronic heart failure and is a major determinant of both operative mortality and long-term survival, particularly after orthotopic cardiac transplantation. Patients with pulmonary artery (PA) systolic pressure > 50 mmHg or pulmonary vascular resistance (PVR) > 3 Wood units (20 dynes/sec/cm$^{-5}$) undergo provocative testing with nitroprusside according to an established protocol. Failure to reduce PA pressure or resistance below the threshold level while maintaining adequate systemic perfusion and blood pressure is considered an absolute contraindication to orthotopic cardiac transplantation. Borderline patients either undergo heterotopic or orthotopic transplantation with a large donor organ, short ischemic time, or "domino" (living) donor heart.

### 4. How are abnormalities in other organ systems evaluated?

Coexisting abnormalities in other organ systems are evaluated carefully to determine the impact on operative mortality, long-term survival, and quality of life after transplantation. Moderate renal, hepatic, or pulmonary dysfunction of recent onset and secondary to poor cardiac function does not necessarily exclude transplantation. However, the presence of severe single-organ dysfunction, multisystem organ failure, or a separate disease that by itself is life threatening or limiting or significantly reduces the chance of a successful outcome normally excludes patients from consideration.

### 5. Why is psychological evaluation important?

The long-term success of cardiac transplantation depends on the patient's ability to comply consistently and reliably with a complex medical regimen. Patients who are clearly unable, unwilling, or unlikely to meet the expected level of self-care are not accepted.

### 6. What are the relative contraindications to heart transplant?

- Advanced age (> 60 yr)
- Active but potentially treatable infection
- Recent pulmonary infarction. Clinical experience has shown that such patients are at high risk for posttransplant pulmonary sepsis. Despite a high morbidity rate, however, successful outcomes have been reported.
- Recent cerebrovascular event. A recent (< 1 week) uncomplicated cerebral infarct increases only slightly the operative risk of cardiac surgery. However, a recent hemorrhagic cerebral infarction or one complicated by substantial cerebral edema and mass effect is considered an absolute contraindication.
- Asymptomatic severe cerebrovascular or peripheral vascular disease
- Insulin-dependent diabetes mellitus without neuropathy, retinopathy, or nephropathy
- Systemic hypertension without secondary vasculopathy
- Symptomatic peptic ulcer disease, cholelithiasis, or diverticulosis
- Lack of psychosocial and financial support mechanisms

### 7. Why is advanced age a factor?

Results are ambiguous in the upper age limit because of the small number of patients over 60 years who have been transplanted. However, operative mortality and morbidity rates and long-term survival rates after other forms of cardiac surgery (e.g., CABG, valve surgery) are adversely affected by older age. Much of the excessive mortality and morbidity appears to be non–cardiac-related. It seems likely that the clinical results of cardiac transplantation also would be affected by age. Older patients who do not appear to have the capacity to tolerate transplant and posttransplant complications are not considered.

### 8. How are patients listed for transplant?

Patients are listed on the national waiting list with the United Network for Organ Sharing (UNOS). They are listed by ABO blood type and date and time of placement on the list.

| | |
|---|---|
| **Status 1A** | Patients who are very ill, in the ICU, and on multiple inotropic medications, ventilator, or ventricular assist device (for less than 30 days) with a life |

expectancy of 7 days or less without a heart transplant. These patients are first offered the donor hearts. If no one in the 1A group can use the donor heart, the Organ Procurement Organization (OPO) offers the heart-lung block to patients waiting for a heart-lung transplant.

**Status 1B**   Patients who are stable on intravenous inotopic medication or a VAD (more than 30 days after placement). They can be either in the ICU or on a telemetry floor.

**Status 2**   Patients who are stable and at home waiting for a heart transplant

## 9. How long are waiting times?
The average waiting time for a status 2 heart transplant candidate is 1.5 –2 years.

## 10. How is the donor heart evaluated?
The donor history is taken from a family member or significant other, and laboratory work is done. An electrocardiogram (ECG) and echocardiogram are reviewed for abnormalities. Cardiac catheterization is done only if necessitated by the history and ECG results. If the donor has coronary artery disease, most programs do not accept the heart. However, some programs use such hearts for older recipients and at the time of transplant also perform CABG.

## 11. How is the donor heart matched to the recipients?
Blood type and weight are the predominant factors. When the patient is listed for transplant, a weight range for acceptable donors is given. The range usually is within 20% of the recipient's weight.

## 12. What are the surgical sites for heart transplantation?
A median sternotomy is performed. Bicaval orthotopic heart transplant is the current standard procedure. The anastomoses involve the inferior and superior vena cava, left atrium, pulmonary artery, and aorta. This procedure has fewer problems with sinus node function and subsequent arrhythmias. Previous heart transplant surgery used anastomoses of the right and left atrium, pulmonary artery, and aorta. A small percentage of patients required permanent pacemakers because of sinus node dysfunction related to atrial anastomoses.

## 13. What medications are used in transplant patients?
1. **Immunosuppression**
   • Induction therapy: either monoclonal or polyclonal antibodies. Polyclonal antibodies include Atgam and antilymphocytic globulin (ALG). Monoclonal antibodies include OKT3 (muromonab-CD3), daclizumab (Zenapax), and basiliximab (Simulect). These medications are given intravenously at the time of transplant surgery and are used at the discretion of each program.
   • Cyclosporine (Sandimmune or Neoral [microemulsion formulation])
   • Solumedrol (intravenous) and prednisone (oral)
   • Mycophenolate mofetil (Cellcept) or azathioprine (Imuran)
2. **Prophylactic antibiotics**
   • Sulfamethoxazole/trimethoprim (Septra DS) to prevent *Pneumocystis carinii* pneumonia; if it is not tolerated, inhaled pentamidine is used once a month
   • Clotrimazole (Mycelex Troche) to prevent yeast infection of the mouth and esophagus
   • Fluconazole (if fungal infections are found during routine cultures)
   • Ganciclovir (Cytovene; intravenous and oral) for prophylaxis against cytomegalovirus (CMV). Some centers also use intravenous human CMV immunoglobulin (CytoGam) in conjunction with ganciclovir for CMV mismatches (CMV-positive recipient, CMV-negative donor or vice versa)
   • Acyclovir (Zovirax) if ganciclovir is not taken for prevention of CMV
3. **Miscellaneous**
   • Terbutaline (Brethine) to maintain an elevated heart rate when patients are weaned from isoproterenol (Isuprel)
   • Antihypertensive agents

• Mineral replacements (magnesium, calcium, potassium)
• Cholesterol-lowering agents

## 14. What are the major complications during the immediate postoperative period?
Decreased cardiac output (CO) and arrhythmias.

## 15. How do you manage decreased CO?
Be aware of the usual problems that cause decreased CO, such as bleeding, cardiac tamponade, and arrhythmias. The donor heart has myocardial dysfunction related to ischemic injury during preservation and transportation. Signs of right-sided heart failure (increased right atrial or central venous pressure, decreased CO, decreased urine output) may result from increased right ventricular afterload due to a preexisting increase in PVR. Nitroprusside (Nipride) is used to reduce PVR. The patient typically requires inotropic and chronotropic support, including infusions of dobutamine or dopamine and isoproterenol (Isuprel). Because the heart has no innervation from the autonomic nervous system, it cannot respond to vagal or Valsalva stimulation; it relies on circulating catecholamines to increase rate and force of contractions. Some patients require temporary pacing wires to maintain adequate heart rate and CO.

## 16. How do you manage arrhythmias?
New-onset arrhythmias (atrial fibrillation, atrial flutter, supraventricular tachycardia, sinus bradycardia) may be a sign of acute rejection. The arrhythmia should be treated, and an endomyocardial biopsy should be performed to rule out rejection.

## 17. What are the primary causes of death in heart transplant patients?
Infection and rejection are the primary causes of death in the first year after heart transplantation. Long-term complications (>5 years) leading to death include coronary artery vasculopathy and post-transplant lymphoproliferative disorder (PTLD).

## 18. What are the essential components of the postoperative nursing assessment?
**Hemodynamics:** blood pressure, heart rate, central venous pressure (CVP), pulmonary artery pressures, and CO.

**Infection:** monitor all invasive lines (IVs, catheters, chest tubes) for redness, tenderness, and discharge. The signs and symptoms of infection are difficult to recognize in immunosuppressed patients. The anti-inflammatory effect of steroids reduces the ability to produce pyrogens; therefore, any temperature ≥ 38° Celsius requires a full work-up, including blood cultures, urine cultures, chest radiograph, and removal and culture of suspicious-looking lines. Infections are caused by bacterial, viral, fungal, and protozoal pathogens.

**Wound healing** is impaired by steroid use. Monitor all wounds for healing and signs of infection. Culture as needed.

**Nutrition.** Patients with severe congestive heart failure develop cardiac cachexia. After transplant the patient needs adequate nutrition to promote wound healing and maintain muscle mass. A dietician should be consulted to ensure adequate nutritional intake.

**Pain.** As with any cardiac surgery patient, pain control is essential to facilitate coughing, deep breathing, and healing.

## 19. What nursing interventions are appropriate in the postoperative period?
| | |
|---|---|
| Universal precautions | Pacemaker management |
| Sternal precautions | Pain control |
| Physical therapy | Teaching |

## 20. What are the signs and symptoms of acute rejection?
**Signs:** hypotension, fever, arrhythmias, elevated jugular venous pulse, rales, peripheral edema, decreased urine output.

**Symptoms:** shortness of breath, dyspnea, malaise, fatigue.

**21. How is rejection monitored?**

Heart transplant patients undergo endomyocardial biopsies to rule out rejection. The procedure is done in the cardiac catheterization laboratory. The right jugular vein is accessed. A bioptome is passed through an introducer and advanced to the right ventricle. Several small pieces of heart muscle are obtained. The heart biopsies are examined by the pathologist for signs of rejection.

**22. How are endomyocardial biopsies graded?**

The International Society of Heart and Lung Transplantation (ISHLT) developed the following grading scale based on endomyocardial biopsy findings:

| | |
|---|---|
| Grade 0 | No rejection |
| Grade 1A | Minimal rejection; focal perivascular or interstitial infiltrates without necrosis |
| Grade 2 | Mild rejection; monofocal perivascular infiltrates of lymphocytes with focal myocyte damage |
| Grade 3A | Moderate rejection; multifocal infiltrates of perivascular lymphocytes with myocyte damage |
| Grade 3B | Borderline severe rejection; diffuse inflammatory process with necrosis |
| Grade 4 | Severe rejection; diffuse aggressive polymorphous infiltrates, edema, hemorrhage, vasculitis with necrosis |

**23. How is acute rejection treated?**

**Grade 1A** and **grade 2** rejection is treated with augmentation of the current immunosuppression regimen.

For **grade 3A**, the first line of treatment is 1 gm/day of intravenous Solu-Medrol for 3 days. Solu-Medrol can be given in a clinic or outpatient infusion center. The patient then is placed on a prednisone taper, starting at 1–1.5 mg/kg total dose. A repeat biopsy is performed in 1 week to evaluate resolution of the rejection episode. If the rejection continues at grade 3A or progresses to grade 3B or 4, OKT3 is used for a 10–14 days. Hospitalization is required because of the potentially severe side effects (e.g., flash pulmonary edema, fevers, arthralgias).

**24. What are the survival rates for heart transplant patients?**

UNOS and ISHLT maintain a registry of all transplants done in the U.S. All transplant centers report to the registry at time of listing, at time of transplant, and yearly thereafter. The 1-year survival rate is 80–90%, the 5-year survival rate is 70–75%, and the 10-year survival rate is 50–60%.

## LUNG AND HEART-LUNG TRANSPLANTATION

**25. What are the indications for lung or combined heart-lung transplant?**

Patients selected for lung transplantation have (1) end-stage lung disease (or combined heart and lung disease) for which there is no other effective medical or surgical therapy and (2) a high likelihood of survival and successful long-term rehabilitation.

Each center has its own criteria for heart-lung transplants. Diseases for which a heart-lung transplant is recommended are unrepairable Eisenmenger's syndrome, pulmonary hypertension, and cystic fibrosis.

**26. What are the signs and symptoms of end-stage lung disease?**

End-stage lung disease usually is characterized by a progressive decline in exercise capacity, worsening shortness of breath, abnormal pulmonary function studies, and increasing dependence on supplemental oxygen. Many patients with end-stage lung disease also develop signs and symptoms of right heart failure due to abnormalities within the pulmonary vasculature. In most cases, right ventricular function reverts to normal after isolated lung transplantation. In some cases, however, either an uncorrectable structural or irreversible functional cardiac defect requires simultaneous replacement of both heart and lungs. The prognosis for survival generally is estimated at less than 24 months and quality of life is severely impaired.

**27. What are the common causes of end-stage lung disease?**
- Obstructive lung disease (e.g., emphysema and alpha-1-antitrypsin deficiency)
- Interstitial lung disease (e.g., idiopathic pulmonary fibrosis)
- Chronic pulmonary disease associated with sepsis (e.g., bronchiectasis and cystic fibrosis)
- Pulmonary vascular disease (e.g., primary pulmonary hypertension and pulmonary hypertension associated with congenital or other forms of heart disease)
- Lymphangiolyomyomatosis (LAM).

**28. What are the absolute contraindications for lung transplant?**
- Presence of another life-threatening or limiting disease in another organ system (e.g., severe coronary, valvular, myocardial, cerebrovascular, or peripheral vascular disease, irreversible renal or hepatic failure).
- HIV or other uncontrollable extrapulmonary infections. Bilateral chronic pulmonary sepsis (e.g., cystic fibrosis) normally requires bilateral rather than single-lung transplantation.
- Irreversible right ventricular dysfunction. Significant, irreversible cardiac disease is a contraindication to isolated lung transplantation but does not exclude combined heart-lung transplantation.
- Neoplasia. Primary lung cancer, pulmonary metastases, or a poorly controlled primary tumor at another site normally exclude patients from consideration. Patients who appear to have been successfully treated for cancer in the past and who are currently judged to be at low risk for recurrence are evaluated on an individual basis.
- Severe cachexia or muscle wasting. Malnutrition with significant loss of muscle mass increases the operative mortality rate and early risk of pulmonary complications and infection.
- Poor rehabilitation potential due to active smoking, drug or alcohol abuse, severe mental retardation, major psychosis, major affective disorder, maladaptive behavior, or noncompliant behavior. Long-term success depends on the patient's ability to comply consistently and reliably with a complex medical regimen.
- Chest wall deformity or neuromuscular disorder affecting the respiratory muscles. Any disorder that limits ventilatory capacity after transplant is normally a contraindication.

**29. What are the relative contraindications for lung transplant?**
- Age greater than 60 years for single-lung transplant or 50 years for bilateral lung or combined heart-lung transplant. At present there is no consensus about the absolute upper age limit, largely because of the small number and limited follow-up of older patients. However, operative mortality and morbidity and long-term survival after other forms of thoracic surgery are adversely affected by older age. Older patients are considered on an individual basis.
- History of major pulmonary resection or pleurectomy. Prior intrathoracic surgery increases technical difficulty and is associated with an increased risk of bleeding, particularly if cardiopulmonary bypass is required.
- Chronic high-dose systemic corticosteroid use (> 0.2 mg/kg/day) that cannot be tapered to a lower dose or discontinued before transplantation. Adverse effects include poor wound healing and increased risk of infection.
- Current ventilator dependence for more than 1–2 weeks. Patients on mechanical ventilators for longer periods are prone to airway colonization with resistant organisms and loss of respiratory muscle function.
- Pulmonary infection or airway colonization with organisms resistant to multiple antibiotics. Such infections in the allograft or pleural space after transplant markedly reduce the chance for a successful outcome.
- Insulin-dependent diabetes mellitus without neuropathy, retinopathy, or nephropathy
- Lack of psychosocial and financial support mechanisms
- Remote cerebrovascular event, asymptomatic cerebrovascular or peripheral vascular disease
- Symptomatic peptic ulcer disease, cholelithiasis, or diverticulosis
- Obesity

### 30. How are patients listed for lung transplant?

Patients are listed on the national waiting list with UNOS. They are listed by ABO blood type and date and time of placement on the list. Patients on the list are either active on the waiting list or inactive. There is no urgent category for lung transplant patients. The only group of patients with priority are those with a diagnosis of idiopathic lung fibrosis (ILF). Because of the rapid decline in lung function, patients with ILF are credited with 90 days of waiting time when they are placed on the list.

### 31. How long do patients wait for lung transplants?

The average waiting time for a lung transplant candidate is 1–1.5 years.

### 32. How are the donor lung or heart-lung evaluated?

The donor history is taken from a family member or significant other, and laboratory work is done. Chest radiographs are reviewed, arterial blood gases are evaluated on 100% and 40% oxygen. On the 100% challenge the transplant team looks for partial pressure of oxygen ($PO_2$) > 400; on the 40% challenge, $PO_2$ should be greater than 100. Sputum cultures also are reviewed, and updates are faxed to the receiving transplant center with culture results at 24 hours and 48 hours after procurement.

### 33. How are the donor lung or heart-lung matched to the recipients?

Blood type and height are the primary matching factors. When the patient is listed, a height range is given, usually within 10% of the recipient's height. In addition, each lung is measured from apex to base at the diaphragm; then the width is measured at the diaphragm and aortic notch.

### 34. What are the surgical sites for single and bilateral lung transplantation?

**Single lung transplantation.** The patient is intubated with a double-lumen endotracheal tube, which allows independent ventilation of the opposite lung during transplant surgery. If the patient cannot be supported with one lung, cardiopulmonary bypass is used. A posterolateral thoracotomy is performed. The anastamoses are the bronchus, pulmonary artery, and cuff of left atruim.

**Bilateral lung transplantation.** A bilateral anterior transverse thoracosternotomy through the fifth intercostal space is performed. As with single lung transplant, patients are intubated with a double-lumen endotracheal tube. Sequential single lung transplants are done, using the opposite lung for ventilation. If the patient cannot be supported with single lung ventilation (especially patients with pulmonary hypertension), cardiopulmonary bypass is instituted. The anastomoses are the same as for single lung transplant, using both right and left lungs.

### 35. What are the surgical sites for heart and lung transplantation?

A median sternotomy is performed. The patient is placed on cardiopulmonary bypass. The anastomoses are the right atrium, trachea, and aorta.

### 36. What medications are used in lung transplant patients?

The medication regimen is the same for lung transplant and heart transplant patients, except for isoproterenol and terbutaline in heart transplant patients. (See question 13.)

### 37. What are the major complications in the immediate postoperative period? How are they recognized?

**Reperfusion edema.** Watch for fever, tachypnea, diffuse pulmonary infiltrates or pulmonary edema on chest radiograph, decreasing $PaO_2$, and increasing $PaCO_2$. Treatment includes aggressive chest physiotherapy and suctioning, aggressive diruesis, and continuation of mechanical ventilation with pressure support.

**Bleeding.** Monitor chest tube outputs.

### 38. What are the major causes of death in the first year after lung transplant?

Infection and rejection.

### 39. What long-term complications may lead to death?

Long-term complications (> 3 years) that may lead to death after lung transplant include obliterative bronchiolitis and posttransplant lymphoproliferative disorder (PTLD).

### 40. What are the essential components of the nursing assessment?

**Oxygenation.** Monitoring of oxygen saturations and use of supplemental oxygen are essential. For single lung transplant patients, the new lung is denervated, but the native lung continues to send poor oxygenation messages to the brain. Patients may complain of shortness of breath and dyspnea while oxygen saturation is in the 90% range.

**Airway clearance.** Lung transplant patients have ineffective airway clearance because of denervation, loss of cough reflex below the tracheal suture line, and slowing of mucociliary clearance. Patients need to be encouraged to cough and breathe deeply to maintain movement of secretions.

**Infection** and **wound healing** are assessed as in heart transplant patients. (See question 18.)

**Nutrition.** Most patients have poor nutrition before transplant because dyspnea and shortness of breath make it difficult to eat. Posttransplant patients need adequate nutrition to promote wound healing and maintain muscle mass. A dietician should be consulted to ensure adequate nutritional intake.

**Pain.** As with any thoracic surgery patient, pain control is essential to facilitate coughing and deep breathing. Epidural catheters are placed at the time of surgery to help with pain control in the postoperative period.

### 41. What nursing interventions are appropriate in the postoperative period?

Universal precautions                Standard chest tube care
Physical therapy                     Pain control (epidural)
Pulmonary therapy

### 42. What are the signs and symptoms of acute rejection?

**Signs:** fever, rales or rhonchi, decreased oxygen saturations.
**Symptoms:** shortness of breath, dyspnea, malaise, fatigue, increased production of sputum.

### 43. How is rejection monitored?

All lung transplant patients undergo transbronchial biopsies to rule out rejection and infection. The procedure is done in the radiology department. After mild sedation is given and the throat is sprayed with anesthetic to suppress the gag reflex, a bronchoscope is passed through the mouth and into the lungs. The pulmonologist inspects the lungs, obtains bronchial lavage for cultures, and performs a lung biopsy. The biopsies are examined by the pathologist for signs of rejection. The cultures are sent to the microbiology laboratory to rule out infection.

### 44. How are lung transplant biopsies graded?

The ISHLT developed the following grading scale, which is divided into three categories:

**Category A:  Acute rejection**

Grade A0       Normal pulmonary parenchyma
Grade A1       Minimal acute rejection: very few perivascular mononuclear infiltrates in alveolated lung parenchyma
Grade A2       Mild acute rejection; presence of perivascular mononuclear infiltrates surrounding venules and arterioles
Grade A3       Moderate acute rejection; cuffing of venules and arterioles by dense perivascular mononuclear cell infiltrates, usually associated with endotheliitis
Grade A4       Severe acute rejection; diffuse perivascular, interstitial, and air space infiltrates of mononuclear cells with alveolar damage

**Category B: Airway inflammation** (lymphocytic bronchitis/bronchiolitis)

Grade B0       No airway inflammation
Grade B1       Minimal airway inflammation
Grade B2       Mild airway inflammation

Grade B3        Moderate airway inflammation
Grade B4        Severe airway inflammation
**Category C: Chronic airway rejection** (bronchiolitis obliterans)
Grade CA        Active bronchiolitis obliterans
Grade CB        Inactive bronchiolitis obliterans

### 45. How do you treat a rejection episode?

**Grade A1** is treated with augmentation of the current immunosuppression.

**Grade A2** is treated with 1 gm/day of intravenous Solu-Medrol for 3 days. Solumedrol can be given in a clinic or outpatient infusion center. The patient then is placed on a prednisone taper, starting at 1–1.5 mg/kg total dose.

**Grade A3 or A4** is treated with OKT3 for 10–14 days. Patients receiving OKT3 must be hospitalized for monitoring of severe side effects (flash pulmonary edema).

### 46. What are the survival rates for patients with lung transplantation?

UNOS and ISHLT maintain a registry of all transplants done in the U.S. All transplant centers report to the registry at time of listing, at time of transplant, and yearly thereafter. The 1-year survival rate is 75–80%; the 5-year survival rate is 50%.

### BIBLIOGRAPHY

1. Becker C, Petlin A: Heart transplantation. Am J Nurs 5(Suppl):8–14, 1999.
2. Billingham ME, Cary NR, Hammond ME, et al: A working formulation for the standardization of nomenclature in the diagnosis of heart rejection. J Heart Transplant 9:587–593, 1990.
3. Gould KA: Tissue and organ transplantation. Crit Care Nurs Clin North Am 4:97–130, 1992.
4. Hosenpud JD, Bennett LE, Keck BM, et al: The registry of the international society for heart and lung transplantation: Sixteenth official report–1999. J Heart Lung Transplant 18:611–626, 1999.
5. Maurer JR, Frost AE, Estenne M, et al: International guidelines for the selection of lung transplant candidates. Heart Lung 27:223–225, 1998.
6. Smith SL: Tissue and Organ Transplantation: Implications for Professional Nursing Practice. St. Louis, Mosby Year Book, 1990.
7. Yousem SA, Berry GJ, Cagle PT, et al: Revision of the 1990 working formulation for the classification of pulmonary allograft rejection: Lung Rejection Study Group. J Heart Lung Transplant 15:1–15, 1996.

# 11. INTRAAORTIC BALLOON PUMP

*Evelyn Taverna*, RN, MS, CCRN

### 1. What are the goals of using an intraaortic balloon pump (IABP)?

The IABP provides mechanical support for patients with inadequate cardiac output and blood pressure. The goals of IABP are to increase myocardial oxygen supply, to decrease myocardial oxygen demand, to rest a diseased heart, and to maintain adequate end-organ perfusion.

### 2. What are the common clinical indications for IABP therapy?

The most common indications for IABP are cardiogenic shock that is refractory to pharmacologic support and unstable angina. Other indications include left ventricular failure, cardiomyopathy, support before and after cardiac surgery, complications after percutaneous coronary intervention (PCI), support after thrombolytic therapy for failed reperfusion or reocclusion, mechanical defects secondary to myocardial infarction (MI), and refractory ventricular dysrhythmias caused by ischemia. IABP also may be used as a bridge to cardiac transplantation.

**3. What are the absolute contraindications for use of the IABP?**
- Aortic aneurysm
- Aortic dissection
- Severe peripheral vascular occlusive disease
- Aortic valve insufficiency.

**4. How is the intraaortic balloon inserted into the patient?**

The balloon may be inserted percutaneously or by direct arteriotomy via the femoral artery. The polyurethane balloon is mounted on a Silastic catheter and inserted percutaneously using an introducer/sheath. The balloon is advanced into the descending thoracic aorta until it is positioned 1–2 cm distal to the left subclavian artery and the end of the balloon is above the renal arteries. The balloon is connected by tubing to the IABP console. The console compressor moves approximately 40 ml of helium or carbon dioxide through the tubing and into the balloon.

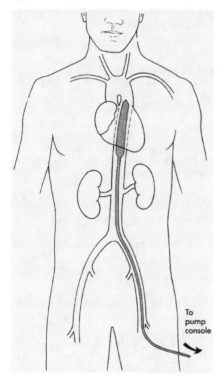

IABP placement. The balloon tip is distal to the left subclavian artery and the balloon end is proximal to the renal arteries. (From Flynn L, Bruce N: Introduction to Critical Care Skills. St. Louis, Mosby, 1993, p 262, with permission.)

To pump console

**5. How is the IABP console programmed?**

The assisted:unassisted augmentation frequency ratio can be set to perform a 1:1, 1:2, or 1:3 augmentation. Every intrinsic cardiac cycle is assisted when the ratio is set at 1:1, providing maximal circulatory support. The 1:3 ratio is used only during weaning when the patient no longer requires IABP support. Balloon inflation and deflation are triggered by (1) the R wave on the electrocardiogram (ECG), (2) ventricular pacemaker spikes on the ECG, (3) upslope of the arterial pressure waveform, or (4) a preset rate. The trigger mode is set by the clinician according to the patient's condition and the monitoring signals available. The R wave on the ECG is the usual choice for triggering the IABP.

**6. What is proper timing of balloon inflation and deflation? How is it checked?**

**Balloon inflation** is timed to begin with the dichrotic notch of the arterial pressure waveform, so that inflation occurs immediately after closure of the aortic valve. Proper timing is determined by observing the arterial pressure waveform. A V-shaped upstroke should occur at the dicrotic notch, producing an augmented diastolic pressure greater than or equal to the preceding systolic pressure.

**Balloon deflation** is timed so that it occurs with the end of diastole on the arterial pressure waveform; the balloon deflates just before the opening of the aortic valve. Proper timing for deflation is determined by observing the arterial waveform. The end-diastolic pressure should be less than the preceding unassisted diastolic pressure, and you should see a V-shaped straight upstroke into the following systolic peak.

IABP waveform. *A,* End-diastolic pressure; *B,* systolic pressure; *C,* dicrotic notch (balloon inflated); *D,* augmented diastolic pressure; *E,* assisted end-diastolic pressure. (From Flynn L, Bruce N: Introduction to Critical Care Skills. St. Louis, Mosby, 1993, p 269, with permission.)

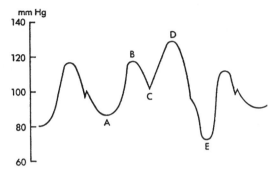

### 7. How does the IABP improve cardiac output?

The increase in diastolic pressure caused by balloon inflation enhances perfusion to the aortic root, coronary ostia, and subclavian arteries. This enhancement is called diastolic augmentation. The augmented diastolic pressure is monitored via a balloon catheter tip. The pressure should be greater than the patient's unassisted systolic pressure. The goal of inflation is to increase perfusion and oxygen delivery to the coronary arteries, as evidenced by decreased chest pain, improvement in mentation, increased urine output, improved skin color, and decreased dysrhythmias.

At the end of diastole, the balloon rapidly deflates, decreasing the resistance/afterload of the left ventricle by creating a vacuum effect. This effect decreases left ventricular workload, reduces oxygen consumption and improves contractility, cardiac output, and end-organ perfusion, as evidenced by improvements in arterial blood gases, cardiac output, and cardiac index and decreases in central venous pressure, pulmonary wedge pressure, and systemic vascular resistance. The assisted end-diastolic pressure should be less than the patient's own diastolic pressure.

### 8. Define counterpulsation.

Balloon inflation during diastole and balloon deflation just before cardiac systole.

### 9. How do you troubleshoot an IABP alarm?

Use the following checkpoints: (1) patient assessment, (2) presence of blood in tubing, (3) presence of condensation, and (4) loose connections or kinks in the IAB tubing.

Balloon pressure waveforms are of great help in troubleshooting. The most common problems that result in poor augmentation are early inflation, late inflation, early deflation, and late deflation. Timing should be assessed at the beginning of each shift, after a change in the patient's condition, and with activation of IABP console alarms.

### 10. What effect do dysrhythmias have on IABP support?

For effective counterpulsation, the pump must receive a trigger signal to identify the beginning of the cardiac cycle. Dysrhythmias can adversely affect the timing of balloon inflation and deflation. Augmentation of tachycardias greater than 120 beats/min is shortened because of the shortened time for diastole. The IABP assist ratio should be decreased to 1:2 during tachycardia to improve mean arterial pressure. In addition, atrial fibrillation reduces the effectiveness of IABP because of the irregular rhythm. During atrial fibrillation the balloon is timed using the ECG trigger so that the R wave triggers deflation.

## 11. What are the proper procedures for cardioversion and defibrillation in patients with an IABP?

Cardioversion and defibrillation for ventricular tachycardia or fibrillation can be performed safely in patients with an IABP. During cardiopulmonary resuscitation, the ECG or arterial pressure trigger should be used; the IABP trigger synchronizes to chest compressions. The balloon should not be immobile for more than 30 minutes because of the potential for thrombus formation.

## 12. What is the most common complication of IABP?

Limb ischemia. The IABP catheter can obstruct blood flow to the extremity and lead to pulse loss, compartment syndrome, and deep vein thrombosis. Pulses, color, temperature, movement, and sensation in the extremities should be monitored every 1–2 hours.

## 13. What other complications may occur with IABP?

Improper positioning of the balloon catheter may result in decreased perfusion to the left arm or renal and mesenteric arteries. Frequent vascular assessments of the left arm and monitoring of urine output are essential. Other vascular complications include thromboembolism, false aneurysm formation, and hematoma/bleeding. Coagulopathies or thrombocytopenia can result from mechanical trauma. Less common complications include infection, aortic dissection, and air embolus due to balloon rupture.

## 14. What are the goals of nursing care in patients with an IABP?

1. Assessment of balloon timing for hemodynamic stability
2. Detection and prevention of complications
3. Patient and family education and support

## 15. How is hemodynamic stability assessed?

A baseline assessment before balloon placement is important. Frequent ongoing assessments focus on the following hemodynamic values:

- Pulmonary artery wedge pressure (no value > 16–18 mmHg)
- Cardiac index (no value < 2.5 L/min/m$^2$)
- Venous oxygen saturation (no value < 50% or a decrease of 10%)
- ECG changes (e.g., ST-segment changes or hemodynamically significant dysrhythmias)
- Urine output (no values < 0.5 ml/kg/hr for 2 hr)

## 16. What are the signs of complications?

Decrease in peripheral pulses, pallor, paresthesias, and coolness of the involved leg should be reported to the physician. A decrease in left radial pulse, an abrupt decrease in urine output, flank pain, decreased or absent bowel sounds, dizziness, and decrease in balloon augmentation are signs of balloon migration and must be treated immediately.

## 17. How should patients and families be supported?

Patients and families need to be informed of the purpose and sensations of IABP insertion and therapy. They should be instructed to keep the affected leg straight and educated about bedrest restrictions and passive foot exercises. They also should be instructed to report any pain, numbness, or tingling in the extremities.

## 18. What are the criteria for weaning and discontinuance of IABP therapy?

Weaning should be considered when hemodynamic stability is achieved, as evidenced by stable heart rate and rhythm, mean arterial pressure > 65 mmHg with minimal or no vasopressor support, cardiac index > 2.5 L/min/m$^2$, adequate urine output, and absence of chest pain or other indicators of myocardial ischemia.

## 19. Describe the method for weaning patients from IABP.

To begin weaning, the assist ratio is changed to 1:3, as tolerated, over 1–6 hours, depending on the patient's response. The heparin infusion is discontinued 4–6 hours before the IABP catheter is removed, or protamine can be given to reverse the effect of heparin immediately before removal. The IABP also can be weaned by reducing balloon volume until the balloon is merely fluttering with each counterpulsation. When this method is used, it is important to inflate the balloon to full volume for 5 minutes of every hour to prevent clot formation.

The balloon must be deflated in the stand-by or off mode to remove the catheter. When the sheath is removed, pressure must be applied to the arterial site for 30–45 minutes until hemostasis is achieved. After the IABP is removed, the patient is monitored for hemodynamic stability, signs of bleeding at the exit site, and perfusion of the affected limb. The patient should continue bedrest with the leg straight for 4–6 hours after the balloon removal.

### BIBLIOGRAPHY

1. Cardiovascular system. In Kinney MR, Dunbar SB, Brooks-Brunn JA, et al: AACN's Clinical Reference for Critical Care Nursing, 4th ed. St. Louis, Mosby, 1998, pp 444–447.
2. Contol System Operation and Troubleshooting. In St. Jude's Medical: Principles of Counterpulsation, St. Jude Medical, Inc, 1992, pp 50-56.
3. Keen JH, Swearingen PL: Intraaortic balloon pump (IABP). In Mosby's Critical Care Nursing Consultant. St. Louis, Mosby, 1997, pp 248–249.
4. Mechanical assist devices. In Thelan LA, Urden LD, Lough ME, Stacy KM: Critical Care Nursing, Diagnosis and Management, 3rd ed. St. Louis, Mosby, 1998, pp 315–319.
5. Quaal SJ: Indications. In Quaal SJ (ed): Comprehensive Intraaortic Balloon Counterpulsation, 2nd ed. St. Louis, Mosby, 1993, pp 118–143.
6. Schell HM: Circulatory assist devices. In Parsons PE, Wiener-Kronish JP (eds): Critical Care Secrets, 2nd ed. Philadelphia, Hanley & Belfus, 1998, pp 83–87.
7. Wojner AW: Assessing the five points of the intra-aortic balloon pump waveform. Crit Care Nurs 6:48–52, 1994.

# 12. VENTRICULAR ASSIST DEVICES

*Ann M. Daleiden, RN, BA*

### 1. What are the components of a ventricular assist device (VAD)?

A VAD system consists of a blood pump (prosthetic ventricle), cannulas, and a pneumatic or electrical drive console.

### 2. What is the basic purpose of a VAD?

A VAD system provides partial or complete mechanical support of the systemic and pulmonary circulatory system. The blood flows from the natural heart to the VAD (prosthetic ventricle), which then pumps blood back to the body. VAD placement can be used for short-term or long-term support.

### 3. How do VADs provide systemic support? Pulmonary support?

Systemic support is provided by insertion of a left VAD (LVAD). Pulmonary support is achieved with a right VAD (RVAD). Concurrent use of both LVAD and RVAD provides complete biventricular (BiVAD) support. The LVAD and RVAD replace the blood pumping function of each respective ventricle.

### 4. What is the goal of short-term VAD placement? How does it work?

Short-term VAD resuscitation is provided when recovery from an acute myocardial event is expected. The RVAD inflow cannula is inserted into the right atrium and diverts blood from the failing right ventricle to the VAD. The outflow cannula is placed in the pulmonary artery and returns blood from the VAD to the pulmonary circulation. The LVAD inflow cannula is inserted into the left atrium, and the outflow is graft-anastomosed to the aorta for return to systemic circulation.

**5. What is the goal of long-term VAD placement? How does it work?**

Long-term support is provided as a bridge to transplantation. It is achieved by placement of either an LVAD or a BiVAD. The LVAD inflow cannula can be inserted into the left atrium or left ventricular apex. The outflow cannula is anastomosed to the ascending aorta. The RVAD inflow cannula is inserted into the right atrium or right ventricular apex and returns blood from the VAD to the pulmonary artery via the inflow cannula. Apical cannulation for long-term support achieves a higher cardiac output with a lower risk for thrombosis in the natural left ventricle.

**6. What is the major contraindication to LVAD support?**

LVAD support is contraindicated in patients with mechanical aortic valves in situ because of the potential for thrombus formation on the valve.

**7. What are the clinical indications for placement of a VAD?**

- Cardiogenic shock refractory to maximal pharmacologic and intraaortic balloon pump (IABP) support
- Inability to wean from cardiopulmonary bypass after cardiac surgery
- Bridge to cardiac transplantation
- For patients with refractory chronic congestive heart failure and contraindications to transplantation, permanent support with the implantable Novacor or Heartmate LVAD is now considered.

**8. What hemodynamic parameters may be used as a guide to initiate VAD support?**

Assuming that maximal pharmacologic support has been instituted to optimize preload and afterload:

- Cardiac index < 2.0 L/min/m$^2$
- Mean arterial pressure < 60 mmHg
- Systolic blood pressure < 90 mmHg
- Pulmonary capillary wedge pressure > 20 mmHg
- Systemic vascular resistance > 2100 dynes/sec/cm$^2$
- Urine output < 20 ml/hr

The goals of VAD support are to decrease myocardial work, to reduce myocardial oxygen consumption, and to maintain perfusion to sustain end-organ function.

**9. Which devices are designed for short-term support?**

Short-term resuscitative circulatory support can be provided by centrifugal nonpulsatile mechanical devices, including the Bio-Medicus VAD, the Nimbus Hemopump, and the Abiomed BVS 5000 VAD.

**10. How does the Bio-Medicus VAD work?**

The Bio-Medicus VAD (Bio-Medicus Inc, Ann Arbor, MI) is a first-generation device designed for use after cardiotomy and can provide left and right ventricular support. Centrifugal pumps provide continuous nonpulsatile flow via an electrically powered magnet located at the base of the pump head. The motor in the console generates the prescribed revolutions per minute (rpms), and through centrifugal force the blood rises from the base of the pump head, forcing a return direction of blood flow. Pump output is proportional to rpms. The Bio-Medicus is capable of generating flow outputs of 2-5 L/min.

**11. What are the advantages and disadvantages the Bio-Medicus VAD?**

**Advantages:** simplicity, low cost, compatibility with standard cannulas used for cardiopulmonary bypass, and ability to provide pediatric support.

**Disadvantages**: limited durability of the pump head (for long-term support), hemolysis, and nonpulsatile flow. An IABP may be inserted to create pulsatile flow.

**12. How does the Nimbus Hemopump work?**

The Nimbus Hemopump (Nimbus Medical Inc, Rancho Cardova, CA) consists of a high-powered intravascular rotor pump contained in a perfusion cannula inserted across the aortic valve into the left ventricle. The rotary action is capable of providing flow rates of up to 4 L/min.

**13. What are the advantages and disadvantages of the Nimbus Hemopump?**

**Advantages:** ease of insertion via the femoral artery, small size, portability, relatively low cost, and ability to provide pediatric support.

**Disadvantages:** inability to provide right ventricular support. Currently it is not approved for bridge to transplant, although a research protocol is under way.

**14. How does the Abiomed BVS 5000 VAD work?**

The Abiomed BVS 5000 VAD (Abiomed Cardiovascular Inc, Danvers, MA) uses a pulsatile pneumatic drive system. The pumping chambers are pole-mounted near the patient. The drive console autoregulates blood flow in response to filling. The Abiomed ejects a fixed volume per beat and responds to preload and afterload.

**15 What are the advantages and disadvantages of the Abiomed BVS 5000 VAD?**

**Advantages:** pulsatile flow, transportability, and ability to provide LVAD and RVAD support. It does not require cardiopulmonary bypass for cannulation.

**Disadvantages:** expense (for short-term use) and increased clotting compared with centrifugal pumps. The Abiomed is used in nontransplant centers that offer cardiac surgery.

**16. Which devices are approved for long-term support as a bridge to transplant?**

Pulsatile VADs, the most advanced forms of mechanical support, provide long-term support as a bridge to transplantation. They can be placed externally or implanted internally. Their advantages include biocompatible blood-contacting surfaces that allow extended use with minimal anticoagulation and hemolysis. Pulsatile perfusion increases oxygen consumption, lowers peripheral artery resistance, and provides maximal renal, cerebral, and myocardial perfusion. Examples include the Thoratec VAD, Novacor LVAD, and Heartmate LVAD.

**17. How does the Thoratec VAD work?**

The Thoratec VAD (Thoratec Medical Inc, Berkeley, CA) is an external pulsatile device. It is placed on the anterior abdominal wall and has percutaneous inflow and outflow cannulas that traverse the abdominal wall and pump blood in parallel with the native circulation. The prosthetic ventricle consists of a smooth, seamless pumping chamber (blood sac) enclosed in a rigid case. Two mechanical valves maintain unidirectional flow through the VAD. A fill switch detects when the VAD is full of blood and signals the console to supply air pressure to eject blood from the VAD into the arterial system. The vacuum line from the console facilitates VAD filling. The blood sac holds 65 ml of blood and can provide outputs of 1.2– 7.2 L/min.

**18. What are the advantages and disadvantages of the Thoratec VAD?**

**Advantages:** ability to provide short-term and long-term univentricular and biventricular support. Because the Thoratec is externally placed, it is adaptable to a wide range of body sizes and can provide pediatric support.

**Disadvantages:** increased risk of infection because of external placement, slight impairment of patient mobility (due to the large pneumatic drive console), and need for anticoagulation (due to the mechanical valves). At present, patients with a Thoratec VAD cannot be discharged from the hospital.

**19. How does the Novacor LVAD work?**

The Novacor LVAD (Novacor Medical Corporation, Oakland, CA) is an electrically driven implantable device. The blood pump provides displacement of blood via an electrically operated dual pusher-plate mechanism that compresses the VAD sac to eject the blood. It is implanted in the abdominal wall anterior to the posterior rectus abdominis sheath. A subcutaneously tunneled cable exits the abdominal wall and serves as the power drive line.

### 20. How does the Heartmate LVAD work?

The Heartmate LVAD (Thermo Cardiosystems, Woburn, MA) comes in a pneumatic and an electrical model. It works much like the Novacor LVAD.

### 21. What are the advantages and disadvantages of implantable devices?

**Advantages:** currently approved as bridges to transplantation. They provide pulsatile flow with high cardiac outputs of 8–9 L/min and allow maximal mobilization of patients. Discharge from the hospital is possible with implantable devices. Long-term support has been provided for more than 2 years with implantable LVADs.

**Disadvantages:** insertion of implantable VADs is technically more complex. They require anticoagulation, and patients are at risk for bleeding complications.Because of lack of space in the abdominal cavity, implantable VADs can provide only left ventricular support. LVAD support is adequate in most cases, however, because the common cause of chronic right ventricular failure is left ventricular failure.

### 22. Why are patients with VADs at risk for bleeding?

Bleeding is the most common postoperative complication associated with VAD insertion. Risk factors for bleeding include (1) preoperative anticoagulation, (2) hepatic and/or renal dysfunction, (3) long cardiopulmonary bypass time, (4) platelet dysfunction, and (5) multiple cannulation sites. It is recommended that type-specific, cytomegalovirus-negative blood products with leukocyte filters be administered for bridge to transplant patients. The purpose is to limit antigen exposure and possible antibody formation.

### 23. How common are VAD-related infections?

The incidence of infections associated with VAD insertion ranges from 30–50%. Infections are most common at cannula sites and drive-line exit sites, in the LVAD insertion pocket and sternal incisions, and inside the VAD device itself.

### 24. How are VAD-related infections treated?

Cannula site infections require aggressive therapy, which includes antibiotic irrigation for tracking along the cannula. Infections of the drive-line exit site and pump pocket are managed conservatively with antibiotics and local wound care until transplantation. Device-related bacteremias are the most challenging infections to manage because removing the device is not a viable alternative in the absence of concurrent transplantation.

A minimal 6-week course of antibiotic therapy is suggested. Pathogens related to the indigenous microflora of nursing care units vary from institution to institution. Sterile dressing changes should be performed at all times. Heart transplantation may be performed before completion of antibiotic therapy if blood cultures become sterile and a donor heart is available.

### 25. Why is management of arrhythmias important for patients on VADs?

Arrhythmia management is important when patients are hemodynamically compromised. Patients receiving univentricular support depend on the diastolic and systolic function of the unsupported ventricle. Most ventricular arrhythmias are short and convert spontaneously. Signs of hemodynamic compromise include hypotension, decreased mental status, shortness of breath, decreased VAD output, and pulmonary edema (which can develop rapidly with RVAD support.) Treatment with antiarrhythmic drugs or cardioversion is recommended for hemodynamic deterioration. Patients receiving BiVAD support tolerate lethal arrhythmias because the VADs have taken over the pumping function of both ventricles.

### 26. What potential complication is unique to patients receiving LVAD support?

Patients with isolated LVAD support should be monitored for right ventricular (RV) failure.

**27. What are the risk factors for RV failure?**
- Pulmonary hypertension
- Lethal arrhythmias
- Bleeding
- Right ventricular septal infarction

**28. What are the symptoms of RV failure?**
- Increased right atrial pressure (central venous pressure)
- Elevated pulmonary vascular resistance (PVR)
- Failure of the LVAD to fill
- Decreased VAD output and cardiac output
- Decreased perfusion
- Atrial arrhythmias
- Liver enlargement
- Jaundice
- Peripheral edema

Pulmonary capillary wedge pressure may decrease or remain unchanged.

**29. Describe the management of RV failure.**
Management includes pharmacologic support with pulmonary vasodilators and inotropes and hyperventilation to decrease the partial pressure of carbon dioxide in arterial blood (in an attempt to decrease PVR). After maximal pharmacologic support has been implemented, nitric oxide therapy (which decreases PVR) or RVAD insertion may be indicated.

**30. When should patients be mobilized and started on an exercise regimen?**
Patients should be mobilized and started on a progressive exercise regimen as early as possible after VAD insertion. Many patients lived with exercise intolerance for a long time before VAD insertion because of their deteriorating cardiac condition. Postoperative exercise protocols need to be individually tailored depending on type of device, insertion site, and prior exercise tolerance. Patients with implantable devices tolerate more aggressive activity than patients with externally placed devices. In the immediate postoperative period, once hemodynamics are stable, patients may be turned from side to side every 2–4 hours. At this time range-of-motion exercises should be initiated. Longer-term patients progress to stationary bike riding and ambulation.

**31. When can patients with a VAD be transferred out of the intensive care unit (ICU)?**
Patients with VADs can be transferred out of the ICU once they are hemodynamically stable with no evidence of life-threatening complications. The following general discharge criteria should be kept in mind: (1) no pulmonary artery catheter, arterial line, or left atrial catheter; (2) no ventilatory support; (3) stable low-dose intravenous inotropic support that does not require titration; and (4) absence of life-threatening ventricular arrhythmias requiring cardioversion. The objectives of transferring patients out of the ICU is gradually to restore a level of physical and mental ability that facilitates self-care.

**32. What psychosocial issues are relevant to patients with VAD support and their families?**
Two common issues are anxiety and powerlessness. In the ICU during the acute phase of VAD support, the primary psychosocial focus is the family. Frequently the device is placed as the result of a life-threatening or emergent situation. Anxiety and fear are common responses. Allowing the patient and family to express their concerns, providing support, and educating them about the VAD device help them to work through such feelings. Powerlessness is a common long-term issue. Uncertainty and lack of control over when a donor heart will become available are major concerns. Promotion of independence, exercise, uninterrupted sleep, and preparation for eventual transfer out of the ICU to a general ward help patients and their families cope effectively.

**33. What additional nursing considerations are relevant to VAD patients?**
Another potential complication of VAD support is **thromboembolism** that results in a neurologic event. Risk factors include inadequate anticoagulation, incomplete VAD ejection, low VAD

output (< 2.0 L/min/m$^2$), a kinked cannula or pneumatic hose, and sepsis. Management includes therapeutic anticoagulation, maintaining adequate VAD output, and observing aseptic technique. With the state-of-the-art devices currently available, the incidence of device-related neurological events in patients treated with VADs is now less than 5% with minimal or no anticoagulation.

**Monitoring of volume status and VAD output** is crucial. The leading cause of low VAD output is hypovolemia. Maintaining right and left filling pressures of 10–16 mmHg is recommended to optimize VAD filling. In the presence of RVAD or BiVAD support, thermodilution cardiac outputs are invalid because of the diverted injectate path through the RVAD pump. With LVAD support thermodilution cardiac output measurements are valid. Thermodilution cardiac output does not always equal the VAD output determined by the VAD console. Certain VADs calculate output based on fixed variables, such as VAD rate and filling capacity, whereas others measure flow rate. Assessment of VAD output vs. native cardiac output is accomplished by subtracting thermodilution cardiac output from VAD output.

### BIBLIOGRAPHY

1. Farrar DJ, Hill JD: Univentricular and biventricular thoracic VAD support as a bridge to transplantation. Ann Thorac Surg 55:276–282, 1993.
2. Lutwick LI, Vaghjimal A, Connolly MW: Postcardiac surgery infections. Crit Care Clin 14:242–245, 1998.
3. Moroney DA, Vaca KJ: Infectious complications associated with ventricular assist devices. Am J Crit Care 4:204–209, 1995.
4. Reedy JE: Transfer of a patient with a ventricular assist device to a non-critical care area. Heart Lung 22:71–76, 1993.
5. Reedy JE, Swartz MT, Lohmann DP, et al: The importance of patient mobility with ventricular assist device support. ASAIO J 38:M151–M153, 1992.
6. Savage LS, Canody C: Life with a ventricular assist device: The patient's perspective. Am J Crit Care 8:340–343, 1999.
7. Schell HM: Circulatory assist devices. In Parsons PE, Wiener-Kronish JP (eds): Critical Care Secrets, 2nd ed. Philadelphia, Hanley & Belfus, 1998, pp 87–89.
8. Scherr K, Jensen L, Koshal A: Mechanical circulatory support as a bridge to cardiac transplantation: Toward the 21st century. Am J Crit Care 8:324–337, 1999.
9. Shinn JA: Nursing care of the patient on mechanical circulatory support. Ann Thorac Surg 55:288–294, 1993.

# 13. DEFIBRILLATION AND CARDIOVERSION

*Lynn Houweling*, RN, MS, CCRN

### 1. What is the difference between defibrillation and cardioversion?

Although both defibrillation and cardioversion use electricity to reset cardiac pacemaker cells, they are used in different circumstances based on the dysrhythmia and the patient's condition.

**Defibrillation**, also known as *unsynchronized* cardioversion, is the emergent use of electric current delivered in large amounts for a brief time. The defibrillation shock causes temporary depolarization in the fibrillating myocardium, followed by a refractory period during which pacemaker cells can reset themselves to normal coordinated activity.

**Cardioversion** is the delivery of a *synchronized* electrical impulse designed to revert dysrhythmia to sinus rhythm. In a process known as synchronization, the defibrillator is set to track the R wave of the QRS complex. The current is delivered at a predetermined point in the cardiac cycle (approximately 30 msec after the R wave), thus avoiding the relative refractory stage (T wave) and resultant deterioration to ventricular fibrillation (R-on-T phenomenon). Cardioversion may be emergent or elective.

### 2. What are the indications for defibrillation?

Defibrillation is an emergency procedure used to convert ventricular fibrillation (VF) or hemodynamically unstable ventricular tachycardia (VT) to a life-sustaining rhythm. In general, rhythms with a pulse are not defibrillated.

### 3. What are the indications for cardioversion?

Cardioversion, which may be emergent or planned, is used to convert hemodynamically stable VTs, supraventricular tachycardias (SVTs) with rapid ventricular response, or stable new-onset SVTs. Rhythms that require cardioversion must be slow enough so that synchronization with a QRS complex is feasible. Some rapid VTs, even with a pulse, are better managed with defibrillation to avoid inadvertent synchronization with the T wave and potential deterioration to VF (R-on-T phenomenon). Generally, hemodynamically stable dysrhythmias are treated initially with medical therapy. If medications fail, cardioversion is often used.

### 4. What are the contraindications to defibrillation?

Defibrillation should be avoided in all but the conditions mentioned in question 2. Defibrillating a heart in a normal rhythm can cause VF. Defibrillation is not indicated or recommended for asystole, because it is ineffective and may inhibit the recovery of the cardiac pacemaker cells, thus making resuscitation impossible. However, because fine VF can mimic asystole, the electrocardiographic (ECG) rhythm should be checked in more than one lead and the electrodes assessed before diagnosing asystole.

### 5. What are the contraindications to cardioversion?

Contraindications to nonemergent cardioversion are relative rather than absolute. Cardioversion is usually futile in patients with long-standing atrial fibrillation or atrial hypertrophy. Bradycardia, VT, or VF can result after cardioversion of a patient with digitalis intoxication. Recent embolic events of questionable etiology are also a relative contraindication to cardioversion. Defibrillation should be used instead of cardioversion if the "sync" button cannot highlight the R wave or if it is thought that the machine is reading the R wave incorrectly (i.e., if the machine reads a pacemaker spike as the R wave).

### 6. What equipment is needed?

- Defibrillator with synchronizing button
- Code cart with emergency medications
- Airway management supplies, including intubation equipment
- Oxygen
- ECG monitor with recording capabilities

### 7. What is the nurse's role during defibrillation?

Because rapidly applied electricity is the key to successful resuscitation, most intensive care units expect nurses who have demonstrated competency to perform defibrillation independently in the setting of cardiac arrest. Refer to your institution's policy and procedure manual.

### 8. What is the nurse's role in cardioversion?

Nurses do not perform routine synchronized cardioversion independently. Routine procedures are usually planned under controlled circumstances. Nursing responsibilities in caring for patients undergoing elective cardioversion include:

- Ensuring that the patient has given informed consent
- Patient teaching, including pre- and post-procedure care
- Establishing intravenous access
- Continuous 3- or 5-lead ECG monitoring
- Obtaining a 12-lead ECG before and after the procedure
- Ensuring that the "sync" button is pressed and the R wave highlighted
- Sedation management, including airway assessment

- Anticoagulation administration, if indicated
- Documentation of the above as well as the number of shocks, energy applied, and patient response

### 9. What are the options for correct paddle placement?

Electrodes should be placed in a position to maximize current flow to the myocardium. Any of the following positions can be used with either traditional paddles or self-adhesive electrodes:

- **Anterior-apex position.** The anterior electrode is placed to the right of the upper sternum but below the clavicle. The apex electrode is placed to the left of the nipple with the middle of the paddle in the midaxillary line.
- **Anterior-posterior position.** One electrode is placed over the left precordium and the other electrode under the left scapula behind the heart.
- **Apex-posterior position.** The anterior electrode is placed over the left apex and the posterior electrode in the left subscapular area.

### 10. How is defibrillation performed?

1. Assess the patient for airway, breathing, and circulation.
2. Assess ECG rhythm.
3. Apply the appropriate conductive material to the electrodes or use electrode pads.
4. Turn on the defibrillator and select the initial energy level.
5. Charge the defibrillator and place the electrodes on the patient's chest.
6. Before discharging the defibrillator, ensure that no personnel are directly or indirectly in contact with the patient by loudly commanding, "Stand clear," and visually checking for compliance.
7. Discharge the defibrillator according to the manufacturer's instructions.
8. Assess the patient's rhythm and pulse. A brief period of asystole may follow defibrillation. If asystole continues longer than 10 seconds and is confirmed in two or more ECG leads and if all leads are intact, resume cardiopulmonary resuscitation (CPR) and initiate pacing or drug therapy.
9. If VF or pulseless VT continues, immediately defibrillate at 200–300 J.
10. If VF or pulseless VT continues, immediately defibrillate at 360 J.
11. Reassess rhythm and pulse. Initiate supportive resuscitation care as indicated.

### 11. How is cardioversion performed?

**Emergent cardioversion** is performed in the same manner as defibrillation except that the synchronization button on the defibrillator is depressed and the R wave becomes highlighted.

For **nonemergent cardioversion**, patients should receive preprocedure teaching and give informed consent. Sedation is mandatory because patients are awake and often anxious. Benzodiazepines such as midazolam or diazepam are common choices. Morphine or fentanyl is administered for pain control. The nurse is responsible for sedation monitoring and management. Sometimes the patient is electively intubated, especially in the presence of borderline hypoxemia, altered mental status, or difficulty in managing secretions.

### 12. What patient safety issues should be kept in mind when either procedure is performed?

- Correct identification of the dysrhythmia and accurate assessment of clinical status are essential; they are the two factors on which choice of therapy is based.
- If the shock of cardioversion causes the rhythm to decompensate to VT or VF, immediate unsyncronized defibrillation at 200 J is indicated.
- Transdermal medicine patches should be removed before defibrillation because the aluminum backing can cause electrical arcing and severe skin burns.
- Application of too much conductive gel can also causes arcing and burns.
- Alcohol can ignite from the defibrillation shock and should be avoided.
- Paddles should be cleaned after each use with soap and water because residual conductive gel can corrode the metal paddle surfaces and cause arcing.
- Patients may experience skin burns after multiple shocks. As with all burns, treatment is based on severity.

### 13. What provider safety issues should be kept in mind?

- Call out "Stand clear" or "All clear" in a loud voice, and make a visual check to ensure that all personnel are clear of the patient, bed, and defibrillator before discharge.
- The nurse should have no contact with the patient except through the defibrillator handles. Anyone in contact with the patient or surroundings may be subject to the shock.
- Handle IV fluids with care. Wet clothing or surroundings can be an electrical hazard.
- The paddles should never be fired into the air or with the paddles together.
- If the paddles are charged but not needed, they should be replaced in their holders and the defibrillator turned off to dissipate the energy.

### 14. How much electrical energy is required for successful rhythm conversion?

Whatever works. The lowest energy level is applied first, with successive shocks increasing in current until a maximum of 360 J is reached. Traditionally, defibrillation begins with 200 J. If this level is unsuccessful, a 300-J shock should be used immediately, followed by 360 J, if needed. Cardioversion begins with 100 J, followed by 200 J, if needed.

### 15. What is transthoracic impedance (TTI)?

TTI is the resistance to passage of current through the chest wall. This resistance can significantly alter the effectiveness of the defibrillation effort.

### 16. What interventions decrease TTI?

1. The use of multiple consecutive shocks is recommended because TTI decreases after each successive shock.

2. Defibrillation should be attempted only at end expiration because air is a poor conductor of electricity. This is usually not a problem in the setting of cardiac arrest because without artificial ventilation the patient is in end expiration.

3. A salt-containing medium is needed between the paddles and the chest wall to reduce interference. Without the gel interface, TTI is increased by 100%.

4. The correct paddle size should be used. Adult paddles can be applied successfully in most patients older than 1 year. Larger paddles decrease TTI and increase the amount of myocardium to be depolarized.

5. The paddles should be held firmly against the skin to improve contact.

6. Paddles should be placed away from bone, which is not a good conductor of electricity.

### 17. Why are defibrillation and cardioversion sometimes unsuccessful?

Successful defibrillation and cardioversion depend on the state of the myocardium and the proper use of the defibrillator. Because acidosis decreases success rates, rapid defibrillation is essential to prevent further acid build-up from the fibrillating heart. Correct paddle size and placement with proper gel and correct energy selection also increase the chances of success.

### 18. Is there any danger to implanted devices during defibrillation or cardioversion?

**Automated implanted cadiac defibrillators** (AICDs) sometimes fail to convert the rhythm or fail completely to fire. External transthoracic defibrillation should be used immediately. AICDs are protected from damage by external defibrillation but need a check for readiness after any external shock. People touching the patient when the AICD discharges will not be adversely affected. They may feel a tingling in the extremity or be completely unaware of the discharge.

**Implanted pacemakers** occasionally fail after defibrillator use. It is wise to have external pacing capabilities available during defibrillation. Many modern defibrillators have built-in pacemaker properties. Place the defibrillator paddles at least 10 cm from the pulse generator, if possible. Pacemaker failure is probably not related to damage to the pulse generator because of built-in protection from countershock. Possibly it is due to endothelial damage or a rise in stimulation threshold.

### 19. What is the role of anticoagulation therapy with cardioversion?

The patient is at risk of thrombus formation secondary to incomplete emptying in the fibrillating atria. An embolus can be released from the atria with the first complete contraction and emptying after successful cardioversion. Therefore, anticoagulation therapy is indicated for atrial dysrhythmias of more than 2 or 3 days' duration, unless the patient has a major contraindication to anticoagulation. Therapy usually consists of warfarin for 2 weeks before the procedure. If the patient is unable to take warfarin, heparin can be substituted.

### 20. What is internal defibrillation? When is it used?

Internal defibrillation is the application of electricity directly to the epicardium by a physician via specially designed paddles. This procedure is used routinely in the operating room when patients are removed from cardiopulmonary bypass. It also can be used in the emergency department or intensive care unit, if needed. The internal paddles are supplied with energy from the same defibrillator machine used for external defibrillation. The usual energy level is 5–40 J.

### 21. What is the role of automated external defibrillators (AEDs) in acute care settings?

AEDs are used increasingly in prehospital settings, and some research suggests that they have a role in acute care. Patients in areas staffed by personnel unfamiliar with ECG interpretation may benefit from AED access, if it is needed. First-responder nurses can be trained in AED use to ensure the earliest defibrillation possible. Patients may arrive in the intensive care unit after successful AED resuscitation.

### BIBLIOGRAPHY

1. Cummins RO (ed): Advanced Cardiac Life Support Textbook. Dallas, American Heart Association, 1994.
2. Eisenberg JS: Fifty years of defibrillation. Ann Emerg Med 6:808–810, 1997.
3. Leith BA: Defibrillation: What nurses should know. J Can Assoc Crit Care Nurs 7:20–22, 1996.
4. Mancini ME, Kaye W: AEDs: Changing the way you respond to cardiac arrest. Am J Nurs 5:26–30, 1999.
5. Rogove HJ, Hughes CM: Defibrillation and cardioversion. Critical Care Clin 8:839–863, 1992.

# 14. DEEP VEIN THROMBOSIS AND PULMONARY EMBOLISM

*Cheryl Hubner,* RN, MS, CCRN

### 1. Define deep vein thrombosis (DVT).

DVT is a blood clot that has formed in a vein. It usually starts as a cluster of platelets and fibrin growing out of a vein valve pocket in an intramuscular venous sinus of the leg or along a vein wall that has been traumatized. The clot grows in the direction of blood flow, with the tail of the clot floating freely in the vein lumen. The clot continues to form, adheres more firmly to the vein wall, and blocks flow. The clot continues to grow both proximally and distally until the next vein branching is reached or until the clotting process is halted by anticoagulation therapy. A thrombus may form in any vein, but it is found most commonly in the lower extremities. Upper-extremity DVTs are more likely in patients who have a central venous catheter, are undergoing chemotherapy, or have a malignancy.

### 2. Define pulmonary embolism (PE).

PE is a free-floating particle that lodges in a pulmonary artery or arteriole. A massive PE usually lodges in a central pulmonary artery. A moderate-sized embolus lodges in an arteriole. Multiple tiny, undetectable emboli can shower the distal pulmonary arterioles, resulting in pulmonary hypertension. Most PEs are fragments of a thrombus originating in the right heart or the deep veins of the upper extremities, thigh, or pelvis. Nonthrombotic causes of PE include amniotic fluid emboli, fragments of a trophoblast, cotton-wool fragments, talcum or starch particles, fat or fat cells, air, megakaryocytes, tumor fragments, and ova of parasites.

### 3. Why is DVT dangerous?

The two most serious consequences of DVT are PE and phlegmasia cerulea dolens (or venous gangrene). PE occurs in approximately 35% of patients with untreated DVT. Venous gangrene is rare, occurring in patients with extensive iliofemoral thrombosis. A late complication of DVT is chronic venous insufficiency, called postphlebitic syndrome. DVT leads to vein valve damage, chronic reflux across the damaged valve, increased venous pressure, chronic leg swelling, and skin ulcerations.

### 4. Why is PE dangerous?

The consequences of PE depend on the size of the embolus. A massive PE is often fatal. It causes severe pulmonary obstruction, which progresses rapidly to acute hemodynamic instability, right-sided heart failure, and hypoxemia. Pulmonary pressures rise only modestly, but right ventricular and atrial pressures rise sharply, resulting in right ventricular dilatation and failure. Most emboli do not obstruct the pulmonary vessel completely but allow some flow around them.

If the patient survives the immediate event, the clot begins to reorganize within a few hours. It becomes partially recanalized, allowing blood flow through it, and shrinks in size. Small fresh pulmonary emboli that lodge in the smaller arterioles dissolve spontaneously through a process called fibrinolysis. The pulmonary endothelium is a reservoir for plasminogen activator, which triggers fibrinolysis. A serious but rare consequence of PE is pulmonary infarction (death of embolized pulmonary tissue). Infarction is more likely if the embolus completely blocks a large artery or if the patient has preexisting lung and heart disease.

### 5. Why are critically ill patients at risk for developing DVT or PE?

Every patient admitted to a critical care unit should be considered at risk for a thromboembolic event and should receive appropriate prophylactic therapy. Critically ill patients frequently have some or all of the three factors that favor clot formation: stasis of blood, alterations in the blood coagulation system, and abnormalities of the blood vessel wall. Bedrest, casts, restraints, paralytic agents, local pressure, increased blood viscosity (from, for example, dehydration, polycythemia vera, sickle cell disease), hypotension, and states of low cardiac output contribute to stasis of blood, especially in the lower extremities. The stasis of blood allows activated clotting factors to accumulate in a localized area and form a clot. Stasis also decreases the liver's ability to filter activated clotting factors from the blood stream. Malignancy, chemotherapy, trauma, pregnancy, oral estrogen therapy, acidosis, sepsis, surgery, induction of anesthesia, and burns activate clotting factors. Injury to the vein wall is caused by local trauma, acidosis, and bacterial endotoxins. Local trauma is caused by intravascular devices, burns, surgery, retractors, and manipulation of local veins during orthopedic surgery.

### 6. What congenital or acquired conditions increase the risk of thrombotic events?

| INHERITED HYPERCOAGULABLE STATES | ACQUIRED HYPERCOAGULABLE STATES | |
|---|---|---|
| Factor V Leiden mutation | Diabetes | Inflammatory bowel disease |
| G20210A prothrombin gene mutation | Surgery, trauma, burns | Nephrotic syndrome |
| Dysplasminogenemias | Prolonged immobilization | Polycythemia vera |
| Dysfibrinogenemia | Malignancy | Acute leukemia |
| Protein C, S, or antithrombin III deficiency | Pregnancy | Sickle cell disease |
| Heparin cofactor II deficiency | Congestive heart failure | Paroxysmal nocturnal hemoglobinuria |
| Lupus anticoagulant disorder | Obesity | Behçet's disease |
| Homocysteinemia | Varicose veins | Oral estrogen therapy |
| | Infection | |

### 7. What are the two most common inherited hypercoagulable states?

The two most common inherited hypercoagulable states are activated protein C resistance, known as factor V Leiden mutation, and G20210A prothrombin gene mutation. Factor V Leiden is usually caused by a mutation that alters the binding site of factor V for activated protein C. It occurs in 5% of the general population and 20–40% of unselected patients with DVT.

### 8. Is a sequential compression device (SCD) more effective than a thromboembolic stocking (TED) in preventing a DVT?

Preventive measures are most successful when matched to the patient's risk for developing a thromboembolic event. Thromboembolic stockings and foot exercises are appropriate prophylaxis in patients at **low risk** for DVT, who are well hydrated and mobile.

In patients at **moderate risk**, SCD prophylaxis is appropriate when initiated before a clot has started to form and when used consistently until the patient is ambulatory.

In patients at **high risk**, prophylaxis is best achieved with a combination of mechanical and pharmacologic therapy. Pharmacologic therapy may consist of an adjusted dose of oral anticoagulant therapy or fixed low-dose unfractionated heparin, 5000 U subcutaneously every 8–12 hours. Mechanical therapy can be provided by foot impulse technology or SCD. Neurosurgical patients are treated with an SCD alone because of the increased risk of bleeding when anticoagulant therapy is used. Low-molecular-weight heparin (LMWH) has been effective in preventing DVT in patients undergoing elective knee replacement. More research is needed to determine the applicability of LMWH to other populations.

### 9. What are the signs and symptoms of DVT?

The manifestations of a DVT vary widely from no symptoms to pain, fever, unilateral extremity swelling, and increased superficial venous patterning. Symptoms depend on the size and location of the thrombus and the adequacy of collateral flow through the superficial veins. Homans' sign (calf pain on dorsiflexion of the foot) is a poor test for DVT because it is positive in about 50% of patients with DVT, and 40% of patients without DVT.

### 10. What are the signs and symptoms of PE?

The most common signs and symptoms of PE are dyspnea, pleuritic chest pain, and tachypnea, which occur in about 97% of patients. Eighty-one percent of patients with PE will have a partial pressure of arterial oxygen ($PaO_2$) < 80%, and 89% have an alveolar-arterial gradient > 20 mmHg. The signs and symptoms of a PE are related to the size of the occluded or partially occluded artery. Massive PEs lodging in a major pulmonary artery cause acute decompensation, hemodynamic collapse, jugular vein distention, shortness of breath, tachypnea, tachycardia, hypotension, and occasionally chest pain. A loud pulmonic second heart sound ($P_2$) may be auscultated. PEs of moderate size may present with pleuritic pain, dyspnea, slight fever, cough with blood-tinged sputum, tachycardia, and possibly a pleural rub. Small emboli are asymptomatic because they gradually oblate the pulmonary capillary bed. In time, they cause pulmonary hypertension, a right ventricular heave, and a loud $P_2$.

### 11. What is compartment syndrome?

In patients with compartment syndrome, elevated pressure within an osteofascial compartment threatens the function of the leg or arm. Intracompartmental pressures are $\geq 30$–40 mmHg. Lower intracompartmental pressures can cause ischemia in patients with low cardiac output. Increased pressure results in decreased perfusion to the extremity muscle, ischemia, and destruction of the muscle.

### 12. What are the symptoms of compartment syndrome?

- Pain in the affected extremity that increases with passive movement of the affected muscle
- Numbness, especially in the web space between the first and second toes
- Taut edema in the affected extremity
- Pulses are usually present in the extremity until the swelling is extreme

### 13. How do you differentiate DVT from compartment syndrome?

Both DVT and compartment syndrome present with similar symptoms: leg pain and swelling specific to the affected extremity. The quality of the pain is difficult to differentiate. The swelling with DVT may not be as tight as the swelling that accompanies compartment syndrome. The tense limb edema caused by compartment syndrome may feel hard like a football. In addition, patients with compartment syndrome may experience loss of sensation and movement in the affected extremity and complain of numbness between the first and second toes, decreased sensation in the foot, and decreased ability to dorsiflex the foot or wiggle the toes. In addition, the risk factors for DVT and compartment syndrome are different. Risk factors for DVT are listed in question 5. Risk factors for compartment syndrome are traumatic injury to the limb, prolonged period of hypoperfusion to the limb followed by reperfusion, and extreme swelling of a limb.

### 14. What tests are used to diagnose DVT?

Tests available to detect DVT are venography, impedance plethysmography (IPG), ultrasonography, and magnetic resonance imaging (MRI). Radionuclide studies, such as I-125 fibrinogen uptake, are rarely used except during research studies. Venography is the most sensitive test for DVT of the calf vein. Compression ultrasonography (duplex ultrasonography with color Doppler imaging) is highly reliable for DVT above the knee. MRI is excellent for detecting pelvic and lower extremity thrombi and for ruling out external compression of the pelvic veins due to other causes (e.g., tumors).

### 15. What tests can be used to confirm the diagnosis of PE?

The gold standard is the **pulmonary angiogram**. An intraluminal filling defect in the contrast-filled pulmonary arteries is considered diagnostic of PE.

**Ventilation-perfusion scintigraphy** (V/Q scan) is a radioisotope lung scan. Technetium-labeled albumin macroaggregates or microspheres are injected intravenously. If perfusion is normal, no emboli are present. An abnormal perfusion scan may indicate PE or diffuse destructive airway disease, such as chronic bronchitis, infection, or areas of emphysema. Multiple perfusion defects are suspicious for PE. To perform a ventilation scan, the patient inhales krypton-81m. In PE the perfusion scan is abnormal, but the ventilation scan is normal.

Two new tests are **magnetic resonance angiography** (MRA) and **contrast-enhanced spiral computed tomography** (CT). MRA has a sensitivity of 75–100% and a specificity of 95–100%. Spiral CT has a sensitivity of 72% and a specificity of 95%; it is able to detect emboli as distal as the lobar or segmental arteries.

### 16. What nonspecific tests help to evaluate patients with possible PE?

An **electrocardiogram** (ECG) is used to identify right ventricular strain and to rule out myocardial infarction.

**Chest films** are rarely helpful in diagnosing PE but help to rule out processes such as pneumonia and pneumothorax. PE sometimes causes distal hemorrhage, atelectasis, parenchymal infiltrates, and pleural effusions. If PE is present, the chest film may show a moderate increase in heart size, localized areas of underperfused lung, and increased density of the main pulmonary artery associated with peripheral cut-off vessels. These findings cannot be seen on a portable film.

**Arterial blood gas analysis** is helpful in documenting hypoxemia.

### 17. Why is it difficult to diagnose PE?

It is difficult to diagnose PE because most patients are too unstable to undergo pulmonary angiography, the most sensitive test, and because the V/Q scan is reported only in probabilities.

### 18. How accurate are V/Q scans?

The V/Q scan is less sensitive and specific, and requires some patient cooperation. Its probability score (high, intermediate, and low) is based on the presence of perfusion defects and the lack of ventilation defects. A high-probability scan correctly predicts the presence of PE in 86% of cases. However, PE is also present in 30–34% of cases with intermediate probability and 14–31%

of patients with low probability. The most reliable indication of a PE is a match between the probability of the V/Q scan and the probability of the clinical setting (history and physical findings). If the clinical setting and V/Q scan are highly probable for PE, the patient should be aggressively treated for PE. If the clinical probability of a PE does not match the V/Q scan results, the diagnosis of PE is correct in about 50% of cases.

**19. What therapies are available to treat DVT in critically ill patients?**

The goals of therapy for acute proximal DVT are to prevent propagation of the thrombus, to limit leg edema, and to reduce symptomatic recurrence of DVT or PE. Therapies to limit thrombus propagation include anticoagulation, thrombolytic therapy, and surgical embolectomy. An infusion of weight-adjusted unfractionated heparin or LMWH is started immediately and continued until warfarin therapy has increased the international normalized ratio (INR) to 2–3 (usually 5 days). Leg elevation and bedrest are recommended to decrease edema and leg pain. Continued anticoagulation and inferior vena caval (IVC) interruption (e.g., IVC filter) are used to prevent recurrence of thromboembolism.

**20. What therapies are available to treat PE in critically ill patients?**

The goals of therapy for patients with PE are hemodynamic stability, oxygenation, and prevention of recurrent PE. Therapies include anticoagulation, thrombolytic therapy, surgical or catheter embolectomy, oxygen, intubation and mechanical ventilation if needed, vasoactive medications, and consideration of vena caval interruption.

**21. Is the INR or prothrombin time (PT) more accurate in determining therapeutic range for oral anticoagulation therapy?**

The INR is a more sensitive and consistent representation of coagulation status. PT measures the effects of oral anticoagulants on the blood's ability to clot. When a blood sample is drawn for PT, the laboratory personnel add a specific amount of calcium to the blood, spin the blood down, and then add a thromboplastin reagent to the serum. Because thromboplastin reagents vary widely from manufacturer to manufacturer, an international sensitivity index (ISI) has been developed for each reagent. The laboratory compares the PT time to the ISI for the specific reagent and reports the results as an INR. The INR is relatively consistent between laboratories and allows the same patient's blood to be tested at more than one laboratory. New point-of-care testing machines are programmed with the ISI score of the reagent and automatically calculate the INR for each test.

**22. Why do some patients require a higher dose of heparin to reach therapeutic range?**

The anticoagulation effect of heparin is affected by many factors. Heparin is a naturally occurring glycosaminoglycan, consisting of alternating residues of uronic acid and glucosamine that are variably sulfated. The sulfation of the residues is a major determinant of the anticoagulation activity of a given heparin preparation. Not all preparations have the same anticoagulant activity. Heparin catalyzes antithrombin III to inactivate prothrombin and activated factor X (fXa). In the presence of a large thrombus, more heparin may be needed to achieve effective anticoagulation (partial thromboplastin time 1.5 × normal) because of the large amount of thrombin in the clot. Body weight, hereditary resistance to anticoagulants, and amount of heparin binding to plasma and endothelial cell proteins also affect heparin dosing.

**23. What are some medications that interfere with the effectiveness of warfarin?**

*Commonly Used Medications that Influence the Anticoagulant Effect of Warfarin*

| INCREASE EFFECT | DECREASE EFFECT |
| --- | --- |
| Allopurinol | Barbiturates |
| Antibiotics | Carbamazepine |
| Amiodarone | Rifampin |
| Aspirin products | Antacids |

*Table continued on following page*

*Commonly Used Medications that Influence the Anticoagulant Effect of Warfarin (Continued)*

| INCREASE EFFECT | DECREASE EFFECT |
| --- | --- |
| Influenza virus vaccine | Sucralfate |
| Isoniazid | Colestipol |
| Phenytoin | Estrogens |
| Phenylbutazone | Adrenal corticosteroids |
| Thrombolytics | Spironolactone |
| Tolbutamide | Vitamin K |
| Vitamin E | |

### 24. What herbal remedies interfere with the effectiveness of warfarin?

Herbal remedies that have bioflavonoids may interfere with platelet aggregation and increase the patient's risk of bleeding. Examples include feverfew, gingko biloba, grape seed extract, bilberry, ginger, garlic, and nettle leaves. In one case report, ginseng may have increased the patient's hypercoagulability by decreasing the INR.

### 25. What medical conditions influence the effectiveness of warfarin

Patients with the following conditions are **more sensitive** to warfarin: cachexia, malabsorption syndromes, malnutrition, cancer, collagen diseases, congestive heart failure, diarrhea, fever, hepatic disorders, hyperthyroidism, pancreatic disorders, radiation therapy, renal insufficiency, thyrotoxicosis, and vitamin K deficiency.

Patients with the following conditions may require **higher doses** of warfarin to reach therapeutic levels: diabetes mellitus, edema, hereditary resistance to anticoagulants, hypercholesterolemia, hyperlipidemia, hypothyroidism, visceral carcinoma, excessive intake of vitamin K, and nephrotic syndrome.

### 26. What parameters should the nurse monitor to detect potential complications of anticoagulant therapy?

The most common complication of anticoagulation therapy is bleeding. The nurse should monitor and report bleeding from the gums, nose, urinary tract, invasive line sites, or surgical wounds as well as easy bruisability and prolonged menses. Pain and swelling in a joint can also be a sign of bleeding. Other parameters to measure include signs of recurrent thrombotic events, thrombocytopenia, and warfarin-induced tissue necrosis. Heparin causes a slight fall in platelet count in about 25% of people, with gradual recovery despite continuation of therapy.

### 27. What is heparin-induced thrombocytopenia (HIT)?

HIT occurs in about 3% of patients receiving heparin therapy. It is a serious immunoglobulin-mediated response to heparin that may cause life- and limb-threatening thrombotic complications. HIT usually occurs 5–8 days after heparin has been started. Although LMWH is significantly less likely to cause HIT, platelet count should be measured every 2–3 days during therapy.

### 28. What patients are candidates for thrombolytic therapy?

Catheter-directed thrombolytic therapy is presently indicated for patients with acute leg pain and edema (duration < 14 days) caused by an iliofemoral DVT. Others who may benefit include young patients with femoropopliteal vein thrombi, patients with phlegmasia cerulea dolens (venous gangrene), and patients with extensive superior vena caval, subclavian, or axillary vein thrombosis. Thrombolytic therapy should not be used for patients with a short life expectancy, low risk of ambulatory venous hypertension (inability to walk), coagulopathies, or contraindications to lytic therapy. Thrombolytic therapy also is indicated for patients with a massive PE causing right ventricular dysfunction.

### 29. What patients are candidates for an IVC filter?

The most common indications for IVC interruption are recurrent thromboembolism despite adequate anticoagulation, complications of anticoagulation (e.g., significant bleeding), and contraindications to anticoagulation. Less agreed upon indications are presence of a free-floating tail of an IVC or iliac vein thrombosis, thromboembolism in a pregnant woman with or without heparin therapy, and preparation for pulmonary embolectomy.

### 30. What special nursing considerations apply to patients with an intravenous filter?

Immediately after filter placement, patients should be monitored for signs and symptoms of air embolism, bleeding from the insertion site, signs of retroperitoneal bleeding from accidental perforation of the inferior vena cava, contrast dye-related renal failure, sepsis, and hemodynamic compromise from migration of the filter. Patients also must be monitored closely for recurrent DVT, because the presence of the filter increases the risk for DVT. Over time the filter may decrease venous return to the right side of the heart, causing edema below the level of the filter. As the filter fills with clot and debris, superficial veins of the abdomen dilate. Enlargement of superficial veins increases the risk that emboli may travel around the filter through the superficial veins and reach the lungs. Most patients with IVC filters are continued on anticoagulation therapy and must be monitored for all associated complications.

### 31. What is the role of LMWH in the prevention and treatment of DVT?

LMWH may replace unfractionated heparin as the anticoagulant of choice for both prevention and treatment of DVT. LMWH safely treats DVT in inpatient and outpatient settings. It has several advantages over unfractionated heparin, including a greater affinity for anti-factor Xa and a longer half-life. It is not affected by heparin-binding proteins in the blood. Because the effects of LMWH are highly predictable, it is dosed on a per kilogram schedule and does not need to be followed with blood tests for partial thromboplastin time.

### 32. What are the special nursing considerations in caring for patients with DVT or PE?

Patients with DVT or PE need detailed instructions about medical therapy, how to administer their medications, signs and symptoms of bleeding or rethrombosis, and the importance of regular follow-up and laboratory testing. They also need emotional support to cope with an acute illness that may have chronic sequelae. Patients usually are encouraged to shave with a safety or electric razor to prevent skin nicks. Dental care is important. Patients are encouraged to brush and floss gently to prevent bleeding. If gum disease is a problem, the patient is encouraged to discuss possible treatments with a dentist. During the acute phase of care, health care providers try to minimize the risk of bleeding by minimizing invasive procedures and monitoring the patient closely for signs of bleeding. Patients with a DVT are measured for knee or thigh-high graduated compression stockings before ambulation but after leg swelling has decreased. They also are encouraged to keep the affected extremity elevated as much as possible to reduce swelling. Warm moist compresses occasionally are used to increase comfort and reduce leg swelling. Care must be taken to prevent skin maceration due to moisture.

### BIBLIOGRAPHY

1. Bick RL, Haas SK: International consensus recommendations. Summary statement and additional suggested guidelines. Med Clin North Am 82:613–633, 1998.
2. Bick RL, Kaplan H: Syndromes of thrombosis and hypercoagulability: Congenital and acquired causes of thrombosis. Med Clin North Am 82:409–458, 1998.
3. Burroughs KE: New considerations in the diagnosis and therapy of deep vein thrombosis. South Med J 92:517–520, 1999.
4. Glisson J, Crawford R, Street S: Review, critique and guidelines for the use of herbs and homeopathy. Nurse Practitioner 24:44–67, 1999.
5. Heit JA, Silverstein MD, Mohr DN, et al: Predictors of survival after deep vein thrombosis and pulmonary embolism: A population-based, cohort study. Arch Intern Med 159:445– 453, 1999.
6. Kahn SR: The clinical diagnosis of deep venous thrombosis: Integrating incidence, risk factors, and symptoms and signs. Arch Intern Med 158:2315–2323, 1998.
7. McEvoy GK (ed): American Hospital Formulary Service Drug Information 1999. Bethesda, MD, American Society of Health-System Pharmacists, 1999, pp 1243–1265.

8. Mehra MR, Bode FR: Venous thrombosis and pulmonary embolism. In Civetta JM, Taylor RW, Kirby RR (eds): Critical Care, 3rd ed. Philadelphia, Lippincott-Raven, 1997, pp 1887–1903.
9. Payne J: Vascular trauma. In Fahey VA (ed) Vascular Nursing, 2nd ed. Philadelphia, W.B. Saunders, 1994, pp 536–557.
10. Pineo GF, Hull RD: Unfractionated and low-molecular weight heparin: Comparisons and current recommendations. Med Clin North Am 82:587–599, 1998.
11. Raphael MJ, Donaldson RM: The pulmonary circulation. In Sutton D (ed): Textbook of Radiology and Imaging, 6th ed. New York, Churchill Livingstone, 1998, pp 577–596.
12. Savage KJ, Wells PS, Schulz V, et al: Outpatient use of LMWH (Dalteparin) for treatment of deep vein thrombosis of the upper extremity. Thromb Haemost 82:1008–1010, 1999.

# 15. ACUTE MYOCARDIAL INFARCTION

Brigid Ide, MS, RN

## 1. Define acute coronary syndrome.

Acute coronary syndrome describes a dynamic spectrum of clinical conditions that begin with the rupture of an atherosclerotic plaque, platelet deposition, and thrombus formation. Arterial injury, extent and type of thrombus, and duration of ischemia determine the clinical presentation. These factors underlie the diagnosis of unstable angina, non–Q-wave, or Q-wave myocardial infarction.

## 2. What is the difference between non–Q-wave and Q-wave infarctions?

Development of a Q wave requires transmural death of the muscle, which permanently alters electrical conduction on the ECG. With subendocardial injury, electrical conduction is not permanently altered, and a Q wave does not develop; hence the term non–Q-wave infarct.

## 3. How are the acute coronary syndromes differentiated?

|  | UNSTABLE ANGINA | NON–Q-WAVE AMI | Q-WAVE AMI |
|---|---|---|---|
| Nonspecific ST segment changes or ST depression | Yes | Yes | Maybe |
| ST segment elevation | No | Maybe | Yes |
| Development of Q waves after infarction | No | No | Yes |
| Elevation of cardiac injury markers (CK-MB enzyme, troponin T or I) | No | Lower elevations | Higher elevations |
| LV function | Return to normal | Less damage | More damage |
| Complications | Few | Low | High |

AMI = acute myocardial infarction, CK-MB = creatine kinase, myocardial-bound; LV = left ventricular.

## 4. What are the diagnostic criteria for acute myocardial infarction (AMI)?

At least **two** of the following criteria must be present:
1. History of ischemic-type chest discomfort
2. Change on serial ECG tracings
    • ST-segment elevation of 0.1 mV in two or more contiguous leads
    • Presence of new left bundle-branch block
3. Rise and fall in serum markers of cardiac injury

**5. When do serum markers of cardiac injury begin to rise? When do they peak? For how long are they elevated?**

| SERUM MARKER | POSITIVE LEVEL | BEGINS TO RISE (HR) | PEAK (HR)* | DURATION (DAYS)* |
|---|---|---|---|---|
| CK-MB | 0–5 μg/L | 4–6 | 10–24 | 2–3 |
| Troponin T | 0.1–0.2 μg/L | 3–5 | 10–24 | 5–14 |
| Troponin I | 1.5–3.1 μg/L | 3–5 | 14–18 | 5–9 |
| Myoglobin | Serum levels double with q 2 hr serial samples | 2–3 | 3–15 | 0.5–1 |

CK-MB = creatine kinase, myocardial-bound.
* Lack of standardized upper reference levels account for variations in values.

**6. What are the current recommendations for emergency department (ED) treatment of patients with AMI?**
- Relief of pain
- Supplemental oxygen (keep oxygen saturation > 90%)
- Assessment of hemodynamic stability
- Assessment of ECG electrical stability
- Identification of reperfusion candidates and rapid delivery of therapy
- Intravenous (IV) thrombolytic therapy started within 30 minutes from arrival at ED
- Percutaneous transluminal coronary angioplasty (PTCA) started within 60 minutes from arrival at ED
- Administration of aspirin, beta blockers, and glycoprotein IIb/IIIa inhibitors (unless contraindicated)
- Administration of IV nitroglycerin in patients with congestive heart failure (CHF), hypertension, persistent pain, or large anterior infarction
- Additional drugs to treat arrhythmias and hypotension (if present)

**7. What early general measures are recommended for hospital care of patients with AMI?**
- Selective ECG monitoring based on infarct location and rhythm
- Relief of pain
- Bedrest with bedside commode for initial 12 hours, and longer if the patient is hemodynamically unstable or pain persists
- Identification and management of high-risk patients
- Pulmonary artery catheter for severe or progressive CHF, shock, hypotension, or suspected mechanical complication (e.g., ventricular septal defect [VSD], mitral regurgitation [MR])
- Intraarterial pressure monitoring for severe hypotension (systolic blood pressure < 80 mmHg) or cardiogenic shock
- Intraaortic balloon counterpulsation for cardiogenic shock refractory to pharmacologic therapy, MR, VSD, incessant ventricular tachycardia, or bridge to PTCA or coronary artery bypass grafting (CABG)
- Arrhythmia management

**8. What drugs may be used during hospital care of patients with AMI?**
1. Continue beta blockers, glycoprotein IIb/IIIa inhibitors, and aspirin.
2. Angiotensin-converting enzyme (ACE) inhibitors within the first 24 hours in selected patients and before discharge for all patients with AMI and left ventricular ejection fractions < 40%.
3. IV heparin for patients receiving tissue plasminogen activator (Alteplase).
4. Unfractionated heparin or low-molecular-weight heparin for patients not treated with thrombolytic therapy and patients with non–Q-wave MI.

### 9. How is the patient with AMI prepared for discharge?

- Exercise, vasodilator stress nuclear scintigraphy, or exercise echocardiography
- Invasive testing for patients with persistent pain or hemodynamic instability
- Management of lipids
- In-hospital cardiac rehabilitation

### 10. How are thrombolytic drugs best administered?

The primary intravenous thrombolytic agents are streptokinase (SK), tissue plasminogen activator (tPA), and anisoylated plasminogen streptokinase activator complex (APSAC). Thrombolytics are augmented by heparin and dosed as follows.

| DRUG | BOLUS | INFUSION | TIME | HEPARIN | INFUSION |
|------|-------|----------|------|---------|----------|
| SK | None | 1.5 million U | 60 min | 6 hr after SK/APSAC and when aPTT is < 2 times control or approximately 70 sec | 1000 U/hr for 48 hr |
| APSAC | 30 mg | | 5 min | As above | As above |
| tPA | 15 mg | 0.75 mg/kg up to 50 mg; then | 30 min | 60 U/kg bolus at start of tPA (maximal bolus of 4000 U) | 12 U/kg/hr |
| | | 0.5 mg/kg up to 35 mg | 60 min | | Maximum of 1000 U/hr |

SK = streptokinase, APSAC = anisoylated plasminogen streptokinase activator complex, tPA = tissue plasminogen activator, aPTT = activated partial thromboplastin time.

### 11. What are the most common complications of AMI? How are they identified?

| COMPLICATION | METHOD OF IDENTIFICATION |
|--------------|--------------------------|
| Postinfarction angina | Ongoing monitoring of ST segment of culprit lesion |
| Arrhythmias | Monitor in lead with diagnostic specificity:<br>• Leads $V_1$ and $V_6$ help to discriminate supraventricular from ventricular beats<br>• Lead II is useful in amplifying atrial contribution |
| Left ventricular failure (size and intensity of infarct are predictive of development of heart failure) | Monitor for early signs of heart failure:<br>• Increased heart rate • Rising BUN, creatinine<br>• Reduced blood pressure • Inappropriate response to<br>• Extra heart sounds (S3)   activity progression<br>• Shortness of breath • Intolerance of beta blockers,<br>• Decreased urine output   nitrates, or ACE inhibitors |
| Rupture of intraventricular septum (e.g., VSD) | Development of new holosystolic murmur at left sternal border<br>Pulmonary artery (PA) mixed venous saturation ($SvO_2$) is elevated by mixture of blood in left and right ventricles |
| Rupture of papillary muscle | Development of new holosystolic murmur starting at apex and radiating to axilla<br>No increase in $SvO_2$ |
| Pericarditis (inflammation of pericardial sac) | Monitor for localized chest pain (may be affected by position) and friction rub<br>Usually manifests 2–4 days after AMI |

BUN = blood urea nitrogen, ACE = angiotensin-converting enzyme, VSD = ventricular septal defect, IABP = intraaortic balloon pump.

### 12. What nursing interventions are appropriate for rupture of the intraventricular septum or papillary muscle?

- Prepare for measures to reduce left ventricular afterload and facilitate forward flow (e.g., intraaortic balloon pump, vasodilators, inotropic support).
- Prepare the patient for surgery.

### BIBLIOGRAPHY

1. American College of Cardiology/American Heart Association 1999 Update: Guidelines for the Management of Patients with Acute Myocardial Infarction: Executive Summary and Recommendations. http://www.americanheart.org/Scientific/statements/l999/hc3499.htr
2. Drew BJ, et al: Multilead ST-segment monitoring in patients with acute coronary syndromes: A consensus statement for healthcare professionals. Am J Crit Care 8:372–386, 1999.
3. Murphy M, Berding CB: Use of measurements of myoglobin and cardiac troponins in the diagnosis of acute myocardial infarction. Critical Care Nurse 19(1):58–66, 1999.

# 16. SHOCK

## Linda M. Couts, RN, MS, ACNP-CS, CEN, MICN

### 1. Define shock.

Shock is an acute clinical syndrome initiated by hypoperfusion (hypotension) and leading to inadequate tissue perfusion and altered cellular metabolism, which result in vital organ dysfunction.

### 2. What are the four classifications of shock? Give examples of each.

1. **Hypovolemic**
   - Hemorrhagic (trauma, gastrointestinal bleeding)
   - Nonhemorrhagic (vomiting, diarrhea, burns, polyuria, third spacing)
2. **Cardiogenic**
   - Myocardial (myocardial infarction or contusion, cardiomyopathy, medication)
   - Mechanical (valvular stenosis or regurgitation, wall defects)
   - Arrhythmias
3. **Obstructive**
   - Pulmonary embolism
   - Aortic dissection
   - Cardiac tamponade
   - Tension pneumothorax
   - Tumors
   - Sickle cell crisis
4. **Distributive**
   - Anaphylaxis
   - Sepsis
   - Spinal trauma
   - Toxic exposure
   - Pharmacology
   - Endocrine disorders

### 3. Is the pathophysiology of shock different for each classification?

No. The primary pathologic defect underlying all acute shock states, regardless of classification, is the same: a reduction of effective blood flow (hypoperfusion/hypotension) that leads to inadequate tissue perfusion and cellular injury or death. The classifications of shock represent various precipitating mechanisms that initiate the low-flow (hypoperfused) state.

### 4. How does hypoperfusion affect cellular metabolism?

In a state of hypoperfusion, the cell does not receive an adequate amount of oxygen. Lack of oxygen causes the cell to shift from aerobic to anaerobic glycolysis (glucose catabolism), resulting in an increase in lactate production and subsequent metabolic acidosis. Hypoperfusion also causes severe impairment of cellular glucose delivery and uptake. With diminishing glucose stores, the liver breaks down glycogen stores to form glucose through the process of glycogenolysis. It also synthesizes new glucose, using amino acids as substrates, through the process of gluconeogenesis. In addition, in a state of anaerobic metabolism, removal of toxic cellular waste products is impaired, further altering cellular metabolism and ultimately leading to cellular injury and/or death.

## 5. What mechanisms precipitate hypoperfusion?
- Decreased venous return to the heart (hypovolemic)
- Decreased ability of the heart to pump volume (cardiogenic)
- Decreased resistance of the vascular bed (distributive)
- Obstruction of circulating volume (obstructive)

## 6. What are the body's early compensatory responses to hypoperfusion?
The effects of hypotension, increasing acidosis, and hypoxemia initiate several of the body's compensatory mechanisms. One of the earliest compensatory responses during shock is activation of the sympathetic nervous system (SNS). Baroreceptors in the aorta and carotid sinus mediate the release of epinephrine and norepinephrine. Cardiac output is improved by increases in heart rate (reflex tachycardia) and systemic vascular resistance (SVR; increased venous tone and arteriole constriction). Activation of the renin-angiotensin system by renal juxtaglomerular cells releases the potent vasoconstrictor angiotensin II. The pituitary gland increases production of antidiuretic hormone, causing an additional increase in SVR and a decrease in urinary output. Respirations increase in an attempt to improve oxygenation and increase ventilation to compensate for metabolic acidosis. Blood is shunted from less critical organs (i.e., skin and intestine) to allow adequate perfusion of the brain and heart. In addition, fluid is shifted from interstitial and intracellular spaces into capillaries to increase circulating intravascular volume.

## 7. Describe the clinical presentation of early (compensated) hypovolemic shock.
Patients in early hypovolemic shock probably manifest the effects of large amounts of circulating catecholamines:
- Tachycardia (110–120 beats per minute[bpm])
- Rapid, shallow breathing
- Cold, pale, and moist skin
- Agitation and restlessness
- Decrease in urine output

Hypotension may not be apparent in early shock, with systolic blood pressure remaining the same or falling slightly. Diastolic pressure may increase (narrowing pulse pressure) secondary to vasoconstriction. A fall in systemic arterial blood pressure is a cardinal sign of progressing (uncompensated) shock.

## 8. What are the classes and clinical signs of hemorrhagic shock?

|                      | CLASS I             | CLASS II   | CLASS III | CLASS IV           |
|----------------------|---------------------|------------|-----------|--------------------|
| Blood loss (ml)      | Up to 750           | 750–1500   | 1500-2000 | > 2000             |
| % Blood volume       | Up to 15%           | 15–30%     | 30–40%    | ≥ 40%              |
| Heart rate (bpm)     | < 100               | 100–120    | 120–140   | >140               |
| Blood pressure       | Normal              | Normal     | Decreased | Decreased          |
| Pulse pressure       | Normal or increased | Decreased  | Decreased | Decreased          |
| Urine output (ml/hr) | > 30                | 20–30      | 5–15      | < 5                |
| Respirations (min)   | 14–20               | 20–30      | 30–40     | > 35               |
| Mental status        | Slightly anxious    | Mildly anxious | Confused | Confused/lethargic |
| Capillary refill     | < 2 sec             | > 2 sec    | > 2 sec   | No filling noted   |
| Skin                 | Cool/pink           | Cold/pale  | Cold/moist | Cyanotic/mottled  |

Adapted from Lanros NE, Barber JM: Shock states and fluid resuscitation. In Lanros NE, Barber JM (eds): Emergency Nursing with Certification Preparation and Review, 4th ed. Stamford, CT, Appleton & Lange, 1997, pp 139–148.

### 9. What are the immediate nursing priorities for a patient in clinical shock?

1. Assess the ABCs (airway, breathing, circulation).

2. Secure an airway, evaluate respiratory effort, and assist as needed. All patients in shock should receive supplemental oxygen.

3. Control any external hemorrhage and establish a minimum of two large-bore intravenous lines for crystalloid/colloid infusions.

4. Insert a Foley catheter to monitor urine output.

5. Obtain laboratory specimens for complete blood count, coagulation studies, type and cross-match, and serum electrolytes.

6. Attach a cardiac monitor, pulse oximeter, automated blood pressure cuff, and patient warming device.

7. Obtain a 12-lead electrocardiogram (ECG) and portable chest film.

8. Review the patient's history and physical exam, and attempt to identify the classification and source of shock.

### 10. Is there a quick bedside assessment technique to determine tissue perfusion status and classification of shock?

Evaluate skin signs. Feeling the skin of the extremities is a fast, helpful tool to assess whether the patient is compensating for early hypoperfusion. Recall that nonessential organs (i.e., skin) shunt blood to more critical organs as an early compensatory mechanism. Often, the first signs of early shock are changes in skin temperature and color. In addition, skin signs help to determine the classification of shock. Warm skin indicates distributive causes of shock, whereas cool skin probably indicates a hypovolemic or cardiogenic cause.

### 11. What type of fluid should you give to a patient in hypovolemic shock? How much?

The type and amount of fluid administered to a patient in shock remain controversial. Literature examining various fluids given in traumatic shock resuscitation has shown that no particular protocol reliably affects patient outcome. IV crystalloids (normal saline, lactated Ringer's solution) are favored by most authorities because of their ability to restore volume and improve microcirculation rapidly. Crystalloids should be given in a 3:1 ratio (300 ml for every 100 ml of fluid or blood loss). Keep in mind that crystalloids lack oncotic properties and produce only transient effects on circulating volume.

### 12. What role do colloids play in shock resuscitation?

Intravenous colloids (plasma proteins, synthetic or blood products) are commonly used after initial fluid resuscitation to sustain intravascular volume. Whole blood or packed red blood cells (PRBCs) are used to replace blood loss and to obtain an optimal hematocrit level (30–48%). Type O-negative PRBCs may be administered if type-specific blood cannot be obtained immediately.

### 13. What is the role of pharmacologic support in shock resuscitation?

Sympathomimetic agents such as dopamine, dobutamine, and norepinephrine are often first-line drugs. They improve perfusion by increasing mean arterial pressure (MAP) and cardiac output. Inotropic agents that increase myocardial contractility may be required to support tissue perfusion, particularly in cardiogenic, obstructive, and distributive shock states. They are rarely used in hypovolemic shock unless the patient responds poorly to crystalloid and/or colloid infusions.

### 14. What is the best position for a patient in shock?

Modified Trendelenburg position (keep the patient's head flat while raising the legs above the level of the heart). Recent literature reports that the head-down (full Trendelenburg) position does not significantly redistribute blood volume centrally.

**15. What are the normal hemodynamic values of cardiac output (CO), systemic vascular resistance (SVR), and central venous pressure (CVP)?**
- CO (heart rate × stroke volume) = 4–6 L/min
- SVR (MAP – CVP divided by CO × 80) = 900–1400 dynes/sec/cm
- CVP = 2–6 mmHg

**16. What hemodynamic patterns are commonly seen in the various classifications of shock?**

|                    | CO        | SVR       | CVP                 |
|--------------------|-----------|-----------|---------------------|
| Hypovolemic shock  | Decreased | Increased | Decreased           |
| Cardiogenic shock  | Decreased | Increased | Normal or increased |
| Obstructive shock  | Decreased | Increased | Normal or increased |
| Distributive shock | Increased | Decreased | Normal or decreased |

### BIBLIOGRAPHY

1. Alspach JG: Shock. In Alspach JG (ed): American Association of Critical-Care Nurses Core Curriculum for Critical Care Nursing, 5th ed. Philadelphia, W.B. Saunders, 1998, pp 323–329.
2. Brar RS, Hullenberg SM: Administering fluid resuscitation effectively for trauma shock. J Crit Ill 11:672–683, 1996.
3. Jimenez EJ: Shock. In Civetta JM, Taylor RW, Kirby RR (eds): Critical Care, 3rd ed. Philadelphia, Lippincott-Raven, 1997, pp 359–383.
4. Kline JA: Shock. In Rosen P (ed): Emergency Medicine: Concepts and Clinical Practice, 4th ed. St. Louis, Mosby, 1998, pp 86–103.
5. Lanros NE, Barber JM: Shock states and fluid resuscitation. In Lanros NE, Barber JM (eds): Emergency Nursing with Certification Preparation and Review, 4th ed. Stamford, CT, Appleton & Lange, 1997, pp 139–148.
6. Rauen CA, Munro N: Shock. In Rodgers-Kinney M et al (eds): AACN's Clinical Reference for Critical Care Nursing, 4th ed. St. Louis, Mosby, 1998, pp 1151–1177.
7. Schwartz GR: Shock: Clinical treatment. In Schwartz GR (ed): Principles and Practice of Emergency Medicine, 4th ed. Baltimore, Williams & Wilkins, 1999, pp 37–45.
8. Tierney L: Hypotension and shock. In Tierney L, et al. (eds): Current Medical Diagnosis and Treatment, 38th ed. Stamford, CT, Appleton & Lange, 1999, pp 481–484.
9. Toto KH: Fluid balance assessment: The total perspective. Crit Care Nurs Clin North Am 10:383–388, 1998.
10. Weil MH, Rackow EC: Shock. In Schwartz GR (ed): Principles and Practice of Emergency Medicine, 4th ed. Baltimore, Williams &Wilkins, 1999, pp 36–37.

# 17. VASOACTIVE DRUGS

*Steven R. Kayser, Pharm D, and Hildy Schell, RN, MS, CCRN*

**1. Define inotropy, chronotropy, and dromotropy.**
**Inotropy** refers to the contractility of the cardiac muscle.
**Chronotropy** refers to the heart rate.
**Dromotropy** refers to the automaticity of the cardiac conduction system.

**2. What do "positive" and "negative" mean when applied to inotropy, chronotropy, and dromotropy?**

Positive refers to an increase and negative to a decrease. For example, dobutamine is a positive inotrope because it increases cardiac contractility and therefore cardiac output. Esmolol is a negative chronotrope because it decreases heart rate.

### 3. Where are the adrenergic receptors? How do they respond to stimulation?

| RECEPTOR | LOCATION | PHYSIOLOGIC RESPONSE TO STIMULATION |
|---|---|---|
| Alpha ($\alpha$) receptors | Blood vessels | Vasoconstriction ($\uparrow$ BP, $\uparrow$ SVR, $\uparrow$ PVR) (of pupil) |
| Beta$_1$ ($\beta_1$) receptors | Heart (sinoatrial node, myocardium) | $\uparrow$ HR (positive chronotropy) $\uparrow$ Contractility (positive inotropy) $\uparrow$ Automaticity (positive dromotropy) $\uparrow$ Cardiac conduction velocity |
| Beta$_2$ ($\beta_2$) receptors | Blood vessels, bronchioles | Vasodilation ($\downarrow$ BP, $\downarrow$ SVR, $\downarrow$ PVR) Bronchodilation |
| Dopaminergic receptors | Blood vessels (renal, splanchnic, and mesenteric) | Vasodilation |

$\uparrow$ = increase, $\downarrow$ = decrease, BP = blood pressure, SVR = systemic vascular resistance, PVR = pulmonary vascular resistance, HR = heart rate.

### 4. What are the hemodynamic effects of commonly used vasoactive medications?

| MEDICATION | HR | BP | CO | SVR/ PVR | RA/ PCWP | USUAL DOSE* | CLASS OF DRUG |
|---|---|---|---|---|---|---|---|
| Dopamine | | | | | | | |
|   Low dose | $\uparrow$ | 0/$\downarrow$ | 0/$\downarrow$ | 0/$\downarrow$ | 0/$\downarrow$ | 0–2 µg/kg/min | Catecholamine |
|   Medium dose | $\uparrow\uparrow$ | $\uparrow$ | $\uparrow\uparrow$ | $\uparrow$ | $\uparrow$ | 2–5 µg/kg/min | (dopamine $\beta$, |
|   High dose | $\uparrow\uparrow\uparrow$ | $\uparrow\uparrow\uparrow$ | $\downarrow$ | $\uparrow\uparrow$ | $\uparrow\uparrow\uparrow$ | 5–20 µg/kg/min | dopamine $\alpha$) |
| Dobutamine | $\uparrow$ | $\uparrow\uparrow$ | $\uparrow\uparrow\uparrow$ | $\downarrow$ | $\downarrow$ | 2–20 µg/kg/min | Catecholamine ($\beta$1) |
| Milrinone | $\uparrow$ | $\uparrow\uparrow$ | $\uparrow\uparrow\uparrow$ | $\downarrow\downarrow$ | $\downarrow\downarrow$ | 50 µg/kg load 0.1–0.75 µg/kg/min | Phosphodiesterase inhibitor |
| Norepinephrine | $\uparrow\uparrow$ | $\uparrow\uparrow$ | $\downarrow$ | $\uparrow\uparrow$ | $\uparrow\uparrow$ | 1–80 µg/min | Catecholamine ($\beta$, $\alpha$) |
| Phenylephrine | 0 | $\uparrow\uparrow$ | $\downarrow$ | $\uparrow\uparrow$ | $\uparrow\uparrow$ | 1–200 µg/min | Catecholamine ($\alpha$) |
| Epinephrine | $\uparrow\uparrow$ | $\uparrow\uparrow$ | $\uparrow\downarrow$ | $\uparrow\uparrow$ | $\uparrow\downarrow$ | 1–30 µg/min | Catecholamine ($\beta$, $\alpha$) |
| Isoproterenol | $\uparrow\uparrow$ | $\downarrow\uparrow$ | $\uparrow\downarrow$ | $\downarrow\downarrow$ | $\downarrow$ | 1–4 µg/min | Catecholamine ($\beta$) |
| Nitroglycerin | $\uparrow$ | $\downarrow\downarrow$ | $\downarrow\downarrow$ | $\downarrow$ | $\downarrow\downarrow$ | 10–200 µg/min | Organic nitrate $\rightarrow$ nitric oxide |
| Nitroprusside | $\uparrow$ | $\downarrow\downarrow$ | $\downarrow\downarrow$ | $\downarrow\downarrow\downarrow$ | $\downarrow\downarrow$ | 0.1–10 µg/kg/min | Prodrug generates nitric oxide |
| Fenoldopam | 0 | $\downarrow$ | $\downarrow$ | $\downarrow$ | $\downarrow$ | 0.01–1.6 µg/kg/min | Dopamine agonist |

$\uparrow$ = increase, $\downarrow$ = decrease, HR = heart rate, BP = blood pressure, CO = cardiac output, SVR = systemic vascular resistance, PVR = pulmonary vascular resistance, RA = right atrial, PCWP = pulmonary capillary wedge pressure.

* Usual dose ranges may be influenced by factors such as other medications, disease states, and mechanical ventilation. They are intended as guidelines and cannot replace individual clinician's judgment.

### 5. Do all patients receiving vasoactive drugs require invasive hemodynamic monitoring?

The answer depends on the type of drug administered and its clinical effects, the desired clinical endpoints, and the clinical stability of the patient. Invasive monitoring of arterial blood pressure (ABP) should be used for patients with shock or hemodynamic instability who are receiving drugs that are titrated according to ABP or mean arterial pressure (MAP) parameters.

ABP monitoring provides continuous assessment data, which are essential when drugs with vasodilatory properties, such as nitroprusside or esmolol, are administered and titrated.

### 6. When should a pulmonary artery catheter be used?

A pulmonary artery catheter (PAC) provides assessment data about cardiac filling pressures (central venous pressure and pulmonary capillary wedge pressure), pulmonary artery pressures, cardiac output, and venous oxygen saturation ($SvO_2$). Indications for PAC use are highly controversial. The PAC provides clinical endpoint data, such as cardiac output measurements, which are crucial for titrating inotropic drugs, and calculations of systemic and pulmonary vascular resistance, which are crucial for titrating systemic or pulmonary vasodilatory drugs. But the reliability of hemodynamic monitoring depends on the patient's condition, supplies and equipment, and the clinician's technical skill. In addition, hemodynamic monitoring data should be evaluated in conjunction with other clinical assessment data (e.g., mental status, urine output, skin perfusion) before diagnosis and treatment.

### 7. Describe the dose-related pharmacologic and hemodynamic effects of dopamine.

Dopamine acts via several different mechanisms and on several different receptors in the body. Pharmacologically it acts as a precursor to norepinephrine and displaces norepinephrine from storage binding sites in the nervous system. Low doses (0.5–2.0 µg/kg/min) stimulate dopamine receptors in selective vascular beds (renal, splanchnic, and mesenteric); moderate doses (2.0–5.0 µg/kg/min) stimulate β-adrenergic receptors; and higher doses (> 5.0 µg/kg/min) stimulate α-adrenergic receptors.

### 8. Are the dose-related effects of dopamine predictable and reliable? Explain.

No. The hemodynamic effects depend not only on the dose but also on the underlying basal sympathetic tone. Because many critically ill patients have higher-than-normal baseline levels of catecholamines, the administration of even low doses of dopamine may result in unpredictable hemodynamic effects, many of which would be anticipated only with higher doses. For example, a critically ill patient receiving 1.0–2.0 µg/kg/min of dopamine (which is not expected to increase heart rate) may develop tachycardia because even a low dose of dopamine results in increased catecholamines and thus increased heart rate. The most important point is that the dose in actual numbers is of relative importance; it is more important to recognize that the observed pharmacologic effect may be due to the drug and that the dose needs to be adjusted to achieve desired hemodynamic endpoints.

### 9. What are the major differences between dopamine and dobutamine?

Whereas dopamine may influence multiple receptors (as described above), dobutamine stimulates predominantly $\beta_1$-adrenergic receptors in the heart and results in a positive inotropic (contractile) effect with minimal chronotropic (heart rate) effect. Dobutamine reportedly stimulates both peripheral α-adrenergic and peripheral $\beta_2$-adrenergic receptors, but this observation is of little clinical relevance because it results in a neutral hemodynamic effect. Both drugs may increase blood pressure, dobutamine by increasing cardiac output (CO) and dopamine by potentially increasing both CO and systemic vascular resistance (SVR).

### 10. How do dobutamine and dopamine affect renal perfusion?

Dopamine in low doses may increase renal perfusion by stimulating dopaminergic receptors in the renal vascular bed as well as by increasing CO; dobutamine may increase renal perfusion and subsequently urine output by increasing CO.

### 11. How do you choose between dopamine and dobutamine?

The selection of dopamine or dobutamine must be individualized, taking into account the goal of therapy as well as the patient's underlying condition. It is important to establish the underlying cause of the hypotension because the use of the wrong drug may worsen the clinical situation. For example, if a patient is admitted with hypotension associated with chronic congestive heart failure, probably CO is depressed and SVR increased; therefore, dobutamine is the appropriate choice.

Dopamine is not appropriate because it may increase SVR, leading to further compromise in CO as well as a potential increase in pulmonary vascular resistance. If the hypotension is associated with inadequate CO and SVR, dopamine is the better choice. Both drugs may increase heart rate, but dopamine generally increases it to a greater degree. Both drugs increase the likelihood of cardiac arrhythmias because an increased myocardial energy expense is associated with increases in CO.

**12. What is the rationale for the combined use of dobutamine and dopamine?**

Low-dose dopamine (0.5–2.0 µg/kg/min) is used most commonly to increase renal perfusion and urine output by selectively stimulating the dopamine receptors in the kidney. In patients with inadequate CO, dobutamine is the preferred agent. Because most patients with congestive heart failure fall into both categories, the combination is often used in an effort to maximize response. Studies comparing the combination of low-dose dopamine plus dobutamine to dobutamine alone have not been performed. If an adequate increase in renal perfusion or urine output is not achieved with dobutamine alone, the combination may be used. Although 1.0–2.0 µg/kg/min of dopamine is considered a low dose, the pharmacologic and hemodynamic effects may be exaggerated in some patients. The initial dose of dopamine should be in the range of 0.5 µg/kg/min, followed by titration if the desired clinical effect is not achieved.

**13. What is the role of epinephrine in the management of shock or other cardiovascular states?**

Epinephrine stimulates both $\alpha$- and $\beta$-adrenergic receptors. At low doses the $\beta$-adrenergic effect—increased heart rate and contractility and vasodilation—predominates. Some authors view epinephrine as superior to other catecholamines in the management of shock. Although it may be of value in certain patients unresponsive to other agents, superiority has yet to be established. In addition, epinephrine may be associated with potentially worrisome side effects, including increases in systemic and regional lactate accumulation, decrease in splanchnic blood flow, hypokalemia, and hyperglycemia. At present, dopamine and norepinephrine remain the catecholamines of choice for hypotension associated with septic shock; epinephrine should be reserved for patients with refractory hypotension. Low-dose epinephrine (0.030 µg/kg/min) has been compared with dobutamine (5 µg/kg/min) for patients recovering from cardiac surgery and reportedly increases cardiac index to the same extent as dobutamine but with less tachycardia.

**14. Does Levophed really "leave-em dead"?**

According to an old critical care belief, patients who take Levophed most likely will not survive. This belief comes from the traditional practice of reserving Levophed as a last resort for severely hypotensive, critically ill patients with predictably poor prognoses. Levophed, also known as norepinephrine, is a synthetic precursor of epinephrine. It has significant alpha- and beta$_1$-adrenergic effects and weak beta$_2$ effects. The alpha effects of norepinephrine lead to marked vasoconstriction of the systemic, pulmonary, renal, and splanchnic circulations. Studies have shown that norepinephrine increases MAP in patients with hypotension refractory to fluids and dopamine. Early use of norepinephrine in doses of 0.01–3 µg/kg/min is recommended in patients with septic shock after sufficient fluid resuscitation.

Contractility is increased but may not manifest as an increased CO if the elevated SVR (afterload) is too great. Caution should be taken when norepinephrine is used in patients with altered renal or GI perfusion and myocardial ischemia. Side effects include tachycardia, arrhythmias, and altered organ function or tissue necrosis related to decreased perfusion.

**15. What are the side effects of nitroprusside?**

Nitroprusside is a balanced vasodilator that reduces venous as well as arterial vascular tone. The resultant hemodynamic effect is a reduction in filling pressures as well as a decrease in pulmonary and systemic resistance. The vasodilation of the pulmonary vascular bed can be significant enough to cause intrapulmonary shunt because of increased blood flow to alveoli that are partially or completely collapsed or fluid-filled. The intrapulmonary shunt manifests as hypoxemia and/or an increase in the alveolar-arterial oxygen gradient. Nitroprusside is useful in treating hypertension as well as congestive heart failure. The dose range for nitroprusside is wide.

Few patients require doses > 1–2 µg/kg/min; however, doses up to 10 µg/kg/min have been administered for short periods.

### 16. Why is prolonged treatment with nitroprusside a major concern?

Concern about prolonged use of nitroprusside centers on its metabolic breakdown products, which can result in significant morbidity and even death. Nitroprusside is broken down into cyanide and subsequently converted to thiocyanate by the liver. Cyanide accumulation occurs most commonly in patients with abnormal liver function, usually associated with decreased hepatic perfusion. Conversion of cyanide to thiocyanate occurs in the liver via the enzyme rhodanase. Thiocyanate is removed via the kidney.

### 17. What are the symptoms of cyanide accumulation?

Symptoms of cyanide accumulation and toxicity include unexplained metabolic acidosis, hypoxemia, coma, absent reflexes, widely dilated pupils, shallow breathing and pink skin color. A sudden loss of response (tachyphylaxis) to the hemodynamic effects despite an increase in the dose may be a harbinger of impending cyanide intoxication. This effect rarely occurs with short-term administration (< 2–3 days).

### 18. What are the symptoms of thiocyanate toxicity?

Symptoms of thiocyanate toxicity include nausea, vomiting, diarrhea, arthralgias, muscle cramps and twitching, irritability, blurred vision, and psychosis. It usually takes at least several days for thiocyanate to accumulate in patients with renal compromise. It can be removed by dialysis.

### 19. How should patients receiving nitroprusside be monitored?

Patients should be monitored closely for signs and symptoms of toxicity while receiving nitroprusside. Routine thiocyanate or cyanide levels are not necessary but should be obtained if unexplained side effects occur. Serum thiocyanate levels < 10 mg/dl (100 mg/L) are rarely associated with serious toxicity. One practical problem is that many critically ill patients have similar symptoms as the side effects of the drug (e.g., altered mental status, hypoxemia). Efforts to prevent cyanide accumulation with the administration of hydroxocobalamin are impractical. Close clinical observation and prompt recognition of adverse effects are of key importance.

### 20. What is the role of nitroglycerin in critical care?

Nitroglycerin is a useful drug in the management of myocardial ischemia, pulmonary edema, or increased filling pressures, as in congestive heart failure. It also has been used postoperatively to reduce blood pressure. Nitroglycerin exerts its pharmacologic action by promoting release of nitric oxide from vascular endothelium. It decreases venous tone, resulting in increased vascular capacitance, reduced venous return, decreased filling pressures, and a subsequent reduction in stroke volume. For patients with normal cardiac output these effects may be well tolerated, but in patients with decreased contractile function cardiac output may be reduced. There also may be an increase in heart rate, which could worsen underlying ischemia. For these reasons, nitroglycerin is not the preferable drug to use if blood pressure reduction is the goal.

### 21. How is nitroglycerin administered?

Intravenous nitroglycerin can be titrated rapidly because it has a fast onset and a half-life of approximately 5 minutes. Common dosing regimens start at 10 µg/min and are titrated upward by 10 µg/min every 10 minutes.

### 22. How and when does tolerance to nitroglycerin develop?

Prolonged (> 24 hour) continuous administration of nitroglycerin may result in tolerance to its hemodynamic effect. The mechanism for the development of tolerance is not clearly known but may involve one or more of the following: decrease in available receptors, decrease in production of cyclic guanosine monophosphate secondary to a decrease in the activity of guanylate cyclase, depletion of sulfhydryl groups at the level of the nitrate receptor, and counterregulatory vasoconstrictor mechanisms such as increased sympathetic activation and stimulation of the renin-angiotensin-aldosterone system.

The actual rate at which patients develop tolerance is variable; therefore, patients should be observed for the loss of the hemodynamic response. Most patients should respond to doses in the range of 10–200 µg/min. If patients require a larger dose, they most likely are tolerant.

### 23. How can tolerance be prevented?

To avoid development of tolerance, patients should be converted to intermittent oral dosing as soon as possible. Tolerance develops with oral, transcutaneous, or other routes of administration unless there is a nitrate-free interval of at least 12 hours.

### 24. What are the maximal doses of vasoactive drugs?

The dose of the drug is not as important as its clinical effect. Many vasoactive drugs are prescribed using weight-based dosages. The typical regimen consists of a starting dose, titration parameters, and possibly a maximal dose. Clinical responses to vasoactive medications vary tremendously.

### 25. Why is titration of vasoactive drugs described as both an art and a science?

Basic science includes knowledge about the actions of the drug, potential side effects and complications, and particular administration procedures. But nurses must have astute assessment skills to monitor accurately the clinical effects and potential complications. Experiential knowledge guides the nurse to increase or decrease the dose based on knowledge of the patient and ability to anticipate how the patient may respond. For example, the nurse may know that blood pressure will drop when dobutamine is started because (1) his or her assessment of the patient's hemodynamics and fluid status identifies fluid depletion; (2) the patient has mottled knees and her blood pressure dropped when 12.5 µg of fentanyl was given; and (3) the nurse has seen the same response in many similar patients.

### 26. What are the general recommendations for titration of vasoactive drugs?

1. Vasoactive drugs should be titrated to clinical endpoints (parameters) that are appropriate to the specific drug. Parameters for vasopressor drugs include blood pressure (MAP), signs of adequate tissue perfusion (urinary output, mental status, skin perfusion, $SvO_2$, lactate levels), and/or related hemodynamic data (CO, SVR, CVP, PCWP), if accessible.

2. Increase the dose until the clinical effect is achieved (usually effects are seen within minutes), and decrease the dose as tolerated.

3. Notify the physician of potentially serious side effects or complications, and titrate downward or discontinue the drug, if warranted. For example, the new onset of multifocal premature ventricular contractions or increased premature atrial contractions on ECG with an increase in the dose of dobutamine may be related to increased myocardial oxygen consumption, which is associated with dobutamine. The intervention may require decreasing the dose, discontinuing the drug, and/or changing to another inotropic drug to prevent myocardial ischemia and/or lethal arrhythmia. If increased or significant tachycardia occurs with initiation or increased titration of dopamine, another drug, such as phenylephrine may be considered to avoid tachycardia in specific at-risk patients.

### 27. What weight should be used in dosing vasoactive drugs?

The various weights used by clinicians to administer drugs with weight-based dosages are "dry weight", weight on admission, usual weight, actual body weight, ideal body weight, or a percentage of actual weight. Methods for determining these weights are not standardized in many ICUs and hospitals. "Dry weight" is used synonymously with both usual weight and weight on admission. Limited data support recommendations for which weight should be used for drug calculations and dosing. According to an informal survey of critical care nurses on a listserv, the weight used to calculate vasoactive drug dosages varies considerably. Many used weight on admission, which was referred to as "dry weight" by some responders. Most reported that they also titrated to clinical effect.

**28. What is the bottom line for calculating weight-based dosages?**

Again, the bottom line is that monitoring of related clinical endpoints and effects is more important than dose, weight- based or not. Empiric weight-based drug dosages are derived from pharmacologic data. The use of weight-based drug dosages without monitoring for clinical effect and adjusting appropriately becomes a particular concern in obese, fluid-overloaded, and critically ill patients. Critically ill patients often have elevated baseline levels of catecholamines.

**29. What is Flolan?**

Epoprostenol (Flolan), or prostacyclin ($PGI_2$), is a potent vasodilator and inhibitor of platelet function produced by the vascular endothelium. Its short half-life (3–5 minutes) requires continuous intravenous administration. It is eliminated by nonenzymatic hydrolysis and does not require dose adjustment for renal or hepatic disease.

**30. What are the indications for use of epoprostenol?**

The primary indication for epoprostenol is the long-term management of primary pulmonary hypertension (PPH). It is also used for short-term management of pulmonary hypertension in the postoperative setting. Epoprostenol has been shown to decrease symptoms, improve exercise tolerance, and prolong survival in patients with PPH.

**31. How is epoprostenol administered?**

Epoprostenol usually is initiated at 0.5–1.0 ng/kg/min and titrated to the desired hemodynamic effect or to a dose that is limited by adverse effects. The typical initial dose range for PPH management is 1–6 ng/kg/min. With prolonged therapy the dose must be increased frequently and may be as high as 50–70 ng/kg/min. Long-term administration is accomplished via a tunnelled or peripherally inserted central line.

**32. What are the side effects of epoprostenol?**

The most common side effects of epoprostenol are nausea, vomiting, headaches, flushing, abdominal discomfort, diarrhea, systemic hypotension, tachycardia, unusual jaw pain, chest pain, and generalized musculoskeletal pain.

**33. What is the role of phenylephrine in the management of critically ill patients?**

Phenylephrine (Neosynephrine) is a synthetic agent that acts as an alpha-adrenergic receptor agonist and produces arterial and venous vasoconstriction ($\uparrow$ SVR). It is easily titrated because of its rapid onset and short duration of action. It is used primarily to treat hypotension. It is also used to increase blood pressure, MAP, and cerebral perfusion pressure in neurologically injured patients. Usage guidelines are limited because few studies have evaluated the clinical use of phenylephrine. It is usually started at doses of 10–50 µg/min and titrated to the desired MAP or systolic blood pressure. Phenylephrine can cause bradycardia related to vagal stimulation as a compensatory response to rapid increase in blood pressure. The drop in HR is rarely seen with doses of 50–200 µg/min via continuous infusion. Studies have shown an increase in MAP, SVR, cardiac index, and stroke volume without significant increases or decreases in HR. Phenylephrine is attractive for use in critically ill patients because it does not increase heart rate and myocardial oxygen consumption like other vasopressors (e.g., dopamine, norepinephrine, epinephrine).

**34. What are amrinone and milrinone? What is their role in management of critically ill patients?**

Amrinone and milrinone are phosphodiesterase inhibitors that block the breakdown of cyclic adenosine monophosphate (cAMP). Thus, the mechanism by which cardiac contractility is increased does not require binding to beta-adrenergic receptors. Amrinone and milrinone are alternatives to agents such as dobutamine in patients with congestive heart failure, in whom beta-receptors may be downregulated. In addition to their positive inotropic effect, both agents cause some degree of systemic and pulmonary vasodilation.

## 35. Which is preferred—amrinone or milrinone? Why?

Amrinone and milrinone are closely related both structurally and hemodynamically, but milrinone has replaced amrinone in most centers because it is associated with a lower incidence of thrombocytopenia, a troublesome side effect of amrinone.

## 36. How is milrinone administered?

Milrinone may be administered with a loading dose of 50 μg/kg, but it is rarely indicated and may result in hypotension in some patients. It can be titrated relatively rapidly when administered in the usual continuous intravenous dose of 0.25–0.75 μg/kg/min. Milrinone has a half-life of 1–2 hours and is eliminated primarily by the kidneys. Dose adjustment may be necessary for patients with renal insufficiency. Because no specific guidelines for dose adjustment in renal insufficiency are available, close hemodynamic observation is recommended.

## 37. Why are two positive inotropes, milrinone and dobutamine, used together?

Although this combination is rarely used, the underlying rationale is that they act by two different mechanisms to increase the intracellular concentration of cAMP. As discussed above, dobutamine binds to beta-adrenergic receptors to increase cAMP, whereas milrinone inhibits the breakdown of cAMP via inhibition of phosphodiesterase. Experience has shown an additive hemodynamic effect with the concomitant administration of amrinone and dobutamine as well as milrinone and dobutamine. Patients should be monitored closely for adverse effects such as ventricular arrhythmias as well as an exaggerated hemodynamic response. Other combinations of catecholamines and inotropes have been used, although few head-to-head comparisons are available. The use of combinations should be guided by a familiarity with their receptor pharmacology, anticipated hemodynamic endpoints, and underlying disease physiology.

## BIBLIOGRAPHY

1. Barst RJ, et al: A comparison of continuous intravenous epoprostenol with conventional therapy for primary pulmonary hypertension. N Engl J Med 334:296–301, 1996.
2. Duranteau J, et al: Effects of epinephrine, norepinephrine, or the combination of norepinephrine and dobutamine in gastric mucosa in septic shock. Crit Care Med 27:893–900, 1999.
3. Elkayam U: Tolerance to organic nitrates: Evidence, mechanisms, clinical relevance, and strategies for prevention. Ann Intern Med 114:667–677, 1991.
4. Gage J, et al: Additive effects of dobutamine and amrinone on myocardial contractility and ventricular performance in patients with severe heart failure. Circulation 74:367–373, 1986.
5. Hollenberg SM, et al: Cardiogenic shock. Ann Intern Med 131:47–59, 1999.
6. Marik P, Varon J: The obese patient in the ICU. Chest 113:492–498, 1998.
7. Martin C, et al: Effects of norepinephrine plus dobutamine or norepinephrine alone on left ventricular performance of septic shock patients. Crit Care Med 27:1708–1713, 1999.
8. McLaughlin VV, et al: Reduction in pulmonary vascular resistance with long-term epoprostenol therapy in primary pulmonary hypertension. N Engl J Med 338:273–277, 1998.
9. Moran JL, et al: Epinephrine as an inotropic agent in septic shock: A dose-profile analysis. Crit Care Med 21:70–77, 1993.
10. Prielipp RC, Butterworth J: Cardiovascular failure and pharmacologic support after cardiac surgery. New Horizons 7:472–488, 1999.
11. Rudis MI, e tal: Is it time to reposition vasopressors and inotropes in sepsis? Crit Care Med 24:525–537, 1996.
12. Rutherford JD: Nitrate tolerance in angina therapy. How to avoid it. Drugs 49:196–199, 1995.
13. Schultz V: Clinical pharmacokinetics of nitroprusside, cyanide, thiosulfate, and thiocyanate. Clin Pharmacokinet 9:239–251, 1984.
14. Task Force of the American College of Critical Care Medicine, Society of Critical Care Medicine: Practice parameters for hemodynamic support of sepsis in adult patients. Crit Care Med 27:639–660, 1999.
15. Tisdale JE, et al: Proarrhythmic effects of intravenous vasopressors. Ann Pharmacother 29:269–281, 1995.
16. Uretsky BF, et al: Combined therapy with dobutamine and amrinone in severe heart failure. Improved hemodynamics and increased activation of the renin-angiotensin-aldosterone system with combined intravenous therapy. Chest 92:657–662, 1987.
17. Veseg CJ, et al: Blood cyanide and thiocyanate concentrations produced by long-term therapy with sodium nitroprusside. Br J Anesth 57:148–155, 1985.

# 18. CENTRAL VENOUS CATHETERS

*Charlene Trouillot, RN, ANP*

### 1. What is a central line?

A central line, commonly called a vascular access device (VAD) or central venous catheter (CVC), is a temporary or long-term intravenous catheter inserted into one of the major veins of the neck, chest, or groin (subclavian vein, superior vena cava, internal or external jugular vein, femoral vein) or peripherally through the brachial or cephalic vein. The distal tip of a central line is located in the superior vena cava (SVC), just above the right atrium. The tip of a pulmonary artery catheter lies in the pulmonary artery. The tip of catheters in the femoral venous system lies in the proximal inferior vena cava.

### 2. For what purposes are central lines used?

1. Administration of intravenous (IV) fluids, antibiotics, chemotherapy, blood products, total parenteral nutrition, and analgesics
2. Laboratory blood sampling, dialysis/pheresis, and continuous renal replacement therapies
3. Large-volume infusions (for bleeding, trauma, surgery, sepsis)
4. Hemodynamic monitoring

### 3. What are the acute and nonacute indications for insertion of a central line?

**Acute indications** in the intensive care unit include central venous or pulmonary capillary wedge pressure monitoring, cardiac output monitoring, rapid infusion of IV fluids or blood products, and/or administration of vasoactive drugs.

**Nonacute indications** include long-term IV medication administration and/or parenteral nutrition in patients with conditions such as human immunodeficiency virus (HIV), cancer, sickle cell disease, Crohn's disease, and osteomyelitis.

### 4. What are the advantages of a central line?

- The high blood flow of the vena cava promotes rapid dilution of IV fluids and concentrated solutions, thereby preventing an inflammatory response and the rapid thrombosis that occurs in smaller peripheral veins.
- A central line provides more stable access to the venous system, decreasing the risk of infiltration and tissue damage when irritating agents are administered.
- A central line provides the ability to infuse two or more incompatible solutions at the same time, through two or more separate lumens.
- CVCs may shorten hospital stays by providing access for therapy in an outpatient setting.
- Central venous access also may be used to overcome physical or psychological factors associated with repeated venipuncture.

### 5. List the different types of central lines.

| | |
|---|---|
| Nontunneled catheters | Peripherally inserted central catheters (PICCs) |
| Tunneled catheters | Implanted ports |

### 6. Which type is used most commonly? What are its major disadvantages?

Nontunneled catheters are the most commonly used central lines. They are available with 1–4 lumens and are inserted into the subclavian, internal jugular, or external jugular vein. The right internal jugular is preferred, because it is a straight line to the SVC. Nontunneled catheters may be changed over a guidewire. Disadvantages include risk for infection, daily flushing, routine sterile dressing changes, and restrictions on activities such as bathing.

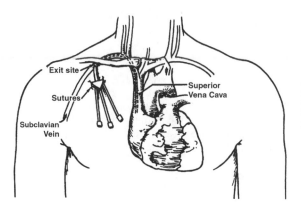

Nontunneled catheter. (Drawing by Mel Drisko; courtesy of Educational Support Services, University of Colorado Health Sciences Center.)

### 7. What optional features are available for nontunneled catheters?

Optional catheter features include heparin, antibiotic, or antiseptic coatings along the catheter. Some catheters have a Dacron and/or antimicrobial cuff that forms a barrier against the inward spread of microorganisms along the catheter wall from the incision.

### 8. When are tunneled catheters indicated? How are they inserted?

Tunneled catheters (Hickman, Broviac, Leonard, and Groshong) are indicated when long-term (several months and longer) therapy is expected. Single-, double-, and triple-lumen catheters are available. Each is placed in a central vein, then tunneled several centimeters under the skin to a suitable exit point and brought out through the skin. Common exit sites include the anterior chest between the sternum and nipple. The subcutaneous portion of the catheter tunneled under the skin has a Dacron cuff.

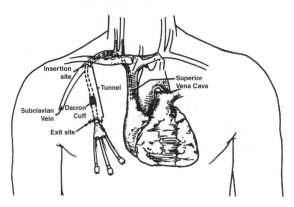

Tunneled catheter. (Drawing by Mel Drisko; courtesy of Educational Support Services, University of Colorado Health Sciences Center.)

### 9. What are the advantages and disadvantages of tunneled catheters?

The major advantage of tunneling the catheter is the lower risk of ascending infection compared with nontunneled catheters. Some catheters have a second antimicrobial cuff. Vita Cuff releases silver ions for 4–6 weeks, which deters infection and further spread of organisms along the tunnel. Disadvantages include site care with dressing changes for the first few weeks, activity restrictions, and regular flushing. Once the exit site of a tunneled catheter has healed (approximately 3–4 weeks), the sterile dressing change is modified to a clean technique, which decreases cost and time. Insertion costs are high, estimated at $2500 –3000, especially if anesthesia and the operating room are used. Most tunneled catheters, however, can be placed under fluoroscopy in the radiology department.

**10. When are PICCs indicated? What are their advantages and disadvantages?**

PICCs generally are indicated when therapy is expected to last for weeks to a few months. Insertion costs are lowest (about $300) of all CVCs. A trained nurse or physician easily inserts the PICC via the basilic or cephalic vein. Other advantages include reduced insertion risks (e.g., pneumothorax) and decreased rate of complications compared with other CVCs. Disadvantages include daily flushing (weekly for the Groshong PICC), sterile dressing changes, and activity restrictions. PICC placement requires adequate peripheral antecubital access, which may be difficult to locate in some patients. Self-care may be difficult or impossible since the patient is required to change the dressing and flush the catheter with one hand.

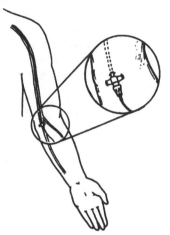

Peripherally inserted central catheters. (Drawing by Mel Drisko; courtesy of Educational Support Services, University of Colorado Health Sciences Center.)

**11. When are implanted ports indicated? How are they inserted?**

Implanted ports (Mediport, Portacath, Cathlink, Groshong, Infusaport) are made of stainless steel, titanium, or plastic. They are indicated for long-term use. Port implantation is usually done in the operating room or radiology suite at a cost similar to that for tunneled catheters. Single- or double-lumen and newer, low-profile ports (placed in the chest of a thin patient) are available. Ports are implanted entirely under the subcutaneous tissue and attached to a catheter, which is threaded into the SVC. Smaller ports also may be implanted peripherally in the forearm and the catheter threaded into the SVC, as with a PICC.

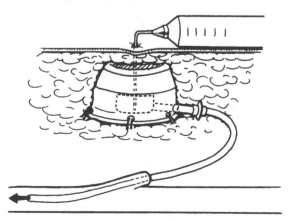

Implanted port. (Drawing by Mel Drisko; courtesy of Educational Support Services, University of Colorado Health Sciences Center.)

## 12.  What are the advantages and disadvantages of implanted ports?

Advantages of implanted ports include minimal site care (no dressing when not accessed) and infrequent flushing (generally once per month when not accessed), which may lead to decreased costs and decreased risk of infection. Other benefits may include an intact body image and unrestricted activity, because the port lies completely implanted under the subcutaneous tissue. Disadvantages include discomfort related to accessing the port with a needle puncture through the skin and the need for a surgical procedure to remove the port when it is no longer needed or becomes infected.

## 13.  How are Groshong catheters different from other catheters?

A Groshong tunneled catheter, Groshong PICC, or Groshong implanted port is a Silastic catheter with two-way, pressure-sensitive valves at the tip. Infusion of fluid opens the valve outward, and aspiration of blood opens the valve inward. When not in use, the two-way valve remains closed to prevent back flow of blood or air into the catheter lumen. Other catheters have a hole or holes at the tip of the lumen. The closed valve can potentially lower the incidence of fibrin sheath formation and eliminates the need to clamp the catheter when injection caps are removed. The distal port of the Groshong catheter can be transduced to monitor central venous pressures. The pressurized flush system keeps the two-way valve open.

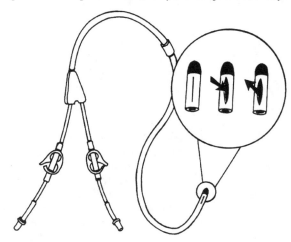

Groshong catheter and valves. (Drawing by Mel Drisko; courtesy of Educational Support Services, University of Colorado Health Sciences Center.)

## 14.  How is a central line selected?

Suggesting a specific type of central venous catheter falls within the domain of nursing care. The choice depends on many factors:
- Type of therapy or monitoring required
- Length of therapy
- Cost
- Benefits and risks related to the catheter and insertion procedure
- Capability of the patient caring for a central line at home (site care and flushing requirements)
- Patient preference (cosmetic appearance, concerns with activity or work limitations, anxiety associated with needle sticks)
- Treatment schedule (daily, intermittent, continuous)

## 15.  What risks are involved when a central line is placed?

The procedural risks of central line insertion include bleeding and hematoma, malpositioned tips and migration, pneumothorax, air embolus, nerve injury, and dysrhythmia. A pneumothorax may occur if the pleura is punctured by a needle on insertion. This complication can generally be avoided if a catheter is placed under fluoroscopy. Rare complications of PICC placement are nerve injury and arterial puncture, most commonly of the ulnar artery, which lies deep in the medial forearm.

### 16. What causes an air embolus? How can the risk be reduced?

An air embolus may be caused by either a catheter tip sheared off by a needle during advancement or by entry of air from the catheter. Entry of air is possible during initial placement, replacement over a guidewire, removal (air tracks along residual catheter track), or removal of injection cap. Risk of air embolus is greatly reduced with use of a Groshong catheter. During CVC insertion, patients should be positioned supine with the head of bed flat or in Trendelenburg position.

### 17. What are the signs and symptoms of an air embolus? How is it managed?

Signs and symptoms of air embolus include a drop in oxygen saturation, shortness of breath, agitation, and mental status changes. If air embolus is suspected, assist the patient into the Trendelenburg position, left side down; cover the CVC exit site with occlusive dressing; apply oxygen, if needed; and notify the physician.

### 18. How soon can a CVC be used after placement?

A central line may be used after fluoroscopy or radiography confirms its position. Implanted ports may be used immediately after placement—perhaps even accessed during surgery. Some surgeons may request that the port not be accessed until postoperative swelling has decreased.

### 19. How common are malpositioned catheter tips? What is the appropriate response?

Malpositioned tips are common and can be especially problematic with catheters placed at the bedside and PICCs (4–38%). Catheters can coil in the SVC or become malpositioned in the jugular vein when the basilic vein is accessed or in the axillary vein when the cephalic vein is accessed. In general, malpositioned catheters should be removed and replaced or repositioned under fluoroscopy.

### 20. What are the signs and symptoms of malpositioned tips?

| SITE OF MALPOSITIONED TIP | SYMPTOMS |
|---|---|
| Internal jugular vein (ipsilateral or contralateral) | Sensation of ear gurgling, headache, swelling, neck pain |
| Axillary vein | Hand and arm swelling, with arm and shoulder pain |
| Azygos vein | Vague back discomfort |
| Innominate or contralateral subclavian vein | Shoulder pain or swelling of contralateral arm |
| Internal thoracic vein | Anterior chest pain or tenderness |
| Right atrium or ventricle | Thrombosis, arrhythmia, or perforation, leading to pulmonary embolus |

### 21. Is bloody drainage at the insertion site of a newly placed central line a worrisome finding?

Not necessarily. It is common for blood to saturate the dressing of a new exit site. Patients with a low platelet count or prolonged bleeding times (e.g., prothrombin time, partial thromboplastin time) should be monitored closely for increased bleeding and hematoma formation. Bloody dressings should be changed frequently to prevent infection. Apply manual pressure, pressure dressing, or sandbag to prevent development of a hematoma.

### 22. What is considered routine care and maintenance of a central line?

Routine care includes cleansing the exit site, changing dressings and caps, and flushing the lumens to prevent clotting. Cleansing solutions, type of dressing, and frequency of dressing changes or flushing are controversial issues. Protocols vary from hospital to hospital.

*Common Maintenance Procedures*

| VAD | DRESSING | FLUSHING* | CAP CHANGE† | BLOOD WITHDRAWAL DISCARD (ml) |
|---|---|---|---|---|
| Central (subclavian) | Transparent dressing every 5–7 days; gauze dressing on alternate days or with catheter change | Heparin, 100 U/ml, 3 ml/day or 2ml/day for each lumen | Weekly | 1–2 |
| PICC lines | 24 hr after insertion, then transparent dressing every 5–7 days or gauze dressing on alternate days | Heparin, 100 U/ml, 3 ml/day or 10 U/ml, 3 ml 3 times/wk | Weekly | 1–2 |
| Tunneled | Transparent dressing every 5–7 days; gauze dressing on alternate days, then clean technique unless myelosuppressed | Heparin, 100 U/ml, 3 ml/day or every other day | Weekly | 3–5 |
| Implanted port | For continuous access, change noncoring needle and transparent dressing every week or gauze dressing on alternate days | Heparin, 100 U/ml 5 ml/month | Weekly | 5 |
| Groshong (Bard Access Systems, Salt Lake City) | Transparent dressing every 5–7 days; gauze dressing on alternate days, then clean technique unless myelosuppressed. | Normal saline, 5–10 ml weekly | Monthly | 3–5 |

\* Heparin solution may be 10 U/ml concentration.
† Change caps more frequently if damaged or used frequently.
From Oncology Nursing Society: Access Device Guidelines, with permission.

### 23. How should the exit site be cleaned?

Common features of all protocols include removal of the old dressing, inspection of the exit site for signs of infection, cleansing the skin, and covering with a dressing. Cleanse with friction, working outward in a circular pattern from the exit site. The 1996 Centers for Disease Control Guidelines make no recommendation for the use of nonsterile vs. sterile gloves during dressing changes. Tunneled catheters have two incisions that require care.

### 24. What solutions or agents are recommended for cleaning the exit site?

- Tincture of isopropyl alcohol (70%) removes skin oils and squamous skin cells that may harbor bacteria. It provides the most rapid and greatest reduction in microbial counts on the skin, but does not have any residual antimicrobial activity. Alcohol prep should be applied first, followed by iodine.
- Tincture of iodine (1–2%) or povidone-iodine (10%) should remain on the skin for at least 2 minutes to enhance antimicrobial activity while drying.
- Chlorhexidine has residual antibacterial activity for up to 6 hours but is not commercially available as single-use packets or swab sticks. In 1991 Maki and colleagues concluded that the use of 2% chlorhexidine for postinsertion site care demonstrated the lowest incidence of infection and bacteremia compared to alcohol and povidone-iodine.

The Centers for Disease Control and Prevention does not recommend routine use of topical ointments. Iodophor ointments have been shown ineffective. Polymicrobial ointments have some benefit but may increase the frequency of candidal growth and infection.

### 25. How often should dressings be changed?

Central line dressings should be changed according to hospital protocol and when the dressing is damp, loose, or soiled. Dressings minimize the build-up of skin microorganisms, provide protection against external contamination, and keep the exit site dry. Immunosuppressed or hospitalized patients should always have a dressing in place to prevent infection. Tunneled catheters do not require a dressing after the cuff has healed (approximately 2–3 weeks after insertion). Dressing changes may consist of either an occlusive, sterile gauze-and-tape covering or a transparent, semipermeable membrane. They should be nonirritating as well as easy to apply and remove and permit convenient examination of the site.

### 26. Is it better to cover the exit site with gauze and tape or a transparent dressing?

A **gauze-and-tape dressing**, in which the tape covers the entire gauze surface and secures all edges, may be preferred for diaphoretic or fragile skin. Because visualization of the site is obstructed, the dressing must be removed for inspection. Gauze-and-tape dressings do not provide a barrier for water and bacteria and have an increased potential for contamination.

Transparent semipermeable membrane dressings permit continuous inspection of the site, adhere well, provide protection against external moisture, and assist in stabilizing the catheter. One limitation of the transparent dressing is moisture retention beneath the dressing, which can significantly increase colonization of the site. Moisture-permeable transparent dressings have been developed to allow evaporation of moisture away from the site. They appear to reduce colonization under the dressing.

### 27. How are central lines flushed?

Heparinized saline, in concentrations of 10–10,000 U/ml, is used as flush solution for most catheters. Groshong catheters require only saline flush. The volume and dose of flush solutions and the frequency of flushing are debatable. Higher concentrations (1000-10,000 U/ml) are generally reserved for dialysis catheters. Frequency of flushing varies from once per week to twice per day. The Intravenous Nursing Society (INS) recommends that the flushing volume of heparinized saline be equal to two times the internal volume of the catheter. It is important to provide a positive-pressure flush to prevent fibrin sheath formation and blood back-up into the lumen. Removing blood from the injection hubs and stopcocks helps to prevent colonization and potential infection. CVCs are designed to withstand various infusion pressures, but the pressure should never exceed 25–40 pounds per square inch (PSI). Smaller sized syringes generate pressures in excess of this amount. Use a different syringe for flushing each lumen. Injection caps should be changed at least weekly, when they are removed for blood drawing, and more often if punctured frequently. Injection hubs are good for approximately 200 punctures.

### 28. Is saline as effective as heparin for routine flushing of unused lumens?

Studies report that use of 0.9% sodium chloride is as effective as heparin in preventing phlebitis and maintaining patency of peripheral catheters; however, it is not routine practice to use only saline for flushing CVCs. Although sodium chloride is cheaper than heparin and may cause less interference with lab tests, use of sodium chloride alone as a flush for central lines may increase the potential for occlusion, phlebitis, and the formation of small clots or fibrin strands. CVCs usually are flushed once daily with heparin and intermittently with normal saline (e.g., between antibiotics). Even low doses of heparin (200–250 U) may be associated with thrombocytopenia and bleeding problems. Low-dose warfarin (1 mg/day orally) may be used prophylactically to decrease the incidence of thrombus.

### 29. What is the proper procedure for drawing blood?

Approximately 5 ml of blood from adults or 3 ml from children is discarded before drawing the sample. There is no need to discard any blood drawn for cultures. All infusions should be stopped for 1 minute, and blood should be drawn through the most proximal lumen through the catheter end or injection hub. Pulling back slowly on the syringe helps to prevent catheter collapse. A Vacutainer or needleless system can be used to minimize risk of a needle stick. Flush with 10–20 ml (20 ml for Groshong catheter) of normal saline after blood withdrawal. It is important to consider what IV solutions and flush solutions are infusing or present in the catheter when lab samples are drawn. Blood samples for measuring partial thromboplastin time (PTT) should be drawn peripherally to avoid contamination with heparin.

### 30. What should be done if blood cannot be aspirated?

If blood cannot be aspirated, the catheter may be kinked, clotted, or no longer in the venous system. Assess the site for:

- Drainage due to catheter damage/obstruction or fibrin sheath forcing backflush of infusate
- Subcutaneous swelling
- Obstructed lumen from constriction of sutures
- Swelling of the neck, throat, arm, or hand
- Loops of tunneled catheter under the skin

Ask the patient to change position, perhaps into the Trendelenburg position, to increase venous flow and to cough or breathe deeply to help move the catheter away from the vein wall. Remove the injection caps and attempt to aspirate. Infuse vigorously with 10–20 ml normal saline while assessing for swelling. In case of implanted ports, try to reposition the needle. If catheter placement is still questionable, confirm position in the SVC by chest radiograph and/or a radiographic dye study.

### 31. When should central line occlusion be suspected?

Occlusion should be considered when it is difficult to infuse, flush, and/or aspirate the catheter. Partial obstruction manifests as resistance with flushing and/or absence of blood return with aspiration.

### 32. What causes central line occlusion?

**Intraluminal thrombus** may be formed as a result of injury to the vein wall during insertion or contact with the catheter tip or from hardened blood in the catheter lumen.

**Fibrin formation** (fibrin sheath or sleeve) at the entrance site to the venous system may impair the ability to flush but not to aspirate.

**Drug precipitate** may be formed by incompatible solutions, inadequate flushing, or calcium-phosphorus complexes (seen with total parenteral nutrition).

**External occlusion** may occur when the Huber needle has not been pushed all of the way through the septum or when the catheter is clamped, kinked, or constricted by sutures.

### 33. What is extravasation? How is it managed?

Extravasation is defined as leakage of infusate from the vein into the subcutaneous space. Although more common in peripheral IV access, it is a potential complication of CVCs. Symptoms of extravasation may include pain, burning or stinging, and perhaps swelling or leaking. Blood return may or may not be present. A chest radiograph or dye study should be performed to confirm catheter placement in the venous system. If extravasation is suspected, stop the drug, aspirate residual, and notify the physician.

### 34. What are the common causes of extravasation?

- Accidental dislodgement of the Huber needle in implanted ports
- Formation of a fibrin sheath along the catheter tract, starting from the exit site and growing toward the catheter tip. When fluid infuses out of the catheter tip, it backtracks along the catheter and leaks out of the exit site.
- Catheter damage: more likely in the presence of a clot when overly vigorous flushing can result in weakening of the catheter wall and perforation.
- Dislodgement or migration of catheter tip out of the venous system. The mechanism for spontaneous migration is unclear, but coughing or sneezing may be factors, especially with softer catheters.

### 35. What is pinch-off syndrome? How is it diagnosed and managed?

Pinch off results from narrowing and shearing of the catheter between the clavicle and first rib. It should be suspected with intermittent lack of blood return or inability to infuse, which usually is exacerbated by sitting, and relieved by raising the arms over the head. Pinch off is diagnosed on chest radiograph and requires catheter removal because of the risk of catheter embolization.

**36. Can a central line be repaired?**

A leaking catheter must be repaired or removed to prevent infection and/or air embolus. Catheter lumens are damaged by overly vigorous flushing, which weakens the catheter wall and eventually causes a hole. If the catheter tears or breaks, fold the remaining end of the catheter in half, cover with gauze, and secure tightly with a rubber band. If a clamp is available, clamp the catheter above the leak. Notify the physician immediately. Some damaged central lines can be repaired, including tunneled catheters and PICCs.

**37. Can a registered nurse remove a central line?**

In accordance with hospital policy and specific State Board of Nursing Practice Acts, nurses may discontinue a noncuffed CVC. A cut-down procedure usually is needed to remove cuffed catheters.

**38. How is a noncuffed CVC removed?**

After obtaining a physician order, remove all sutures, and lay the patient flat. To prevent an air embolus, instruct the patient to perform a Valsalva maneuver or hold his or her breath while the catheter is withdrawn. If the patient cannot cooperate or is on mechanical ventilation, remove the catheter during the expiratory phase of the respiratory cycle. Apply pressure with a sterile gauze for several minutes. Because air may enter the vein through a subcutaneous tract, apply an occlusive dressing for 24–72 hours. Once the catheter is removed, inspect the tip to ensure that it is intact.

**39. What complications are associated with central lines?**
- Infection
- Occlusion
- Pinch off
- Sepsis
- Migration
- Extravasation

**40. What are the signs of central line infection?**

Erythema, pain, and purulence at the exit site or along the tunnel are the most consistent indicators of infection. Daily assessment for fever, redness, tenderness, edema, and drainage is necessary. Immune suppression may diminish or completely mask these signs.

**41. List the risk factors for central line infection.**
- Type of catheter material
- Number of lumens
- Duration of manipulation
- Age < 1 yr or > 60 yr
- Emergent vs. elective placement
- Altered host defenses (dermatitis, burns, HIV infection, neutropenia, immunosuppression)
- Skill of operator inserting the catheter
- Absence of maximal barrier precautions during placement (sterile gloves, gown, drape, masks)
- Failure to maintain aseptic technique during routine care
- Sepsis or infection at time of placement

**42. What is the difference between local and systemic catheter-related infections?**

**Local catheter-related infections** occur at the exit site, tunnel, or port pocket. Erythema that extends 2 cm from the exit site, warmth, tenderness, and swelling are suggestive of exit site infection. Sometimes it is difficult to distinguish an exit site infection from irritation due to tape, adhesives, cleansing agents, or transparent dressings.

**Systemic catheter-related infections** present with bacteremia or sepsis. Sepsis is defined as clinical evidence of infection plus two or more of the following systemic responses: body temperature > 38°C or < 36°C, tachycardia, increased respiratory rate, partial pressure of carbon dioxide in arterial blood < 32 mmHg, or leukocytosis.

**43. What are tunnel infections and port pocket infections?**

A tunnel infection is defined as inflammation along the subcutaneous tract extending > 2 cm from the exit site. A port pocket infection is characterized by inflammation or necrosis of the skin over an implanted device or purulence and infection in the pocket containing the device. Port pocket infections closely resemble tunnel infections and respond to similar treatment plans. It is important to avoid cannulating an implanted port when a port pocket infection is suspected.

**44. Define systemic catheter-related blood stream infection (CR-BSI).**

CR-BSI is defined as isolation of the same organism from a catheter culture and a peripheral blood culture with clinical symptoms of a blood stream infection. Semiquantitative blood cultures, simultaneously drawn peripherally and through the catheter, compare the concentration of organisms in the catheter vs. the peripheral sample. Criteria that implicate the catheter as the source of infection include semiquantitative cultures showing 5–10 times more of the organism in the line than in the peripheral blood.

**45. What are the sources for central line infection?**
- Skin insertion site (bacteria may gain easy access along the subcutaneous tract toward the catheter tip)
- Catheter hub (microorganisms may be introduced into the catheter and blood stream through the hub or injection ports and stopcocks)
- Secondary catheter infection through bloodstream seeding (rare)
- Infusate contamination

**46. How are central line infections treated?**

Management depends on the causative organisms and extent of infection. Treatment decisions include choice of antimicrobial agent, need for removal of indwelling line, and need for hospital admission. Aggressive local site care and oral antibiotics may treat local infections in the absence of neutropenia. Tunnel infections and sepsis require parenteral antibiotics and/or removal of the catheter. It is important to alternate the lumens of the catheter through which the antibiotic is infused if the catheter is not removed. If the patient shows no clinical response to antibiotics within 48 hours, removal of the catheter is suggested.

**47. What can be done to prevent catheter-related infections?**

Infection prevention strategies include hand washing, strict aseptic technique, daily assessment, appropriate site care, and replacement of administration sets and IV fluids at adequate intervals. Routine replacement of nontunneled CVCs is recommended. Special catheter designs include those with antimicrobial substances to prevent colonization and heparin coatings that decrease formation of fibrin sleeves, thereby decreasing the colonization of bacteria. CVCs with a collagen cuff impregnated with silver ions, which exert an antimicrobial effect for 4–6 weeks, serve as a barrier to organism migration.

**48. What is mechanical phlebitis? What are the signs and symptoms?**

Mechanical phlebitis is the most common complication of PICC insertion (incidence rate: 2.5–23%) and generally occurs within the first week after insertion. It may be caused by trauma to the endothelial lining of the vein during insertion and consequent vasoconstriction. Signs and symptoms include a palpable venous cord, skin temperature change, and tenderness.

**49. How is mechanical phlebitis treated? Should the PICC be removed?**

Immediate removal is not always necessary. A warm pack should be applied for 24 hours at the first sign of redness and swelling along the vein. Immobilization and elevation of the affected arm and nonsteroidal anti-inflammatory drugs (NSAIDs) may be of benefit. If symptoms do not improve within 24 hours or resolve in 72 hours, the catheter should be removed.

**50. What should be suspected if a PICC is resistant to removal?**

The most likely cause of resistance to removal is venospasm. A hard cord may be palpated along the arm vein. A thrombus or fibrin sheath also may cause difficulty with removal.

**51. How can venospasm be prevented?**

Spasm can be prevented by removing the catheter at moderate speed with gentle traction. Aggressive pulling is not recommended. Do not apply pressure at or near the length of the vein during removal.

## 52. How is venospasm managed?

Warm compresses may be helpful in dilating the vein. Attempt removal 20–30 minutes after interventions to abate the spasm. If resistance persists, wait an additional 12–24 hours before another attempt. Infusing warmed IV fluids for 5–15 minutes to vasodilate the vein and increase blood flow may help ease catheter removal.

## 53. What type of needle should be used to access an implanted port?

A noncoring (Huber) needle should be used to access an implanted port, because it helps to preserve the life of the port septum. In an emergency, a straight needle may be used. The viscosity of the infused solution and the depth of port placement under the subcutaneous tissue determine the gauge and length of the needle. Huber needles are available in various configurations. The 90°-angled needle is used most frequently because it is more easily secured with a dressing. A straight Huber needle may be used for withdrawing blood samples or giving bolus injections. Always attach the needle to a short extension set that has been primed with normal saline.

## 54. Describe the procedure for accessing an implanted port.

1. Locate the port by palpating the subclavian area.
2. Using sterile technique, clean the skin with povidone iodine or Hibiclens, using spiral motion over the port and moving outward.
3. Stabilize the port with your fingers, and insert the needle through the skin, pushing it through the septum until it touches the bottom of the port.
4. Verify needle position by aspirating for blood return. If neither irrigation nor aspiration is possible, the needle may need to be pushed further into the septum or repositioned.

## 55. How often should Huber needles be changed?

Needles typically are changed every 7 days when kept in place for continuous infusions.

## 56. How is the needle changed?

A folded 2-× 2 gauze pad can be used to stabilize the needle if it is not close enough to the skin or chest wall. Huber needles may come with attached extension tubing, wings, and even foam padding. Cover the insertion site with an occlusive dressing. Before needle removal, flush with normal saline, followed by heparin flush according to hospital procedure.

## 57. How can patient discomfort be minimized during port access?

Topical anesthetics, such as Emla cream (lidocaine 2.5%, prilocaine 2.5%) may be applied to the skin over the port site at least 1 hour before needle placement. Application of ice or ethyl chloride spray also may be helpful.

### BIBLIOGRAPHY

1. Baranowski L: Central venous access devices: Current technologies, uses and management strategies. J Intraven Nurs 16:167–194, 1993.
2. Berlam C: Vascular access devices. In Oncology Nursing Secrets. Philadelphia, Hanley & Belfus, 1997.
3. Brown JM: Polyurethane and silicone: Myths and misconceptions. J Intraven Nurs 18:120–122, 1995.
4. Camp-Sorrell D (ed): Access Device Guidelines: Recommendations for Nursing Practice and Education. Pittsburgh, PA, Oncology Nursing Society, 1996.
5. Eastridge BJ, Lefor AT: Complications of indwelling venous access devices in cancer patients. J Clin Oncol 13:233–238, 1995.
6. Eyer S, Brummitt C, Crossley K, et al: Catheter-related sepsis: Prospective, randomized study of three methods of long-term catheter maintenance. Crit Care Med 18:1073–1079, 1990.
7. Intravenous Nursing Standards of Practice. J Intraven Nurs 21(15), 1998.
8. Maki DG, Ringer M, Alvarado CJ: Prospective randomized trial of povidone-iodine, alcohol, and chlorhexidine for prevention of infection associated with central venous and arterial catheters. Lancet 338:339–342, 1991.
9. Maki DG, Stolz SS, Wheeler S, Mermel LA: A prospective, randomized trial of gauze and two polyurethane dressings for site care of pulmonary artery catheters: Implications for catheter management. Crit Care Med 22:1729–1737, 1994.

10. Public Health Service, U.S. Department of Health and Human Services, Centers for Disease Control and Prevention: Guidelines for prevention of intravascular device-related infections. Am J Infect Control 24:262–293, 1996
11. Raad I, Davis S, Becker M, et al:Low infection rate and long durability of nontunneled silastic catheters. Arch Intern Med 153:1791–1795, 1993.
12. Reynolds MG Tebbs SE, Elliot TSJ: Do dressings with increased permeability reduce the incidence of central venous catheter related sepsis? Intens Crit Care Nurs 13:26–29, 1997.
13. Ryder MA: Peripherally inserted central venous catheters. Nurs Clin North Am 28:937–971, 1993.
14. Wickham R, Purl S, Walker D: (1992). Long term central venous catheters: Issues for care. Semin Oncol Nurs 8:133–147, 1992.

# 19. PRIMARY PULMONARY HYPERTENSION

*Brigid Ide, MS, RN*

**1. What is pulmonary hypertension?**

Pulmonary hypertension is defined as mean pulmonary artery pressure (MPAP) > 25mmHg at rest or > 30 mmHg during exercise.

**2. What mechanisms may contribute to high pulmonary pressures?**

| MECHANISM | DUE TO | EXAMPLE |
|---|---|---|
| Passive | Increase in left atrial or left ventricular pressures | Myocardial infarction with stiff ventricle, congestive heart failure, left atrial myxoma, mitral stenosis |
| Hyperkinetic | Increased blood flow | Atrial or ventricular septal defect, Eisenmenger's physiology |
| Obstructive | Impaired blood flow | Pulmonary embolism |
| Vasoconstrictive | Alveolar hypoxia | Vasospasm, hypoxemia |
| Obliterative | Diminished vascular capacity | Collagen vascular diseases (e.g., scleroderma), primary pulmonary hypertension |
| Polygenic | Arising from two or more mechanisms | |

**3. What distinguishes primary pulmonary hypertension from other forms?**

Primary pulmonary hypertension (PPH) is considered "precapillary" because the pathophysiology occurs before the blood is oxygenated. It is a rare disease of unknown cause. Extensive changes in the pulmonary vascular endothelium lead to vasoconstriction and thromboses.

**4. Who is affected by PPH?**

The disease afflicts primarily young women, with a female-to-male ratio of 2:1. Approximately 400 persons are diagnosed annually.

**5. What is the prognosis for PPH?**

Poor. The median survival time in the National Institute of Health Registry of PPH is 2.5 years after diagnosis.

**6. Describe the pathophysiology of PPH.**

Sustained increases in pulmonary pressures and pulmonary vascular resistance lead to increases in right ventricular afterload. Eventually right ventricular hypertrophy and dilatation fail to compensate for the high pulmonary pressures. Cardiac function deteriorates, and right heart failure develops, resulting in a low, fixed left ventricular cardiac output.

### 7. What are the signs and symptoms of PPH?
Signs and symptoms become extreme and include fatigue, dyspnea, syncope, edema, chest pain, and palpitations.

### 8. What are the hemodynamic findings on initial evaluation?
- High MPAP
- Normal pulmonary capillary wedge pressure (PCWP)
- Normal mean arterial pressure (MAP)
- Low cardiac output (CO)
- High pulmonary vascular resistance (PVR)
- Normal-to-high systemic vascular resistance (SVR)

### 9. How is PVR calculated?

$$PVR = \frac{MPAP - PCWP}{CO}$$

where PCWP is a substitute for actual measurement of pulmonary vein pressure.

### 10. What is the normal value for PVR?
0.25–1.5 Woods units (resistance units).

### 11. How else can PVR be expressed?
PVR can be expressed in dynes/sec/cm$^{-5}$ by using the following equation:

$$PVR = \frac{MPAP - PCWP}{CO} \times 80$$

In other words, resistance units are multiplied by a factor of 80. The normal value for PVR using this method is 20–120 dynes/sec/cm$^{-5}$.

### 12. How is PPH treated?
Treatment of PPH is directed primarily at the treatment of right ventricular failure; digoxin, diuretics, vasodilators, and oxygen (if hypoxemia is present) are used. Specific treatment of PPH includes a combination of warfarin to diminish occurrence of thromboembolic events, high-dose calcium channel blockers to relax the vascular endothelium, and prostacyclin to provide vasodilatation and reduce platelet aggregation. Exercise must be modified to avoid symptoms, and pregnancy should be avoided.

### 13. What brings a patient with PPH to the intensive care unit (ICU)?
Because of their delicate hemodynamic balance, patients with PPH come to the ICU for initial evaluation and treatment with vasoactive drugs. In addition, factors that increase blood flow or cause significant changes in hemodynamic status (e.g., pregnancy, surgery, increased heart failure) lead to deterioration and require hemodynamic and respiratory monitoring. Swift intervention with oxygen, mechanical ventilation, and inotropic support and adjustments of prostacyclin therapy may be necessary.

### 14. What is epoprostenol? How soon does it work?
Epoprostenol (Flolan), a prostacyclin used to treat PPH, is a potent vasodilator and inhibits platelet aggregation. It is an intravenous preparation with a short half-life (6 minutes). Drug induction may show minimal hemodynamic effect; the optimal therapeutic benefit occurs in 2–3 months.

### 16. What is the usual dosage of epoprostenol? How is it administered?
Dosage begins at 2 ng/kg/min and is titrated every 30 minutes to the maximal tolerated dose. The average discharge dose is 6–8 ng/kg/min. Central line administration is preferred because of

its high alkaline properties (pH = 10.2–10.8). The drug can be safely administered for short periods through a large-bore peripheral line. No other drugs can be administered in the same IV line.

### 17. How often should infusion lines be changed?

Because it is an unstable agent, epoprostenol and its infusion lines must be changed every 8 hours at room temperature. It is stable for 48 hours when reconstituted and chilled to 36–46° F.

### 18. What are the signs of excessive and insufficient doses?

**Excessive doses:** flushing, headache, nausea, diarrhea, and symptomatic hypotension.
**Insufficient doses:** cool extremities and pallor, return of PPH symptoms.

### 19. What are the long term side effects?

Jaw pain and tolerance.

### 20. How long is epoprostenol used?

It is a life-long therapy, often used as a bridge to lung or heart-lung transplant. Patients are taught to mix, administer, and manage their own continuous intravenous infusions through ambulatory pumps and a network of home care services and medical oversight.

### BIBLIOGRAPHY

1. Barst RJ, et al: A comparison of continuous intravenous epoprostenol (prostacyclin) with conventional therapy for primary pulmonary hypertension. N Engl J Med 334:296–301, 1996.
2. Cheever KH, et al: Epoprostenol therapy for primary pulmonary hypertension. Crit Care Nurse 19(4):20–27, 1999.
3. Rich S: Medical treatment of primary pulmonary hypertension: A bridge to transplantation? Am J Cardiol 75:63A–66A, 1995.
4. Rubin L: Pathology and pathophysiology of primary pulmonary hypertension. Am J Cardiol 75:51A–54A, 1995.
5. Rubin L: Primary pulmonary hypertension. ACCP Consensus Statement. Chest 104:236– 250, 1993.

# II. Respiratory System

## 20. RESPIRATORY ASSESSMENT

*Christine L. Nelson, RN, BSN, CCRN, and Hildy Schell, RN, MS, CCRN*

### 1. Is respiratory assessment different in the intensive care unit (ICU)?

The physical exam of a critically ill patient focuses on the same basic components used to assess the respiratory system of any patient: inspection, auscultation, palpation, and percussion. The ICU has equipment that provides additional assessment data, including pulse oximetry, capnography, arterial blood gases (ABGs), and ventilator data. Respiratory assessment can be slightly limited or enhanced when patients have endotracheal or tracheal tubes and/or are receiving mechanical ventilation support.

### 2. What factors are important in general observation of the patient?

The mental status of the patient provides information about oxygenation and ventilation status. Assess for shortness of breath (dyspnea). Does the patient complain of difficulty with breathing? Can the patient complete a full sentence without pausing to catch his or her breath? Note any audible snoring and/or stridor. Restlessness, diaphoresis, and anxiety are early signs of respiratory distress related to hypoxemia. Observe the patient's skin and visible mucous membranes for cyanosis. The presence and characteristics of cough, sputum production, pain with respiration, and/or nasal drainage are also assessed during general observation and inspection.

### 3. What factors are important in inspection of the patient

Note the shape and general condition of the thorax. Observe the chest for asymmetry and intercostal retractions or bulging. To evaluate the patient's work of breathing (WOB), observe respiratory rate and pattern, and look for nasal flaring, pursed-lip breathing, and use of accessory muscles of respiration. Respiratory rate and rhythm assessment should be compared with the monitor count and respiratory waveform for accuracy. Respiratory rhythm waveforms are derived from the chest wall movement detected by the electrocardiographic (ECG) leads. They provide valuable data related to the depth of inspiration and pattern of breathing.

### 4. What factors are important in auscultation?

Auscultating breath sounds provides information related to air movement through the airways and alveoli. Normal and abnormal breath sounds can be identified and trended in relation to changes in the patient's clinical condition or therapeutic interventions. For example, if the patient suddenly complains of shortness of breath and diminished breath sounds are noted on the right, early interventions for diagnosing and treating a possible pneumothorax can be instituted. Trending the presence and degree of crackles provides information that helps to evaluate the effectiveness of diuretic or renal replacement therapy. The stethoscope should be moved from one side of the chest to the other, starting at the top and moving downward. The anterior and posterior chest should be auscultated unless repositioning leads to instability or is otherwise contraindicated.

### 5. What factors are important in palpation?

Palpation of the thorax and neck area provides assessment data related to chest wall expansion and symmetry. Subcutaneous (SQ) air (crepitus, SQ emphysema) can be detected by palpation and indicates a communication between the subcutaneous tissue and airway, mediastinum, or a pneumothorax. A "popping" sensation is felt when the fingertips are pressed into the tissue where air is present. SQ air may be localized and due to a small leak around a chest tube, or it may be an early sign of pneumothorax or cardiac tamponade due to increased mediastinal air. Patients at high risk for SQ air include those with chronic obstructive pulmonary disease (COPD), asthma, or acute respiratory distress syndrome (ARDS) who are receiving positive-pressure ventilation.

### 6. What factors are important in percussion?

Percussion provides assessment data that helps to differentiate the cause of lung consolidation (e.g., atelectasis, pleural effusions, pneumothorax, hydrothorax, fluid). Percussion is not routinely performed by critical care nurses.

### 7. How are breath sounds described?

**Crackles or rales** have been described as sounding like "strands of hair being rubbed together next to the ear." Crackles are caused by air passing through fluid-filled airways or collapsed alveoli that snap open on inspiration. They typically do not clear with coughing and often are heard in patients with pneumonia, pulmonary edema, chronic bronchitis, or emphysema.

**Rhonchi** have a coarse and low-pitched sound created by air movement though excessive mucus or fluid or inflamed airways. They clear with coughing and typically indicate significant secretions.

**Wheezes** are a result of air passing through narrowed or obstructed airways. They are high-pitched and have a musical, squeaking quality. They frequently are heard in patients with reactive airway disease, bronchospasm, or bronchitis.

### 8. What are abnormal breathing patterns?

**Apnea** is complete cessation of air movement that lasts longer than 15 seconds. It can be caused by neurologic disorders, overuse of narcotics and sedatives, and obstructions to the airway.

**Bradypnea** is a respiratory rate < 10 breaths/minute and is related to oversedation, analgesia, or neurologic disorders.

**Tachypnea** is a respiratory rate > 20 breaths/minute and is caused by increased metabolism, pain, fever, hypoxemia, and early hypercapnia.

**Kussmaul breathing** is tachypnea with a regular and deep pattern. It is associated with metabolic acidosis because the compensatory result is increased carbon dioxide removal.

**Biot's breathing** is an abnormal pattern in which irregular periods of apnea are interspersed with bursts of a few rapid breaths.

**Cheyne-Stokes respirations** manifest as periods of shallow to deep to shallow breaths followed by apnea. These periods repeat in a fairly regular pattern. Cheyne-Stokes respiration is associated with neurologic disorders and heart failure, and may be seen during sleep in some people.

### 9. What are the normal and accessory muscles of respiration?

The normal muscles of respiration are the intercostal muscles and diaphragm. Use of accessory muscles is abnormal. The sternocleidomastoid muscle helps to increase the anterior-posterior diameter of the thorax. The scalene muscles of the neck help to lift up the rib cage. These accessory muscles aid the inspiratory phase of ventilation. The abdominal muscles facilitate the exhalation phase of ventilation during respiratory distress.

### 10. What determines oxygenation status? How is it assessed?

Oxygenation is determined by how well oxygen can reach arterial blood so that it can be delivered to tissues. It is assessed as follows:

1. Assess the patient's baseline respiratory rate, mental status, breath sounds, and pulse oximetry ($SpO_2$), if available.

2. Assess for stridor, shortness of breath, fatigue, and ability to speak full sentences.

3. Inspect for alterations in mental status, anxiety, pallor or cyanosis, abnormal respiratory rate or pattern, diaphoresis, and productive cough.

4. Auscultate for abnormal breath sounds.

5. Monitor $SpO_2$ via pulse oximetry and partial pressure of oxygen in arterial blood ($PaO_2$) by ABG analysis.

6. Evaluate $SpO_2$ and $PaO_2$ in relation to delivered oxygen concentration, flow, and/or level of positive end-expiratory pressure (PEEP), if the patient is ventilated. Hypoxemia is a decreased amount of oxygen in arterial blood ($PaO_2 < 60$ mmHg, $SpO_2 < 90\%$).

**11. What is intrapulmonary shunt?**

Intrapulmonary shunt (IPS) is the percentage of cardiac output that does not participate in gas exchange because of collapsed or fluid-filled alveoli (perfusion without ventilation). Normal IPS is ~ 5%. IPS is a major cause of hypoxemia in critically ill patients. Atelectasis, pneumonia, pulmonary edema, and pulmonary hemorrhage can cause hypoxemia due to IPS.

**12. How is IPS quantitated?**

The degree of IPS is quantitated in the clinical setting with various oxygen tension-based indices: alveolar-arterial oxygen gradient (A-a$DO_2$), arterial-alveolar (a-A) ratio, and the ratio of $PaO_2$ to the fractional concentration of oxygen in inspired air ($FiO_2$) referred to as the $PaO_2/FiO_2$ ratio. These indices can be calculated with an ABG and known $FiO_2$.

$$\text{Alveolar air equation: } PAO_2 = FiO_2(PB - PH_2O) - PaCO_2/RQ$$

where $PAO_2$ = alveolar oxygen partial pressure, PB = barometric pressure, $PH_2O$ = partial pressure of water vapor, $PaCO_2$ = partial pressure of carbon dioxide in alveolar gas, and RQ = respiratory quotient.

$$\text{A-a}DO_2 = PAO_2 - PaO_2 \text{ (normal = 5–20 mmHg)}$$

Normal a/A ratio: 0.75–1.0 (75–100/104)

Normal $PaO_2/FiO_2$ ratio: > 300 mmHg (75–100/0.21 on room air)

**13. What determines ventilation status? How is it assessed?**

Ventilation is determined by how well the patient can move air in and out of the lungs and rid the body of carbon dioxide. Assessment of ventilatory status includes respiratory rate and rhythm, chest expansion, and work of breathing. The physical exam is evaluated along with the $PaCO_2$/pH relationship from the ABG analysis. Hypoventilation results in a $PaCO_2 > 45$ mmHg and hyperventilation in a $PaCO_2 < 35$ mmHg. Capnography measures end-tidal carbon dioxide ($ETCO_2$), which also contributes to assessment of ventilation.

**14. What is minute ventilation?**

Minute ventilation ($V_E$) is the volume of air moved in and out of the lungs in 1 minute. It is calculated by multiplying respiratory rate (RR) times tidal volume ($V_t$):

$$V_E = RR \times V_t$$

Normal $V_E$ is 4–6 L/min. $V_E$ is assessed for evaluating readiness to wean from mechanical ventilation.

**15. What is deadspace?**

Deadspace, also called wasted ventilation (ventilation without perfusion), is the percentage of minute ventilation that is not perfused and therefore does not participate in gas exchange. Normal deadspace is 30% because the nasooropharynx and airways are normally ventilated but do not participate in gas exchange. Pulmonary emboli, low cardiac output states, ARDS, and pulmonary hypertension can increase the amount of deadspace. The level of exhaled carbon dioxide ($P_ECO_2$) obtained from collection over 3 minutes and $PaCO_2$ from ABG analysis are required to calculate the deadspace ratio.

**16. What assessment data provide information about lung compliance and resistance?**

Resistance to air flow can be assessed in ventilated patients by evaluating the peak inspiratory pressures (PIPs) and the relationship to the plateau pressure ($P_{plt}$). Compliance (distensibility) of the lungs and chest wall can be assessed by evaluating lung volumes and related lung pressures. Static compliance ($C_{st}$) can be calculated for patients receiving mechanical ventilation as follows:

$$C_{st} = V_t/(P_{plt} - PEEP)$$

Measurements of compliance and resistance are helpful when they are monitored regularly for trends.

### 17. How is sputum assessed?

Sputum should be assessed for quantity (scant to copious amounts) and characteristics (color, consistency/viscosity, smell, and presence of blood). The respiratory system and submucosal glands normally produce approximately 100 ml/day of clear, thin mucus. Mucus production increases and can change characteristics with clinical conditions that cause infection, inflammation, fluid overload, bleeding, or capillary leak. Sputum samples can be analyzed for protein levels to differentiate cardiogenic and noncardiogenic pulmonary edema and for the presence of organisms. Sputum samples for Gram stain and culture tests should be obtained from endotracheal and tracheal tubes with sterile technique to avoid contamination. Nonintubated patients can rinse their mouth with water before they cough and expectorate the sputum sample. The Gram stain is done quickly and can detect the shape of any organisms and determine whether they are gram-positive or gram-negative. This distinction helps to guide antibiotic therapy. Some cultures take up to 5 days to grow organisms. Once culture and sensitivity information is available, more specific antibiotic therapy can be initiated.

### BIBLIOGRAPHY

1. Ahrens T: Changing perspectives in the assessment of oxygenation. Crit Care Nurs 4:78–83, 1993.
2. Ahrens T, Rutherford K: Essentials of Oxygenation: Implication for Clinical Practice. Boston, Jones & Bartlett, 1993.
3. Bordow RA, Moser KM: Manual of Clinical Problems in Pulmonary Medicine, 4th ed. Boston, Little, Brown, 1996.
4. Brooks-Brunn JA, Sakallaris BR: Respiratory disorders. In Bucher L, Melander S (eds): Critical Care Nursing. Philadelphia, W.B. Saunders, 1999, pp 353–445.
5. Chulay M, Dossey B, Guzzettta C: AACN Handbook of Critical Care Nursing. Stamford, CT, Appleton & Lange, 1997.
6. Guyton A: Textbook of Medical Physiology, 8th ed. Philadelphia, W.B. Saunders, 1991.
7. Luce JM, Pierson DJ, Tyler ML: Intensive Respiratory Care, 2nd ed, Philadelphia, W.B. Saunders, 1993.
8. O'Hanlon-Nichols T: Basic assessment series: The adult pulmonary system. Am J Nurs 2:39–45, 1998.
9. Pierce LNB: Guide to Mechanical Ventilation and Intensive Respiratory Care. Philadelphia, W.B. Saunders, 1995.
10. St. John RE: The pulmonary system. In Alspach J (ed): Core Curriculum for Critical Care Nursing. Philadelphia, W.B. Saunders, 1998, pp 1–84.
11. Stacey KM: Pulmonary alteration. In Thelan LA, Davie JK, Urden LD, Lough ME (eds): Critical Care Nursing: Diagnosis and Management, 2nd ed. St. Louis, Mosby, 1994, pp 369–476.
12. Stone KS: Respiratory physiology. In Clochesy J M, Breu C, Cardin S, et al (eds): Critical Care Nursing, 2nd ed. W.B. Saunders, 1996, pp 561–582.

# 21. AIRWAY MANAGEMENT

Lisa M. Boulais, RN, MS, CCRN, CEN

### 1. How does one identify actual or potential airway obstruction?

**Look** for evidence of trauma about the face and neck. Examine the airway for blood, secretions, vomitus, a relaxed tongue, dislodged teeth, or other foreign body. Observe for agitation or altered consciousness. A decreasing level of consciousness may be an indication of hypoxia as a result of airway compromise.

**Listen** for noisy or absent breathing. Partial airway obstruction may be characterized by labored or noisy respirations such as snoring, gurgling, or stridorous breathing. Hoarseness may indicate laryngeal obstruction or injury. Absent breath sounds may be a manifestation of complete airway obstruction.

**Feel** for exhaled air from the mouth and nose. In cases of trauma, palpate for facial instability, tracheal position, and subcutaneous emphysema.

## 2. What is the first step in obtaining a patent airway?

The first step in obtaining a patent airway is to position the airway properly, using the head-tilt, chin-lift maneuver. In unconscious patients, the relaxed muscles of the oropharynx allow the tongue to fall posteriorly, occluding the airway. The head-tilt, chin-lift maneuver elevates the tongue away from the posterior pharynx and opens the airway. If trauma is suspected, the jaw thrust or chin lift maneuver should be used. These techniques pull the tongue away from the posterior pharynx while maintaining the cervical spine in a neutral position.

## 3. When should an oral airway be used instead of a nasal airway?

An oral pharyngeal airway (OPA) is used to maintain a patent airway in unconscious patients. Because OPAs stimulate the gag reflex, a nasopharyngeal airway should be used in conscious or semiconscious patients.

An OPA also may be used in conjunction with a bag-valve-mask device to assist with ventilation. The effective use of a bag-valve-mask device necessitates an open airway. An OPA may be inserted to assist in maintaining an open airway by removing the tongue from the posterior pharynx. Finally, an OPA may be used for patients with endotracheal tubes. With an OPA properly inserted in the mouth, the patient is prevented from biting on the endotracheal tube and occluding airflow.

## 4. What is a laryngeal mask airway (LMA)? How is it used?

The LMA is a device that may be used temporarily when attempts at endotracheal intubation have been unsuccessful. The device should not be used as a definitive airway. The LMA consists of a tube similar to that of an endotracheal tube. However, the distal end is made of a small mask encircled by an inflatable cuff. When inserted into the airway, the mask sits in the lower hypopharynx. The device seals the laryngeal opening when the cuff is inflated. Positive-pressure breaths are delivered through the laryngeal opening into the lungs. Unlike endotracheal intubation, the LMA does not protect the patient against aspiration of gastric contents.

## 5. What are the indications for obtaining a definitive airway?

**Resuscitation** is one of the most common indications for obtaining a definitive airway. Patients in cardiac or respiratory failure should be intubated to facilitate adequate oxygenation and ventilation with positive-pressure ventilation. In head-injured patients, a definitive airway with mechanical ventilation can be used as a method of controlling levels of carbon dioxide ($CO_2$).

**Airway protection** is necessary in patients who are unable to protect their own airway, typically because of an altered level of consciousness as a result of stroke, drug overdose, or head injury.

Patients undergoing **surgical procedures** may need a definitive airway. This is particularly true in operations lasting more than 2 hours or for surgical procedures involving the airway.

## 6. Why are some patients intubated nasotracheally?

Nasotracheal intubation is an alternative to endotracheal intubation for patients who may have contraindications to oral intubation, such as oral trauma, anatomic abnormalities, cervical spine injury, or seizure activity. Nasotracheal intubation typically is performed using a blind technique. The tube is placed without direct visualization of the patient's airway. The patient is sedated, and topical anesthetic is used in the nasooropharynx. A topical vasoconstrictor such as phenylephrine or cocaine may be used to minimize bleeding in the nose.

## 7. What is rapid-sequence intubation (RSI)?

RSI provides optimal conditions for intubation and minimizes potential complications. RSI begins with preoxygenating the patient with 100% oxygen. Then a rapid-acting sedative such as midazolam or thiopental is administered. The patient is mask-ventilated. The sedative is followed by a rapid-acting neuromuscular blocker, such as succinylcholine or rocuronium. Once pharmacologic relaxation and paralysis are achieved, oral intubation can be accomplished. Head-injured patients may be premedicated with lidocaine to minimize increases in intracranial pressure. Because of the potential adverse effects of the drugs involved in RSI, the patient should be observed closely. Monitoring must include blood pressure, heart rate, pulse oximetry, and end-tidal $CO_2$.

**8. Should the Sellick maneuver (cricoid pressure) be used to assist with intubation?**

Yes. It is performed by applying slight posterior pressure to the cricoid cartilage with the thumb and index finger. This light pressure pushes the esophagus against the vertebral column, occluding the esophageal passage and thus minimizing gastric insufflation and potential regurgitation. In addition, the Sellick maneuver may assist intubation efforts by improving visualization of the airway. Pressure should be maintained on the cricoid cartilage until the endotracheal tube has been successfully inserted and the balloon inflated.

**9. Describe the techniques used to confirm endotracheal tube placement.**

The gold standard for validation of proper endotracheal intubation is visualization of the tube passing through the vocal cords. Other verification techniques include the presence of breath sounds over the lung fields, visualization of chest movement with ventilation, the absence of stomach gurgling with respirations, and chest radiograph. In confirming tube placement by auscultating breath sounds, it is best to listen over the epigastric area before listening to the lung fields. If gurgling sounds are heard, the tube can be removed before unnecessary air is directed into the stomach.

A disposable, colorimetric end-tidal $CO_2$ monitoring device may assist in confirming proper tube placement by detecting $CO_2$ in exhaled air. An appropriate color change on the device suggests proper tube placement.

Pulse oximetry should be monitored throughout the intubation procedure. Maintenance of an appropriate oxygen saturation suggests proper tube placement.

Assessment of the patient's clinical status and response to intubation is an important tool in determining proper endotracheal tube placement. However, this method of verifying tube placement can be erroneous. Therefore, a variety of techniques should be used to confirm endotracheal tube placement.

**10. What is an esophageal obturator airway?**

An esophageal obturator airway (EOA) is a large-bore tube that is inserted blindly into the esophagus. The tube has multiple holes positioned proximally in the pharynx area. When oxygen is applied, it passes into the tube, through the holes, and into the larynx, trachea, and lungs. The device has a large cuff at the end of the tube that is inflated in the esophagus to prevent gastric regurgitation and insufflation. The EOA is used with a mask that seals the mouth and nose. Because of the length of the tube, the EOA should be used in adults only. Although endotracheal intubation is the preferred method of definitive airway management, the EOA may be used as an alternative if endotracheal intubation proves unsuccessful or not feasible.

**11. When is retrograde intubation considered?**

Retrograde intubation is a historical name for the translaryngeal guided-intubation technique. This procedure is used to obtain an airway when attempts at endotracheal intubation have been unsuccessful or when visualization of the vocal cords is not feasible. Indications include secretions or foreign body obstructing the airway, anatomic abnormalities, cervical spine fracture, or trauma to the airway.

**12. How is retrograde intubation performed?**

Retrograde intubation is performed by inserting a needle with syringe into the cricothyroid membrane. Once access into the tracheal lumen is achieved, air is drawn into the syringe to confirm placement. A guidewire is then threaded through the needle, into the trachea, past the vocal cords, into the oropharynx, and out through the mouth. The guidewire is used to position an endotracheal tube. The endotracheal tube is placed over the guidewire, into the mouth, and through the glottic opening. After proper positioning of the endotracheal tube in the trachea, the guidewire is removed.

### 13. What is a needle cricothyrotomy?

Needle cricothyrotomy is an emergent procedure to provide oxygen for a short time. It is performed in the presence of airway obstruction or when other airway techniques have failed. Needle cricothyrotomy involves the insertion of a 12- or 14-gauge, over-the-needle catheter into the cricothyroid membrane. A syringe is used to aspirate as the catheter is advanced. The trachea has been entered when air is drawn into the syringe. The catheter is held in place as the needle is removed. This technique provides a small airway that may save a patient's life. A cricothyrotomy is temporary and should be used only until a definitive airway is obtained.

### 14. How is oxygen delivered through a needle cricothyrotomy?

Oxygen is delivered through a needle cricothyrotomy with transtracheal jet ventilation. The key components include a high-pressure oxygen supply, noncompliant tubing attached to the oxygen source, and the ability of the patient to exhale passively through the glottic opening.

The oxygen source must be able to deliver 50 psi. Most hospital wall outlets have this capability. The rigid, noncompliant tubing is used to deliver oxygen to the transtracheal catheter. The Shrader blowgun is ideal for this purpose. If it is not available, standard pressure tubing may be used with a regulator valve. These components, combined with a large transtracheal catheter, can provide access for adequate oxygen delivery and ventilation. Although commonly available in hospitals, these supplies should be gathered before the airway technique is required. Once the system is established, breaths can be delivered at an appropriate rate.

### 15. How does a surgical cricothyrotomy differ from a needle cricothyrotomy?

A surgical cricothyrotomy allows a larger-bore, more effective airway. It is performed by making a small incision in the cricothyroid membrane. After the incision is dilated, an endotracheal tube or tracheostomy tube is advanced into the trachea. The tube can then be connected to a manual resuscitation bag or ventilator.

### 16. Should an emergency tracheostomy be attempted?

No. In most instances, if emergent airway access is required, a cricothyrotomy should be performed. Because of potential complications and the time required to complete a tracheostomy, this procedure should be done in a controlled environment by an experienced person. The operating room is the ideal place for performing a tracheostomy.

### BIBLIOGRAPHY

1. American College of Surgeons: Advanced Trauma Life Support for Doctors, 6th ed. Chicago, American College of Surgeons, 1997.
2. American Heart Association: Advanced Cardiac Life Support. Dallas, American Heart Association, 1997.
3. American Heart Association: Basic Life Support for Healthcare Providers. Dallas, American Heart Association, 1997.
4. Dailey RH, Simon B, Young GP, Stewart RD: The Airway: Emergency Management. St. Louis, Mosby, 1992.
5. Hanowell LH, Waldron RJ: Airway Management. New York, Lippincott-Raven, 1996.
6. Macleod BA, Heller MB, Gerard J, et al: Verification of endotracheal tube placement with colorimetric end-tidal CO2 detection. Ann Emerg Med 20:267–270, 1991.
7. York D: Laryngeal mask airway. In Proehl JA: Emergency Nursing Procedures, 2nd ed. Philadelphia, W.B. Saunders, 1999, pp 15–18.
8. York D: Percutaneous transtracheal ventilation. In Proehl JA: Emergency Nursing Procedures, 2nd ed. Philadelphia, W.B. Saunders, 1999, pp 48–51.

# 22. ACID-BASE DISORDERS AND ARTERIAL BLOOD GASES

*Vicki Casella-Gordon*, RN, MS, CCRN

### 1. Define acid and base.

An acid is a substance that donates hydrogen ions in solution, and a base is a substance that accepts hydrogen ions.

### 2. How are acids produced in the body?

Acids are constantly produced through the cellular metabolism of carbohydrates, fats, glucose, and protein. Cellular metabolism produces two types of acids: carbonic acid and metabolic acids. Carbonic acid ($H_2CO_3$) is generated from the metabolism of carbohydrates and fats. It is produced when carbon dioxide ($CO_2$) combines with water ($H_2O$). Metabolic acids are produced primarily from the metabolism of phosphate-containing compounds and amino acids that contain sulfur. Sulfuric and phosphoric acid are examples of metabolic acids. During cellular metabolism small amounts of base are also produced as bicarbonate ions ($HCO_3^-$). $HCO_3$ results from the oxidation of small organic anions such as citrate.

### 3. How are acids regulated in the body?

Many physiologic processes require a delicate balance of hydrogen ion concentration between intracellular fluid (ICF) and extracellular fluid (ECF). The hydrogen ion ($H^+$) concentration or degree of acidity of body fluids is calculated and reported as the pH. The higher the concentration of unbound $H^+$, the lower the pH. Conversely, the lower the concentration of $H^+$, the higher the pH. The pH is the negative logarithm of $H^+$ concentration. A pH of 7 is neutral. The blood is normally slightly alkaline with a normal pH range of 7.35–7.45. Normal cellular metabolism continually produces acids, which can lead to dangerous acidemia if the closely regulated processes by which the body neutralizes or excretes acids and maintains a normal pH are not functioning.

### 4. How does the acid-buffering system work?

Buffers are located in the ICF, ECF, blood, and bone. The buffer system neutralizes acids by combining with excess hydrogen ions. Bases become neutralized by releasing $H^+$. The major buffer system is the carbonic acid-bicarbonate-carbon dioxide buffer system (commonly referred to as the bicarbonate buffer system). The weak acid, $H_2CO_3$, pairs with $HCO_3^-$ and then combines with strong acids, such as hydrochloric acid (HCl), to weaken them. The lungs regulate carbonic acid production ($CO_2 + H_2O = H_2CO_3$), and the kidneys regulate bicarbonate production. Below is the chemical equation for the bicarbonate buffer system:

$$CO_2 + H_2O \leftrightarrow H_2CO_3 \leftrightarrow H^+ + HCO_3^-$$

The body also buffers acids with the phosphate-buffer system and proteins. Hemoglobin and other serum proteins serve as buffers.

### 5. What are the compensatory mechanisms that regulate acid-base disturbances?

Acid excretion mechanisms are necessary to maintain acid-base balance. The lungs play a role in $H_2CO_3$ excretion, and the kidneys excrete metabolic acids. When a primary acid-base disturbance occurs, the lungs and/or kidneys respond to regulate $H^+$ concentration. Compensation by the lungs or kidneys restores the acid-base balance toward a normal pH but does not correct the problem that originally caused the imbalance.

**6. Discuss the role of the lungs in regulating acid-base balance.**

Carbonic acid is excreted in the form of $CO_2$ and $H_2O$. When the rate and depth of ventilation are increased, more carbonic acid is excreted. When alveolar ventilation decreases, less carbonic acid is excreted. Central chemoreceptors in the medulla are stimulated by increased or decreased $H^+$, and peripheral chemoreceptors in the carotid and aortic bodies are stimulated by increased or decreased partial pressure of carbon dioxide ($PaCO_2$) and oxygen ($PaO_2$). An increase in $PaCO_2$ results in increased alveolar ventilation so that excess carbonic acid can be eliminated. Conversely, a decrease in $PaCO_2$ or an increase in pH causes a decrease in alveolar ventilation. A decreased pH (increased acid in the body) causes the production of ammonia, which facilitates retention of acid in the body. Normally, alveolar ventilation responds rapidly to changes in $PaCO_2$ so that carbonic acid is effectively excreted to maintain acid-base balance.

**7. Discuss the role of the kidneys in regulating acid-base balance.**

The kidneys excrete metabolic acids or hydrogen ions in the form of ammonium chloride and sodium dihydrogen phosphate. Bicarbonate is the major buffer of metabolic acids. A decreased pH (increased acid in the body) causes the kidneys to reabsorb $HCO_3^-$ and excrete $H^+$ with ammonia or phosphate in the urine. This process begins within 2–4 hours but may take several days to achieve maximal effectiveness. The serum bicarbonate level indicates how much metabolic acid is present. A decrease in serum bicarbonate level indicates increased amounts of metabolic acid.

**8. Explain base excess (BE)/base deficit (BD).**

BE/BD is an indirect measure of all the buffer systems in the blood. It is calculated and reported on the arterial blood gas analysis. It reflects the amount of base that needs to be added to 1 liter of arterial blood to achieve a normal pH (7.40). The normal range of BE/BD is –2 to +2. BE/BD can be used to assess trends in metabolic acidosis and alkalosis and to monitor response to therapies.

**9. What are the primary acid-base disorders?**

Three major processes are generally involved in an acid-base disturbance: acid production, ventilation, and renal acid excretion. Acidosis and alkalosis are classified as metabolic or respiratory.

During periods when lung function is altered, **respiratory acid-base disorders** occur. For example, respiratory acidosis occurs when ventilation is impaired. During hypoventilation $PaCO_2$ is retained, leading to increased production of $H_2CO_2$ (carbonic acid), which subsequently increases $H^+$ concentration in the plasma, resulting in a low pH. Conversely, during periods of hyperventilation when $PaCO_2$ decreases, the plasma concentrations of $H_2CO_3^-$ and $H^+$ also decrease, resulting in increased pH or respiratory alkalosis.

**Metabolic acid-base disorders** occur when the buffering of hydrogen ions is not balanced by renal bicarbonate reabsorption and retention. When acid production or intake exceeds bicarbonate generation, metabolic acidosis develops. When base intake or renal generation of bicarbonate is greater than acid production, metabolic alkalosis develops.

**10. Define acidemia and acidosis.**

**Acidemia** occurs when the pH of the blood is below the normal range (7.35–7.45). **Acidosis** is the process or condition that causes an accumulation of acid or loss of base in the blood. Acidemia presents when compensatory mechanisms are insufficient for the degree of acidosis. A pH below 6.9 affects myocardial contractility, cardiac rhythm, and mental status; it can be life-threatening. Acidosis is classified as respiratory or metabolic, depending on what type of acid ($CO_2$ or $HCO_3$) is present in excess.

**11. What is respiratory acidosis?**

Respiratory acidosis occurs with any process that decreases the rate of $CO_2$ gas exchange in alveolar ventilation. When the elimination of $CO_2$ by the lungs decreases, $PaCO_2$ increases, thus increasing the concentration of dissolved $CO_2$ in the ECF. This causes an increase in carbonic acid and $H^+$ formation and a decrease in pH.

**12. What is the difference between acute and chronic respiratory acidosis?**

**Acute respiratory acidosis.** With an acute rise in $PaCO_2$, the immediate responses are buffering with nonbicarbonate ions and stimulation of ventilation. Initially the kidneys compensate by excreting more than the usual amount of metabolic acids. This helps to shift the pH toward normal. As more metabolic acids are excreted and $HCO_3$ is reabsorbed, the bicarbonate ion concentration increases. Uncompensated respiratory acidosis in the acute setting manifests as pH < 7.35, $PaCO_2$ > 45 mmHg, and little or no increase in $HCO_3^-$. In this setting, ventilation must be assisted (e.g., mechanical ventilation) to facilitate the exhalation of $CO_2$ and the restoration of pH and $PaCO_2$ to normal.

**Chronic respiratory acidosis.** When a chronic condition such as chronic obstructive pulmonary disease (COPD) is present, the kidneys compensate for the elevated $PaCO_2$ by increasing plasma $HCO_3$ concentration. This process usually takes 3–5 days to be fully effective. Chronic or compensated respiratory acidosis is characterized by normal pH, $PaCO_2$ > 45 mmHg, and $HCO_3$ > 26 mEq/L.

**13. What are the signs and symptoms of respiratory acidosis?**

Signs and symptoms of respiratory acidosis are related to the effect of $CO_2$ on the central nervous system (CNS) and cardiovascular system. When $CO_2$ diffuses through the meninges, the pH of cerebrospinal fluid decreases and causes CNS depression, which is manifested clinically as decreased mentation, disorientation, restlessness, lethargy, or somnolence. Increased $CO_2$ levels can lead to headaches caused by vasodilation of cerebral vessels. Patients may experience neuromuscular symptoms such as fatigue, muscle weakness, tremors, diminished reflexes, and incoordination. Cardiovascular symptoms may include tachycardia and cardiac arrhythmias (possibly due to an increase in circulating catecholamines), and hypotension related to vasodilation of peripheral blood vessels.

**14. What causes respiratory acidosis?**

Respiratory acidosis results from any condition that impedes ventilation and elimination of $CO_2$ by decreasing central respiratory drive, impairing gas exchange at the capillary/alveolar level, or impairing chest wall expansion. Conditions that impede respiratory drive include over-sedation, lesions of the medulla, obesity, anesthesia, and respiratory arrest. Airway obstruction caused by a foreign object, emphysema, asthma, or bronchiectasis can cause respiratory acidosis. Neuromuscular disorders that decrease ventilation include Guillain-Barré disease, myasthenia gravis, and poliomyelitis. Conditions that impair chest wall expansion include kyphoscoliosis, abdominal distention, diaphragmatic injury, mechanical hypoventilation, and chest wall injury. Impaired gas exchange may result from increased pulmonary dead space and interstitial lung disease.

**15. What is metabolic acidosis?**

Metabolic acidosis is defined as a decrease in plasma bicarbonate concentration and pH related to an accumulation of acid or a loss of base in the ECF. Characteristic lab values of uncompensated metabolic acidosis include pH < 7.35, $HCO_3$ < 22 mEq/L, BD < –2, and normal $PaCO_2$. The lungs respond quickly by increasing ventilation to excrete carbonic acid. The kidneys respond by excreting acid and reabsorbing $HCO_3$ (base).

**16. What causes metabolic acidosis?**

Metabolic acidosis is due to a gain of acid or loss of base. Acids accumulate with an increase in intake or rate of metabolism, production of unusual acids due to altered metabolic processes, or decreased renal excretion. Bicarbonate ions lost through excessive diuresis with potassium-sparing diuretics, diarrhea, and pancreatic fistula drainage can cause metabolic acidosis. An accumulation of lactic acid from anaerobic metabolism during shock and ischemia can cause metabolic acidosis. Specific causes include the following:

- Ingestion of acid (aspirin, methanol, paraldehyde)
- Increased acid production (hyperthyroidism, hypermetabolic states, lactic acidosis, shock)
- Abnormal or incomplete metabolic pathways (ketoacidosis due to diabetes, alcohol, or starvation)

- Impaired acid excretion (acute renal failure, severe hypovolemia, hypoaldosteronism)
- Primary loss of bicarbonate by GI tract (severe diarrhea, intestinal decompression, uretero-sigmoidostomy, fistula drainage, vomiting)

### 17  What are the signs and symptoms of metabolic acidosis?
Signs and symptoms of metabolic acidosis include nausea/vomiting, abdominal pain, cardiac arrhythmias, increased respiratory rate and depth (Kussmaul breathing), headache, and CNS depression (confusion, drowsiness, lethargy, stupor, coma).

### 18.  What is the anion gap?
The anion gap (AG) is a measurement of the difference between the body's major cations (positive charge) and anions (negative charge). Sodium (Na) is the major cation, and chloride ($Cl^-$) and $HCO_3^-$ are the major anions. AG is calculated as follows:

$$AG = Na - (HCO_3 + Cl^-)$$

The normal value is 8–14 mEq/L. AG is useful in differentiating the potential causes of metabolic acidosis and can be calculated when metabolic acidosis is diagnosed by arterial blood gas analysis. An increase in AG (> 14 mEq/L) indicates an increase in acid load or production (e.g., lactic acidosis). A normal AG indicates a loss of base/$HCO_3^-$, hyperchloremia, or renal tubular acidosis.

### 19.  Define alkalemia and alkalosis.
Alkalemia occurs when pH is above normal (> 7.45). Alkalosis, defined as relative excess of base or relative deficit of acid, results from loss of acid or accumulation of base. A pH above 7.8 is usually fatal. The cause of alkalosis is classified as either respiratory or metabolic.

### 20.  What is respiratory alkalosis?
Respiratory alkalosis is the result of hyperventilation and hypocapnia. As ventilation increases, $PaCO_2$ decreases, leading to a decrease in carbonic acid and increase in pH. Respiratory alkalosis typically presents as a pH > 7.45 and $PaCO_2$ < 35 mmHg. The lungs compensate for respiratory alkalosis by decreasing the drive to breathe. The kidneys compensate by excreting bicarbonate ions, but this response may not take place for several days.

### 21.  What causes respiratory alkalosis?
Respiratory alkalosis is caused by hyperventilation, which is stimulated by hypoxemia, hypotension, intrinsic pulmonary reflexes, or direct stimulation of the respiratory center. Common causes include
- Hyperventilation syndrome (anxiety)
- Hypoxemia (pulmonary disease, anemia, left ventricular failure, high altitude)
- Pulmonary disorders (pneumonia, asthma, acute respiratory distress syndrome, fibrosis, pulmonary embolism)
- CNS disorders (cerebrovascular accident, tumors, infection, trauma)
- Drugs/hormones (aspirin, theophyllines, catecholamines, progesterone, alcohol intoxication)
- Cardiovascular disorders (acute myocardial infarction, congestive heart failure)
- Others (pain, thyrotoxicosis, early sepsis, excessive mechanical ventilation, exercise, hepatic insufficiency)

### 22.  What is metabolic alkalosis?
Metabolic alkalosis is defined as an excessive gain of base (from bicarbonate or anions metabolized to form bicarbonate) or a loss of hydrogen ions.

### 23.  What lab values suggest metabolic alkalosis?
Laboratory values that reflect uncompensated metabolic alkalosis include pH > 7.45, $HCO_3$ > 26 mEq/L, BE > +2, and normal $PaCO_2$. Compensated metabolic alkalosis is characterized by normal pH, $HCO_3$ > 26 mEq/L, and $PaCO_2$ > 45 mmHg. The lungs hypoventilate to increase

$PaCO_2$, thus increasing carbonic acid in the blood. However, the increase in $PaCO_2$ is limited to 55–60 mmHg. Hypoventilation, as a compensatory mechanism, is limited because of other overriding stimuli. The kidneys increase excretion of $HCO_3$, water, and electrolytes.

### 24. What are the signs and symptoms of metabolic alkalosis?

Signs and symptoms of metabolic alkalosis are often related to the decreased calcium ionization that results from the low $H^+$ level. Increased calcium ionization leads to overexcitability of the peripheral and central nervous system, resulting in tetany, irritability, disorientation, and seizures. Cardiac arrhythmias may result from fluid and electrolyte disturbances. A shift in the oxygen dissociation curve results in an increased affinity of hemoglobin for oxygen. Signs and symptoms associated with metabolic alkalosis include dizziness, agitation, confusion, seizures, paresthesias, tetany, hypertonic muscles, nausea, vomiting, diarrhea, hypokalemia, cardiac dysrhythmias, cardiac ischemia, coronary vasospasm, and hypoventilation.

### 25. What causes metabolic alkalosis?

Metabolic alkalosis may be chloride-responsive or chloride-resistant.

In **chloride-responsive disorders**, the kidney's ability to respond to loss of $H^+$ or addition of base is impaired by chloride deficiency, ECF depletion, decrease in glomerular filtration rate, or activation of the renin-angiotensin system. Specific causes include use of potassium-wasting diuretics, loss of gastric secretions (HCl) with vomiting, or nasogastric suctioning.

**Chloride-resistant disorders** are less common and usually associated with mineralocorticoid excess, which leads to hypokalemia, Hypokalemia causes the kidneys to conserve potassium, which results in excessive $H^+$ excretion. Examples of mineralocorticoid excess include Cushing's syndrome, primary and secondary hyperaldosteronism (e.g., cirrhosis, congestive heart failure, and renal failure), diarrhea, and hypomagnesemia.

### 26. What are mixed acid-base imbalances?

At times two or more acid-base disturbances occur simultaneously. Mixed acid-base imbalances usually are seen in patients who are extremely ill and have a concomitant underlying disease process such as COPD or renal disease.

### 27. How do I recognize mixed acid-base imbalances?

If a patient has coexisting primary acidosis and alkalosis, the pH may be near normal because the two imbalances cancel one another out. However, the combination of primary metabolic alkalosis and primary respiratory alkalosis can cause the pH to approach the fatal limit. If lab values that reflect compensation are higher than predicted, it is prudent to suspect a superimposed acid-base disorder. For example, when the $HCO_3^-$ is <10 mEq/L, one should suspect primary metabolic acidosis because a compensatory reduction in $HCO_3^-$ rarely reaches this level. Conversely, if the $HCO_3^-$ is > 40 mEq/L, a primary metabolic alkalosis should be suspected because, even with chronic hypercapnia, the compensatory response does not reach this level.

### 28. Give examples of mixed acid-base disorders.

- Cardiac arrest (metabolic acidosis/respiratory acidosis)
- Emesis with COPD (metabolic alkalosis, respiratory acidosis)
- COPD and diarrhea (respiratory acidosis/metabolic acidosis)
- Renal failure and emesis (metabolic acidosis/metabolic alkalosis)
- Salicylate poisoning (metabolic acidosis/respiratory alkalosis).

### 29. What information does an arterial blood gas (ABG) analysis provide?

ABG monitoring is used to evaluate the body's acid-base balance, ventilation, and oxygenation. ABGs tell us whether the compensatory mechanisms of the lungs and kidneys are successful at maintaining a normal pH. The body's acid-base balance is indicated by pH (normal value: 7.35–7.45). The effect of the lungs on pH is indicated by the $PaCO_2$ (normal value: 35–45 mmHg). A lower $PaCO_2$ denotes respiratory alkalosis, and a higher $PaCO_2$ denotes respiratory acidosis. Metabolic influences on pH are reflected by the level of bicarbonate (normal value: 22–26 mEq/L). An $HCO_3$ level > 26 mEq/L denotes metabolic alkalosis; an $HCO_3$ level < 22 mEq/L denotes metabolic acidosis.

Oxygen tension in arterial blood is reported as $PaO_2$, which reflects the amount of dissolved $O_2$ in plasma and accounts for only 3% of the total $O_2$ content in blood. The normal range of $PaO_2$ is 80–100 mmHg. The majority of $O_2$ in blood is attached to hemoglobin, as reflected by oxygen saturation ($SaO_2$). The normal range of $SaO_2$ is 95–100%.

## 30. Describe a systematic way to analyze ABG results.

1. Determine whether the pH is normal or abnormal. A pH < 7.35 indicates acidosis, and a pH > 7.45 indicates alkalosis.

2. Determine whether the $PaCO_2$ is normal or abnormal. During hypoventilation, $PaCO_2$ is > 45 mmHg and reflects respiratory acidosis. If $PaCO_2$ is < 35 mmHg, respiratory alkalosis is present.

3. Determine whether $HCO_3$ is normal or abnormal. If $HCO_3$ is < 22 mEq/L, metabolic acidosis is present. If $HCO_3$ is > 26 mEq/L, metabolic alkalosis is present.

4. Determine whether compensation has occurred. When both $PaCO_2$ and $HCO_3^-$ are abnormal, one is the primary acid-base disorder and the other is the compensating disorder. To decide which is which, check the pH to see if it is alkalotic or acidotic. The primary disorder causes the abnormal pH. For example, if pH is 7.25, $PaCO_2$ is elevated, and $HCO_3^-$ is elevated, the primary disorder is respiratory acidosis; the kidneys compensate with retention of $HCO_3^-$. The three states of compensation include noncompensation (reflected by an alteration in pH and $PaCO_2$ or $HCO_3$); partial compensation ($PaCO_2$, $HCO_3^-$, and pH are abnormal); and complete compensation ($PaCO_2$ and/or $HCO_3^-$ are abnormal, but pH is normal).

5. Assess oxygenation. Mild hypoxemia is indicated by a $PaO_2$ of 60–80 mmHg, moderate hypoxemia by a $PaO_2$ of 40–60 mmHg, and severe hypoxemia by $PaO_2$ < 40 mmHg. The normal value for $SaO_2$, which measures saturation of hemoglobin, is 95–100%.

6. Record the degree of compensation, the primary disorder, and oxygenation status. The relationship between oxygen content in plasma and oxygen content in hemoglobin is explained below.

## 31. What is the oxyhemoglobin dissociation curve?

The oxyhemoglobin dissociation curve describes the relationship between $PaO_2$ and $O_2$ saturation. $O_2$ saturation, which refers to the percentage of hemoglobin molecules that are fully saturated with oxygen, depends on $PaO_2$ and the amount of hemoglobin available. As $PaO_2$ levels drop, the percentage of fully saturated hemoglobin molecules decreases. When oxygen is combined with hemoglobin, oxyhemoglobin is formed. This process occurs in the lungs, where the pressure of oxygen is high. When oxyhemoglobin reaches tissues in which oxygen pressure is low, oxygen is released by hemoglobin. A fully saturated hemoglobin molecule tends to resist releasing oxygen at the tissue, where it is needed for cellular activity. Thus, when $O_2$ availability is decreased, the percentage of hemoglobin saturation drops more rapidly than $PaO_2$ levels. When a lower percentage of fully saturated hemoglobin molecules is available, the hemoglobin releases oxygen at the cell where it is needed.

## 32. What causes a shift to the right or left of the oxyhemoglobin dissociation curve?

$SaO_2$ does not fall in direct proportion to $PaO_2$ levels. It falls only slightly until the $PaO_2$ drops below 60 mmHg. Thus, $PaO_2$ is a more sensitive measure of gas exchange status than $SaO_2$. For example, a "small" decrease in $SpO_2$ (pulse oximetry) from 95% to 90% means that $PaO_2$ has decreased more significantly.

Certain factors modify the relationship between hemoglobin saturation and $PaO_2$ and change the normal relationship of the oxyhemoglobin dissociation curve. Factors that increase hemoglobin affinity for oxygen shift the curve to the left, whereas factors that decrease hemoglobin affinity for oxygen shift the curve to the right. Examples of such factors include body temperature, pH, and use of banked blood or blood that has been stored for more than 72 hours.

A **shift to the right** is caused by a low pH, fever, and increased levels of 2,3-diphosphoglyc-erate (2,3-DPG), an enzyme that decreases rapidly in old blood. With a shift to the right, the per-centage of fully saturated hemoglobin is below normal for a given $PaO_2$ level. Decreased saturation means that $O_2$ is released more readily at the cellular level, which is desirable when the $O_2$ supply is low.

A **shift to the left** is caused by a decrease in body temperature, decreased levels of 2,3-DPG, and an increase in pH. These factors increase hemoglobin affinity for oxygen, thereby decreasing availability of oxygen to tissues.

### BIBLIOGRAPHY

1. Anderson S: ABGs: Six easy steps to interpreting blood gases. Am J Nurs Aug:42–45, 1990.
2. Beachy W: Oxygen equilibrium and transport. In Roche J (ed): Respiratory Care: Anatomy and Physiology Foundations for Clinical Practice. St. Louis, Mosby, 1998, pp 134–152.
3. Czekaj LA: Promoting acid-base balance. In Kinney M, Dunbar S, Brooks-Brunn J, et al (eds): AACN's Clinical Reference for Critical Care Nursing, 4th ed. St. Louis, Mosby, 1998, pp 135–144.
4. Felver L: Acid-base balance and imbalances. In Woods SL, Sivarajan-Froelicher ES, Halpenny CJ, Underhill-Motzer S (eds): Cardiac Nursing, 3rd ed. Philadelphia, Lippincott, 1995, pp 139–146.
5. Marino PL: Acid–base interpretations. In Zinner SR (ed): The ICU Book, 2nd ed. Baltimore, Williams & Wilkins, 1997, pp 581–591.
6. Mays DA: Turn ABGs into child's play. RN Jan:36–39, 1995.
7. Stringfield YN: Back to basics: Acidosis, alkalosis, and ABGs. Am J Nurs Nov:43–44, 1993.
8. York K, Moddeman G: Arterial blood gases as easy as ABG. Assoc Operat Room Nurs J 49:1308–1329, 1989.

# 23. ENDOTRACHEAL AND TRACHEOSTOMY TUBE MANAGEMENT

*Theresa Lynn Griffin, RN, MS*

## ENDOTRACHEAL TUBES

### 1. What are the nursing responsibilities during the intubation process?

In most hospitals nurses are not responsible for intubating patients, even though they may be certified in Advanced Cardiac Life Support (ACLS) or have other certifications. Nurses in the in-tensive care unit (ICU) and nurses on hospital code teams are responsible for assisting with intu-bations. The assisting nurse should be knowledgeable about the type of equipment necessary for intubation, where it is located, and how to set it up.

### 2. What supplies and equipment are used during the intubation process?

- Endotracheal tube (ETT)
- Stylet
- Laryngoscope handle with functioning light
- Macintosh and Magill laryngoscope blades (MaC [C for curved blade] and MagiLL [L for straight blade)
- Syringe for checking and inflating the pilot balloon for the cuff
- Tape and benzoin for securing the ETT after placement

In addition, intravenous (IV) access and IV fluids should be available before the procedure is started. It is also essential to have a stethoscope for auscultating breath sounds after intubation, a suction set-up, and an ambu bag with face mask and oxygen to ventilate and hyperoxygenate the patient before intubation and between unsuccessful attempts. Pulse oximetry should be monitored throughout the procedure. It is recommended that two people tape the ETT after placement, one to hold and secure the ETT while the other tapes it.

**3. What are the nursing responsibilities immediately after the ETT is secured?**

The nurse is responsible for assessing even chest expansion, auscultating for equal breath sounds, and obtaining chest radiographs to evaluate ETT placement. If the ETT needs repositioning, the physician typically writes an order to advance or pull back the ETT a specified length in centimeters. The nurse should document the ETT position (e.g., right/left nostril or lip at 21 cm, as noted on the ETT) after intubation and per policy or hospital standard. If the ETT needs to be repositioned, suction the ETT and the back of the pharynx before deflating the cuff to minimize the chance of secretion aspiration. Reassess ETT location at lip or nostril, and auscultate breath sounds after repositioning the ETT.

**4. What are the nursing responsibilities for ETT maintenance?**

1. Monitoring and recording the ETT size and cm mark where the tube exits the patient's lip, teeth, or nostril, which help to detect accidental advancement or dislodgement of the ETT.

2. Assessment for and prevention of skin breakdown related to ETT pressure or the securing device, which include repositioning the ETT and changing the securing tape or device on a routine basis and applying topical antibiotic ointments for actual breakdown.

3. Maintaining a patent ETT by suctioning as needed and providing warm and humidified gases.

4. Providing comfort measures and minimizing anxiety with analgesia, sedation, repositioning, and ongoing communication with the patient.

**5. What are the common causes of unplanned extubations?**

Unintentional extubation (UE) is a serious and partially avoidable complication of mechanical ventilation. The main causes of UE are (1) inadequate ETT fixation, (2) improper ETT length, (3) improper ETT cuff inflation, (4) excessive weight and traction from ventilator tubing, (5) release of ETT fixation system during oral care, (6) inadequate use of restraints, (7) inadequate use of sedation, and (8) lack of staff education.

**6. What can nurses do to prevent UEs?**

A Holter type ETT fixation system is most effective for securing ETTs. To reduce traction from head turning, a swivel adapter can be incorporated into the ventilator circuit. Once the post-intubation chest radiograph has verified the proper ETT position, the excessive ETT can be cut to 1 inch beyond the mouthpiece. Excessive ETT length can act as a fulcrum and result in UE as well as in reduction in ETT lumen kinking. Proper adjustment of the ventilator side arm as well as removal of excessive water in the tubing can help to prevent the excess weight and risk of UE. Nurses can work with respiratory therapists to ensure routine assessment and management of the ETT.

UE due to agitation or coughing during oral care and retaping or repositioning of the ETT can be avoided by asking a second person to hold the ETT during the procedure. Sedation also may be necessary to minimize the patient's anxiety and restlessness. The confused or agitated patient must be adequately sedated and restrained to prevent harm due to UE and to provide comfort. Most UEs occur during weaning and are due mainly to inadequate sedation. Sedation scales make assessment of level of sedation more objective and management more consistent. Performance improvement projects using sedation scales have decreased the incidence of UEs.

**7. What complications are associated with ETTs?**

**Early complications** include cervical spine injury, ventilatory obstruction, aspiration (despite the inflated cuff), bleeding, pneumothorax, and rupture of the trachea (rare). Extubation may cause trauma to the glottis if the cuff is not deflated, and airway obstruction may result from edema.

**Late complications** include sore throat; dysphagia; hypoglossal or lingual nerve injury; vocal cord paralysis; pressure-related ulcerations of the lips, mouth, or pharynx; laryngitis; sinusitis; respiratory tract infection; stricture of the nostril from a nasal tube; laryngeal edema; and tracheal stenosis.

**8. What can nurses do to prevent complications?**

Careful attention to ETT cuff pressures and tube size, proper oral care, routine ETT care, and suctioning as needed can reduce the incidence of complications.

**9. What are advantages of oral ETTs?**

Oral ETTs are generally placed in emergency situations. It is easier to insert the ETT accurately because the vocal cords are directly visualized during the procedure. Placement of an oral ETT is generally less traumatic than placement of a nasal ETT, and epistaxis is avoided. Larger sized ETTs, which can be inserted orally, reduce the work of breathing because of less resistance to flow. A larger ETT is less difficult to suction and reduces the chance of mucus plugging or obstruction. Oral placement is preferred over nasal placement in patients with face and head trauma to avoid brain intubation when fractures are present.

**10. What are the disadvantages of oral ETTs?**

A major disadvantage of oral ETTs is the discomfort caused by pressure on the lips and in the mouth. The presence of the ETT in the mouth increases the production of oral secretions. Oral care can be more difficult. Oral ETTs are difficult to stabilize because the patient's lip, tongue, and lower jaw movements manipulate the tube. The chemical components of the ETT (polyvinyl chloride or silicone), as well as the pressure of the tube, can irritate the lips, tongue, and laryngeal areas, causing inflammation and pressure ulcers. The risk of airflow obstruction related to biting of the ETT is a potentially serious problem. Bite blocks can be used to prevent this complication.

**11. What are the advantages of nasotracheal tubes (NTTs)?**

Because NTTs are passed blindly without the use of a laryngoscope, the conscious patient is less likely to gag during insertion. The architecture of the nasal passages secures the tube better than the mouth does, and dislodgement is less likely. NTTs cause fewer laryngeal ulcerations due to the friction of frequent movement. The NTT allows the stable patient who is being weaned from the ventilator to eat soft foods and swallow oral secretions. Oral care is more efficient with an NTT, and communication is easier because the patient can move his or her lips more freely. Ulceration and trauma to the tongue, lips, teeth, and mouth are avoided. Usually, the NTT is more comfortable and better tolerated than the oral tube. NTTs are preferred for patients with seizures, tetanus, masseter muscle spasms, oral trauma, and jaw fractures.

**12. What are the disadvantages of NTTs?**

The major disadvantage of NTTs is the smaller size of the tubes. Smaller tubes have increased resistance to airflow, can be difficult to suction, and are at greater risk of mucus plugging. In addition, the location of the NTT increases the risk of frontal sinusitis and otitis media. Pain in the ear or sinus area with a slight fever may indicate infection. Sinusitis manifests as copious, colored nasal discharge that may have a foul odor. A sinus radiograph, computed tomography (CT) scan, and/or culture may be done to diagnose the infection. Nasal necrosis can develop as a result of mucosal irritation. Nurses can help to prevent this complication by limiting manipulation of the ventilator tubing with turning, suctioning, and general care. Supporting the NTT tubing with pillows or towel rolls helps to minimize the traction and pull on the tube.

**13. What are the nursing responsibilities throughout the extubation process?**

1. Immediately after extubation, the patient's mouth should be suctioned and the appropriate oxygen device applied.

2. Postextubation assessment includes observation for signs of airway obstruction and respiratory failure (e.g., audible or auscultated stridor, dyspnea, abdominal/chest paradoxical breathing, accessory muscle use, tachypnea, or bradypnea). Breath sounds should be auscultated to ensure adequate air movement and to detect any changes from baseline.

3. Ask the patient to say something to assess air movement and vocal cord function.

4. Assess the patient for pulmonary edema, which may result from changes in thoracic pressures.

5. Obtain and assess a postextubation arterial blood gas sample within the ordered time frame (i.e., 15–30 minutes) or if clinically indicated.

6. If the patient appears to have a compromised airway or respiratory distress, insert an oral airway; ventilate with a face mask (Ambu bag) at 100% oxygen, if indicated; and obtain assistance from a registered nurse, respiratory therapist, and physician.

7. Anticipate reintubation if the patient does not respond quickly to interventions.

## TRACHEOSTOMY TUBES

### 14. What are the indications for tracheostomy tubes?

A tracheotomy is a surgical opening into the trachea through which a tracheostomy tube can be passed. Indications for tracheostomy tubes are airway obstruction, ventilatory support, and/or removal of tracheobroncheal secretions. Although other routes of tracheal intubation may be easier, tracheostomy has certain distinct advantages, especially when long-term intubation and mechanical ventilation are needed. The algorithm below is an example of an approach to considering tracheotomy in respiratory patients with long-term intubation.

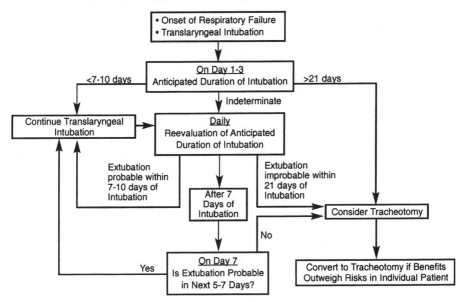

An approach to timing of tracheotomy in patients intubated and mechanically ventilated for respiratory failure. (From Godwin JE, Heffner JE: Airway management in the critically ill patient. Clin Chest Med 12:622, 1991, with permission.)

### 15. When should a tracheostomy tube be placed for ventilator weaning?

The ideal duration of translaryngeal intubation before elective tracheotomy remains controversial. The use of ETTs with high-volume, low-pressure cuffs has dramatically decreased the incidence of tracheal injury. Such tubes allow clinicians to maintain translaryngeal ETTs for longer periods without laryngeal ulceration, fistulas, or other complications associated with high-pressure cuffs. Factors to consider in deciding whether to perform a tracheotomy include the trade-off between the specific risks and benefits of each therapy. Numerous investigations since 1970 have compared patient outcomes with tracheotomy and prolonged translaryngeal intubation. Limitations of study designs and varying results among institutions prevent absolute recommendations for the timing of tracheotomy.

**16. What are the comparative benefits of tracheotomy and translaryngeal intubation?**

*Commonly Cited Benefits of Tracheotomy and Translaryngeal Intubation*

| TRACHEOTOMY | | TRANSLARYNGEAL INTUBATION | |
|---|---|---|---|
| BENEFITS | DISADVANTAGES | BENEFITS | DISADVANTAGES |
| Spares direct injury to larynx | Surgical complications | Provides reliable airway in urgent | Bacterial airway colonization |
| Facilitates nursing care | Expense | intubations | Inadvertent decannulation |
| Enhances patient mobility | Surgical scar | Well tolerated by | tion |
| Provides secure airway | Stomal stenosis | most patients | Tracheal stenosis at |
| Facilitates transfer from ICU | Tracheal stenosis at cuff site | for 1–3 wk | cuff site |
| Improves patient comfort | Tracheal erosion into adjacent structures | | Chronic laryngeal dysfunction |
| Permits speech | Bacterial airway colonization | | Purulent sinusitis (nasotracheal route) |
| Facilitates oral nutrition | nization | | |
| Provides psychological benefit | | | |

From Godwin JE, Heffner JE: Airway management in the critically ill patient. In Clin Chest Med 12:612, 1991, with permission.

**17. What are the two common types of tracheostomy tubes in the ICU? How are they used?**

Most tracheostomy tubes have **low-pressure, high-volume cuffs**. The outer cannula is inserted through the tracheotomy incision, and the wings are secured with cloth ties or a manufactured tie that is secured around the patient's neck. Some tracheostomy tube holders use Velcro® for easy adjustments. The inner cannula is either disposable or nondisposable. It is secured to the outer cannula by a turn/lock connection (nondisposable) or a clip connection (disposable).

The **fenestrated tracheostomy tube** has fenestrations (holes) in the curved part of the outer cannula that allow air to move upward through the vocal cords and to exit the mouth and nose, resulting in speech and phonation. The inner cannula must be removed for phonation, or the fenestration will be blocked. The tube cuff should be deflated to permit additional airflow around the tube as well as through the fenestrations when the patient exhales.

**18. Describe the routine care of patients with a tracheostomy tube in the ICU.**

Routine care includes assessment and documentation of the type and placement of the tracheostomy tube, the tracheotomy site and surrounding skin, and any secretions or drainage from the tube or site. Standard care also includes routinely cleaning the inner cannula to keep secretions from building up and potentially obstructing the airway.

**19. What are the components of standard skin care?**

Standard skin care includes removing the old pad, noting the quality and quantity of drainage, cleansing the stoma site with a sterile Q-tip or gauze pad soaked with normal saline or one-half strength hydrogen peroxide, and placing a $4 \times 4$ sterile pad under the tube wings.

**20. How are drainage and secretions assessed?**

It is not uncommon to have a small-to-moderate amount of tenacious secretions from the tracheotomy site. Usually they result from nasopharyngeal drainage above the tube cuff. The physician should be notified if the drainage becomes foul-smelling, the quality changes, or the skin is not intact. Treatment typically consists of topical antibiotic ointments or systemic antibiotics, as needed.

**21. How is the inner cannula cleaned or changed?**

The inner cannula should be cleaned (nondisposable type) or changed (disposable type) with aseptic technique. The patient should be hyperoxygenated and suctioned, if needed, in advance. The procedure should be done quickly (< 15 seconds) to avoid compromising the patient's oxygenation status. Explain the procedure to the patient before and during care. The nurse can minimize the torque at the tracheotomy site by supporting and positioning the ventilator tubing close to the site with a rolled towel.

**22. What techniques and devices are available to assist communication for patients with a tracheostomy tube?**
- Slow deflation of the cuff to allow speech during exhalation
- Specialized tracheostomy tubes that direct pressurized air or oxygen over the vocal cords, independent of the respiratory cycle
- Electrolarynx
- Fenestrated tracheostomy tubes (see question 17)
- Passey-Muir valve

**23. How does slow deflation of the cuff allow speech during exhalation?**
    Slow deflation of the cuff allows air movement around the cuff. This technique can be used for patients with a stable respiratory status and low minute ventilation requirements. It is important to suction the tracheostomy tube and oropharynx above the cuff to eliminate risk of aspiration when the cuff is deflated. Patients learn to time speech during exhalation and often can whisper short phrases. Brief "speaking" periods can be arranged for family visits or rounds with the team, as tolerated by the patient. The nurse should remain with the patient during these sessions and monitor for respiratory distress or hypoventilation. The cuff should be reinflated afterward. Applying 2–5 cmH$_2$O of positive end-expiratory pressure (PEEP) to ventilation adds a continuous air leak that helps to coordinate speech with the respiratory cycle.

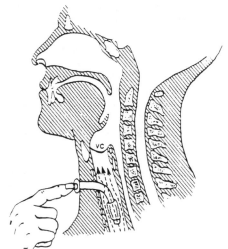

Tracheostomy tube with the cuff deflated. Expired gases can flow across the larynx. VC = vocal cords. (From Godwin JE, Heffner JE: Airway management in the critically ill patient. Clin Chest Med 12:576, 1991, with permission.)

**24. Describe the specialized tracheostomy tubes that allow speech independent of the respiratory cycle.**
    One type has Y-connector tubing that, when occluded during speaking, forces air through the top of the tracheostomy tube and the vocal cords. Problems with these devices include misdirection of the pressurized air flow and occlusion of the tube exit port with secretions or tissue. Such devices should be avoided during the first 5–7 days after tracheotomy because the air flow may cause subcutaneous and mediastinal emphysema. Vocal cord inflammation and hoarseness may result from the pressurized air. Tone generators assist speech by establishing an audible vibration that is transmitted through an air-filled cannula positioned in the posterior pharynx. The tone generator can be controlled by the patient with a hand-held button or forehead-mounted "butterfly" switch that is activated by wrinkling the brow.

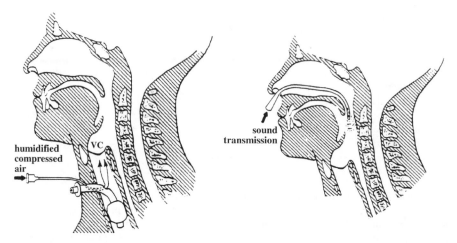

*Left,* Tracheostomy tube for speaking. With occlusion of the Y-port, an external cannula directs a flow of gas through the wall of the cannula and into the trachea, allowing speech. *Right,* Tone-generator catheter positioned in the posterior pharynx. (From Godwin JE, Heffner JE: Airway management in the critically ill patient. Clin Chest Med 12:575, 1991, with permission.)

### 25. Describe the electrolarynx.

The "electrolarynx," which has been available since 1942, consists of a hand-held vibrator that is applied midway between the mandible angle and the notch of the thyroid cartilage. It works like the larynx as an amplifier of speech. Similar to the electrolarynx are devices that emit a buzzing tone through a catheter placed in the mouth. Major problems with these devices include induction of excessive salivation and clogging of the mouth tube with secretions.

### 26. How are fenestrated tracheostomy tubes used?

Fenestrated tracheostomy tubes allow spontaneous speech in patients who are being weaned from mechanical ventilation and are able to manage periods of spontaneous ventilation. Some designs have an inner cannula that is in place during mechanical ventilation with the cuff inflated. For sessions of speech communication, the inner cannula is removed, and the tracheostomy tube is buttoned or plugged with a finger. The cuff should be deflated to allow more airflow through the vocal cords. Limitations of fenestrated tubes include occlusion of the fenestrations as granulating tissue grows into the orifice and blocks air passage.The fenestrations also may be occluded if the tube's greater curvature (location of fenestrations) does not match the patient's anatomy.

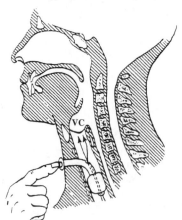

A fenestrated tracheostomy tube with the inner cannula removed allows spontaneously breathing patients to occlude the port and speak through the native airway. VC = vocal cord. (From Godwin JE, Heffner JE: Airway management in the critically ill patient. Clin Chest Med 12:576, 1991, with permission.)

### 27. How does the Passey-Muir valve work?

A Passey-Muir valve is a one-way valve that allows air to pass through the tracheostomy tube during inspiration but closes during expiration, promoting airflow through the fenestrations, around the deflated cuff, and through the vocal cords. The Passey-Muir valve fits on standard tracheostomy tubes. It is important that the cuff be deflated and that the fenestrations not be occluded. The nurse should remain with the patient to monitor for respiratory distress and tolerance of the valve.

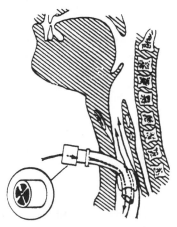

Placement of a Passey-Muir valve on a fenestrated tracheostomy tube allows spontaneous speech. (From Godwin JE, Heffner JE: Airway management in the critically ill patient. Clin Chest Med 12:577, 1991, with permission.)

### 28. What is a "buttoned" tracheostomy tube? When and how is it used?

As part of weaning from the tracheostomy tube and/or mechanical ventilation, the tracheostomy tube may be "buttoned" for increasing lengths of time until the patient is ready for decannulation. The button snaps onto the end of the tube after the cuff is deflated so that the patient can begin to breathe around the tube through the oral pharyngeal airway. The tracheostomy tube remains in place to access periods of mechanical ventilation or suctioning during weaning.

### 29. What early complications are associated with tracheotomies?

Prompt recognition and management of complications are essential to achieve positive outcomes. **Intraoperative complications** associated with tracheotomies include hemorrhage (incidence of 1–37%), pneumothorax (0–4% in adults), pneumomediastinum, tracheoesophageal fistula, recurrent laryngeal nerve injury, and cardiopulmonary arrest. Cardiopulmonary arrest is related to vasovagal reflex, failure to obtain an airway, tension pneumothorax, postoperative pulmonary edema, or misplacement of the tube into the soft tissues or main stem bronchus.

**Immediate postoperative complications** include hemorrhage, wound infection, subcutaneous emphysema, tube obstruction, displacement of the tube, and swallowing problems. Displacement of the tracheostomy tube is the most likely complication during the first 72 hours.

### 30. What causes early bleeding? How is it managed?

Bleeding may occur when a vessel with previously undetected weakness opens up with straining, coughing, or movement after the vasoactive effect of the anesthetic wears off or when the tube erodes a vessel. Prolonged oozing or oozing that starts 48–72 hours after the procedure suggests a coagulation defect. Minor oozing may be controlled with light packing. Brisk bleeding requires wound exploration. Significant bleeding 48 hours after the surgery should make the nurse suspect erosion of the innominate artery. If massive hemorrhage occurs, pressure should be applied to the innominate artery until emergency surgery can be performed to ligate the vessel. The physician can manually occlude the artery by inserting an index finger through the tracheotomy stoma to compress the artery against the sternum.

### 31. How are wound infections managed?

Postoperative tracheostomy site infection is rare because of open wound drainage. Prophylactic antibiotics are not recommended because they are ineffective in diminishing bacteria colonization and may promote resistance. True infection responds well to local treatment. Systemic antibiotics are indicated if cellulitis is present around the tracheostomy site.

### 32. What causes subcutaneous emphysema? How is it treated?

Subcutaneous emphysema (air in the soft tissue) has an incidence of 9% in the early postoperative period. It usually is caused by positive-pressure ventilation or coughing against a tight occlusive dressing or a sutured or packed wound. Subcutaneous emphysema can be noted by crepitus over the chest and neck area and is usually mild, although it can be massive and include the entire body. Treatment includes reassurance to the patient that it is a self-limited process, use of a cuffed tube, and removal of any stitches or packing around the tube. The trapped air is reabsorbed by the body within days. It is vital to obtain a chest radiograph to rule out pneumothorax.

### 33. What causes tube obstruction? How is prevented and treated?

Tube obstruction can be caused by a blood clot, mucus plugs, false passage into the soft tissues, or positioning of the opening of the cannula against a tracheal wall. Proper nursing care, suctioning, and humidification can prevent some of these complications. The inner cannula should be removed and cleaned or exchanged with a disposable inner cannula during every shift to prevent the formation of crusts that may occlude the airway.

### 34. What causes displacement of the tracheostomy tube? How is it prevented?

The tube ties can loosen with patient movement, coughing, or tension from the ventilator tubing. To prevent these complications, it is recommended that the tube ties or Velcro® straps be tied such that only one or two fingers can be placed between the tape and the neck before the dressing is applied. Suturing the tracheostomy plate to the peristomal skin after the procedure is an additional safety feature performed by some surgeons. These sutures are removed around 72 hours after the procedure when a tracheocutaneous tract has formed. In some institutions, orders are written for ear-nose-throat physicians to change the initial tube ties when they remove the sutures.

### 35. How is tube displacement recognized and treated?

Signs of tube displacement are similar to those of an obstructed airway. It also may manifest as a sudden ability of the patient to speak or the inability to pass a suction catheter through the tube. If decannulation accidentally occurs in a fresh tracheotomy patient, the nurse should support the patient's airway, ventilate with a face mask at 100% oxygen, and call the appropriate emergency team for translaryngeal intubation. If trained physicians are available, they may reintubate the trachea if they can directly visualize the tracheal rings. Unsuccessful attempts at reintubation through the trachea can lead to tube misplacement in the pretracheal fascia ("false tract"), with resultant tracheal compression and respiratory arrest.

### 36. How can a tracheostomy tube aid in nutrition?

A significant benefit of tracheostomy tubes for mechanically ventilated patients is the potential for oral nutrition. Oral consumption of food increases the patient's sense of well-being as well as helps to diminish the risks associated with parenteral and enteral feedings (e.g., infection and aspiration). Candidates for oral feedings must be clinically stable and alert. Because of aspiration risks, patients must be evaluated carefully for ability to swallow, usually by a speech therapist. Risk of aspiration is increased when a tracheostomy tube is present because the tube interferes with normal glottic function. The anchoring effect of the tube tethers the larynx, preventing the upward motion during swallowing that normally assists glottic closure. Initial feedings consist of ice chips, followed by semisoft foods. Thin liquids should be avoided. Suction equipment should be readily available.

### 37. What complications may be seen after removal of the tracheostomy tube?

After removal of the tracheostomy tube, the stoma is dressed with loose-fitting dry gauze. Most wound tracts seal within several days, although occasionally poor wound healing or stomal infection prevents closure and necessitates a stomaplasty procedure. Several factors combine to place the patient at risk after extubation. The larynx becomes desensitized during long periods of intubation and may not detect liquid or small particles around the glottis after airway decannulation. Swallowing is less than adequate for the same reason. Vocal cords also may be affected. As many as 90% of patients experience hoarseness. Speech therapy may accelerate improvement in laryngeal function, but surgical procedures may be needed in patients with severe hoarseness. Patients are also at risk for vocal cord paralysis and should be monitored for up to 6 months for signs of abnormal function.

### BIBLIOGRAPHY

1. Cook DI, Reeve BK, Guyatt GH, et al: Stress ulcer prophylaxis in critically ill patients: Resolving discordant meta-analysis. JAMA 275:308–314, 1996.
2. Godwin JE, Heffner JE: Special critical care considerations in tracheostomy management. Clin Chest Med 12:573–583, 1991.
3. Grap MJ, Munro CL: Ventilator-associated pneumonia: Clinical significance and implications for nursing. Heart Lung 26:419–429, 1997.
4. Holzapfel L, Chevret S, Madinier G, et al: Influence of long-term oro-nasotracheal intubation on nosocomial maxillary sinusitis and pneumonia: Results of a prospective, randomized, clinical trial. Crit Care Med 2:1132–1138, 1993.
5. Maguire GP, DeLorenzo LJ, Moggio RA: Unplanned extubation in the intensive care unit: A quality-of-care concern. Crit Care Nurs Q 17(3):40–47, 1994.
6. Myers EN, Carrau MR: Early complications of tracheotomy. Clin Chest Med 12:589–595, 1991.
7. Pesiri AJ: Two-year study of the prevention of unintentional extubation. Crit Care Q 17(3):35–39, 1994.
8. Pfister S, Bullas J: Caring for a patient with an endotracheal tube. Crit Care Nurse 4:29, 56–61, 1984.
9. Sanders AB, Kern KB, et al: End-tidal carbon dioxide monitoring during cardiopulmonary resuscitation. JAMA 262:1347–1351, 1989.
10. Torres A, Serra-Batles J, Ros E, et al: Pulmonary aspiration of gastric contents in patients receiving mechanical ventilation: The effect of body position. Ann Intern Med 116:540–543, 1992.

# 24. SUCTIONING

*Kristina J. Carson, RN, MS*

### 1. Define suctioning.

Suctioning is the mechanical aspiration of oral and pulmonary secretions for the purpose of maintaining a patent airway. The three types of airway suctioning are oropharyngeal, nasotracheal, and endotracheal.

### 2. Distinguish among the three types of airway suctioning.

| TYPE | SPECIFIC EQUIPMENT | TECHNIQUE | COMMENTS |
|---|---|---|---|
| Oropharyngeal | Yankauer (tonsil) or soft suction catheter Oropharyngeal airway | Clean technique Avoid: • Dislodging artificial airway • Stimulating gag reflex • Contact with uvula or open lesions • Blind suctioning Administer oral care with suctioning | Assess: • Mucous membrane integrity • Swallow • Gag reflex Oropharyngeal airway: • Holds tongue anteriorly • Aids secretion removal • Useful in cardiac arrest if intubation is not imminent |

*Table continued on following page*

| TYPE | SPECIFIC EQUIPMENT | TECHNIQUE | COMMENTS |
|---|---|---|---|
| Nasotracheal (nonintubated patient) | Soft suction catheter Water-based lubricant Nasopharyngeal airway | Suction only as needed Aseptic technique Hyperoxygenation Insert catheter on inspiration when glottis is open Nasopharyngeal airway prevents mucosal trauma with frequent suction | Contraindications • Absolute: epiglottitis, croup • Relative: nasal bleeding, occluded nasal passages, coagulopathy, head/facial/ neck trauma, laryngospasm Blind procedure with high risk of mucosal trauma May provide enough airway clearance to avoid intubation |
| Endotracheal (via ETT or tracheostomy tube) | Sterile suction catheter (either open suction or closed/in-line system) | Aseptic technique for hospitalized patients Hyperoxygenation Hyperinflation Negative pressure of –80 to –150 mmHg | Artificial airway prevents glottic closure, thus compromising cough Suction ETT/tracheostomy tube and oropharynx thoroughly before deflating cuff or extubating Most blind suctioning results in right main bronchus catheterization |

ETT = endotracheal tube.

### 3. Which critical care team members share the responsibility for suctioning?

Respiratory therapy and nursing staff commonly share the responsibility for maintaining a patent airway. Communication about patient goals, assessments related to suctioning, and specific suctioning techniques with all team members is crucial for cohesive patient care.

### 4. What concerns are of particular importance when suctioning is done outside the intensive care unit (ICU)?

Communication is especially important when nurses and respiratory therapists care for critically ill patients outside the ICU. For example, suctioning equipment may be unfamiliar or less than ideal during transport or response to cardiopulmonary arrest. The keys to maintaining a patent airway, wherever you and the patient may travel, are to know the equipment, to prepare the patient for the trip (i.e., assess, suction, and intervene accordingly), and to anticipate the sequence of necessary interventions in case of a respiratory emergency. What initially appears to be excessive preparation by the critical care team may later be life-saving.

### 5. When should patients be suctioned?

Suctioning is indicated whenever a patient is unable to clear secretions independently. Frequency of suctioning should not be based on a routine schedule but on clinical signs and symptoms. Other indications for suctioning include preparation for extubation, assessment of airway patency, cough reflex stimulation, and sputum specimen collection. Suctioning is not indicated for peripheral crackles, which are either far beyond the large central airways or caused by interstitial processes not associated with secretions.

### 6. What are the signs and symptoms of excessive secretions?

• Visible or audible secretions in the airway
• Adventitious breath sounds on auscultation (especially expiratory crackles in the central airways)
• Ineffective cough
• Increased work of breathing
• Increased peak inspiratory pressures (with volume-controlled mechanical ventilation)

• Decreased tidal volumes (with pressure-controlled mechanical ventilation)
• Suspected aspiration of gastric or upper airway secretions
• Deteriorating arterial blood gas values
• Decreasing oxygen saturation
• Radiologic changes consistent with retention of pulmonary secretions

7. **What are the potential complications of endotracheal suctioning?**

• Increased mucous production
• Mucosal trauma
• Interruption of mechanical ventilation
• Bronchospasm
• Atelectasis
• Pulmonary bleeding or hemorrhage
• Infection
• Nosocomial pneumonia
• Hypoxemia

• Respiratory arrest
• Hypotension
• Hypertension
• Cardiac dysrhythmias or arrest (especially bradycardia or asystole due to mechanical stimulation of the vagus nerve)
• Increased intracranial pressure
• Pain
• Anxiety

8. **What are the contraindications for endotracheal suctioning?**

Despite the long list of potential negative effects of endotracheal suctioning, there are no absolute contraindications. Avoidance of suctioning may result in potentially lethal complications. Therefore, the risks of endotracheal suctioning need to be balanced against the benefits of pulmonary secretion clearance for the patient's current clinical condition.

9. **What type of catheter should be used for suctioning?**

Suction catheters are made of polyvinylchloride, a clear material that allows visualization of aspirated secretions and is soft enough to insert into the endotracheal tube (ETT) without lubricant. The suction catheter should be no larger than half of the internal diameter of the artificial airway (i.e., usually 12–16 French). For example, a 14-French catheter has a 4-mm outer diameter for use with an 8.0-mm ETT, thus allowing gas flow around the catheter during suctioning. The catheter must be long enough to extend approximately 2 inches (5 cm) beyond the end of the ETT. More than one hole ("eye") at the catheter tip allows greater contact with secretions, facilitates removal, and minimizes mucosal trauma caused by catheter adherence. Some catheters have directional tips to aid in entering the left or right bronchus selectively.

10. **What other equipment is needed for suctioning?**

A collection cannister is attached to both the suction catheter and the vacuum source using connective tubing. A calibrated, adjustable regulator is used to set the negative suction pressure at –80 to –150 mmHg. The goal of clearing secretions without mucosal trauma can be difficult to achieve in some patients because pressures of –50 to –100 mmHg may be too low for adequate vacuum through the catheter but still damage the mucosa.

Sterile supplies necessary for tracheal suction, available in prepackaged kits, include a single-use, disposable suction catheter, a reservoir for water/saline to clear the catheter, and gloves. The health professional should exercise universal precautions, using goggles, mask, and other protective equipment. Additional equipment for suctioning includes an oxygen source, manual resuscitation bag (if the ventilator is not used), stethoscope, and monitoring equipment.

11. **Why is hyperoxygenation with tracheal suctioning important?**

Research has shown that hyperoxygenation before tracheal suctioning mitigates the hypoxemia, increased mean arterial pressure (MAP), increased peak inspiratory pressure (PIP), changes in cardiac output, and heart rate variations associated with suctioning and aggravated by successive suction passes. To prevent such negative outcomes of suctioning and to maximize arterial partial pressure of oxygen ($PaO_2$) and arterial oxygen saturation ($SaO_2$), researchers consistently recommend using hyperoxygenation with the mechanical ventilator. Another method to prevent postsuctioning hypoxemia is hyperinflation with a manual resuscitation bag (MRB) or the sigh function on the ventilator.

### 12. What is hyperoxygenation?

Hyperoxygenation is the delivery of 100% oxygen given in 3–5 breaths before, between, and after passes of the suction catheter to minimize suction-induced decreases in $PaO_2$.

### 13. How is hyperoxygenation achieved during tracheal suctioning?

To deliver 100% oxygen, turn the flowmeter up to 10–15 L/min. If the patient is unable to breathe spontaneously, hyperoxygenation can be accomplished with either an oxygen-enriched MRB or the temporary oxygen-enrichment program available on microprocessor ventilators. Two minutes of "washout time" are required to prime the ventilator tubing with 100% oxygen. The resident lung gas is exchanged for 100% oxygen to offset what is lost through catheter aspiration and metabolic consumption during suctioning. Many facilities discourage a manual change in the ventilator setting for fraction of inspired oxygen ($FiO_2$) in fear that the $FiO_2$ will not be reset to baseline level after suctioning.

### 14. Which is better for hyperoxygenation—the MRB or the ventilator?

Mastery of the MRB depends on operator skill and hand size; administering specific and consistent tidal volumes with the MRB is difficult. Although some clinicians prefer to "feel" the secretions in the airway and coordinate hyperinflation with the patient's inspiratory efforts, research supports the use of the ventilator over the MRB. In select pulmonary populations, higher $PaO_2$, higher $SaO_2$, and lower PIP levels were noted when the ventilator was used instead of the MRB to hyperoxygenate before suctioning.

### 15. Why is hyperinflation important during tracheal suctioning?

Hyperinflation improves oxygenation by increasing functional residual capacity (FRC), which minimizes intrapulmonary shunt.

### 16. How is hyperinflation achieved during tracheal suctioning?

Hyperinflation involves administering tidal volumes greater than the patient's baseline (usually 150% times normal). If the patient is unable to breathe deeply when asked, hyperinflation can be accomplished by using an MRB or the manual inspiration/sigh function on a ventilator. Care must be exercised in administering hyperinflation breaths to avoid barotrauma or decreased venous return.

### 17. What technique is recommended for tracheal suctioning?

1. The suction catheter is placed through the artificial airway into the trachea and intermittent negative pressure is applied only as the catheter is withdrawn. This process constitutes one suction pass.

2. To ease insertion during nasotracheal suction, lubricate the catheter with a small amount of water-soluble lubricant.

3. To prevent aspiration of mucosa, withdraw the catheter approximately 1 cm before applying suction.

4. Twirl or rotate the catheter in a smooth, constant motion so that the "eyes" of the catheter are exposed to a larger surface area; this motion is believed to remove the largest amount of secretions and to prevent mucosal aspiration.

5. Although both continuous and intermittent suction may cause mucosal trauma, intermittent suction may not effectively clear the airway. For these reasons, clinical experts no longer recommend intermittent suction over continuous suction.

6. Each pass should be no more than 10 seconds, because the fall in $PaO_2$ is related to suction duration.

7. Limit suction passes to the minimal number necessary to clear the airway; do not use more than three passes. Because research indicates a stepwise increase in intracranial pressure

(ICP) with each suction pass, patients with increased ICP should be suctioned only if necessary and then with no more than two passes.

8. Minimal recovery time between suction passes should be 20–30 seconds.

9. Clear thick secretions out of the suction catheter between passes and afterward with sterile water or saline. In the closed system, squirt the solution directly into the catheter while applying suction to clear the catheter.

### 18. What nursing interventions facilitate tracheal suctioning?

1. Before suctioning, position the patient to facilitate coughing (semi-Fowler's to high Fowler's position, if tolerated) and explain the procedure.

2. Research has shown that suctioning is a painful procedure for many patients. Therefore, pain should be assessed and treated accordingly, preferably before suctioning.

3. Because the goal is independent airway maintenance, encourage the patient to take deep breaths during hyperoxygenation and to cough when suction is applied, if possible.

4. Assess tube patency during suctioning, and do not apply suction during catheter insertion.

5. Difficulty with introducing the suction catheter, excessive coughing, and localized expiratory wheeze may be caused by tenacious secretions. In association with bilateral decreased breath sounds, these signs may indicate low tube placement at the level of the carina.

6. Maintain aseptic technique and use universal precautions, especially eye protection, during suctioning.

7. After suctioning the lower airway with aseptic technique, use the same catheter with clean technique for oropharyngeal care. Suction the oropharynx to remove secretions that pool in the mouth and on top of the ETT cuff in the back of the throat.

### 19. How does patient assessment relate to suctioning?

The patient should be assessed before, during, and after suctioning. Know where and why you are suctioning, and assess the patient appropriately beforehand. Assessments include:

- Respirations (rate, depth, pattern, changes)
- Work of breathing
- Breath sounds on auscultation (clear, normal, adventitious)
- Cough (character, ability to expectorate)
- Sputum (amount, color, character, odor, changes)
- Oxygen saturation
- Vital signs (including cardiac rhythm)
- Intracranial pressure
- Arterial blood gases
- Skin (color, temperature, diaphoresis)

Because suctioning is a noxious stimulus, it is relevant to the neurologic examination. In unconscious patients, monitor for decorticate/decerebrate posturing with suctioning, and assess the gag reflex (cranial nerves IX and X). Any changes in assessments during suctioning may require cessation of the procedure, hyperoxygenation, and subsequent intervention. Ensure that vital signs have returned to baseline before a subsequent suction pass. Assess breath sounds by auscultating before and after suctioning; document any changes.

### 20. Describe the components and proper use of a closed tracheal suction system.

A closed tracheal suction system includes a suction catheter housed in a plastic sheath, an irrigation port for solution instillation, and a thumb-activated suction control valve. Adapters attach the system to the ventilator circuitry; the resulting in-line system is designed to maintain oxygenation during suctioning. When the suction catheter is not in use, it is completely withdrawn into the plastic sleeve. If the closed suction system is disconnected, cover the open end with a sterile barrier to prevent contamination or change the catheter. Although the in-line suction system is closed, health care providers still need to wear gloves.

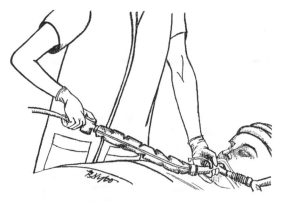

In-line tracheal suction.

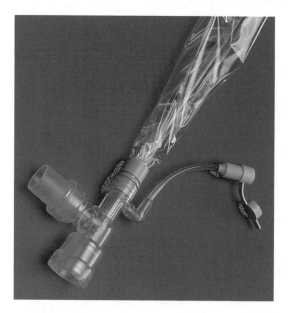

T-piece design of the TRACH CARE®
closed suction system. This product is
manufactured by Kimberly Clark-Ballard,
Draper, Utah 84020.

## 21. What are the advantages and disadvantages of a closed tracheal suction system?

The closed tracheal suction system maintains an uninterrupted oxygen supply, positive end-expiratory pressure (PEEP), and positive-pressure ventilation. Maintenance of positive-pressure ventilation and PEEP are cited as advantages of closed suctioning, but if suction flow rates are not lower than ventilator flow rates, excessive negative airway pressure may result. Other advantages include the ease of suctioning copious secretions and containment of blood or contaminated airborne particles (e.g., tuberculosis). Studies have recorded fewer dysrhythmias, increased $SaO_2$, and increased mixed venous oxygen saturation ($SvO_2$) with closed tracheal suction compared with decreased $SaO_2$, decreased $SvO_2$, and increased MAP with open suction.

## 22. How often should in-line catheters be changed?

Current research demonstrates that nosocomial pneumonia occurs no more frequently in patients whose in-line suction catheters are changed daily than in patients whose catheters are changed only when they are soiled or damaged. Eliminating daily changes of in-line catheters is safe for patients and health care workers, who thus minimize exposure to secretions. Cost estimates vary, but eliminating daily catheter changes saves both catheter costs and nursing time.

### 23. Why is saline lavage no longer recommended during endotracheal suctioning?

Current research has not demonstrated that normal saline lavage before endotracheal suctioning liquefies pulmonary secretions or enhances secretion clearance. The saline is in contact with secretions too briefly and in amounts too small to affect viscosity, and it is no more effective than a suction catheter in inducing a cough reflex. Although the saline does not disperse far beyond the mainstem bronchi, the flow of saline may dislodge bacteria colonized along the artificial airway and wash these potential contaminants into lower airways. Using pulse oximetry and $SvO_2$ to evaluate small samples of critically ill patients before, during, and after endotracheal suctioning, researchers have documented decreases in oxygen saturation with slower return to patient baseline as a result of saline lavage.

### 24. What is recommended instead of saline lavage to mobilize secretions?

Artificial airway humidification, systemic hydration, mucolytic agents, and nebulizer treatments.

### 25. What are the potential consequences of not suctioning?

The primary consequence of not suctioning is retained pulmonary secretions; their accumulation eventually alters gas exchange in the patient's pulmonary passages or in the artificial airway lumen. An artificial airway is a foreign body that impairs ciliary movement and stimulates increased production of mucous. Inspired air that is inadequately humidified irritates delicate pulmonary membranes and dries out secretions. Retained pulmonary secretions become a medium for bacterial growth. Potential outcomes include dyspnea, atelectasis, increased work of breathing, hypoxemia, hypercapnea, infection, and airway occlusion.

### BIBLIOGRAPHY

1. American Association for Respiratory Care (AARC) clinical practice guideline: Endotracheal suctioning of mechanically ventilated adults and children with artificial airways. Respir Care 38:500–504, 1993.
2. American Association for Respiratory Care (AARC) clinical practice guideline: Nasotracheal suctioning. Respir Care 37:898–901, 1992.
3. Dettenmeier PA: Invasive techniques for improving oxygenation and ventilation. In Pulmonary Nursing Care. St. Louis, Mosby-Year Book, 1992, pp 312–317.
4. Grap MJ, Glass C, Corley M, et al: Endotracheal suctioning: Ventilator vs. manual delivery of hyperoxygenation breaths. Am J Crit Care 5:192–197, 1996.
5. Johnson K, Kearney P, Johnson S, et al: Closed versus open endotracheal suctioning: Costs and physiologic consequences. Crit Care Med 22:658–666, 1994.
6. Luce J, Pierson D, Tyler M: Methods of airway maintenance. In Intensive Respiratory Care, 2nd ed. Philadelphia, W. B. Saunders, 1993, pp 127–133.
7. Pierce L: Lung expansion therapy and bronchial hygiene. In Guide to Mechanical Ventilation and Intensive Respiratory Care. Philadelphia, W.B. Saunders, 1995, pp 130–135.
8. Raymond SJ: Normal saline instillation before suctioning: Helpful or harmful? A review of the literature. Am J Crit Care 4:267–271, 1995.
9. St. John RE: The pulmonary system. In Alspach JG (ed): AACN Core Curriculum for Critical Care Nursing, 5th ed. Philadelphia, W.B. Saunders, 1998, pp 1–136.
10. Stone KS: Ventilator versus manual resuscitation bag as the method for delivering hyperoxygenation before endotracheal suctioning. AACN Clin Issues Crit Care Nurs 1:289–299, 1990.

# 25. STATUS ASTHMATICUS

Lisa M. Boulais, RN, MS, CCRN, CEN

**1. What is status asthmaticus?**

Status asthmaticus is an unstable, life-threatening illness in which severe asthmatic symptoms fail to respond to conventional therapeutic interventions. Patients with status asthmaticus experience extreme airway obstruction, ventilatory compromise, and potential respiratory failure. They require aggressive treatment, which may include admission to an intensive care unit, a complicated medication regimen, tracheal intubation, and mechanical ventilation.

**2. How does an acute asthma exacerbation progress to status asthmaticus?**

Many asthmatic patients progress to this level of disease as a result of a diminished sensation of dyspnea and respiratory deterioration. In addition, they possess a greater tolerance to airflow obstruction. Combined, these phenomena allow the patient to delay seeking medical treatment until symptoms become severe.

Some patients who progress to status asthmaticus may have experienced a rapid onset of symptoms. Typically, asthma symptoms develop over a period of 24–48 hours. In status asthmaticus, acute symptoms may develop over a few hours. When symptoms progress over such a short time, it is often difficult to gain control with traditional therapy.

**3. What risk factors predispose an asthmatic patient to status asthmaticus?**

- History of two hospitalizations or three emergency department visits over the past 12 months.
- Sudden onset of symptoms
- History of intubation
- Multiple antiasthmatic drugs
- Psychiatric or socioeconomic challenges

**4. Describe the typical clinical presentation of patients with status asthmaticus.**

Patients in status asthmaticus experience bronchospasm, increased mucus production, and impaired gas exchange. The clinical presentation demonstrates severe airflow obstruction. The patient may report dyspnea, difficulty in breathing, chest tightness, and nonproductive cough. Clinical findings may include use of accessory muscles, tachypnea, fragmented speech, diaphoresis, tachycardia, and pulsus paradoxus. Depending on the degree of air flow, wheezing may or may not be heard. Signs of impending respiratory failure include decreased air sounds, diminished oxygen saturation, decreased respiratory effort, and an altered level of consciousness.

**5. Which tests help to guide therapy?**

**Peak expiratory flow rates** (PEFRs) should be monitored to determine the severity of airflow obstruction and to assess the effectiveness of therapy. PEFRs should be compared with the patient's baseline. Less than 60% of the baseline for PEFR is an indication of severe airway obstruction.

**Arterial blood gas** (ABG) sampling identifies acid-base status, arterial oxygen tension and degree of hypoxemia, and arterial $CO_2$ tension and adequacy of ventilation. With severe airflow obstruction, ABGs generally exhibit an increasing $PaCO_2$. However, repeat ABGs are not necessary.

**Chest radiographs** are *not* done on a routine basis but may be considered if pneumonia, pneumothorax, or atelectasis is suspected.

**Electrocardiography** (ECG) is *not* done on a routine basis but may be considered for patients who are at risk for cardiac disease. The ECG should be examined for cardiac ischemia, axis deviation, and atrial or ventricular ectopy.

Clinical deterioration or improvement can be determined through frequent assessments.

**6. Should a sputum sample be obtained?**

A sputum sample may be obtained if infection is suspected. The sputum from an asthmatic patient may look purulent. However, it is typically composed of eosinophils, epithelial cells, and bronchiolar casts. If the patient does not improve with aggressive treatment or exhibits signs of infection such as fever or abnormal chest radiograph, a sputum sample should be collected.

**7. What are the goals of therapy for status asthmaticus?**

The goals of therapy for status asthmaticus are to reverse severe airflow obstruction and to improve the exchange of oxygen and carbon dioxide. Methods include reduction of airway inflammation and relief of bronchospasm through aggressive use of pharmacologic agents. If drug therapy is not effective, tracheal intubation and mechanical ventilation may be required.

**8. Which medications are helpful in treating status asthmaticus?**

To prevent respiratory failure, the treatment of status asthmaticus must be rapid and intense. Standard therapy includes oxygen, bronchodilators, and anti-inflammatory agents. In some instances, an anticholinergic medication is added to the therapeutic regimen.

**9. What is the goal of oxygen therapy?**

Because of bronchospasm, airway inflammation, and sputum production, profound hypoxemia and ventilation/perfusion mismatch are common findings in patients with status asthmaticus. Supplemental oxygen should be administered to improve systemic oxygen delivery. The goal of oxygen delivery is to maintain $SaO_2 > 90\%$.

**10. Which agents may be used as bronchodilators?**

Beta$_2$ agonists are used to reverse bronchoconstriction in status asthmaticus. Inhaled beta$_2$ agonists such as albuterol should be delivered in a wet, nebulized form. The onset of action is rapid. Nebulized treatments may be given at 20–30-minute intervals or continuously, as the clinical picture demands. In ventilated patients, nebulized beta$_2$ agonists can be delivered through the ventilator tubing. However, for optimal bronchodilatory effects, higher doses are typically required.

**11. Which anti-inflammatory agents may be used?**

Corticosteroids are used in status asthmaticus as adjunctive therapy to reduce airway inflammation and to allow bronchodilators to work more effectively. An intravenous steroid such as methylprednisolone should be administered as soon as possible and every 6 hours over a 24-hour period.

**12. What is the role of anticholinergic agents?**

Anticholinergics are not considered first-line drugs in the treatment of status asthmaticus. The onset of bronchodilatory action is slower and less significant than that of beta$_2$ agonists. However, if symptoms fail to respond to bronchodilators and anti-inflammatory therapy, ipratropium bromide may be added to the treatment regimen. Given in a wet, nebulized form, anticholinergics may augment the bronchodilatory effects of beta$_2$ agonists and improve airflow.

**13. Is theophylline still used in the treatment of status asthmaticus?**

Theophylline is not recommended for the treatment of status asthmaticus. Because of its narrow therapeutic margin, theophylline has been replaced with beta agonists as the drug of choice for bronchodilation. However, many practitioners continue to use theophylline for the treatment of status asthmaticus. If theophylline is used, drug levels must be monitored closely. Children, elderly people, and patients with liver or cardiac disease are particularly susceptible to theophylline toxicity.

**14. What other pharmacologic agents are used to manage status asthmaticus?**

Several unproven pharmacologic agents are used in the treatment of status asthmaticus. Although they are not first-line drugs, they may benefit patients who are slow to respond to previously described therapies.

The use of **magnesium sulfate** is controversial. However, because of its ability to relieve bronchospasm, magnesium sulfate may be beneficial to patients with status asthmaticus. The drug may be given intravenously or by inhalation.

**Heliox,** a mixture of helium and oxygen, may be used to increase ventilation and minimize the effort required for breathing. Because it is less dense than air, heliox decreases airway resistance and enhances gas flow. It can be administered by non-rebreathing face mask or through mechanical ventilation.

Inhaled **furosemide** may be used not for its diuretic effects, but for its protective abilities. Furosemide weakens the ability of stimuli to induce bronchoconstriction. It also may prevent the release of cells participating in the bronchoconstrictor cascade.

**Isoflurane** is an inhalational anesthetic that can be used to provide sedation and bronchodilation for patients with severe asthma. It is administered via the ventilator circuit or an anesthesia ventilator and machine.

### 15. When is assisted ventilation indicated?

Clearly, the patient who becomes apneic or experiences a significant decrease in respiratory rate should be intubated. Of course, not all patients exhibit this obvious clinical picture. In the alert, conscious patient, tracheal intubation and mechanical ventilation may be required if aggressive therapy results in no improvement.

It is important to consider the clinical picture and general appearance of the patient. A decreasing level of consciousness, increasing work of breathing, rising $PCO_2$, and respiratory fatigue are strong indications for tracheal intubation. Anticipating the need for intubation is crucial. It is best to intubate semielectively rather than emergently.

### 16. How does mechanical ventilation for status asthmaticus differ from mechanical ventilation for other conditions?

Patients with status asthmaticus are at particular risk for developing barotrauma as a result of positive-pressure ventilation. The disease process creates an airflow obstruction that affects both inspiratory and expiratory air movement. Because of expiratory airflow obstruction, the alveoli become hyperinflated as a result of gas trapping (auto-PEEP). Positive-pressure ventilation can produce significant airway pressures, reduce alveolar emptying, and exacerbate hyperinflation.

### 17. What measures reduce the risk of barotrauma?

The expiratory time may be lengthened to allow additional time for the alveoli to empty. In addition, the tidal volume may be lowered from the normal level of 10–12 ml/kg to a level of 7–9 ml/kg to minimize alveolar hyperinflation and barotrauma.

### 18. What other measures facilitate mechanical ventilation and prevent associated complications?

- Minimal or no PEEP
- High inspiratory flow rates
- Routine assessment for auto-PEEP
- Monitoring for signs of gas trapping
- Adequate sedation, analgesia, and/or neuromuscular blocking agents, if necessary

### 19. Why has the mortality rate from asthma increased?

Despite improved understanding of asthma pathophysiology and advances in therapeutic modalities, the mortality rate from asthma is on the rise. The reason is unclear. However, it has been suggested that undertreatment and inappropriate treatment play a key role.

Outpatient pharmacologic treatment can be complicated. Patients may not fully understand the disease process, their drug regimen, or the severity of their symptoms. In addition, patients may lack social support and financial resources for medication supply and routine follow-up care. Consequently, they may delay seeking medical care in the face of acute symptoms. Early and intensive treatment of symptoms is crucial.

## BIBLIOGRAPHY

1. Corbridge TC, Hall JB: The assessment and management of adults with status asthmaticus. Am J Respir Crit Care Med 151:1296–1316, 1995.
2. Cohen NH, Eigen H, Shaughnessy TE: Status asthmaticus. Crit Care Clin 13: 459–476, 1997.
3. Freichels TA: Managing mechanical ventilation in status asthmaticus. Dimens Crit Care Nurs 17:2–10, 1998.
4. Kavuru MS, Pien L, Litwin D, et al: Asthma: Current controversies and emerging therapies. Cleve Clin J Med 62: 293–304, 1995.
5. Leatherman J: Life-threatening asthma. Clin Chest Med 15:453–478, 1994.
6. Levy KD, Kitch B, Fanta CH: Medical and ventilatory management of status asthmaticus. Intens Care Med 24:105–117, 1998.
7. National Institutes of Health, National Heart, Lung, and Blood Institute: Practical guide for the diagnosis and management of asthma (NIH Publ. No. 97-4053). Washington, DC, National Institutes of Health, 1997.

# 26. NONINVASIVE POSITIVE-PRESSURE VENTILATION

*Brian M. Daniel, RCP, RRT*

### 1. What is noninvasive positive-pressure ventilation (NPPV)?

NPPV is the use of mechanical ventilation without an endotracheal tube or tracheostomy in place. During NPPV air enters the nose, mouth, or both by way of a nasal mask, mouthpiece, or face mask that covers the nose and mouth, respectively, each of which is connected to a positive-pressure machine. NPPV provides bilevel or biphasic (BiPAP) positive pressure. The use of this strategy dates back to the 1960s when NPPV, in the form of intermittent positive-pressure breathing (IPPB), was successfully used to lower carbon dioxide levels in patients with chronic obstructive pulmonary disease (COPD) and acute or chronic carbon dioxide retention.

### 2. How does NPPV differ from continuous positive airway pressure (CPAP)?

NPPV differs from CPAP in that it provides ventilatory assistance, whereas CPAP provides only constant positive pressure, usually through the nose.

### 3. What are the advantages of NPPV?

The primary advantage of NPPV is avoidance of the complications associated with an artificial airway tube, such as injury to the larynx and trachea. Nosocomial pneumonia (1–3% incidence every day that a patient is intubated) and sinusitis also can be avoided with NPPV. In addition, the patient feels less isolated and, depending on the interface (nasal vs. oronasal), may be able to drink, eat, and phonate.

### 4. What are the disadvantages of NPPV?

Whether by NPPV or conventional mechanical ventilation, positive-pressure ventilation is still evolving. The patient is at risk for all of the hazards and complications associated with increasing intrathoracic pressure. At least one study suggests that NPPV may lead to an increased incidence of myocardial infarction. Another disadvantage is related to the selection criteria. NPPV may delay appropriate intubation in patients who are medically unstable, cannot fit the mask, or have excessive secretions.

### 5. Which clinical conditions most benefit from NPPV?

Most of the success observed to date with NPPV has been in patients with various forms of hypercapneic respiratory failure. Examples include COPD exacerbations, neuromuscular disorders, chest wall deformities, and nocturnal hypoventilation. Compelling data also suggest that patients with hydrostatic pulmonary edema, a form of hypoxemic respiratory failure, benefit from NPPV, particularly when hypoxemia is accompanied by hypercapnea.

### 6. What are the selection criteria for NPPV?

*Guidelines for the Use of Noninvasive Ventilation for Acute Respiratory Failure*

---

1. Acute respiratory failure with at least two of the following:
   • Acute respiratory acidosis
   • Respiratory distress
   • Accessory muscle use
2. Partial pressure of carbon dioxide in arterial blood ($PaCO_2$) > 55 mmHg
3. Baseline arterial pH > 7.22
4. Hemodynamic stability
5. No evidence of upper airway obstruction
6. No excessive secretions

---

### 7. What is the role of NPPV in hypoxemic respiratory failure?

Hydrostatic pulmonary edema, acute respiratory distress syndrome (ARDS), pneumonia, and postoperative hypoxemia fall into the category of hypoxemic respiratory failure. Affected patients may not have carbon dioxide retention. Several controlled studies suggest that CPAP is highly effective in patients with hydrostatic pulmonary edema. In patients who remain uncomfortably dyspneic or begin to retain carbon dioxide, NPPV is a reasonable option that has been shown to be effective. Further studies are needed to determine whether NPPV is useful in patients with pneumonia or ARDS.

### 8. What equipment is necessary for noninvasive positive NPPV?

A ventilator and patient-ventilator interface are essential components of the NPPV system. The ventilator may be pressure-targeted or volume-targeted and can be set to assist and/or control ventilation. The therapist should select a ventilator that will achieve the goals of decreasing the work of breathing and correcting gas exchange abnormalities. Ventilator selection depends largely on the disease process and where the therapy will be provided (intensive care unit [ICU] or acute ward).

Available patient-ventilator interfaces include nasal mask, nasal pillows, and oronasal mask. Different types of interfaces should be available because facial contours vary and the interfaces fit individual patients differently. The interface must fit comfortably with minimal leak. If signs of pressure breakdown are noted, it is helpful to alternate types of interfaces. To date, no data suggest an advantage to one interface over the others. Patient comfort and cooperation with therapy should be considered in selecting the type of ventilator and interface. (See figures at top of following page.)

### 9. Is there an advantage to using an ICU ventilator as opposed to the BiPAP machine commonly used on regular wards?

Various ventilators have been used for NPPV. The choice of ventilator should depend on the type of respiratory failure and the capabilities of the particular ventilator. ICU ventilators offer better monitoring and more sophisticated alarms. They also allow the therapist to control precisely high levels of fractional concentration of oxygen in inspired air ($FiO_2$). In patients with hypoxemic respiratory failure the ability to deliver 100% oxygen is important. ICU ventilators (particularly the newer ones) use algorithms to allow adjustments in the rate of rise to pressure (rise time) and termination of inspiratory flow. However, the gap between ICU ventilators and conventional BiPAP machines is closing. BiPAP machines are beginning to incorporate similar types of enhancements.

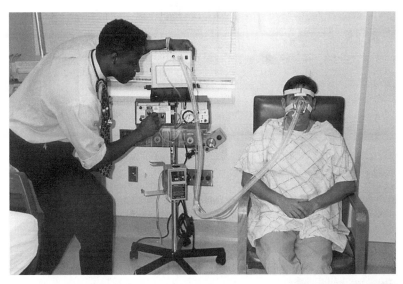

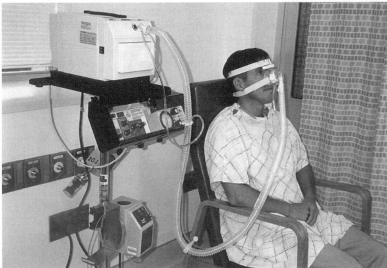

Demonstration of NPPV with a nasal mask. The respiratory therapist adjusts the inspiratory pressure support level and checks for proper mask fit. The nasal mask is less claustrophobic than the full-face mask. Both types of masks must be fitted properly to achieve minimal air leak and minimal pressure on the skin. (From Parsons PE, Wiener-Kronish JP (eds): Critical Care Secrets, 2nd ed. Philadelphia, Hanley & Belfus, 1998, with permission.)

## 10. What are the potential complications of NPPV?

Most of the potential complications associated with NPPV have been linked to the mask:
- Pressure sores on the bridge of nose
- Nasal and mucosal drying
- Corneal irritation from air blowing into the eyes
- Skin irritation due to tight mask fit or, occasionally, allergy
- Claustrophobia (usually with full-face mask)
- Patient-ventilator dyssynchrony (excessive leak around the mask makes flow termination difficult)
- Gastric distention from swallowing air
- Increased risk of aspiration
- Difficulty in wearing corrective lenses

### 11. What is involved in the care of patients receiving NPPV?

Monitoring depends on where NPPV is instituted and the severity of illness. Patients on the regular ward probably should be close to the nursing station so that alarms can be easily heard. Alternatively, the machine may have some type of remote alarm to alert the nurse to problems. Continuous pulse oximetry is a reasonable option for monitoring, particularly for patients receiving NPPV because of hypoxemic respiratory failure. Patients in the ICU have the benefit of sophisticated monitoring (e.g., telemetry).

No device takes the place of an experienced practitioner in ensuring patient cooperation and hence a successful outcome. Verbal and nonverbal communication is key to success. Inexperience and lack of confidence on the part of the practitioner are communicated rapidly to the patient.

### 12. How is the effectiveness of NPPV assessed clinically?

Successful initiation of NPPV requires clinical expertise and a moderate amount of time for monitoring and management. The respiratory therapist or nurse can spend as long as an hour providing reassurance and adjusting the machine to meet the patient's needs. Clinical assessment of the effectiveness of NPPV includes the following:

1. Observe the patient for synchrony with the ventilator.
2. Evaluate patient comfort.
3. Assess vital signs, including respiratory rate and oxygenation. Respiratory rates should be < 25 breaths/minute.
4. Adjust tidal volumes in the range of 4–8 ml/kg or until good chest movement is observed.
5. Auscultate breath sounds.
6. Look for signs of improved dyspnea scores.
7. Assess the patient for increased work of breathing (paradoxical breathing and accessory muscle use).
8. Monitor arterial blood gases for changes in oxygenation and ventilation. A decrease in $PaCO_2$ of 5–12 mmHg in the first hour is desirable and suggests that the patient is effectively ventilated.

### 13. What ventilator settings are prescribed for NPPV?

The prescribed NPPV settings depend on the type of machine and interface. In general a pressure-targeted mode (i.e., pressure support ventilation [PSV]) is tolerated well because inspiratory flow varies to meet patient demand. A volume-targeted mode may be used, but because the inspiratory flow is "fixed," dyssynchrony between patient and ventilator usually is increased. Inspiratory pressure (peak inspiratory pressure [PIP], PSV, or inspiratory positive airway pressure [IPAP]) should be ordered to achieve a tidal volume of 4–8 ml/kg.

Peak inspiratory pressures > 25 $cmH_2O$ should be avoided for patients using the full-face mask because of complications associated with gastric distention and aspiration. If gastric distention becomes a problem, a nasogastric tube can be inserted for decompression. However, be aware that the tube interferes with mask fit and may cause a leak.

Positive end-expiratory pressure (PEEP) of 4–8 $cmH_2O$ should be prescribed to counterbalance auto-PEEP, which commonly occurs in patients with respiratory failure due to COPD exacerbation. In patients using a full-face mask, PEEP also helps to prevent the rebreathing of carbon dioxide by lavaging the mask. Set the inspiratory time to match closely the patient's inspiratory effort when the assist or control, volume or pressure modes are used. Inspiratory times are usually short (≤ 1.0 seconds).

Acclimate the patient to the system by gradually adjusting the settings to meet the goals of therapy. It is prudent to start with low pressures (PEEP of ~3 $cmH_2O$ and inspiratory pressure of ~ 6 $cmH_2O$) and gradually increase until effective ventilation is achieved.

### 14. Where does the use of NPPV stand at the present time?

To date, at least 850 patients have been enrolled in various phases of clinical trials with both positive and negative results. These studies assess safety, efficacy, and outcome. According to one phase-3, multicenter study, NPPV is the modality of choice in patients with acute respiratory failure due to COPD exacerbation. Patients with restrictive lung disease due to thoracic cage abnormalities, slowly progressive neuromuscular conditions, or nocturnal hypoventilation derive some benefit from NPPV. Recently interest has increased in instituting NPPV in patients with ARDS and similar forms of hypoxemic respiratory failure (without hypercapnea). However the data in such patients (with the exception of cardiogenic pulmonary edema) have not been conclusive.

Crucial questions for future research include the following: Is there a cost benefit to NPPV? What physiologic indicators are important in determining benefit? Can we determine optimal initiation and follow-up strategies? Although these and other questions remain unanswered, NPPV is an important technology that will increase in use over the next decade. Efficacy will depend largely on evolving specific selection criteria (see question 6).

### BIBLIOGRAPHY

1. Antonelli M, Conti G, Rocco M, et al: A comparison of noninvasive positive-pressure ventilation and conventional mechanical ventilation in patients with acute respiratory failure. N Engl J Med 39:429–435, 1998.
2. Brochard L, Mancebo J, Wysocki M, et al: Noninvasive ventilation for acute exacerbations of COPD. N Engl J Med 333:817–822, 1995.
3. Criner GJ, Brennan K, Travaline JM, Kreimer D: Efficacy and compliance with noninvasive positive pressure ventilation in patients with chronic respiratory failure. Chest 116:667–675, 1999.
4. Kramer N, Meyer TJ, Meharg J, et al: Randomized, prospective trial of noninvasive positive pressure ventilation in acute respiratory failure. Am J Respir Crit Care Med 151:1799–1806, 1995.
5. Meecham-Jones DJ, Paul EA, Jones PW: Nasal pressure support ventilation plus oxygen compared with oxygen therapy alone in hypercapneic COPD. Am J Respir Crit Care Med 152:538–544, 1995.
6. Mehta S, Jay GD, Woolard RH, et al: Randomized, prospective trial of bilevel versus continuous positive airway pressure in acute pulmonary edema.. Crit Care Med 25:620–628, 1997.
7. Strumpf DA, Millman RP, Carlisle CC, et al: Nocturnal positive-pressure ventilation via nasal mask in patients with severe chronic obstructive pulmonary disease. Am J Respir Crit Care Med 144:1234–1239, 1991.
8. Wood KA, Lewis L, Von Harz B, Kollef M:. The use of noninvasive positive pressure ventilation in the emergency department: Results of a randomized clinical trial. Chest 113:1339–1346, 1998.
9. Wysocki M, Tric L, Wolff MA, et al: Noninvasive pressure support ventilation in patients with acute respiratory failure. A randomized comparison with conventional therapy. Chest 107:761–768, 1995.

# 27. OXYGEN DELIVERY SYSTEMS

*Jeffrey L. Tarnow, RRT*

### 1. What is the difference between $FDO_2$ and $FiO_2$?

$FDO_2$ refers to the fraction of *delivered* oxygen. The amount of oxygen that a system delivers is regulated by the settings on the delivery apparatus (i.e., a nasal cannula set at 2 L delivers 28% oxygen). However, the amount that the patient actually receives is variable.

$FiO_2$ refers to the fraction of *inspired* oxygen or the amount of oxygen that the patient inspires into the lungs. The patient's respiratory rate, inspiratory effort, and underlying medical condition can cause a variance in the amount of $FiO_2$.

### 2. What is the most commonly used oxygen delivery device?

The nasal cannula is the most commonly used low-flow oxygen delivery device. Developed around 1929 by Barach, it was designed initially as a dual nasal catheter and later as a bifurcated metal cannula. Currently nasal cannulas are made of plastic, which is more economical, more comfortable, and associated with good patient compliance. They are available in adult, pediatric, and infant sizes. When nasal flows > 4 L/min are administered, the nasal cannula should be connected to a bubble humidifier to minimize drying of the nasal mucosa and avoid patient discomfort.

### 3. What $FiO_2$ levels can be achieved with the nasal cannula?

The range of $FiO_2$ levels depend on the patient's ventilatory pattern, oxygen flow rate, and respiratory dead space. Normally, $FiO_2$ levels of 24–44% are achieved with flow rates of 1–6 L/min.

### 4. What complications are associated with use of nasal cannulas?

Complications related to the nasal cannula include skin breakdown, nares and ear irritation, and nasal bleeding. Displacement of the cannula or disconnection from the oxygen source results in a drop in $FDO_2$.

### 5. If a patient becomes slightly hypoxemic on a nasal cannula, how can you administer a higher $FiO_2$?

The simple mask is used to administer slightly higher (moderate) $FiO_2$ than the nasal cannula. Estimated values range from 40–60% with flow rates between 5 and 10 L/min. A minimal oxygen flow of 5 L/min is recommended to prevent carbon dioxide build-up within the mask. As with the nasal cannula, the $FiO_2$ is influenced by the patient's ventilatory pattern.

### 6. If the patient becomes more hypoxemic, how can you administer an even higher $FiO_2$?

The partial rebreather mask provides an even higher $FiO_2$ by adding a reservoir bag to the simple mask. These masks use oxygen flow rates of 10–15 L/min to maintain partial inflation of the reservoir bag during inspiration. The reservoir is filled during expiration by a portion of the patient's exhaled gas. The $FiO_2$ in the bag remains high, because the exhaled dead-space gas is composed primarily of oxygen. The gas in each inhaled tidal volume is derived from the oxygen in the reservoir and from the mask, typically providing an $FiO_2$ in the range of 60–80%. The minimal flow rate is 10 L/min to prevent carbon dioxide build-up. As with the nasal cannula and the simple mask, the partial rebreather mask is influenced by the patient's ventilatory pattern.

### 7. What is the difference between the partial rebreather mask and nonrebreather mask?

The nonrebreather mask is similar to the partial rebreather mask except for the addition of three one-way valves. One valve is placed between the reservoir bag and mask to prevent exhaled gas from returning into the bag. Exhaled gas is diverted through two valves, one on either side of the mask. During inspiration, the valve between the reservoir bag and mask opens to allow gas flow from the reservoir bag in addition to the set gas flow. The valves on either side of the mask close to decrease the entrainment of room air and to maintain the delivered $FiO_2$. The nonrebreather mask can deliver an $FiO_2$ of 80% and higher if the flow rate is 15 L/min or greater. Nonrebreather masks should be used for the short-term emergency administration of high concentrations of oxygen.

### 8. Summarize the approximate values for $FiO_2$ provided by low-flow devices at normal minute ventilation.

| LOW-FLOW DEVICE | 100% OXYGEN FLOW (L/MIN) | $FiO_2$ |
|---|---|---|
| Nasal cannula | 1 | 24% |
| | 2 | 28% |
| | 3 | 32% |
| | 4 | 36% |
| | 5 | 40% |
| | 6 | 44% |
| Simple oxygen mask | 5–7 | 40–50% |
| | 8–10 | 50–60% |
| Partial rebreather mask | 7 | 65% |
| | 8–15 | 80% |
| Nonrebreather mask | 15-flush | 90%+ |

**9. Can other medical gas mixtures be used with the nonrebreather mask?**

The nonrebreather mask also is recommended for the administration of other medical gas mixtures such as heliox (helium/oxygen) and carbogen (carbon dioxide/oxygen). It is easy to use, conserves gas flow (compared with high-flow systems), and provides the highest concentration of inspired gas of all simple oxygen devices.

**10. What type of mask is used for patients with a high inspiratory flow demand and high $FiO_2$ requirement?**

The aerosol mask, which uses air entrainment and incorporates large-volume nebulizers and large-bore tubing. Two types of aerosol mask delivery systems are available: nondisposable and disposable nebulizers. The nondisposable nebulizers are preset to deliver an $FiO_2$ of 40%, 70%, and 100%. The disposable nebulizers provide a wider range of $FdO_2$ settings (28–100%). Disposable nebulizers may have flow rates of 12–35 L/min.

**11. Can you use a similar system with other devices?**

The large-bore tubing can be attached to a number of devices, including a tracheotomy collar, a "T" piece, or an aerosol mask.

**12. Why would you place 6-inch tubing in the openings on the mask?**

Six-inch, large-bore tubing, also called "horns" or "whiskers," may be placed in the openings on either side of the mask. The horns or whiskers act as a reservoir in an effort to maintain a high $FiO_2$ in a tachypneic patient.

### BIBLIOGRAPHY

1. American Thoracic Society: Standards for the diagnosis and care of patients with chronic obstruction lung disease (COPD) and asthma. Am Rev Respir Dis 136:225–244, 1987.
2. Branson RD: The nuts and bolts of increasing arterial oxygenation devices and techniques. Respir Care 38:672–686, 1993.
3. Jesen AG, Johnsen A, Sandstedt S: Rebreathing during oxygen treatment with face mask: The effects of oxygen flow rates on ventilation. Acta Anaesthesiol Scand 35:289–292, 1991.
4. Leigh JM: The evolution of the oxygen therapy apparatus. Anaesthesia 29:4, 1974.
5. Ooi R: An evaluation of oxygen delivery using nasal prongs. Anaesthesia 47:591,1992.
6. Scanlan CL, Wilkins RL, Stoller JK (eds): Medical gas therapy. In Egan's Fundamentals of Respiratory Care, 7th ed. St. Louis, Mosby, 1999, p 739.
7. Wilson BG, Bone RC: Administration of oxygen and other medical gases. In Eubanks DH, Bone RC (eds): Principles and Applications of Cardiorespiratory Care Equipment. St. Louis, Mosby, 1994, p 35.

# 28. MECHANICAL VENTILATION AND WEANING

*Suzanne M. Burns*, RN, MSN, RRT, ACNP-CS, CCRN

**1. What is the difference between volume and pressure ventilation?**

With **volume ventilation** the desired tidal volume is delivered, regardless of the pressure required to do so. Thus airway pressure varies with changing resistance (airways) or compliance (lung and chest wall). Airway pressure reflects the pressure required to move gases down the airways (resistance) and to distend the lungs and chest wall (compliance).

**Pressure ventilation** ensures a preselected pressure with each breath, but volume varies with resistance and compliance.

**2. Define PEEP and CPAP.**

**PEEP** (positive end-expiratory pressure) is the term used when the patient receives positive-pressure breaths, whereas **CPAP** (continuous positive airway pressure) is the term used when the patient is breathing entirely on his or her own. Both options are used in mechanically ventilated patients to restore functional residual capacity (FRC)—the volume left in the lungs at the end of a resting exhalation.

### 3. When is PEEP used?

In patients with restrictive (noncompliant) diseases, FRC is reduced and the work of breathing is greatly increased. By restoring FRC, PEEP decreases the work of breathing and makes the lungs more compliant. Generally, a small amount (5 cmH$_2$O) of PEEP is considered physiologic and is applied in most cases. PEEP levels are increased to "recruit lung" (see question 10) and to reduce the required fractional concentration of oxygen in inspired gas (FiO$_2$) in patients with high oxygenation requirements. In adults, PEEP is adjusted in increments of 5 cmH$_2$O, as tolerated, to lower FiO$_2$ to 50% or less during mechanical ventilation.

### 4. When is CPAP used?

CPAP often is used to restore FRC during spontaneous breathing trials. It also is used in patients with sleep apnea to provide a pneumatic splint during sleep so that apneic episodes secondary to airway occlusion are prevented.

### 5. What volume modes are available? Describe the appropriate use of each.

**Control ventilation** is used only when the patient is unable to initiate spontaneous inspiration (i.e., sedated and paralyzed). In reality, however, all ventilators have the ability to sense patient-initiated efforts (i.e., trigger sensitivity). Thus the control modes require simply that a rate be selected. Trigger sensitivity is set between –1 and –2 cmH$_2$O so that the patient can breathe, if necessary.

With the **assist-control (A/C) mode**, the clinician selects a control rate, inspiratory time, volume, sensitivity, FiO$_2$, and PEEP (if desired). When the patient initiates a breath between control breaths, the ventilator delivers a full tidal volume (just as with control breaths). Weaning with A/C is not possible because the patient receives full tidal volume breaths with spontaneous effort. For weaning, the patient must be switched to a different mode or to a spontaneous breathing method such as T-piece or CPAP.

With **synchronized intermittent mandatory ventilation** (SIMV), tidal volume, mandatory rate, inspiratory time, sensitivity, and FiO$_2$ are set. PEEP is selected if desired. When the patient initiates a breath, the ventilator senses the effort and delivers air flow to the patient. The patient can breathe at his or her own rate and volume between the mandatory tidal volume breaths. "Synchronized" refers to the the ventilator's attempts to deliver the mandatory breaths within a certain period in synchrony with the patient's spontaneous breaths. In earlier ventilators, which lacked the synchronized feature, this mode was called IMV.

### 6. How are patients weaned with the SIMV or IMV mode?

Weaning is done by decreasing the SIMV rate and allowing the patient to assume more of the work of breathing. Unfortunately, as the mandatory rate decreases to the 4–6 range, the effort associated with spontaneous breathing through the circuit becomes excessive. Current practice offsets this complication with the addition of flow-by or pressure support ventilation between the mandatory breaths. Flow-by ventilation makes continuous flow available to the patient during spontaneous breathing, thus decreasing the effort. Pressure support ventilation is described in question 7.

### 7. What pressure modes are available? How are they used?

**Pressure support ventilation (PSV)** requires that the clinician select a pressure level and set the sensitivity. PEEP may be selected if desired. The patient must have a spontaneous respiratory drive. Once the patient initiates a breath, the machine delivers a high flow of gas at the preselected pressure level. The patient determines his or her own rate, inspiratory time, and tidal volume. Weaning generally is done by decreasing the pressure level in stages as the patient is able to assume more of the work of breathing. PSV decreases the work associated with high breathing rates and small endotracheal tubes and circuits. Thus it is often used in combination with IMV. The combination of IMV and PSV has been associated with longer weaning times in one study.[9]

**Pressure control/inverse ratio ventilation (PC/IRV)** consists of two modes used in combination in patients with acute respiratory distress syndrome (ARDS) or conditions associated with decreased compliance. PCV allows control of the plateau pressure while providing a decelerating flow pattern during inspiration. The inverse ratio is 1:1, 2:1, 3:1, or 4:1. In patients with ARDS the inverse ratio prevents the collapse of alveoli during expiration. A desirable outcome of the prolonged inspiratory times is auto-PEEP. With PC/IRV, inspiratory pressure, control rate, inspiratory time, and PEEP are selected.

### 8. Why were volume modes of ventilation initially more popular?

For over 20 years volume modes were preferred because they ensured a preselected tidal volume regardless of the patient's condition. If a tidal volume was selected and a rate determined, minute ventilation was guaranteed. This guarantee was especially desirable in critically ill patients.

### 9. Why are pressure modes increasing in popularity?

**Decelerating flow pattern.** With pressure ventilation, the speed of gas delivery (flow) is initially high. As the breath is delivered and the lungs fill, the flow tapers (slows) until the ventilator cycles off and exhalation begins. In volume ventilation, the flow pattern is steady; flow rate is the same at the beginning of the breath as at the end. The decelerating flow pattern of pressure modes is believed to be more conducive to optimal gas distribution.

**Volutrauma.** When stiff (noncompliant) lungs are ventilated with traditional tidal volumes of 10–20 ml/kg, they incur injury. In fact, such large volumes result in high distending pressures. Distending pressure, or the pressure required to keep the lung open, is also called static pressure, plateau pressure, and alveolar pressure. When plateau pressures > 35 $cmH_2O$ are sustained for longer than 72 hours, alveolar fractures occur. Lung water increases, and ARDS is exacerbated. As a result, it is important to control plateau pressures in patients with noncompliant lungs. To accomplish this goal, however, resultant tidal volumes must be significantly lower and hypercarbia is expected (called permissive hypercarbia or permissive hypercapnia).[7,11,15] Pressure modes of ventilation, unlike volume modes, control pressure and thus may afford better lung protection.

### 10. What are lung protective strategies?

Lung protective strategies refer to ventilatory applications designed to protect the lung from high plateau pressures (especially in patients with ARDS). As noted above, plateau pressures > 35 $cmH_2O$ for greater than 72 hours result in lung injury. Plateau pressure can be controlled with either volume or pressure ventilation. Pressure ventilation often is used because the clinical goal is easily accomplished by selecting the inspiratory pressure. With volume ventilation, frequent measurement of plateau pressure is necessary because tidal volume is adjusted to attain the desired plateau pressure (see table below). Another protective strategy is the optimal reccuitment of lung with PEEP, which has been associated with improved outcomes (morbidity and mortality). Optimal PEEP levels are determined by performing an inflection pressure maneuver. The maneuver seeks to determine the PEEP level at which the lung is most compliant (greatest volume change for a given pressure).[1] The optimal inflection pressure is generally between 14 and 16 $cmH_2O$.

*Measurement of Plateau Pressure with Volume Ventilation*

1. Push the inspiratory "hold" button on the ventilator at peak inspiration (the end of inspiration on a volume breath).

2. Watch the airway pressure manometer during the inspiratory hold.

3. The manometer will drop to the plateau pressure (the pressure it takes to distend the lungs).

4. The normal gradient between peak airway pressure and plateau pressure is 10–15 $cmH_2O$. If the gradient is greater, airway resistance is present.

## 11. How do I select a mode of ventilation for individual patients?

The selection of mode of ventilation depends on clinician preference and comfort. No mode has been found to be superior, although common sense considerations apply. It is important to keep in mind the clinical goal (see questions 11, 12, and 21) and to avoid complications (see questions 14–20).

## 12. What are the options for initial ventilation?

Initially, especially when the patient is experiencing hypercarbic respiratory failure, the mode choice is volume ventilation at a rate high enough to perform most of the work of breathing. Thus A/C, high-rate IMV, or IMV with PSV may be used to determine the minute ventilation requirements. The rate should be high enough that patient effort ceases but not so high that the patient becomes extremely alkalotic. Most patients readily relax with the combination of sedatives and mechanical ventilation.

## 13. What are the options for resting the respiratory muscles?

Respiratory muscle rest varies, depending on the mode used. With volume ventilation, respiratory muscle effort must cease; that is, ventilator rate must be high enough to avoid spontaneous effort. With PSV the level must be high enough that the respiratory rate is ≤ 20 breaths/minute, tidal volume is 8–12 ml/kg, and accessory muscles are not used. Full rest generally requires 12–24 hours on these settings.

## 14. What are the potential complications of mechanical ventilation and the different modes?

The complications associated with mechanical ventilation include respiratory muscle fatigue, barotrauma, volutrauma (see question 9), hypotension, auto-PEEP, dynamic hyperinflation, and patient-ventilator dyssynchrony. These complications have less to do with mode per se and more to do with mode application.

## 15. Who is at risk for respiratory muscle fatigue? What are the signs and symptoms?

Patients at risk include those who are weak, hypermetabolic, or malnourished and those with chronic obstructive pulmonary disease (COPD). Signs and symptoms include dyspnea, tachypnea (rapid shallow breathing), chest abdominal asynchrony, and elevated partial pressure of carbon dioxide in arterial blood (a late sign). When these signs and symptoms emerge, the prudent approach is to provide respiratory muscle rest for 12–24 hours.

## 16. What is barotrauma? Who is at risk? What are the signs and symptoms?

Barotrauma refers to all air-leak phenomena; tension pneumothorax is the most dreaded example in mechanically ventilated patients. Barotrauma is common in patients who have required prolonged ventilation, especially at high distending pressures. It is important to keep plateau pressures low. Signs and symptoms include high peak and plateau pressures, tachycardia, hypotension, agitation, diaphoresis, and drop in oxygen saturation.

## 17. Who is at risk for hypotension?

Positive pressure may result in decreased venous return, especially in patients with decreased intravascular volume status. In addition, patients with compliant lungs (e.g., emphysema) are especially at risk. Any mode of mechanical ventilation as well as PEEP can result in hypotension.

## 18. Who is at risk for auto-PEEP? How is it measured and treated?

Auto-PEEP results from inadequate expiratory time. It is common in patients with high minute ventilation requirements, small endotracheal tubes, bronchospasm, long inspiratory times, and high respiratory rates. Auto-PEEP may be associated with any mode of ventilation and must be anticipated and measured (see table below) because it is occult and may result in dynamic hyperinflation (see question 19). Interventions to offset auto-PEEP include shortening inspiratory times, decreasing respiratory rates, treating bronchospasm, using larger endotracheal tubes, and sedating agitated patients.

### Measurement of Auto-PEEP

1. Push the end-expiratory button on the ventilator at the end of expiration just prior to the next inspiration.

2. Watch the airway pressure manometer while holding the button.

3. The manometer will register the level of set PEEP and gradually rise to the level of auto-PEEP (if present). Auto-PEEP is the level above set PEEP.

4. Auto-PEEP is difficult to measure in spontaneously breathing patients, especially those with rapid respiratory rates.

**19. Who is at risk for dynamic hyperinflation? What are the signs and symptoms? How is it treated?**

Dynamic hyperinflation is a result of auto-PEEP. Patients with asthma are particularly at risk because bronchospasm prevents adequate alveolar emptying. Since the abnormality in asthma is airways resistance rather than lung compliance, it is easy to distend the alveoli. They quickly become overdistended with vigorous "bagging" and mechanical ventilation. The result is compression of the alveolar capillaries and hypotension. Simultaneously, the airway pressure increases (as does plateau pressure), and the patient becomes increasingly hard to ventilate. These signs and symptoms mimic pneumothorax. Unfortunately, many a chest tube has been inserted over the years as a result. In fact, the treatment of dynamic hyperinflation is to disconnect the patient from the ventilator briefly or to decrease the ventilator rate to allow alveolar decompression. If dynamic hyperinflation is present, hypotension resolves immediately, along with other signs and symptoms.

**20. What causes patient-ventilator dyssynchrony? How is it corrected?**

Patient-ventilator dyssynchrony may result from any of the above complications or from inappropriate or inadequate ventilator settings. For example, if ventilator inspiratory time does not match the patient's inspiratory flow demand, the patient appears dyssynchronous. In this case, the inspiratory time is too long, the flow is too slow, or the patient's inspiratory demand is extremely high and cannot be met by the ventilator. To correct these problems, flow may be increased by shortening the inspiratory time, additional flow may be delivered, or the patient's demand may be decreased with sedatives and, in some cases, muscle relaxants.

**21. How do I know when the patient is ready to wean?**

In **patients ventilated less than 3 days,** the reason for mechanical ventilation should be resolved and the patient should be hemodynamically stable with normal acid-base status, able to protect the airway, and strong enough to provide adequate spontaneous ventilation. Often, especially in surgical cases, the criteria for extubation include ability to lift the head off the pillow, good negative inspiratory pressure value, and adequate minute ventilation and acid–base status on CPAP.

In **patients ventilated longer than 3 days**, the criteria are less easily defined. In fact, weaning criteria are poor positive predictors but good negative predictors. No single factor appears to be responsible for the inability to wean. Thus, a comprehensive approach to weaning assessment is important. Ability to wean does not depend solely on respiratory factors but also on improvement of general factors such as hemodynamic status, hematocrit, nutrition, comfort, anxiety, and mobility.[4,14] Patients who require prolonged mechanical ventilation should be assessed at regular intervals so that trends are observed and impediments to weaning are corrected in a timely fashion. The table below lists some clinical weaning indices and thresholds. To learn more about the indices and how to calculate them, refer to the citations at the end of the chapter.

*Weaning Indices*

---

**Standard criteria (traditional)**
• Negative inspiratory pressure (NIP) :< –20 cmH$_2$O
• Positive expiratory pressure (PEP) > +30 cmH$_2$O
• Spontaneous tidal volume (SVt) > 5ml/kg
• Vital capacity (VC) 15 ml/kg
• FiO$_2$ < 50%

**Integrated indices (pulmonary-specific)**
• Rapid shallow breathing index (fx/Vt)[16] < 105
• Compliance, rate, oxygenation, and pressure (CROP)[16] >13
• Weaning index (WI)[12] < 4

**Integrated indices (comprehensive)**
• Morganroth instrument[17] (ventilator score plus adverse factor score) < 60
• Burns Wean Assessment Program (BWAP)[4] >65%

---

### 22. Which modes or methods for weaning work best?

To date, no mode or method appears superior. Two large, well-designed studies reported disparate findings.[2] Brochard and colleagues suggested that PSV resulted in shorter weaning trial duration. Conversely, Esteban and colleagues demonstrated shorter weaning times with once-and twice-daily spontaneous breathing trials of short duration (2 hours only).[10] The important factor appears to be the manner in which the modes and methods were applied. In both cases, the weaning methods were applied using protocols with noninvasive criteria for entry, discontinuance (intolerance), successful completion, and rest between trials. Although no mode or method appears superior, it is increasingly obvious that systematic approaches decrease variation and may result in shorter weaning times.

### 23. Are protocols the best way to wean patients?

Weaning traditionally has been the domain of physicians and respiratory therapists. Unfortunately, wide variations in practice have been the norm, and results of the various practices were not routinely monitored. Now institutions are aware of the high costs and long hospital stays incurred by patients requiring prolonged mechanical ventilation. Attention is paid to which methods decrease the cost burden while improving patient outcomes. Multidisciplinary methods that decrease variation, keep care planning on target, and make efficient use of resources and time are obvious solutions. Protocols are a logical approach because they are designed to be used in a specific way without variation. Reports of faster weaning times are emerging with protocol-driven approaches.[8,13]

### 24. What are the elements of a good weaning protocol?

Protocols must be easy for all caregivers to understand. Long protocols that have numerous steps and look like algorithms have little chance of being applied accurately. The essential protocol elements include criteria for entry, intolerance, rest, protocol progression, and successful protocol completion. Many studies use noninvasive criteria (e.g, few arterial blood gas analyses), relying instead on clinical signs and symptoms.

### 25. Are outcomes better for patients who are managed in a systematic manner?

Any systematic approach to weaning is likely to decrease variation and improve efficiency and outcomes. However, because systematic approaches include multiple interventions, it is difficult to attribute the effects to any one element. Multidisciplinary approaches appear safe and promote quality care. Examples reported in the literature include "wean teams" and "outcomes managed approaches."[3,5,6]

### 26. What are wean teams?

Wean teams generally include representatives of key disciplines, such as physicians, nurses, and respiratory therapists. In a study by Cohen and colleagues,[5] the team evaluated the patient's weaning potential, designed a weaning plan, and monitored its progress. The multidisciplinary approach was compared with care rendered by critical care fellows during the previous year. Care by the wean team resulted in statistically significant decreases in blood gas analyses, arterial lines, and ventilator days. Cost savings were considerable.

## 27. What are outcomes managed approaches?

Outcomes managed approaches employ a case manager to manage and coordinate the care of mechanically ventilated patients assigned to a multidisciplinary clinical pathway. This approach has been associated with improved clinical and cost outcome. Systematic approaches to weaning appear to be effective and efficient and, in fact, may be superior to individualized approaches.

### BIBLIOGRAPHY

1. Amato MB, Barbas CSV, Medeiros DM, et al: Effect of a protective-ventilation strategy on mortality in acute respiratory distress syndrome. N Engl J Med 338:347–354, 1998.
2. Brochard L, Benito S, Conti G, et al: Comparison of three methods of gradual withdrawal from ventilatory support during weaning from mechanical ventilation. Am J Respir Crit Care Med 150:896–903, 1994.
3. Burns SM, Marshall M, Burns JE, et al: Design, testing and results of an outcomes-managed approach to patients requiring prolonged mechanical ventilation. Am J Crit Care 7:45–57, 1998.
4. Burns SM, Burns JE, Truwit JD: Comparison of five clinical weaning indices. Am J Crit Care 3: 342–352, 1994.
5. Cohen IL, Bari N, Strosberg MA, et al: Reduction of duration and cost of mechanical ventilation in an intensive care unit by use of a ventilatory management team. Crit Care Med 19:1278–1284, 1991.
6. Douglas SL, Daly BJ, Brennan PF, et al: Outcomes of long-term ventilator patients: A descriptive study. Am J Crit Care 6:99–105, 1997.
7. Dreyfuss D, Saumon G: Ventilator-induced lung injury: Lessons from experimental studies. Am J Respir Crit Care Med 157:294–323, 1998.
8. Ely EW, Baker AM, Dunagan DP, et al: Effect on the duration of mechanical ventilation of identifying patients capable of breathing spontaneously. N Engl J Med 335:1864–1869, 1996.
9. Esteban A, Alia I, Ibanez J, et al: Modes of mechanical ventilation and weaning: A national survey of Spanish hospitals. Chest 106:1188–1193, 1994.
10. Esteban A, Frutos F, Tobin MJ, et al: A comparison of four methods of weaning patients from mechanical ventilation. N Engl J Med 332:345–350, 1995.
11. Hickling KG, Wright T, Laubscher K, et al: Extreme hypoventilation reduces ventilator-induced lung injury during ventilation with low positive end-expiratory pressure in saline-lavaged rabbits. Crit Care Med 26:1690–1697, 1998.
12. Jabour ER, Rabil DM, Truwit JD, Rochester DF: Evaluation of a new weaning index based on ventilatory endurance and efficiency of gas exchange. Am Rev Respir Dis 144:531–537, 1991.
13. Kollef MH, Shapiro SD, Silver P, et al: A randomized, controlled trial of protocol-directed weaning from mechanical ventilation. Crit Care Med 25:567–574, 1997.
14. Morganroth ML, Morganroth JL, Nett LM, Petty TL: Criteria for weaning from prolonged ventilation. Arch Intern Med 144:1012–1016, 1984.
15. NHLBI ARDS Clinical Network: ARDS Network Study of Ventilator Management in ARDS Report. Presented at the Meeting of the American Thoracic Society in San Diego, April 26, 1999. HYPERLINK: http://hedwig.mgh.harvard.edu/ardsnet http://hedwig.mgh.harvard. edu/ardsnet.
16. Yang KL, Tobin MJ: A prospective study of indexes predicting the outcome of trials of weaning from mechanical ventilation. N Engl J Med 324:1445–1450, 1991.

# 29. CHEST TUBE REVIEW AND MANAGEMENT

*Debbie L. Dempel,* RN, BSN, CCRN

### 1. Describe a chest tube.

Chest tubes are made of clear plastic with distance markers, multiple drainage holes, and a radiopaque strip that outlines the proximal drainage hole. The tube diameter ranges from 20–40 French for adults. Smaller catheters, such as pigtail catheters, also may be used. Small catheters are more effective for air removal.

### 2. What is the purpose of chest tubes?

A chest tube is inserted into the pleural space to drain air, blood, or fluid and to reestablish negative intrapleural pressure so that the lung can re-expand. The pressure in the pleural space is normally subatmospheric (–4 to –10 mmHg). Chest tubes also are inserted in the pericardium after cardiac surgery to remove residual blood from the mediastinum.

### 3. How does the chest tube drainage system work?

The various drainage systems use the principles of gravity, end-expiratory pressure, and suction to drain air and/or fluid from the pleural space. Chest tube suctioning is based on a traditional three-chamber system. The first chamber is connected directly to the chest tube for fluid collection. The second chamber contains approximately 2 cm of water that creates a water seal. Any incoming air travels upward through the water, which acts as a one-way valve to prevent backflow through the system. The air then enters the suction control chamber. This third chamber regulates the amount of negative pressure that can be applied to the pleural space. The typical amount of suction is –20 cmH$_2$O for chest tube systems in adults.

### 4. What is the difference between wet and dry chest tube drainage systems?

In **wet systems** the suction control chamber in wet systems is filled with sterile water. The amount of water added to the chamber corresponds to the amount of suction desired. If –20 cmH$_2$O suction is ordered, the chamber is filled to the 20-cm mark. The suction control chamber has a vent to atmospheric air that prevents generation of excessive suction. The wall suction is adjusted until the water in the suction control chamber bubbles gently and continuously. Excessive suction and vigorous bubbling create excessive noise and cause the water to evaporate rapidly. The water level should be checked during each shift and refilled as necessary.

In **dry systems** no water is added to the suction control chamber. The amount of suction is determined by a dial on the dry unit and wall suction. The dial is turned to the prescribed level of suction in centimeters of water. The chamber then is connected to wall suction. An indicator shows when enough suction has been applied to operate the system. Most dry units have a floating disc or indicator that becomes visible in a window when enough suction has been applied. Dry systems use one of two methods to limit the amount of negative pressure: (1) restrictive orifice mechanism, which is an opening in the suction control chamber that can be made larger or smaller to increase or decrease the amount of negative pressure, or (2) a regulator that adjusts automatically to changes in negative pressure.

### 5. How much suction is typically applied to a chest tube?

Under most circumstances –20 cmH$_2$O is applied to chest tubes in adults. Suction levels range from –10 to –40 cmH$_2$O. Low-pressure suction (–10 to –20 cmH$_2$O) is the standard amount reported in the literature and community practice. High-pressure suction (> –20 cmH$_2$O) is associated with persistent pleural air leaks, lung tissue entrapment, and re-expansion pulmonary edema.

**6. What are the indications for chest tube placement?**
- Spontaneous pneumothorax
- Tension pneumothorax
- Penetrating chest injuries
- Hemothorax
- Parapneumonic effusions (empyema)
- Pleurodesis for intractable effusions
- Chylothorax
- Postthoracic surgery
- Bronchopleural fistula

The most common indication is a pneumothorax with greater than 15% of total lung volume.

**7. Define pneumothorax.**
A pneumothorax occurs when air accumulates between the two pleurae of the lung. It may lead to partial or total lung collapse. Pneumothoraces are classified as spontaneous or traumatic.

**8. What are the signs and symptoms of pneumothorax?**
- Dyspnea
- Chest pain
- Hypoxemia
- Tachycardia
- Ipsilateral hyperresonance
- Decreased or absent breath sounds

**9. What is a tension pneumothorax?**
A tension pneumothorax occurs when air enters the intrapleural space but cannot escape through the chest wall or airway. The pressure created in the pleural cavity compresses the lung, leading to collapse. A large tension pneumothorax can cause decreased venous return, decreased cardiac output, diaphragm depression, and a mediastinal shift to the contralateral side.

**10. What are the signs and symptoms of tension pneumothorax?**
- Dyspnea
- Labored breathing
- Tachycardia
- Hypotension
- Tracheal deviation away from the affected side
- Cyanosis

**11. When does pneumothorax require placement of a chest tube?**
Chest tube treatment is based on the patient's clinical status and size and type of pneumothorax. Generally, a pneumothorax of less than 20–25% of total lung volume with minimal symptoms does not require chest tube placement but is followed closely.

**12. How are chest tubes used for treatment of pneumothorax?**
The chest tubes inserted for pneumothoraces are generally smaller (16–20 French) and placed toward the lung apex. A water seal system may be sufficient to evacuate air from the pleural space, but suction can be applied to enhance removal. It is important to assess the water seal chamber for bubbling on expiration, which indicates removal of air from the pleural space. The amount of bubbling should decrease over time as the pneumothorax resolves. Any increase in the air leak should be noted, investigated, and reported to the physician.

**13. What assessments are appropriate in caring for patients with a chest tube?**
- Thorough and complete assessment of hemodynamic and respiratory status is essential.
- The amount, color, and consistency of the chest tube drainage should be assessed and documented. A permanent marker is recommended to date and time the drainage in the collection chamber. The frequency of documentation for chest tube drainage is dictated by the clinical status of each patient and hospital procedure. Chest tube assessment should be done at least once a shift and with any sudden change in drainage or clinical status of the patient.
- The chest tube insertion site should be assessed during every shift or as clinically indicated.
- Note the fluctuation/tidaling of the fluid in the water seal chamber as the patients breathes. Suction may need to be turned off briefly. The fluid rises on inspiration and falls on expiration; the reverse occurs if the patient is on positive-pressure ventilation (PPV). If tidaling stops, the lung has fully expanded or there is an obstruction in the unit.

• Monitor the water seal chamber for bubbling. Intermittent bubbling occurs on expiration when air is present in the pleural cavity. Continuous bubbling during inspiration and expiration indicates a leak in the system.

## 14. What is "dumping"?

Increased drainage may correspond to patient activity as a result of evacuation of old drainage. This phenomenon, which occurs frequently the first time a patient gets out of bed after open-heart surgery, is called "dumping."

## 15. What should you look for in assessing the chest tube insertion site?

Note any signs of infection, such as redness, warmth, foul odor, or purulent drainage. Assess the surrounding area for signs of air infiltration (subcutaneous emphysema) by palpating the skin. An air leak or gas trapping may cause swelling and subcutaneous emphysema (crepitus). A small amount of crepitus is not dangerous, but if the area of subcutaneous emphysema grows or travels to the neck or face, the physician should be notified. Extensive subcutaneous emphysema of the face and neck may be an early sign of pneumothorax and can lead to a compromised airway.

## 16. How do you locate the leak in a chest tube drainage system?

Briefly clamp the chest tube in sequential increments, starting from the exit site and moving downward to the drainage unit. If the bubbling stops when the clamp is next to the chest, a pleural leak may be present. If the bubbling continues, the leak is distal to the clamp and outside the patient. Check all connections, and continue the search. The drainage unit itself may have a leak; if so, it must be replaced.

## 17. How are chest tubes maintained?

All chest tube connections should be taped and secured. The drainage unit should be below the level of the chest tube insertion site, ideally 2–3 feet below chest level. The tubing should be kept free of dependent loops and kinks that impede drainage or obstruct flow. The optimal position of the tubing is straight or coiled. Placement of the drainage unit below the foot of the bed with the tubing along the side of the patient and slight elevation of the head of the bed enhance proper drainage.

Chest tube dressings should be clean, dry, and occlusive. Note any drainage on dressings, and reinforce as needed. Follow hospital procedure for frequency of dressing change. Traditionally, the chest tube insertion site was surrounded with petroleum-laden gauze to prevent air leaks. In recent years, however, this practice was found to cause maceration of the skin and to predispose to infection; it is no longer recommended. All chest tubes should be securely anchored to the chest wall to prevent accidental dislodgement.

## 18. Should chest tubes be stripped or milked?

Many studies have investigated the assumption that stripping and milking promote drainage and patency. Stripping is not recommended because it produces high negative pressures (–100 to –400 cmH$_2$O) in the pleural space and may cause lung entrapment. Milking requires gently squeezing and releasing the tubing between the palms of the hands or fingers. Milking is not necessary but may be useful when a clot or other obstructive drainage is visible in the tubing.

## 19. Is it safe to clamp a chest tube?

Clamping chest tubes is not recommended because it may lead to a life-threatening complication such as a tension pneumothorax. Patients with air leaks have an increased risk for this complication. During patient transport, the suction tubing should be disconnected and the drainage unit kept at water seal. If the chest tube becomes disconnected from the drainage unit, do not clamp it. Instead, submerge the distal end in a container with sterile water to form a temporary water seal. The chest tube should be reconnected to a drainage unit as soon as possible.

## 20. What situations require clamping of the chest tube?

1. Assessing the system for the source of an air leak. Brief, sequential clamping of the chest tube is necessary to identify the source of the leak and is not harmful to the patient.

2. Changing the drainage unit requires that the chest tube be momentarily clamped.

3. A physician may order clamping of the chest tube to assess how the patient will tolerate removal. The tube may be clamped for 12–24 hours to assess recurrence of pneumothorax. Close monitoring of respiratory status is imperative during this time.

### 21. Why are mediastinal chest tubes used?

After open heart surgery chest tubes are placed in the mediastinum to remove residual blood or drainage. Generally, two large-bore (36-French) chest tubes are used. An angled chest tube is inserted between the diaphragmatic pericardium and inferior wall of the heart, and a straight tube is placed on the anterior surface of the heart. Both exit the chest below the xiphoid process.

### 22. How are mediastinal chest tubes assessed?

Mediastinal chest tubes are closely assessed for the amount, color, and consistency of drainage in the collection chamber. Drainage must be encouraged to flow into the collection chamber and not to build up in the mediastinum. Proper suction, correct placement of the drainage unit, and loop-free tubing facilitate drainage. Milking also facilitates flow of drainage. Elevating the head of the bed at least 30° enhances drainage and is recommended unless the patient is hemodynamically unstable. Tubing connections may require gentle tapping to dislodge particularly large clots.

### 23. What is the most serious complication of mediastinal chest tube placement?

Cardiac tamponade, which occurs when blood or other fluid collects in the pericardial sac and compresses the heart. Tamponade can lead to life-threatening cardiac dysfunction.

### 24. What type of drainage unit is used for mediastinal chest tubes?

Any drainage unit can be used for mediastinal chest tubes. Special units allow the blood in the collection chamber to be autotransfused into the patient.

### 25. How does autotransfusion work?

Autotransfusion works in a variety of ways, depending on the system used. In continuous autotransfusion, tubing connected to the bottom of the collection chamber is fed through a pump and connected to the patient, thereby regulating the hourly amount infused. Other products allow a specified amount of drainage to accumulate in the collection chamber before it is evacuated into a special vacuum-pressured bag. The bag is hung, and the contents infuse by gravity into the patient. Similarly, certain systems have breakaway bags connected to the collection chamber. When the specified amount of drainage is collected, the bag is simply disconnected and hung for reinfusion.

The Centers for Disease Control requires blood to be transfused within 4 hours when it is kept at room temperature. Keep this guideline in mind when autotransfusing drainage that has collected over time.

### 26. What are the potential complications of chest tubes?

- Bleeding and internal laceration of organs may occur at the time of insertion.
- Infection at the entry site or in the pleural cavity may lead to development of empyema. It is important to maintain a closed, sterile system and to use aseptic techniques during tube manipulations and dressing changes. Occasionally, prophylactic antibiotics are prescribed for the duration of chest tube placement, but this practice remains controversial.
- Mechanical failure to drain air or fluid can lead to further respiratory compromise. This complication can be lessened by diligent assessment of the chest tube and drainage system.
- Re-expansion pulmonary edema is a rare complication but has a mortality rate up to 20%. Unilateral pulmonary edema develops on the side of the chest from which a pleural effusion or pneumothorax is evacuated.

### BIBLIOGRAPHY

1. Carroll P: Chest tubes made easy. Regist Nurse 58:46–55, 1995.
2. Edmunds LH, Norwood WI, Low DW: Atlas of Cardiothoracic Surgery. Philadelphia, Lea & Febiger, 1990.

3. Gordon PA, Norton JM, Merrell R: Refining chest tube management: Analysis of the state of practice. Dimens Crit Care Nurs 14:6–16, 1995.
4. Halow KD, Peters RA: Chest tubes. In Parsons PE, Wiener-Kronish JP (eds): Critical Care Secrets, 2nd ed. Philadelphia, Hanley & Belfus, 1998, pp 70–74.
5. Hanley ME: Pneumothorax. In Parsons PE, Wiener-Kronish JP (eds): Critical Care Secrets, 2nd ed. Philadelphia, Hanley & Belfus, 1998, pp 392–396.
6. Humphrey EW, McKeown DL: Manual of Pulmonary Surgery. New York, Springer-Verlag, 1982.
7. Miller KS, Sahn SA: Chest tubes: Indications, technique, management and complications. Chest 91:258–263, 1987.
8. O'Hanlon-Nichols T: Commonly asked questions about chest tubes. Am J Nurs 96:60–64, 1996.
9. Pettinicchi TA: Trouble shooting chest tubes. Nursing 98 28:58–59, 1998.

# 30. ACUTE RESPIRATORY FAILURE

*Gabull Abdullah*, RN, MS, ACNP

## 1. Define acute respiratory failure.

Acute respiratory failure (ARF) occurs when the body cannot adequately oxygenate tissues and remove carbon dioxide ($CO_2$). ARF is a laboratory diagnosis that can be made only if an arterial blood gas (ABG) reveals hypoxemia (partial pressure of oxygen in arterial blood [$PaO_2$] < 60 mmHg), hypercapnia (partial pressure of carbon dioxide in arterial blood [$PaCO_2$] > 45 mmHg), and/or hypocapnia ($PaCO_2$ < 45 mmHg). ARF superimposed on chronic respiratory failure is manifested by sudden deviations in $PaCO_2$ of 5 mmHg or more from baseline.

## 2. What are the two types of ARF?

1. ARF in which hypoxemia (with hypocapnia) is present in the context of acute, diffuse lung injury

2. ARF in which both hypoxemia and hypercapnia are present

The two types differ significantly in pathogenesis, pathophysiology, and management. The first type is commonly called acute respiratory distress syndrome (ARDS) and is discussed in chapter 33. This chapter focuses on hypoxemic-hypercapnic ARF, which often is called alveolar hypoventilation. The hallmark of hypercapnic ARF is an elevated $PaCO_2$, which signals that pulmonary clearance of carbon dioxide ($CO_2$) is inadequate. More $CO_2$ is produced by body metabolism than the respiratory system can clear by ventilation.

## 3. List and describe the six mechanisms of hypoxemia.

1. Decrease in the ambient concentration of inspired oxygen ($P_IO_2$). Examples: high altitude, flying in a nonpressurized airplane cabin, or breathing expired gases (as in a paper bag or closed space).

2. Hypoventilation: Normal movement of gas in and out of alveoli is disrupted and results in hypercapnia, which leads to hypoxemia. Examples: choking, chronic obstructive pulmonary disease (COPD), asthma, respiratory muscle paralysis, and central nervous system (CNS) impairment.

3. Diffusion abnormality: An increased alveolar-capillary diffusion gradient impairs oxygen transport from the alveoli to the capillaries. Diffusion abnormality alone does not account for significant hypoxemia. Example: diffuse interstitial pulmonary fibrosis.

4. Ventilation-perfusion (V/Q) mismatch: Ventilation is impaired by partially collapsed or partially fluid-filled alveoli. Hypoxemia from V/Q mismatch is responsive to oxygen therapy and positive end-expiration pressure (PEEP) in intubated patients. V/Q mismatch is the most common cause of hypoxemia in ARF.

5. Intrapulmonary shunt (IPS): Perfusion of nonventilated alveoli. The alveoli are completely collapsed or filled with pus, water, or blood. IPS is not responsive to increases in oxygen and PEEP therapy. Examples: pneumonia, pulmonary edema, and intrapulmonary hemorrhage.

6. Low mixed venous oxygen tension ($PvO_2$) with IPS: The mixed venous oxygen tension is an important determinant of $PaO_2$ as IPS fraction increases. Examples: low cardiac output state (congestive heart failure) with IPS (pulmonary edema or pneumonia).

### 4. What are the potential causes of hypoxemic-hypercapnic ARF?

The causes can be thought of in terms of patients who *will not* breathe and patients who *cannot* breathe. Patients who will not breathe may have normal lung mechanics but develop respiratory failure when neuromuscular strength and endurance are markedly decreased. Altered ventilation is due to a CNS or neuromuscular cause. Patients who cannot breathe have normal neuromuscular function but develop ventilatory failure in the face of markedly altered lung mechanics, resulting in an increase in the work of breathing. A wide variety of alterations may increase the mechanical load or decrease the effectiveness of neuromuscular strength and endurance.

*Common Conditions That May Cause Ventilatory Failure with Hypercapnia*

| PATIENTS WHO CANNOT BREATHE<br>CONDITIONS THAT INCREASE VENTILATORY LOAD | PATIENTS WHO WILL NOT BREATHE<br>CONDITIONS THAT DECREASE VENTILATION |
|---|---|
| **Increased airway resistance** | **Depressed respiratory drive** |
| Upper airway obstruction | Sedative drugs |
| Increased bronchial secretions and edema | Hypothyroidism |
| Dynamic airway obstruction | Brainstem lesion |
| **Decreased lung compliance** | **Altered neuromuscular transmission** |
| Increased lung water | Poliomyelitis |
| Pneumonia | Myasthenia gravis |
| Atelectasis | Guillain-Barré syndrome |
| Interstitial fibrosis | Amyotrophic lateral sclerosis |
| Acute lung injury | Spinal cord or phrenic nerve injury |
| Infarction | Drugs: neuromuscular-blocking agents, |
| Intrinsic positive end-expiratory pressure | aminoglycosides, steroids |
| **Decreased chest wall compliance** | **Muscle weakness** |
| Chest wall trauma | Myopathies |
| Pleural effusion | Muscular dystrophy |
| Pneumothorax | Malnutrition |
| Kyphoscoliosis | Hypokalemia |
| Ascites | Hypocalcemia |
| Peritoneal dialysis | Hypophosphatemia |
| Upper abdominal surgery | Hypomagnesemia |
| Obesity | |

### 5. What are the signs and symptoms of ARF?

Signs and symptoms of ARF are those of the underlying disease mixed with those of hypoxemia and hypercapnia. The cardinal symptom of hypoxemia is dyspnea. Signs of hypoxemia include cyanosis, restlessness, confusion, anxiety, delirium, tachypnea, tachycardia, hypertension, cardiac arrhythmias, and tremor. Dyspnea and headache are considered the cardinal symptoms of early hypercapnia; however, not all patients present with these symptoms. Other signs and symptoms of hypercapnia include peripheral and conjunctival hyperemia, hypertension, tachycardia, tachypnea, irritability, impaired consciousness, papilledema, and asterixis. These signs and symptoms are insensitive and nonspecific.

### 6. What are the two primary goals of managing hypercapnic respiratory failure?

The two primary goals of management in hypercapnic ARF are (1) restoration of adequate gas exchange to provide oxygen for delivery to vital organs and (2) treatment of the underlying disorder(s). Prompt action must be taken to revert or avoid hazardous levels of hypoxemia, hypercapnia, and acidosis.

### 7. What are the most serious complications of ARF?

Severe hypoxemia is the greatest danger to survival and requires immediate attention. $PaO_2$ levels below 40 mmHG are poorly tolerated by adults and commonly are associated with cardiac arrhythmias and functional abnormalities of the heart, brain, kidney, liver, and other organs. Severe hypercapnia can result in altered mental status and inability to protect the airway, which in turn may lead to respiratory or cardiopulmonary arrest. A pH level below 7.20 should be avoided or corrected. Acidosis potentiates the functional abnormalities induced by hypoxemia, such as pulmonary hypertension, cerebral vasodilatation, and depression of myocardial contractility.

### 8. What are the two greatest dangers related to oxygen administration?

**Respiratory depression** with oxygen administration is confined to patients with chronic hypercapnic failure in whom normal stimuli of ventilation are compromised and in whom hypercapnia has been present for several days. Retention of bicarbonate by the kidneys in chronic respiratory failure leads to moderation of the acidosis caused by acute hypercapnia. Acidosis provides a strong drive for respiration. In hypercapnic ARF, this drive is present, and oxygen is not a hazard for respiratory depression. However, in chronic hypercapnic states in which the patient is obtunded or sedated, hypoxemia is the major drive of ventilation. With oxygen administration, this drive is blunted; the patient ventilates less, and $PaCO_2$ rises. Recent investigations indicate that the process of exaggerating hypercapnia with excessive oxygen administration is much more complex than the simple "blunting" of the hypoxic drive. However, the fact remains that excessive oxygen administration may induce hypercapnia in a hypoxemic patient. Oxygen therapy should not be withheld for fear of causing progressive respiratory acidemia. Artificial ventilation (invasive or noninvasive) can be used to treat hypercapnia, if needed.

**Direct lung injury** is a well-established danger of oxygen therapy. Excessive oxygen leads to excessive $O_2$ free radicals, which cause cellular damage. The two major determinants are (1) inspired oxygen concentration ($FiO_2$) and (2) duration of oxygen administration. Therefore, to avoid this potentially lethal form of oxygen-induced lung injury, the general rule is to use the lowest $FiO_2$ that will maintain adequate oxygenation for the shortest time possible.

### 9. What are the options for rapid administration of oxygen?

An established secure airway is of primary importance for the delivery of oxygen and treatment of ARF. **Soft nasal prongs**, through which oxygen is delivered at the required flow rate, are the most widely used method. Some prongs deliver oxygen continuously; others contain a small reservoir and deliver a more concentrated form of oxygen during inspiration, thereby economizing on oxygen utilization.

An alternative method is the use of masks designed to deliver fixed oxygen concentrations. Such masks include the **nonrebreather (reservoir bag) masks**. When the need for oxygen necessitates a nonrebreather mask, the patient has experienced a significant change in condition and requires reassessment.

**Noninvasive positive-pressure ventilation** (NPPV) is commonly used to treat respiratory failure as an alternative to tracheal intubation. For more information, see chapter 26.

### 10. What problems are common in patients with obstructive lung disease and ARF?

Accumulation of secretions, infection, and bronchospasm. Secretions are best removed by encouraging the patient to cough and by adequate hydration. Chest percussion and vibration may enhance sputum mobilization in some patients (e.g., those with cystic fibrosis or bronchiectasis). If necessary, catheters inserted by the nasal or oral route into the trachea can be used to suction secretions. Occasionally, fiberoptic bronchoscopy is performed to visualize and remove secretions. Use of bronchodilators to treat bronchospasm has proved successful because bronchoconstriction is to some degree reversible. Infection is a common complication of chronic hypercapnic failure. Treatment with broad-spectrum antimicrobial agents is usually initiated on the presumption that infection is present.

## 11. Describe various treatment regimens for ARF.

All treatment regimens for ARF must start with a conversation between the clinician and the patient, family, and/or caregivers about the patient's desire for resuscitation and mechanical ventilation. The clinician can provide a clear picture of the patient's condition based on history, physical exam, and other diagnostic data. Options of treatment and prognosis must be discussed.

Treatment consists of controlling hypoxemia with respiratory support, using nonventilatory and ventilatory measures. Oxygen therapy is essential to relieve hypoxemia, but oxygen should be administered to achieve a $PaO_2$ in the range of 50–60 mmHg, corresponding to an oxygen saturation of approximately 90%. Monitor $PaO_2$ and the $PaCO_2$ closely during oxygen therapy.

Control of infection, bronchoconstriction, and secretions is also part of the treatment regimens. Management of treatment-related complications, such as cardiac arrhythmias, left ventricular failure, pulmonary emboli, and gastrointestinal hemorrhage, is also necessary. The final aspect of a complete treatment regimen is weaning from mechanical ventilation (see chapter 28).

## 12. What is the role of corticosteroids in ARF?

Corticosteroids are commonly given, usually in high doses during the first few days of therapy, for treatment of bronchospasm and inflammation. Empiric trials suggest that corticosteroid therapy has a modest impact on the course of hypercapnic ARF.

## 13. How important is nutrition in patients with ARF?

Many patients with COPD are malnourished because of increased metabolic needs and inadequate intake. Correction of nutritional depletion and minimizing further depletion during an episode of ARF can enhance recovery and forestall further episodes. Patients require consultation with a dietician or nutritionist for a thorough nutritional assessment. Early intervention with oral and/or enteral feeding is preferred. Parenteral nutrition is considered when the enteral route is absolutely contraindicated.

### BIBLIOGRAPHY

1. Beers M: Acute respiratory failure. In Fishman AP (ed): Pulmonary Diseases and Disorders: Companion Handbook, 2nd ed. New York, McGraw-Hill, 1994, pp 411–418.
2. Chestnutt M, Prendergast T, Stauffer J: Acute respiratory failure. In Tierney L, McPhee S, Papadakis M (eds): Current Medical Diagnosis and Treatment, 38th ed. Stamford, CT, Appleton & Lange, 1999, pp 334–336.
3. George R: Approach to the patient with acute respiratory failure. In Kelley WN (Ed): Textbook of Internal Medicine, 3rd ed. Philadelphia, Lippincott-Raven, 1997, pp 1932–1937.
4. Hall J, Schmidt G, Wood L: Principles of critical care for the patient with respiratory failure. In Murray J, Nadel J (eds): Textbook of Respiratory Medicine, 2nd ed. Philadelphia, W.B. Saunders, 1994, pp 2545–2588.
5. Honig E, Ingram R: Chronic bronchitis, emphysema, and airway obstruction. In Fauci AS, Braunwald E, Isselbacher KJ, et al (eds): Harrison's Prinicples of Internal Medicine, 14th ed. New York, McGraw-Hill, 1998, pp 1458–1460.
6. Meyer T, Hill N: Noninvasive positive pressure ventilation to treat respiratory failure. Ann Intern Med 120:760–770, 1994.
7. Tobin M: Mechanical ventilation. N Engl J Med 330:1056–1061, 1994.
8. Tobin M, Luce J: Update in critical care medicine. Ann Intern Med 125:909–916, 1996.

# 31. PULSE OXIMETRY AND CAPNOGRAPHY

*Theresa Lynn Griffin, RN, MS*

### 1. What is pulse oximetry?

Pulse oximetry is a noninvasive device used to measure the percentage of oxygen bound to hemoglobin in pulsating vessels. It provides an oxygen saturation value ($SpO_2$). Pulse oximetry allows assessment and detection of hypoxemia in real time and can alert the nurse to changes in oxygenation status.

### 2. How does pulse oximetry work?

Pulse oximetry detects the percentage of dissolved oxygen that is attached to the hemoglobin of a red blood cell by using a probe with a light source and photodetector. Oximeters function by placing a pulsatile vascular bed between a light-emitting diode (LED) and a detector. Two lights are emitted from the source, red and infrared light, each with different wavelengths. Hemoglobin with oxygen attached (oxyhemoglobin) and hemoglobin without oxygen attached (reduced hemoglobin) absorb the emitted light differently. The difference in absorption of the light wavelengths is calculated in the probe sensor to give the $SpO_2$ value.

### 3. Where is the best place to put the pulse oximetry probe?

The oximetry probe is routinely placed on the finger over the pulsating nail bed. Extremity perfusion may be diminished by hypothermia and vasoconstriction. In such cases, seen routinely in trauma patients, elderly patients, and postoperative patients, warm fluids or warming blankets can help perfusion and improve pulse detection. In the presence of hypoperfusion (i.e., poor cardiac output caused by hypovolemia, myocardial infarction, shock states, or some other factor), the body shunts blood to the core organs, and pulses are diminished or absent in the extremity digits. In trying to resolve these issues, the nurse may try to move the probe to other sites, such as toes, ear lobes, or bridge of the nose. The last two sites necessitate a specific nose or ear probe from the oximeter manufacturer, or the finger probe can be customized to fit these areas, if needed. Nurses can be creative and try to optimize the light source emitting and absorption by covering the probe with a cut-off glove finger or by slipping the digit into an alcohol wrap.

### 4. How accurate is pulse oximetry?

In lab studies, pulse oximetry is accurate within 2–3% of oxyhemoglobin levels measured in arterial blood gas samples. Commercially available pulse oximeters maintain this accuracy rate over a range of 70–100% oxygen saturation.

### 5. How are placement and function of the oximeter probe routinely assessed?

Oxygen saturation data are displayed digitally on a monitor screen as a numeric value and waveform. The waveform reflects the pulsatile flow of the monitored vascular bed between the sensing probe. If the displayed numeric value does not seem to reflect the patient's clinical picture, the nurse can assess the pulsatile waveform on the monitor screen and troubleshoot the functioning of the probe if it appears abnormal. A normal wave looks like an arterial waveform with regular cycles of peaks and valleys. If it is flat or irregular and the patient is stable, the probe may have been misplaced, or the patient may have poor perfusion. The probe should be repositioned or moved to another pulsatile site. Alarms for oximetry should be adjusted to patient-specific limits and be turned on to pick up clinical trends or acute episodes of respiratory failure (e.g., pneumothorax, mucous plugs, pulmonary edema, pulmonary emboli).

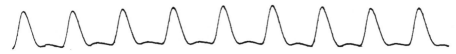

Normal oximetry waveform.

**6. What are the nursing responsibilities in caring for the patient with pulse oximetry?**

Nursing responsibilities include applying the oximetry probe and monitoring the $SpO_2$ and waveform. If a patient is monitored with oximetry for extended periods, probe and skin integrity should be assessed, and the probe should be replaced as needed or according to protocol. If placement of the probe on the face or fingers seems to bother the patient, the nurse can move the probe to a toe to keep it out of the patient's sight. If the probe is not sensing appropriately, the nurse is responsible for troubleshooting the patient, probe, and oximeter. Nail polish should be removed before placing the probe to avoid problems with saturation detection. The nurse is responsible for accurately assessing real and significant changes in $SpO_2$ values and intervening appropriately.

**7. How often should pulse oximetry be documented?**

$SpO_2$ is considered a vital sign and should be documented with other vital signs according to standards of care or as prescribed. Any change in the patient's condition warrants reassessment and documentation of $SpO_2$ and vital signs. $SpO_2$ also should be documented with arterial blood gas analyses to correlate $SaO_2$ with $SpO_2$.

**8. What factors affect pulse oximetry measurements?**

Many factors can greatly affect the accuracy and reliability of pulse oximetry. As discussed above, most inaccurate values of oximetry result from poor signal quality due to hypoperfusion or motion artifact (i.e., restless patients). Other reasons for optical interference are extraneous lights, such as fluorescent, intravenous dyes, and nail polishes (especially green, blue or black). Patients with dependent venous pooling or vascular insufficiency may have falsely low $SpO_2$ readings because the venous pulsations dilute the arterial readings. In general, oximetry during cardiopulmonary resuscitation is unreliable because of simultaneous pulsations of arterial and venous circulation.

**9. What is capnography?**

Capnography is the noninvasive measurement of exhaled carbon dioxide ($CO_2$), expressed either as a percentage (%) or as partial pressure in mmHg. The displayed waveform of capnography is called a capnogram. The numeric value that is displayed is termed end-tidal $CO_2$ ($ETCO_2$). This exhaled measurement closely reflects the arterial partial pressure of carbon dioxide ($PaCO_2$). $ETCO_2$ is usually 1–6 mmHg lower than $PaCO_2$ in patients without significant ventilatory disease or circulatory problems.

**10. When is capnography used?**

Capnography is used most commonly in intubated patients in the intensive care unit (ICU), emergency department, or surgical recovery unit and during anesthesia in the operating room. It can be used to assess placement of the endotracheal tube during intubation. $CO_2$ is not detected if the tube is placed in the esophagus. Capnography provides additional assessment data related to respiratory and metabolic trends and can alert clinicians to acute and episodic changes.

**11. What are indications for capnography in the ICU?**

Capnography is commonly used during weaning from mechanical ventilation. Capnography and oximetry provide essential assessment data to guide ventilator weaning. Capnography also alleviates the need to draw frequent arterial blood gases, especially with ventilator adjustments. These noninvasive data should be evaluated along with the clinical examination. Arterial blood gas samples should be drawn at initiation of capnography for correlation and with any decline in the patient's condition. Capnography trends are used to guide clinical care when accurately interpreted.

### 12. How does capnography work?

Capnography measures the amount of $CO_2$ produced during a respiratory cycle. $ETCO_2$ reflects the $CO_2$ that is expired with each respiratory cycle. Most capnography systems use infrared spectrometry. The exhaled gas passes through an analyzer that releases an infrared light beam absorbed by $CO_2$ molecules. By measuring how much is absorbed, the analyzer determines the concentration of the gas, then transmits the data to a monitor, where it is displayed in digital numerics and as a waveform. In-line sensors are either mainstream or side stream. Regardless of the type of sampling technique, the airway adaptor or sampling port should be placed as close as possible to the patient's airway. $ETCO_2$ also may be measured using a special caloric pH-sensitive indicator that changes color in response to different concentrations of carbon dioxide, like litmus paper. One such model is Nellcor's Easy Cap™ $ETCO_2$ detector. The $ETCO_2$ device is attached between the endotracheal tube and manual resuscitation bag. Such equipment is helpful in assessing tube placement after intubation and effectiveness of ventilation and can be useful in the prehospital field or emergency department when monitors and cables are not available.

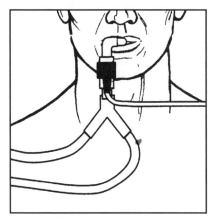 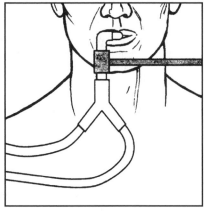

In mainstream sampling *(left)*, the sensor that measures $CO_2$ is attached to the ET tube. In sidestream sampling *(right)*, the exhaled gas travels to the sensor located in the monitor. (From Witta KN: When gauging respiratory status is critical. RN 56(11):40–46, 1993, with permission.)

### 13. How is a capnogram read and interpreted?

The numeric display on the monitor represents the highest concentration of $CO_2$ reached at the end of exhalation. On the capnogram, the X (horizontal) axis reflects time, whereas the Y (vertical) axis represents the concentration of exhaled $CO_2$. Depending on the equipment, $ETCO_2$ is expressed either as a percentage (normal value = about 5%) or in mmHG (normal value = about 38 mmHg). Each waveform represents a single respiratory cycle. The A-B phase represents the beginning of exhalation with $CO_2$-free gas from anatomic dead space (oropharynx, trachea, and bronchioles). Phase B-C is a rapid sharp upstroke, rising at a nearly 90° angle. It represents mixed dead space and alveolar air. Phase C-D is the alveolar plateau. At this point in the respiratory cycle, the graph is nearly horizontal and alveolar exhalation is nearly complete. $ETCO_2$ is measured at end expiration, point D on the graph, when $CO_2$ is at its maximal concentration. Recognizing and interpreting changes in the shape of the capnogram are crucial when capnography is used to assess ventilatory status.

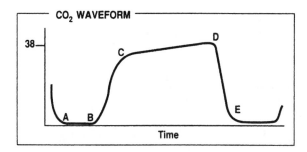

Normal capnogram waveform. *A–B:* baseline, indicating $CO_2$-free gas exhaled first from dead space—air from portions of the mouth, trachea, and bronchi that does not participate in gas exchange. *B–C:* $CO_2$ levels rise rapidly as air leaves the larger airways of the lungs. *C–D:* The alveolar plateau reflects the empyting of $CO_2$ at the end of exhalation. The levels rise slowly as the gas is expelled from distal alveoli. *D:* end-tidal point, when capnography measures maximal $CO_2$ exhalation. *D–E:* $CO_2$ declines rapidly with inhalation of carbon dioxide-free gas. (From Sinclair S: Dispelling myths of capnography. Dimens Crit Care Nurs 17:48–55, 1998, with permission.)

**14. What are the most common abnormal capnogram waveforms? What do they reflect about the patient's condition?**

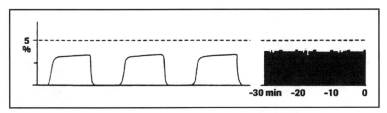

A waveform that has a normal shape but a lower than normal plateau reflects a deficiency of $CO_2$ resulting from hyperventilation.

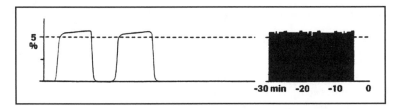

The sudden absence of a waveform usually means that the ventilator has become disconnected from the airway. It also may indicate complete airway obstruction.

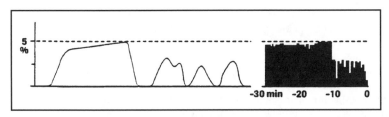

If the waveform drops suddenly and loses its shape but still remains above zero, there may be a partial disconnection in the ventilator circuit or airway, a leak at the ET tube cuff, or the ET tube may be dislodged.

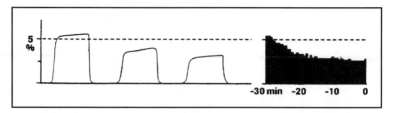

A waveform that drops abruptly over a period of several breaths but maintains its shape may indicate a ventilator malfunction, pulmonary embolism with lack of perfusion to the alveoli, cardiac arrest with no pulmonary perfusion, or severe bleeding resulting in pulmonary hypoperfusion.

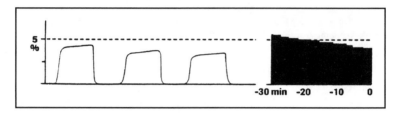

A gradual fall in the waveform may be caused by increased minute ventilation, leading to hyperventilation, or a decrease in cardiac output, resulting in diminished pulmonary perfusion.

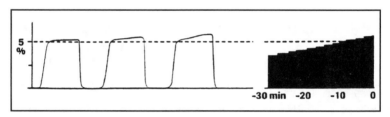

A gradual rise in the waveform may indicate decreased minute ventilation or an increase in the production of $CO_2$, as may be seen with fever or an increased metabolic rate from other causes. Or it may be caused by an accumulation of secretions in the airway that are impairing ventilation.

**Note:** Drawings of abnormal waveforms are reprinted with permission from Carroll P: Evolutions in capnography. RN 62(5):69–71, 1999.

## 15. When is ETCO$_2$ monitoring not appropriate?

ETCO$_2$ monitoring may not be appropriate for critically ill patients with ventilation/perfusion (V/Q) mismatch or intrapulmonary shunt. Patients with normal V/Q matching should have ETCO$_2$ values 1–5 mmHg lower than PaCO$_2$ from blood gas analysis. If the gap falls outside this range, V/Q mismatch should be suspected. Clinical conditions with decreased or absent perfusion despite adequate ventilation are pulmonary embolism, systemic hypovolemia, cardiac arrest, or high levels of positive end-expiratory pressure (PEEP). Once the clinical problem is identified, the nurse can monitor the efficacy of the treatments or the change in the clinical problem by following the difference between the ETCO$_2$ and the PaCO$_2$. Clinical conditions such as atelectasis, pneumonia, lung tumors, mucus plugging, or right main-stem intubation are associated with oxygenation deficits; therefore, oximetry may be more useful than capnography.

## 16. What are the nursing responsibilities for accurate capnography monitoring?

Nurses should follow institutional and manufacturer guidelines in setting up the system and routinely checking the accuracy and calibration of the sensors. Nurses also should be knowledgeable about how capnography works and be able to recognize clinical situations in which ETCO$_2$ may not accurately reflect arterial $CO_2$. It is important to remember that capnography is only a gauge or monitor of trends. If a patient becomes unstable, an invasive arterial blood gas analysis should be done to obtain definitive $CO_2$ values.

**17. How is capnography helpful during cardiopulmonary resuscitation (CPR)?**
A number of studies have demonstrated the value of capnography during CPR. Immediately after cardiac arrest, $ETCO_2$ falls rapidly. The fall in perfusion results in a decrease in circulation to the pulmonary beds and therefore decreased elimination of $CO_2$ from the lung. Because blood flow is returned during adequate compressions and/or spontaneous cardiac function, $ETCO_2$ rises. A rise in $ETCO_2$ during CPR has been associated with increased chances of survival, whereas a decrease in $ETCO_2$ (< 10 mmHg) has been associated with an unsuccessful resuscitation and death.

**18. Is capnography cost-effective?**
Capnography can be a cost-effective measure in the ICU when it is used during weaning instead of blood gas analysis with each ventilator change. Capnography, which reflects $PaCO_2$, and oximetry, which reflects arterial oxygen saturation, are usually used together in the ICU to follow ventilatory and oxygenation status in ventilated patients.

### BIBLIOGRAPHY

1. Ayres SM, Grenvik A, Holbrook PR, Shoemaker WC: Textbook of Critical Care, 3rd ed. Philadelphia, W.B. Saunders, 1995.
2. Carroll P: Evolutions in capnography. RN 62(5):69–71, 1999.
3. Napolitano LM: Capnography in critical care: Accurate assessment of ARDS therapy? Crit Care Med 27(5):862–863, 1999.
4. Sinclair S: Dispelling myths of capnography. Dimens Crit Care Nurs 17:48–55, 1998.
5. St. John RE: Protocols for practice: Applying research at the bedside. Crit Care Nurse 18(6):88–93, 1998.
6. Szaflarski NL, Cohen NH: Use of capnography in critically ill adults. Heart Lung 20:363–374, 1991.
7. Szaflarski NL, Cohen NH: The use of pulse oximetry in critically ill adults. Heart Lung 18:444–453, 1989.
8. Ward KR, Sullivan RJ, Zelenak RR, Summer, WR: A comparison of interposed abdominal compression CPR and standard CPR by monitoring end-tidal $CO_2$. Ann Emerg Med 18:831–837, 1989.
9. Witta KN: When gauging respiratory status is critical. RN 56(11):40–46, 1993.

# 32. POSITIONING FOR OPTIMAL PULMONARY FUNCTION

*Kathleen M. Vollman, MSN, RN, CCNS, CCRN*

**1. How frequently do people turn in their sleep?**
Most people shift position every 11.6 minutes while sleeping.

**2. Describe the effect of body position on the distribution of air flow.**
The intrapleural pressure gradient affects how air is distributed. In the upright position, gravity and the weight of the lung create differences in intrapleural pressure from the apices to the base of the lung, resulting in distribution of more air to the bases. In the supine, lateral, or prone position, the distribution of air becomes more uniform with greater ventilation in dependent than nondependent lung regions. These alterations result from gravitational changes in pleural pressure and the impact of geometric reconfiguration of chest wall structures.

**3. Describe the effect of body position on the distribution of blood flow.**
Position change has a similar effect on perfusion. In the upright position, blood flow increases as it moves from the apical region to the base of the lungs. This gradient is created by the

effect of gravity on a low-pressure system. In the supine or lateral position, blood flow distribution becomes more uniform with greater gravity-dependent perfusion.

**4. What is the overall goal of alterations in distribution of air and blood flow?**

To match ventilation and perfusion in each position so that gas exchange can take place.

**5. What is the effect of the supine position on oxygenation in critically ill patients?**

Ventilation and perfusion matching may worsen because of a reduction in overall lung volumes in moving from a sitting to a supine position. Functional residual capacity decreases by approximately 800 ml in the supine position. This decrease may be caused by pressure of the abdominal contents on the diaphragm, which affects dependent lung ventilation. When the match between ventilation and gravity-dependent perfusion diminishes, gas exchange may worsen. In healthy people the diaphragm acts as a shield, forcibly contracting and pushing the abdominal contents away from the lungs to allow expansion. In critically ill patients, who are often sedated, mechanically ventilated, or paralyzed, the shielding function of the diaphragm is decreased or lost, resulting in restricted lower lung ventilation due to the pressure of abdominal contents. Most intensive care patients lie in the supine position, and many have large abdomens. Both factors may contribute significantly to abnormal gas exchange.

**6. What is the best position for patients with a consolidated type of unilateral lung disease?**

Position the healthy lung downward! The goal is to match alveoli with perfused capillaries. Despite mechanical restriction in the downward position, the healthy lung has an adequate number of functioning alveoli to match gravity-dependent perfusion and thus promote effective gas exchange. This benefit may be more prominent in mechanically ventilated patients than in spontaneously breathing patients.

**7. What are the advantages of continuous lateral rotation therapy (CLRT) compared with turning the patient every 2 hours?**

CLRT reduces the incidence of nosocomial pneumonia and atelectasis as well as time on the ventilator and length of stay in the intensive care unit (ICU). Optimal benefit depends on early placement and > 18 hours of rotation per day. Research has not yet determined whether the degree or the frequency of rotation is the crucial factor.

**8. When should table-based CLRT be used instead of cushion-based CLRT?**

Table rotation should be used if the patient has multiple injuries and requires traction or spinal stabilization.

**9. What criteria are used to determine placement and removal of CLRT?**

Clinical practice varies considerably. To date, only one tool is available to determine placement and removal. The Patient Identification for Rotational Therapy (PIRT) criteria were tested for reliability and validity in a small, 20-patient retrospective analysis. In other studies, diagnostic-related groups have been used to determine placement and removal. Most clinicians who use CLRT develop physiologic criteria to help identify candidates. Reversal of the criteria for 48–72 hours can be used to determine the appropriate time for removal. A good rule of thumb is to discontinue CLRT when the patient can be mobilized effectively with other techniques (e.g., time out of bed).

*Criteria for Placement on Continuous Lateral Rotation Therapy*

---

- Oxygenation problems: partial pressure of oxygen in arterial blood ($PaO_2$) < 60 mmHg on > 40% oxygen in inspired gas ($FiO_2$) and 5 cmH$_2$O of positive end-expiratory pressure (PEEP)
- At-risk mechanically ventilated patients (e.g., patients with septic shock, gastric aspiration, multiple trauma, severe closed head injury, or chemical or functional paralysis for > 24 hours)
- Hemodynamic instability (defined as a sustained drop in blood pressure, decrease in oxygen saturation, or significant increase or decrease in heart rate) with manual turning
- Patients who require frequent bronchoscopy, suctioning for more than 1 hour, or chest physiotherapy for more than 1 hour to remove secretions

---

**10. Why is a protocol important for placement and removal of CLRT?**

Many clinicians use CLRT arbitrarily or as a last resort. Patients may remain on bed systems for extended periods without evidence of benefit. The cost of CLRT beds can mount significantly if their use is not monitored routinely. Clearly, defined criteria for placement and removal are necessary to achieve cost-effective clinical benefit. Other factors that should be included in the protocol are methods of placement, daily monitoring of frequency and degree/percentage of rotation, and outcomes. If the patient demonstrates significant hemodynamic or oxygenation changes with manual turning, the rotational pattern should be increased gradually when CLRT is initiated. Start with small degrees/percentages at low frequency and work toward achieving the percentage of turn that the patient can tolerate at maximal frequency.

**11. When should prone positioning be used in patients with acute lung injury?**

Prone positioning should be initiated when oxygenation worsens despite optimal use of conventional ventilation strategies with adequate sedation. The goal of prone positioning is to improve oxygenation so that $FiO_2$ and PEEP levels can be decreased to prevent further ventilator-induced lung injury. As a rule of thumb, a trial of prone positioning is appropriate when PEEP therapy has been maximized and the $FiO_2$ level has not been reduced below 60%. These criteria should be met relatively early in the course of acute lung injury or acute respiratory distress syndrome.

**12. What kind of improvement in gas exchange is seen when the patient is placed in the prone position?**

Studies have shown an average increase in $PaO_2$ of 20–69 mmHg. Improvements in $PaO_2$ as high as 200 mmHg have been been reported after a single turn.

**13. What percentage of patients respond to prone positioning?**

On average, 70% respond with an increase in $PaO_2$.

**14. Define positive response to prone positioning.**

An increase in $PaO_2 > 10$ mmHg.

**15. When does $PaO_2$ improve in the prone position? How long does the improvement last?**

The response usually occurs within the first 30–60 minutes, but it may take as long as 4–6 hours to determine whether the patient is a responder or nonresponder. Approximately 60% of patients maintain the improvement when they resume the supine position. The duration of improvement is highly patient-dependent. Determination of individual response helps to design the patient's positioning schedule.

**16. What prone positioning schedule should be used in critically ill patients?**

Unfortunately, there are no set guidelines. Some studies have shown a decline in $PaO_2$ after 4–8 hours in the prone position. In addition, the complication rate appears to increase after more than 12 hours in the prone position. With these reports in mind, the practitioner must weigh the positive and negative consequences of leaving the patient in a stationary position for an extended period. A frequency of every 6 hours often is recommended as safe. This schedule also has been combined with CLRT so that when the patient is returned to the supine position, he or she is not stationary. About 40% of patients returned to the supine position lose the improvement in $PaO_2$. Thus, they may need to be returned to the prone position sooner than every 6 hours.

**17. What has limited the use of prone positioning in the critical care setting despite significant improvements in oxygenation?**

Fear! Often considerable fear is associated with the thought of turning upside down a critically ill patient attached to multiple tubes and lines. The process can be safe and relatively easy if you follow a set procedure. The incidence of complications (e.g., hemodynamic instability, extubation, line dislodgement, kinked tubes) is extremely low.

## 18. How is a critically ill patient placed in the prone position?

There are four ways to turn and maintain a patient in the prone position. The first two methods require the use of a specialized bed. The CircOlectric® and Stryker Frame® beds use a bed frame that turns in a circular motion to achieve the prone position. If the practitioner wishes to suspend the abdomen, pillow supports should be placed manually.

The third method is manual positioning using sheets and pillows to turn and maintain the patient in a prone position. This method usually requires 4–6 people, depending on the size and complexity of the patient.

The fourth method is to use the Vollman Prone Positioner, a support frame that facilitates turning and maintaining the patient in a prone position with the abdomen suspended. Only three people are needed. The key concepts for the manual procedure (listed in the table below) are the same with or without the support frame.

### Manual Procedure for Turning Patients from Supine to Prone Position

1. Always turn toward the ventilator.
2. Turn the patient's face away from the ventilator, and loop the ventilator tubing above the patient's head.
3. Place lines inserted above the waist over the shoulders and lines inserted below the waist at the end of the bed. The only exception is chest tubes, which are placed toward the foot of the bed.
4. Using a draw sheet, move the patient to the side of the bed that is farthest from the ventilator. Use a half-step technique for turning. For example, turn to a 45° lateral position, do a safety check, and then complete the rest of the turn.
5. Position the head, arms, and feet correctly to prevent skin, nerve, and joint damage.
6. The procedure is done in reverse to return to the supine position.

## 19. Are patients fed in the prone position?

Yes. The risk for aspiration is highest during the actual turning process. Turn off the feeding tube 45–60 minutes before the turn, and resume feeding once the patient is in the prone position. Some practitioners place the bed in a reverse Trendelenburg position, hoping to minimize the risk for aspiration, but in fact the opposite effect occurs because the esophagus and trachea are in closer proximity. When the head of the bed is flat, drainage is facilitated. This position may prevent aspiration.

## 20. What complications are associated with prone positioning?

Dependent facial edema is the most common complication associated with prone positioning. Pressure ulcers were reported in studies where patients remained in the prone position for more than 12 hours. The most serious complications reported to date are corneal abrasion requiring corneal transplantation and permanent contractures. Other complications are rare but may include the following:

- Hemodynamic instability
- Extubation
- Reduced oxygen saturation
- Apical atelectasia
- Obstructed endotracheal tube
- Kinked esophageal tubes
- Obstructed chest tube
- Dislodgement of central venous catheter or femoral hemodialysis catheter
- Compression of tubing infusing a vasoactive drip
- Transient episode of supraventricular tachycardia

## 21. What are the contraindications to CLRT and prone positioning?

**Contraindications to table-based CLRT:** severe uncontrolled claustrophobia, severe uncontrolled diarrhea, weight > 500 lb.

**Contraindications to cushion-based CLRT:** unstable spinal injuries, marked uncontrollable agitation, severe uncontrollable diarrhea, skeletal traction, weight > 300 lb.

**Relative contraindications to prone positioning:** inability to tolerate head-down position, unstable spine (manual turning with or without a frame), weight > 300 lb (with use of Vollman Prone Positioner), and limitations of bed size, patient size, or number of personnel able to assist.

**22. Is hemodynamic instability an important factor in deciding to turn critically ill patients?**

Hemodynamic instability is the number-one reason that critically ill patients remain in the supine position for extended periods. When you consider the factors affecting tolerance of position change, critically ill patients are clearly at risk. When the patient's gravitational plane is changed, the cardiovascular system attempts to adjust in two ways: (1) The shift in plasma volume may cause messages to be sent to the autonomic nervous system to change vascular tone, and (2) an inner ear or vestibular response probably affects the cardiovascular system with position change. Critically ill patients often have poor vascular tone, a dysfunctional autonomic feedback loop, or low cardiovascular reserve; in addition, they have established equilibrium in a single position over time. Development of hemodynamic instability with a manual turn may be an indication for CLRT, which can gradually train the patient to tolerate turning.

### BIBLIOGRAPHY

1. Basham KR, Vollman KM, Miller A: To everything turn turn turn: An overview of continuous lateral rotation therapy. Respir Care Clin North Am 3:109–132, 1997.
2. Brazzi L, Ravagnan I, Pelosi P, Gattinoni L: Prone position in anaesthesia and intensive care. Care Crit Ill 15:5–8, 1999.
3. Chatte G, Sab JM, Dubois JM, et al: Prone position in mechanically ventilated patients with severe acute respiratory failure. Am J Respir Crit Care Med 155:473–478, 1997.
4. Choi S, Nelson L: Kinetic therapy in critically ill patients: Combined results based on meta-analysis. J Crit Care 7:57–62, 1992.
5. Curley MAQ: Prone positioning of patients with acute respiratory distress syndrome: A systematic review. Am J Crit Care 8:397–405, 1999.
6. deBoisblanc B, Castro M, Everset B, et al: Effects of air-supported, continuous, postural oscillation on the risk of early ICU pneumonia in nontraumatic critical illness. Chest 103:1543–1547, 1993.
7. Pelosi P, Yubiolo D, Mascheroni D, et al: Effects of the prone position on respiratory mechanics and gas exchange during acute lung injury. Am J Respir Crit Care Med 157:387–393, 1998.
8. Shapiro R, Broccard A: Patient positioning in pulmonary disease. Clin Pulmon Med 4:45–52, 1997.
9. Vollman KM: Prone positioning for the ARDS patient. Dimens Crit Care Nurs 16:184–193, 1997.
10. Vollman KM, Bander JJ: Improved positioning utilizing a prone positioner in patients with acute respiratory distress syndrome. Intens Care Med 22:1105–1111, 1996.

# 33. ACUTE RESPIRATORY DISTRESS SYNDROME

*Kathleen M. Vollman*, MSN, RN, CCNS, CCRN

**1. How is acute respiratory distress syndrome (ARDS) defined?**

In 1967 Ashbaugh, Bigelow, Petty, and Levine described the clinical and physiologic characteristics of 12 adult patients who developed severe hypoxemic respiratory failure from various causes. They defined the condition as "a syndrome of acute lung injury in adults, characterized by non-cardiogenic pulmonary edema, manifested by severe hypoxemia caused by right to left shunting through collapsed or fluid filled alveoli." In 1993 a European and American Consensus Conference specified criteria for the diagnosis of ARDS:

- Ratio of partial pressure of oxygen in arterial blood ($PaO_2$) to fractional concentration of oxygen in inspired gas ($FiO_2$) < 200, regardless of positive end-expiratory pressure (PEEP)
- Bilateral infiltrates on chest radiograph
- No evidence of left atrial hypertension

These criteria are evaluated for patients with one or more of the common predisposing risk factors for the development of ARDS.

## 2. What conditions predispose patients to the development of ARDS?

Various disease states or conditions that directly injure the lung or indirectly insult the body place patients at risk for the development of ARDS. Sepsis and gastric aspiration, the two most common predisposing conditions, are associated with a 30–40% chance of developing ARDS.

| DIRECT INJURY | INDIRECT INJURY |
| --- | --- |
| Inhalation injuries: acid aspiration, near drowning, smoke | Sepsis |
| Pneumonitis: bacterial, viral, or fungal origin | Multisystem trauma |
| Pulmonary contusion | Multiple transfusions |
| Oxygen toxicity | Pancreatitis |
| Radiation | Disseminated intravascular coagulation |

## 3. What is acute lung injury (ALI)?

Patients who demonstrate evidence of mild or early injury to the lung and meet the following criteria are diagnosed with ALI:

- $PaO_2/FiO_2$ ratio of < 300, regardless of PEEP
- Bilateral infiltrates on chest radiograph
- No evidence of left atrial hypertension

## 4. What is the $PaO_2/FiO_2$ ratio? Can it be used in everyday practice?

The $PaO_2/FiO_2$ ratio is a user-friendly tool that provides information about the severity of lung injury. This equation places all of the crucial information right at the clinician's fingertips. Simply divide the $PaO_2$ (derived from arterial blood gas analysis) by the $FiO_2$. For example, if the $PaO_2$ is 70 mmHg with a $FiO_2$ of 60% (0.60), the ratio is 70/0.60 = 117. This tool that can be used daily at the bedside for crude assessment and trending of the severity of lung injury.

## 5. What is the mortality rate of ARDS?

The mortality rate of ARDS varies considerably, depending on the specific risk-producing conditions involved. When ARDS was initially reported in the late 1960s and early 1970s, mortality rates ranged between 50% and 70%. Fortunately, over the past 10 years, the general mortality associated with ARDS has declined steadily to the current rate of 40–50%. The improvement most likely is related to progressive advances in many supportive areas.

## 6. What triggers the massive inflammatory insult seen in ARDS?

Various hypotheses have been proposed to explain the pathogenesis of ARDS, but no single theory satisfactorily explains the complex pathophysiologic mechanisms of acute lung injury in ARDS. Experimental and clinical findings suggest that the cooperation, interaction, and amplification of various mediators and mediator systems orchestrate the defect in alveolar capillary permeability and activation of the endothelium, both within the lungs and systemically. Mediators released from activation of the complement, kallikrein-kinin, and coagulation/fibrinolytic systems probably play an important role. These systems are involved in the activation of mediator-forming and mediator-liberating cells, such as neutrophils, macrophages, monocytes, mast cells, endothelial cells, and fibroblasts. The cells of the inflammatory response are involved in the production and secretion of potent mediators. Examples include tumor necrosis factor (TNF) or interleukin-1 (IL-1), proteases, eicosanoids, and reactive oxygen products. However, because research has yet to define the exact path and products of injury, it is difficult to prevent or treat ARDS.

## 7. What pathophysiologic derangements within the lung and systemic circulation create the clinical picture of ARDS?

Four basic pathophysiologic changes associated with ARDS contribute to the clinical picture of severe hypoxemia, pulmonary shunting, bilateral infiltrates, pulmonary hypertension, and additional organ injury:

1. Permeability defect, described as a diffuse, nonuniform injury to the alveolar epithelium and alveolar capillary membrane created by mediators and ventilator-induced injury

2. Acute changes in the caliber of smaller airways

3. Direct injury to pulmonary circulation, created by vasoconstriction and obstruction with microemboli

4. Apparent defect in the body's ability to transport and utilize oxygen at the tissue level

### 8. What normally keeps fluid from entering the lung?

In the normal lung, fluid fluctuations are controlled via hydrostatic pressure, colloidal osmotic pressure, and integrity of the capillary membrane. Disruption of one of these factors can overwhelm the lymphatic drainage system within the pulmonary interstitium and result in flooding of the interstitium and eventually the alveolus itself. In ARDS, the capillary membrane is disrupted, resulting in movement of fluid and high-molecular-weight substances from inside the capillary to the interstitium and alveolar space.

### 9. How does the leaky membrane seen in ARDS affect gas exchange?

Fluid and protein accumulation in the lung results in injury to the gas-exchanging cells and inactivation of surfactant, which enhances collapse of alveoli. The end results of the endothelial defect are decreased lung volumes, severely reduced lung compliance, and impaired gas exchange through the creation of intrapulmonary shunts and ventilation/perfusion (V/Q) mismatching.

### 10. How does damage to the pulmonary vasculature affect gas exchange and oxygen delivery to tissues?

When the vessels are injured, both pulmonary artery pressures and pulmonary vascular resistance increase. The consequences of injury to the pulmonary circuit are twofold:

1. Damage to vascular tone impairs the compensatory mechanism of hypoxic vasoconstriction. Vascular areas previously constricted to prevent perfusion of nonventilated regions dilate, contributing to an increased shunt and worsening hypoxemia.

2. Abrupt increases in pressure within the pulmonary vascular bed place excessive work on the right ventricle, resulting in dilation and hypertrophy. The right ventricle and left ventricle compete for available space within the pericardial sac. Acute right heart dilation, which occurs in an attempt to manage increased pressure from the pulmonary vascular bed, produces a leftward shift of the interventricular septum. As a result of the shift, the potential filling volume of the left ventricle is reduced, causing a fall in cardiac output and, ultimately, a reduction in oxygen delivery to tissues.

### 11. Describe the classic presentation of ARDS.

**Refractory hypoxemia** is the hallmark clinical sign of ARDS. Administration of 100% oxygen concentration leads to little or no change in the $PaO_2$ because of significant intrapulmonary shunting. Another clinical sign is abnormal lung mechanics, with elevations in peak airway pressures and decreased compliance. The change in lung mechanics makes it difficult to move air in and out of the lungs; this phenomenon is often called "stiff lung."

The classic **"white-out" on chest radiographs** is characteristic of ARDS and aids in the diagnosis. However, recent findings suggest that the diffuse homogenous picture of interstitial and alveolar infiltrates seen on radiographs is actually unequal. The consolidation is more patchy, regional and gravity-dependent.

The other two signs and symptoms are **pulmonary hypertension**, reflected in high pulmonary artery pressures, and **additional organ failures**.

### 12. What are the major goals of treatment for ARDS?

The three major goals in treating ARDS are to prevent further injury to the lung, to maintain pulmonary oxygenation, and to optimize oxygen delivery to the tissues.

**13. Is there an easy way to remember the different types of supportive therapy necessary to increase the chance of survival for patients with ARDS?**

The working plan of care for patients with ARDS depends on the six Ps of supportive therapy: prevention, PEEP, pipes, pump, paralysis, and positioning.

**14. What role does the critical care nurse play in the prevention of pneumonia?**

Basic infection control practices minimize bacterial burden and colonization and thus decrease the incidence of ventilator-associated pneumonia (VAP). Effective techniques to reduce the risk of colonization and to prevent infection include the use of sterile technique during endotracheal suctioning, careful handling of the ventilator tubing to prevent backflow of pooled condensation with resultant contamination, lateral rotation therapy, strict handwashing, and appropriate glove use.

Methods to prevent aspiration of colonized secretions should be incorporated in the plan of care. Examples include suctioning of oropharyngeal secretions, routine hygiene of the oral cavity, ensuring adequate endotracheal balloon inflation, maintaining a patent nasogastric tube, avoiding gastric distention, and positioning the head of the bed at > 30°.

**15. How can ventilation strategies help to prevent further injury to the lungs?**

Based on a significant amount of animal research and visualization of the ARDS-affected lung on computed tomography scan, it is clear that ARDS involves small areas of normally functioning lung and areas of complete shut-down. This pattern is called "baby lungs." If "baby lungs" are ventilated at normal tidal volumes of 10–12 ml/kg, hyperinflation and overdistention occur in the functioning areas. Several research studies have associated such overdistention with diffuse alveolar injury. Therefore, ventilating with lower tidal volumes may help to reduce ventilator-induced injury.

**16. What lung-protective strategies are used to ventilate patients with ARDS?**

The new approach to mechanical ventilation for patients with ARDS fully encompasses the following lung-protective strategies:
- Limiting ventilator pressures to prevent barotrauma and alveolar stress injury
- Reducing tidal volumes in response to the reduced lung capacity and regional differences in compliance associated with the "baby lung" model of ARDS, thereby preventing volutrauma
- Administering PEEP at levels high enough to maintain alveolar distention throughout the entire respiratory cycle
- Reducing the $FiO_2$ level below 60% to prevent oxygen toxicity

**17. Describe the rationale behind the new strategies.**

The aim is to adjust tidal volumes based on the patient's lung mechanics instead of normalizing arterial blood gases. Studies show evidence of improved outcome when lower tidal volumes (5–7 ml/kg) are used. The consequence of this lung-protective strategy is hypercapnia. **Permissive hypercapnia** is the technique of deliberate hypoventilation to protect the lung, with emphasis on controlling airway pressures instead of maintaining a normal value for the partial pressure of carbon dioxide in arterial blood ($PaCO_2$). Reports in the literature show that patients tolerate $PaCO_2$ in the range of 50–120 mmHg. The key to this strategy is to allow carbon dioxide levels to rise gradually by slowly reducing minute ventilation. This technique allows the kidneys to compensate for the resultant respiratory acidosis. However, judicious use of bicarbonate replacement may be necessary if the pH falls below 7.20.

**18. Where do alternative ventilation modes fit into the picture?**

Many different ventilator strategies have been attempted over the past 20 years. Examples include pressure control alone or in conjunction with inverse ratio ventilation, extracorporeal membrane oxygenation, extracorporeal removal of carbon dioxide with low-volume pressure ventilation, and high-frequency jet ventilation. However, sufficient randomized controlled clinical trials have not been performed to support their efficiency over standard methods. Therefore, most authors suggest use of these strategies when conventional methods have failed to achieve the desired outcome.

### 19. Should patients with ARDS be kept dry?

Many nurses have played the fluid bolus/Lasix game with patients with ARDS. Fluid management can be compared with walking a tight rope. The goal is to achieve a normovolemic state that allows maintenance of blood volume to ensure adequate cardiac output. However, the issue remains controversial. Some authorities advocate fluid restriction to minimize alveolar flooding, whereas others support maximization of oxygen delivery to the tissues through volume loading to reduce the incidence of multiorgan dysfunction syndrome. So which is the correct answer? Consider aiming for sufficient blood volume to obtain an adequate cardiac output that ensures oxygen delivery to the tissues.

### 20. How important is maintaining the balance between oxygen delivery and tissue demand in patients with ARDS?

Balance is extremely important. In patients with ARDS, oxygen consumption depends on delivery. If demand increases without subsequent improvements in delivery, an oxygen debt develops. Therefore, the plan of care must not only incorporate adequate pharmacologic therapy to limit oxygen consumption due to agitation, it also must include interventions to minimize the impact of various nursing activities on oxygen consumption.

### 21. What strategies help to minimize oxygen consumption?

Time for sufficient oxygen recovery must be included in plans for routine nursing therapy. Recommendations about suctioning, positioning, and temperature control also should be incorporated into the plan of care. A closed technique, explanation of the procedure, reassurance, and hyperoxygenation before and after the procedure can minimize the impact of suctioning on oxygen consumption. Nursing interventions to reduce a fever above 38.5°C are important because, for every 1-degree Centigrade increase in body temperature, oxygen consumption ($VO_2$) increases by 10%. Routine activities such as bathing, dressing change, and weighing also increase oxygen consumption in studies of populations other than patients with ARDS. Further examination of acceptable methods and timing of these interventions needs to be conducted with the ARDS population.

### 22. What role does sedation or sedation plus paralysis play in the management of excessive oxygen consumption caused by agitation and/or asynchrony with the ventilator?

Choice of the appropriate agent for sedation should be based on the diagnosis of pain, anxiety, delirium, or ventilator asynchrony; therapeutic goals; and the half-life, duration of action, and pharmacologic side effects of the agent. The key to effective sedation is a consistent approach to administration of the drug, evaluation of response, and achievement of therapeutic endpoint. Random administration of sedatives and analgesic on as-needed basis can result in a wide spectrum of patient response, from excessive agitation to lethargy. The use of guidelines or protocols for the management of agitation in mechanically ventilated patients allows greater consistency of care, faster response time to ventilator asynchrony, and achievement of therapeutic doses before additional agents are added. If sedation is ineffective in reducing episodes of excessive muscle work and asynchronous ventilation, pharmacologic paralysis with scheduled sedation may be warranted. Paralytics are rarely necessary if sedation is managed effectively.

### 23. What role does positioning play in the treatment of patients with ARDS?

Continuous lateral rotation therapy (CLRT) has been advocated for use in patients with acute lung injury. It appears to be effective in reducing the incidence of nosocomial pneumonia, atelectasis, ventilator time, and length of stay in the intensive care unit. The earlier the patient is placed on the therapy during the acute illness, the better the response. CLRT has some beneficial effect on oxygenation variables over time, but more studies are necessary to verify this finding. The absolute answer about the degree and frequency of rotation that improves outcome is not yet available.

**24. Which position has been found to be most beneficial for patients with ARDS?**

Studies have shown average increases in $PaO_2$ of 20–69 mmHg when patients are placed in the prone position. Improvements in $PaO_2$ as high as 200 mmHg have been seen with a single turn. In one study, the prone position improved gas exchange in 70% of patients with ARDS. The earlier the position is used, the more likely the positive response (see chapter 32).

**25. What new therapies are under investigation for future treatment of ARDS?**

In the future, we may serve a **cocktail of pharmacologic agents** with the potential to block many or all of the significant mediators involved in ARDS. Pharmacologic studies have been directed toward inhibiting substances released by endotoxins, neutrophils, and macrophages, such as oxygen radicals, proteolytic and lysosomal enzymes, metabolites of arachidonic acid metabolism, and cytokines. However, research has not progressed to the point of widespread clinical application.

In a number of small studies, **inhaled nitric oxide** is associated with improved oxygenation and reduced pulmonary artery pressures in ARDS via selective vasodilatation of the pulmonary vasculature. In a phase III trial of nitric oxide use in patients with ALI, no difference in mortality was seen The use of **inhaled surfactant** has been studied extensively in adults. Early studies revealed limited success in improving gas exchange and/or outcome, in part because of problems with surfactant delivery. New trials with improved delivery methods may give a clearer indication of the benefit of surfactant administration.

Finally, the use of **partial liquid ventilation** is under investigation as a mechanism to improve gas exchange. It appears to enhance recruitment of atelectatic lung regions in the dependent zones. An additional mechanism may be the lavaging of exudate by perfluorocarbon from the peripheral airways to a more central location, where suctioning is effective.

**26. If the patient lives, will he or she have permanent lung damage?**

Most survivors of ARDS have significant abnormalities in pulmonary function at the time of discontinuation of mechanical ventilation. Substantial improvement occurs within the first 3 months, and gradual improvement continues for up to 6 months. Chest radiographs and arterial blood gases are normal for most patients, but many continue to experience dyspnea. At the 6-month benchmark, approximately 50% of survivors return to baseline pulmonary function. The other half continues to have alterations in pulmonary function, particularly a reduction in diffusion capacity and/or changes in self-reported physical and psychological well-being.

BIBLIOGRAPHY

1. Amato MB, Barbas CS, Medeiros DM, et al: Effect of a protective-ventilation strategy on mortality in the acute respiratory distress syndrome. N Engl J Med 338:347–354, 1998.
2. American Thoracic Society: Hospital-acquired pneumonia in adults: Diagnosis, assessment of severity, initial antimicrobial therapy: A consensus statement. Am J Respir Crit Care Med 153:1711–1725, 1995.
3. ARDS Network: Ventilation with lower tidal volumes as compared with traditional tidal volumes for acute lung injury and the acute respiratory distress syndrome. N Engl J Med 342:1301–1308, 2000.
4. Artigas A, Bernard GR, Carlet J, et al: The American-European Consensus Conference on ARDS, Part 2. Am J Respir Crit Care Med 157:1332–1347, 1998.
5. Ashbaugh DG, Bigelow DB, Petty TL, Levine, BE. Acute respiratory distress in adults. Lancet 2:319–323, 1967.
6. Basham KR, Vollman KM, Miller A: To everything turn turn turn: An overview of continuous lateral rotation therapy. Respir Care Clin North Am 3:109–132, 1997.
7. Cawley MJ, Skaar DJ, Anderson HL, Hanson CW: Mechanical ventilation and pharmacologic strategies for acute respiratory distress syndrome. Pharmacotherapy 18:140–155, 1998.
8. Dreyfuss D, Saumon G: Ventilator-induced lung injury. Am J Respir Crit Care Med, 157:294–323, 1998.
9. Marini JJ: Evolving concepts in the ventilatory management of acute respiratory distress syndrome. Clin Chest Med 17:555–575, 1996.
10. Marini JJ, Evans TW: Round table conference: Acute lung injury. Am J Respir Crit Care Med 158:675–679, 1998.
11. Nahum A, Shapiro R: Adjuncts to mechanical ventilation. Clin Chest Med 17:491–511, 1996.
12. Vollman KM, Aulbach RK: Acute respiratory distress syndrome. In Kinney M, Brooks-Brunn J, Dunbar S, et al (eds): AACN's Clinical Reference for Critical Care Nursing, 4th ed. St Louis, Mosby, 1998, pp 529–564.

# 34. EXTRACORPOREAL LIFE SUPPORT AND EXTRACORPOREAL MEMBRANE OXYGENATION

*Dianne L. Sodt-Davitt, RN, BS*

### 1. Define extracorporeal life support (ECLS) and extracorporeal membrane oxygenation (ECMO).

ECLS is a therapy that includes continuous extracorporeal cardiopulmonary bypass via extrathoracic cannulation for patients with acute, reversible cardiac or respiratory failure refractory to conventional medical or pharmacologic management. ECLS allows time for the native lungs to rest under low ventilatory pressures while providing adequate oxygen delivery and carbon dioxide ($CO_2$) removal. ECLS also allows lower fractionated concentrations of oxygen ($FiO_2$) and lower volume delivery via the mechanical ventilator, thereby reducing risk of oxygen toxicity and barotrauma. ECLS includes ECMO and ECMO with cardiac extracorporeal support.

### 2. Which patients require ECLS?

The most common indication for ECLS is severe acute respiratory failure in newborn and adult patients. The use of ECLS for cardiovascular support has been extended to other conditions, including perioperative cardiac failure, primary myocardial failure, bridge to transplantation, and emergency cardiopulmonary resuscitation. Acute respiratory distress syndrome (ARDS) continues to be the primary indication for use of ECLS. Although inciting events may be diverse, injury to the alveolar-capillary membrane, which leads to obliteration of the gas-alveolar interface, appears to be a final common pathway for the development of ARDS.

### 3. Is ECLS considered a first-line treatment for acute respiratory failure?

In newborns ECLS is the standard treatment, with > 10,000 applications per year and an 80% survival rate. In adults, alternative modes of ventilation and pharmacologic intervention should be exhausted before implementation of ECLS. Alternative modes of ventilation include low tidal volume ventilation (permissive hypercapnia), proning, inverse ratio ventilation, and high-level positive end-expiratory pressure (PEEP). Pharmacologic interventions include neuromuscular blocking agents, sedatives, and opioids, which facilitate mechanical ventilation and minimize oxygen consumption.

### 4. What are the components of the extracorporeal circuit used for ECLS?

Membrane lung circuit, roller pump, and heat exchanger.

### 5. What are the main features of the membrane lung circuit?

The extracorporeal volume of the circuit is an important feature. Priming volume increases in larger circuits, and platelet consumption increases in proportion to the surface area of the membrane lung. Circuit volumes of 400–3000 ml can be used in neonates and adults.

The membrane lung is connected to a gas mixer (oxygen and $CO_2$) that can be adjusted to meet the patient's gas exchange needs. Pressure monitor and safety devices are located along the circuit. Continuous mixed venous saturation ($SvO_2$) is measured in the venous drain of the circuit. An $SvO_2$ value of 75% is the goal and indicates that perfusion and oxygen delivery are adequate. It also decreases the need for obtaining frequent systemic and circuit blood gases.

### 6. What are the main features of the roller pump?

The bladder and a "bladder box" microswitch act as the servoregulator for the roller pump. The pump is turned off whenever pump flow exceeds venous blood return. Once the bladder has refilled, the pump automatically restarts. This safety mechanism prevents the pump from pulling excessively on the right atrium or a major vessel that may be cannulated. Anticipated blood flow rates are 70–90 ml/kg/min in adults, 80–100 ml/kg/min in children, and 120–170 ml/kg/min in neonates.

## 7. What is the purpose of the heat exchanger?

The heat exchanger is essential to prevent hypothermia caused by the large extracorporeal volume.

## 8. How are vascular access and cannulation configured?

Cannulation configurations vary according to the needs of the patient. The standard is a **veno-venous (V-V) cannulation** that drains blood from a large vein, pumps it through the oxygenator, and returns it to the patient through another large vein. V-V is the preferred access method if cardiac function is adequate. The femoral vein or right internal jugular is the usual access site; the return sites are the right atria via the right internal jugular or femoral veins. In some cases, two venous drains may be necessary to provide adequate pump flow to meet the patient's oxygen requirements.

**Venoarterial (V-A) cannulation** is used in patients with profound cardiac and pulmonary failure. V-A ECMO drains blood from a large vein, pumps it through the oxygenator, and returns it via the femoral or common carotid artery.

## 9. What is the optimal catheter size?

Blood flow through the extracorporeal circuit is limited by the size of the venous catheter. Resistance to blood flow is related directly to the length and diameter of the catheter. Cannula diameters range from 16 to 32 French for adult access. Under optimal circumstances, you should use catheters with the shortest and largest internal diameter that can be placed.

## 10. How are cannulas accesssed?

Percutaneous technique is typically used to place access cannulas; if problems are encountered, a cutdown procedure may be performed.

## 11. Is anticoagulation required during ECLS?

Systemic anticoagulation is maintained with continuous heparin infusion and a target activated clotting time (ACT) of 180–200 seconds for whole blood. In the presence of bleeding, the heparin dose may be decreased and the target ACT lowered to 160–180 seconds. ACTs are measured hourly, and the heparin dose is adjusted according to protocol. Platelets are monitored and transfused to keep the count at 80,000–100,000/mm$^3$. In the presence of bleeding, a higher platelet count may be desired. Platelet counts and function can be affected by heparin, uremia, and the synthetic ECLS cirucuit.

## 12. How should temperature regulation be managed?

The bedside nurse monitors the patient's temperature, and the heat exchanger is altered as needed by the perfusionist/technician. Because ECLS can mask a fever by altering blood temperature, close monitoring of other signs and symptoms of infection is required.

## 13. How does the ECLS circuit affect the hemodynamic profile?

Depending on cannulation sites and amount of flow, cardiac function greatly affects the ability to obtain conventional hemodynamic profiles. Traditional values, such as central venous pressure (CVP), pulmonary capillary wedge pressure (PCWP), and pulmonary arterial diastolic and systolic (PAD/PAS) pressures, may not reflect true pressures and volume status, especially with V-A ECLS.

## 14. What is the role of SvO$_2$ monitoring?

SvO$_2$ is invaluable for monitoring critically ill patients. On ECLS the SvO$_2$ readings from the pulmonary artery catheter are not useful or valid because the oxygen provided to the patient from the ECLS circuit is infused into the venous system. SvO$_2$ measured on the venous side of the circuit (preoxygenator) does not reflect changes in the patient's status due to the recirculation factor.

**15. What factors should be considered in troubleshooting a clinical presentation that does not match the hemodynamic profile?**

Cannula access and the potential effects of ECLS on hemodynamic values (see question 13). Evaluation of the hemodynamic profile can be augmented by a physical examination to inspect for edema, monitoring of the patient's weight, and use of echocardiography to evaluate myocardial function and fluid status.

**16. Explain "cutting out." What is its significance?**

"Cutting out" signals an alarm from the bladder box that the venous drainage is not adequate to meet pump settings. "Cutting out" from the bladder box is an indicator of volume status and typically signifies hypovolemia or inadequate flow. It may be related to volume status, position of cannula (agitation), or bed height.

**17. What are typical ventilator settings for a patient receiving ECLS?**

One goal of ECLS is to allow the native lung to rest by supporting systemic oxygenation and ventilation. The typical settings are a low $FiO_2$ (< 50%), peak inspiratory pressure of < 35 $cmH_2O$, PEEP of 10 $cmH_2O$, respiratory rate of 4–6 breaths/min, and an inspiratory/expiratory (I:E) ratio of 2–4:1. Spontaneous respirations are an important parameter to follow and document, because they provide information about readiness for weaning.

**18. How is the airway managed?**

Tracheostomy allows a stable and secure long-term airway. Usually it is performed early in the course of ECLS, if needed. The expected course of the disease helps to determine whether a tracheostomy should be performed. The advantages of early tracheostomy are well established for patients on ECLS. Some bleeding around the tracheostomy site should be expected because of the anticoagulated state of the patient.

**19. When and how are patients weaned from ECLS?**

Chest radiographs, blood gases, and pulmonary compliance are assessed for improvement and stability before initiation of weaning. The ECLS flow is weaned until flow rates approximate 10–25% of total cardiac output. The oxygen flow to the membrane lung is weaned when V-V ECLS is used to assess gas exchange of the native lung. It is important to assess and document pulse, blood pressure, tidal volumes, $SvO_2$, pulse oximetry, and end-tidal $CO_2$ during weaning. Sedation is typical throughout a trial off ECLS, systemic arterial blood gases are checked, and the patient is observed clinically for tolerance. Multiple weaning trials are attempted, and it may take approximately 2–4 days before the patient is decannulated.

**20. Why is sedation given during ECLS?**

Sedation and analgesia are used to facilitate tolerance of the procedure, to maximize oxygen delivery, to promote patient comfort, and to increase cannula security. Dislodgement of the cannulas can lead to patient death and may occur despite the presence of sutures and dressings and personnel at the bedside. Other protective measures, such as use of restaints, may be necessary.

**21. Which sedative agents are used?**

Various sedatives may be used during ECLS. **Propofol** is an excellent choice because of its short half-life, which allows periodic assessment of neurologic status. Triglycerides should be monitored, and adjustment of caloric intake may be necessary.

**Neuromuscular blockers with continuous opioid coverage**, alone or with sedatives, are often necessary to achieve adequate venous drainage from the cannulas and to reduce oxygen consumption. Lorazepam can be used, but patients take a while to awaken after receiving large doses and it is difficult to assess neurologic status. Drug holidays should be scheduled on a daily basis to assess neurologic function.

**22. How often should neurologic status be assessed?**

Neurologic checks should be performed every 4–8 hours to monitor for cerebral bleeding. We expect patients to awaken daily and to follow simple commands.

**23. What other key areas should the nurse assess during ECLS therapy?**

- **Cardiac parameters:** heart rate, blood pressure, central venous, pulse oximetry, urine output, and circuit $SvO_2$ levels.
- **Respiratory and ventilator parameters:** respiratory rate, $FiO_2$, PEEP, and peak inspiratory pressure. It is important to note and report any changes in assessment parameters with repositioning. Patients in the prone position may have increased tidal volumes and pulmonary drainage.
- **Lab values:** Electrolytes and hemoglobin/hematocrit should be assessed every 4–8 hours. Liver function tests and measurements of blood urea nitrogen and creatinine usually are done daily to assess organ function. Some centers maintain hematocrit at 45–48% to maximize oxygen-carrying capacity and oxygen delivery.

**24. When is treatment considered futile?**

ECLS extends life far longer than conventional therapies. As difficult as it is, ECLS should be stopped when there is no hope for recovery. Futility as well as family desires are considered in making the decision to cease therapy. Indications for withdrawal include advancing multiple organ failure, confirmation of fibrosis on open lung biopsy, refractory septic shock, uncontrollable pulmonary hemorrhage, irreversible brain damage, and demonstrated lack of neurologic function. Careful screening of potential ECLS patients is paramount in minimizing the continuance of futile interventions.

**25. What can be done to support the families of patients receiving ECLS?**

ECLS is highly stressful for the family as well as the patient. Use of written material in lay terms can help families to understand the procedure and share their understanding with others. Frequent, short visits of a few people at once help the staff to answer questions and provide patient care. Family members should be encouraged to be close to the patient as long as they are careful of the circuitry. Guiding them to the side of the bed opposite the ECLS circuitry is helpful. Daily communication between the family and health care team is essential so that the family receives an update on changes in the patient's condition. The development of a trusting relationship between family and care providers offers tremendous support.

## BIBLIOGRAPHY

1. Bartlett RH: Crititcal Care Physiology. Boston, Little Brown, 1995.
2. Cornish JD, Clark RH: Principles and practice of venovenous extracorporeal membrane oxygenation. J Intens Care Med 11:289–301, 1996.
3. Dirkes S, Dickinson S, Valentine J: Acute respiratory failure and ECMO. Crit Care Nurse Oct :39–47, 1992.
4. Hirschl RB, Bartlett RH: Extracorporeal membrane oxygenation support in cardiorespiratory failure. Adv Surg 21:189–212, 1987.
5. Kolla S, Awad S, Rich P, et al: Extracorporeal life support for 100 adult patients with severe respiratory failure. Ann Surg 226:544–566, 1997.
6. Kolla S, Lee W, Hirschl R, Bartlett R: Extracorporeal life support for cardiovascular support in adults. J ASAIO 42:M809–M819, 1996.
7. Matthay MA: The adult respiratory distress syndrome: New insights into diagnosis, pathophysiology and treatment. West J Med 150:187–194, 1989.
8. Rich PB, Bartlett RH,. et al: An Approach to the Treatment of Severe Adult Respiratory Failure. Philadelphia, W.B. Saunders, 1997.
9. Sandber M, Singh A, Graves P: Exracorporoeal membrane oxygenation as therapy in refractory, reversible myocarditis. Crit Care Nurse Dec:53–58, 1995.

# III. Infection Control, Hematology, Oncology, and Immunology

## 35. INFECTION CONTROL

*Marilyn Jordan, RN, MPH*

**1. What are the most common nosocomial (hospital-acquired) infections?**

Urinary tract infection (UTI) is the most common nosocomial infection and often is related to use of indwelling catheters. Of patients with UTI, 1–2% may develop bacteremia. Blood stream infection (BSI) is the second most common nosocomial infection. Most BSIs are due to infection at another site (secondary infections). Approximately 30% of BSIs are primary infections and often are associated with a vascular device such as a central intravenous (IV) catheter.

**2. What can be done to decrease the incidence of UTIs and BSIs?**

Always use sterile supplies and solutions. Use aseptic technique during insertion of catheters, maintain closed systems, wash hands, avoid touch contamination during necessary manipulations, and follow hospital procedures for dressing, catheter, supply, and/or site changes. Peripheral IV catheter sites and IV tubing sets can be maintained safely for 72 hours. Arterial line dressings and transducer set-ups can be maintained up to 96 hours. Multilumen catheters should be avoided if possible, because the risk for infection is greater. Removal of indwelling catheters as soon as possible also minimizes risk of infection.

**3. What is the most deadly nosocomial infection?**

Pneumonia is the most deadly nosocomial infection, especially in the critical care setting, where the mortality rate may exceed 50%. The progression from colonization with either normal or "hospital" flora to miniaspiration, followed by development of an actual infection with or without infiltrates, has been well described. Patients on ventilators are at a 5–10-fold higher risk than patients who are not ventilated.

**4. How can nosocomial pneumonia be prevented?**

The 1994 CDC guidelines recommend the following prevention strategies:
- Standardized processing of reusable circuits and equipment used for ventilation
- Use of sterile fluids for nebulization and medications
- Handwashing and task-oriented gloves for handling ventilator circuitry and suctioning
- Prevention of microaspiration through patient positioning, pulmonary toilet, and pain management to promote adequate respiratory effort
- Judicious use of antibiotics
- Pathogen-specific recommendations for *Legionella* and *Aspergillus* species

In addition, many centers improve patients' immunization status with vaccination for *Streptococcus pneumoniae* (Pneumovax) and influenza (flu vaccine).

**5. What factors put critical care patients at risk for acquiring infections?**

Approximately 10 of 100 patients in the intensive care unit (ICU) or 25 infections per 1000 patient days in the ICU account for more than 50% of all serious nosocomial infections. Patient risk factors include extremes of age, invasive procedures and devices, underlying disease, metabolic dysfunction, and use of antibiotics. In addition, prolonged exposure to intubation or cardiovascular and other monitoring devices, as well frequent emergent events, may lead to breach of aseptic/sterile technique. Compromise of natural barriers to infection, such as skin and normal gastrointestinal tract, and changes in immunologic and nutritional status increase the risk, particularly as the patient's stay is prolonged.

### 6. What is the difference between colonization and infection?

In **colonization**, an organism is present (positive culture), but signs and symptoms of an active infection are absent. Colonized organisms typically live on the surface of the skin, mucosa, or device (e.g., IV catheter, tracheostomy tube). The culture result is still important because it may indicate the organism that later causes a serious infection (e.g., colonization with methicillin-resistant *Staphylococcus aureus* [MRSA] or vancomycin-resistant enterococci [VRE]). In fact, sometimes colonization is treated, especially in immunocompromised patients.

**Infection** is associated with signs and symptoms such as fever, drainage, and changes in white blood cell count. The organism has invaded tissue and provoked a local or systemic inflammatory response.

### 7. What are the common sources of organisms in the clinical area?

Skin organisms such as *S. aureus* and *Staphylococcus epidermidis* are transmitted from patients and staff. Water organisms such as *Pseudomonas* sp. are found in patient fluids (e.g., respiratory secretions and other fluids, especially if left standing), solutions (even antiseptics), urine or other waste containers, or ventilator circuit tubings. VRE, *Clostridium difficile*, and other bowel flora often are found on commodes, electronic thermometers (rectal), or almost any equipment or surface contaminated by gloved or soiled hands. Some immunocompromised patients are at risk from the water supply or ceilings open for work or remodeling.

### 8. Does any evidence indicate that short-staffing contributes to the problem of nosocomial infections?

Staffing fluctuations, particularly with an increase in patient acuity, may undermine aseptic technique and lead to less compliance with handwashing, task-oriented glove use, and other standard infection control practices. Clusters of infection are seen when less-than-optimal conditions exist. However, we need to discover ways to increase staff compliance with infection control practices at all times—not just when staffing is tight.

### 9. What should be used for handwashing in the critical care setting?

Follow your hospital's handwashing policy. Most centers provide both a general soap and at least one antimicrobial agent, such as chlorhexidine or iodine, for handwashing. A thorough wash with soap, using friction, rinsing, and drying, takes about 10–15 seconds. An antimicrobial agent often lowers counts of skin organisms for a longer time and should be used before performing invasive procedures, such as starting IV lines, or in caring for high-risk or immunocompromised patients. In addition, use of antimicrobial soap is recommended after caring for patients known to have resistant organisms such as MRSA or VRE. Waterless cleaners (most of which are alcohol-based) in liquid, foam, or wipes are popular in Canada and Europe and are considered good adjuncts to regular handwashing for dealing with patients with resistant organisms.

### 10. Is it safe to care at the same time for a patient with an infectious disease or antibiotic-resistant infection and an immunocompromised patient?

There must be an invisible line that is never crossed without removal of gloves, handwashing, and proper cleaning and disinfection of shared equipment. The method of isolation depends on the disease involved and hospital policy. Standard precautions used faithfully have made a significant difference in preventing cross-contamination. Common sense should be the basic principle. When an outbreak or possible cluster of infections occurs, it may be necessary to cohort infected patients with designated staff as a short-term intervention.

**11. What are the most important steps in caring for a patient with possible pulmonary tuberculosis (TB)?**

1. Be aware of TB. If diagnosis is delayed, the risk of exposure is increased.

2. Wear the correct respiratory protection. Clinicians should be fit-tested for either a N95 or other respirator mask. An OSHA regulation requires that these safety devices be available at all medical centers.

3. Patients should wear a well-fitting surgical mask if they are transported from the room. All visitors should wear surgical masks as well.

4. Place the patient in a private room with negative-pressure airflow and a minimum of 6 air exchanges per hour. A high-efficiency particulate air (HEPA) machine, running continuously, removes bacilli from the environment and air.

5. Follow safety precautions for all coughing patients and during cough-producing procedures. If diagnosis of TB or other airborne infections is delayed, you will have prevented exposure by instructing patients to cover their cough or by using some sort of mask to protect yourself if patients cannot cover their cough.

**12. What is the relationship between the environment and infectious disease?**

The environment reflects the flora within it—both friends and enemies. Of course, the typical ICU environment is well populated with worrisome pathogens: *C. difficile*, *S. aureus* (both sensitive and resistant to various antibiotics), gram-negative water organisms (e.g., *Pseudomonas* and *Stenotrophomonas* spp.), and many others. Keeping patient areas clear (free of clutter, such as extra supplies and linen) facilitates cleaning and maintenance of the environment. Using a hospital-grade disinfectant at the correct dilution can prevent excessive contamination in patient areas. The detergent/disinfectant should be left wet on the surface for a minimum of 30 seconds—or better yet, 1 or 2 minutes—to break up organic material and kill organisms. Disposable germicidal wipes (not those used for hands) also work, but contact time is often limited. Frequent glove changes and handwashing can also prevent environmental contamination. If gloves are required as part of isolation or other procedures, be aware of what else besides the patient you are touching as you work.

**13. What are the guidelines for supplies used for or by patients with VRE or other resistant organisms?**

1. Keep supply levels in the patient room to a minimum.

2. Keep packages closed and intact. Protect them from contamination and glove contact. Supplies that are open or in some way nonintact should not be considered for use with other patients.

3. Sending questionable items out of the unit with the patient may be a way to avoid waste. Patients may be able to use them during the rest of their hospitalization.

4. Check your hospital policy, and arrange for equipment to be properly disinfected before use on the next patient. Some hospitals have a system whereby commodes, pumps, and other equipment are clearly labeled as cleaned before they are put back into service. Electronic thermometers and other shared equipment have been implicated in outbreaks.

**14. What are the most important steps to protect the nurse from infection and exposure?**

The most important step is use of Standard Precautions (e.g., handwashing, task-oriented glove use, barrier use, including protective face-wear when you may be exposed to body substances). Splashes to mucous membranes of the eyes, nose, and mouth are regularly reported by staff who do not use protective face-wear when working with intubated patients and helping with procedures or during crisis situations. Needlesticks and other sharps injuries are declining because of the introduction of needleless systems and safety devices. It should be a goal of all clinicians to avoid needle use. It is important to use safety devices properly and whenever possible.

**15. What immunizations are recommended for hospital employees?**

Vaccines for hepatitis B, chickenpox (Varivax), if susceptible, and flu (annually) are recommended for nurses. Recent follow-up data about hepatitis B vaccination indicate that once the series of three shots is completed and a positive serum antibody response is obtained, there is no need for revaccination.

**16. Where is the line drawn for employees who come to work with illnesses?**

Be aware that good health provides protection for you and that a simple upper respiratory infection can be deadly for critically ill patients. Direct patient care is hazardous to others when you have fever, draining wounds, or other signs and symptoms indicating a high viral or bacterial load, even when barriers are used. If you are in doubt, get advice from the manager, employee health officer, or infection control practitioner before caring for patients.

### BIBLIOGRAPHY

1. CDC Guidelines for Prevention of Transmission of Tuberculosis in Health Care Facilities, MMWR 43:RR13:1–132, 1994.
2. Cohen F, et al: Microbial resistance to drug therapy: A review. Am J Infect Control 25:51–64, 1997.
3. Lai KK: Safety of prolonging peripheral cannula and IV tubing use from 72 hours to 96 hours. Am J Infect Control 26:66–70, 1998.
4. Levy S: The challenge of antibiotic resistance. Sci Am March:46–53, 1998.
5. Olmstead R (ed): APIC Infection Control and Applied Epidemiology: Principles and Practice. St. Louis, Mosby, 1996.
6. Rutala W: WAAP Infection Control Guidelines for Selection and Use of Disinfectants. Am J Infect Control 18:99–117, 1990.
7. Tablin O, et al: Guidelines for prevention of nosocomial pneumonia. Infect Control Hosp Epidemiol 15:587–627, 1994.
8. U.S. Department of Labor: Occupational Exposure to Bloodborne Pathogens. Washington, DC, U.S. Department of Labor, 1992.

Nurses also are advised to consult Statements of the Advisory Committee on Immunization Practices, which are published periodically in MMWR.

# 36. CHANGING ECOLOGY OF INFECTIONS AND ANTIBIOTIC USE

*Marilyn Jordan*, RN, MPH

**1. What is the number-one cause of community and hospital-acquired infections?**

*Staphylococcus aureus* is a gram-positive organism with which all people are colonized. Newborns become colonized shortly after birth. *S. aureus* causes 12% of all nosocomial infections, 20% of nosocomial pneumonias, and close to the same number of skin and blood stream infections (BSIs). It contains enzymes and toxins that increase its ability to cause severe illness and even death.

**2. Should we be concerned about antibiotic resistance?**

Yes. Since the 1950s, *S. aureus* has developed resistance to penicillin, nafcillin, methicillin, and oxacillin. Recently there have been reports of some vancomycin-resistant strains in critically ill patients exposed to several courses of antibiotic therapy. Currently 10–30% of *S. aureus* infections in the U.S. are nafcillin-resistant (NRSA) or methicillin-resistant (MRSA). This percentage is much higher ( > 50%) in parts of Asia. Infection with resistant organisms may fail therapy, resulting in longer illnesses, longer periods of infectivity, and greater danger to others. This potential exists in both community and hospital and is extremely problematic in the critical care setting.

### 3. How does antibiotic resistance develop?

Numerous organisms, including bacteria, fungi, parasites, viruses, and newer agents such as prions, are responsible for infectious diseases. Antimicrobial agents such as penicillin, amphotericin, and acyclovir combat infection, forcing the microbe to "adapt or die," which usually alters the course of infection. However, surviving microbes may adapt and even develop resistance genes. They may transfer this survival trait to other organisms.

### 4. What is the best strategy to combat antibiotic resistance?

Containment and prevention are the best strategies rather than addition of more antibiotics to the regimen.

### 5. Give two examples of antibiotic-resistant organisms found in the community.

*Mycobacterium tuberculosis* (MTB) is the classic example of an organism developing resistance over time. Resistance made it necessary to treat MTB with a combination of antibiotic therapies. Patients newly diagnosed with MTB may be prescribed four drugs: isoniazid, rifampin, pyrazinamide (all three of which are bactericidal), and ethambutol (a bacteriostatic agent that merely slows the organism). Incomplete treatment was the major contributor to the multidrug resistant tuberculosis (MDRTB) that emerged in the United States in the 1980s.

*Streptococcus pneumoniae* is among the top three organisms responsible for ear infections in children and community-acquired pneumonia in elderly people and chronically ill patients of all ages. Penicillin was the drug of choice for many years. In the mid 1990s, however, resistant strains appeared. Depending on region, 20–30% of pneumococcal organisms are somewhat resistant to penicillin, and a smaller percentage is highly resistant. Recently, programs have been implemented to encourage physicians to temper use of antibiotics for respiratory infections and to vaccinate elderly and chronically ill patients with Pneumovax.

### 6. How serious are resistant organisms in the hospital environment?

The presence of resistant gram-positive organisms, such as *Staphylococcus epidermidis* and *S. aureus*, continues to rise both in critical care and medical surgical settings. The rapid emergence of VRE is of great concern. Recent isolates of vancomycin-resistant *S. epidermidis* and *S. aureus* are part of a disturbing trend.

Many gram-negative organisms also show resistance. Imipenem-resistant *Pseudomonas aeruginosa* is increasing, particularly in intensive care patients with nosocomial pneumonia. Although the initial resistance often follows antibiotic use in a seriously ill patient, potential transmission to others poses a real threat. Restricting some antibiotic agents may help to alleviate the problem temporarily, but often other resistance patterns arise, particularly in gram-negative organisms. The National Nosocomial Infections Surveillance (NNIS) data from 1990 show significantly more resistance in intensive care patients compared with acute ward patients. This trend and the incidence of resistant infections continue to grow; for example, VRE increased from 0.4% of infection in 1989 to > 14% in 1995.

### 7. What can be done to prevent transmission of multidrug resistant organisms (MROs) in the critical care setting?

Although each hospital may have somewhat different policies and procedures, the basic principles are consistent:

- Early recognition of patients who are colonized with resistant organisms
- Consistent use of standard precautions with all patient activities
- Contact precautions for VRE (CDC recommendation)
- Cleaning and disinfecting of patient equipment and environment
- Some centers have a standard isolation approach for all patients, which includes handwashing with an antimicrobial soap, such as chlorhexidine, before and after each patient contact and after removing gloves and use of handwashing adjuncts (e.g., wipes or alcohol foam).
- Gloves may be required for all activities in patients with MRO infections, or task-oriented glove use may be emphasized.

• Individual patient equipment (e.g. stethoscope, blood pressure cuff, thermometer) and all reusable equipment should be disinfected immediately after use.

It has been shown that the next patient to occupy a room after a patient with VRE is at increased risk of colonization. Thus, special attention to housekeeping of patient areas after transfer is essential, no matter how urgent the need to bring another patient into the room.

## 8. Once a patient is colonized or infected with MRSA or VRE, does he or she ever clear the organism?

Although occasionally it is cleared, MRSA usually becomes part of the patient's flora and reappears with future cultures, often in the respiratory tract. For VRE, colonization in the gastrointestinal tract appears to be prolonged. Perirectal swabs can be done to check for clearing of VRE (minimum of 1 week between swabs for a total of 3 consecutive negatives). Most hospitalized patients with VRE remain colonized for the duration of their hospital stay.

## 9. How can staff be alerted that a patient with a previously identified MRO is in their unit?

Many centers have written prompts or other messages in the electronic record of identified patients to alert staff when the patient returns to the hospital. However, this system is far from perfect. Common sense techniques and standard precautions for all patients should be followed. In other words, what we did the day before we knew about the VRE or MRSA counts most!

## 10. Why are so many critical care patients prescribed more than one antibiotic?

Often empiric therapy is initiated early while evaluation for a specific pathogen is in progress. Therefore, coverage for both gram-positive organisms, such as *S. aureus,* and gram-negative organisms, such as *Enterobacter* sp., is standard. However, as soon as information about a specific organism is known, antibiotic therapy should become pathogen-specific, and other drugs should be discontinued. Patients generally receive more antibiotics early in their illness to prevent deadly complications such as gram-negative sepsis, disseminated intravascular coagulation, or multiorgan failure. However, the fallout of this practice is that many of the most resistant bacteria are seen in the most severely ill patients.

## 11. What can nursing staff do to prevent so much antibiotic exposure?

Previously described measures to prevent hospital-acquired infections can decrease the need for antibiotics, although not all infections are preventable. It is essential for nurses to maintain aseptic technique and follow hospital infection control guidelines and procedures.

### BIBLIOGRAPHY

1. CDC Guidelines for Prevention of Transmission of Tuberculosis in Health Care Facilities, MMWR 43:RR13:1–132, 1994.
2. Cohen F, et al: Microbial resistance to drug therapy: A review. Am J Infect Control 25:51–64, 1997.
3. Levy S: The challenge of antibiotic resistance. Sci Am March:46–53, 1998.
4. Olmstead R (ed): APIC Infection Control and Applied Epidemiology: Principles and Practice. St. Louis, Mosby, 1996.

# 37. FEVER

*Jill N. Howie,* RN, CS, MS, ACNP

### 1. How is fever defined?

Fever is a controlled elevation of body temperature resulting from an upward shift in the hypothalamic temperature set-point. However, the level of elevation is arbitrary. Some sources define fever as a core body temperature > 38.0°C (100.4°F), whereas others define it as two consecutive elevations > 38.3°C (101°F). Normal body temperature is generally accepted to be 37.0°C and varies by 0.5–1.0°C. It is influenced by circadian rhythm, phase of menstrual cycle, and exercise. The actual body temperature varies by method and site of measurement.

### 2. What factors influence alterations in body temperature?

Environmental factors, drugs, and central nervous system disorders cause alterations in body temperature. Environmental factors include air conditioning, heat losses from surgery, mattresses and beds, lights, cardiopulmonary bypass, peritoneal lavage, dialysis, respiratory gases from a ventilator, and continuous renal replacement therapies. Drugs that affect body temperature include antipyretics and immunosuppressants. Thyroid disease can influence body temperature through its effect on the central nervous system.

### 3. How is hyperthermia defined?

Hyperthermia is an elevation of body temperature resulting from overload of central thermoregulatory mechanisms. It is manifested by the inability to dissipate peripheral heat and distinguished from fever in that it is an unregulated rise in core temperature. An example is malignant hyperthermia, a rarely seen complication of inhaled anesthetic gases. It occurs most often in the operating room but also may occur in the intensive care unit (ICU).

### 4. What is the significance of hypothermia?

Hypothermia is found in a variety of critically ill patients. Often the cause is obvious, such as surgery or exposure, but it also is seen in patients with large abdominal wounds or burns, patients on extracorporeal membrane oxygenation, and patients taking certain drugs. Less obvious causes may signal a serious infection and require thorough investigation. A substantial number of infected patients, the elderly, and patients with the above conditions may not mount a fever.

### 5. Describe the mechanism of fever.

Infection, inflammation, immunologic processes, exercise, and stress stimulate macrophages in the body, including glial and astrocyte cells in the brain, to produce endogenous pyrogens. Pyrogens are heat-labile proteins that act on the hypothalamus to increase the thermoregulatory set-point. Endogenous pyrogens, or cytokines, include interleukins, interferons, tumor necrosis factor, and others. Interleukin-1 and interleukin-6 appear to be the most prominent cytokines that act centrally to increase body temperature. The sites and mechanisms of cytokines remain poorly understood, but it is thought that they work at the organum vasculosum laminae terminalis. This area is outside the blood-brain barrier and causes synthesis and release of prostaglandins that modify activity of the preoptic anterior hypothalamus. At the same time, endogenous cryogens are released to prevent an exaggerated increase in temperature. Dissipation of heat takes place through vasodilation and sweating. (See figure at top of following page.)

### 6. What causes fever?

Fever has numerous causes, and virtually every body system can provide a source for fever. Several approaches can be used to identify the cause, including the infectious vs. noninfectious approach, the 102°F (38.9°C) rule, and the four Ws (see question 9).

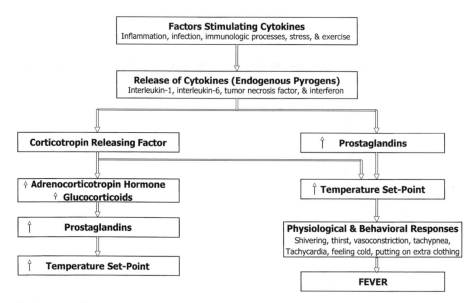

Mechanisms of fever. (From Rowsey PJ: Pathophysiology of fever. Part 1: The role of cytokines. Dimens Crit Care Nurs 16:202–207, 1997, with permission.)

## 7. Describe the infectious vs. noninfectious approach.

**Infectious causes** of fever in hospitalized patients are intravascular therapy sepsis, infected prosthesis, nosocomial bacteriuria, lower respiratory infection associated with ventilator therapy, aspiration pneumonia, surgical wound infection, and postperfusion syndrome.

**Noninfectious causes** of fever in hospitalized patients are drug reaction,s arthritis, ischemia, anesthesia-induced fever, atelectasis after surgery, phlebitis due to intravascular therapy, transfusion reaction, pulmonary embolus, postcardiotomy syndrome, and neoplastic disease.

## 8. What is the 102°F rule?

Certain disorders, usually noninfectious, cause fevers that are < 102°F (< 38.9° C). This rule is best used to exclude noninfectious causes of fever. The common causes of fever using the 102°F rule are listed in the table below.

*Causes of Fever Using the 102°F Rule*

| < 102°F (< 38.9°C) | > 102°F (> 38.9°C) |
| --- | --- |
| Acute myocardial infarction | Nosocomial pneumonia |
| Gastrointestinal bleed | IV-line infections |
| Acute pancreatitis | Antibiotic-associated colitis |
| Hematomas | Drug fever |
| Phlebitis | Blood product transfusion |
| Pleural effusions | Invasive infectious diseases |
| Uncomplicated wound infections | Transient bacteremia related to manipulation |
| Atelectasis | of a colonized/infected mucosal surface |
| Dehydration | |
| Tracheobronchitis | |
| Antibiotic-associated diarrhea | |

9. **What are the four Ws?**
   - Wound (infected wound site)        • Water (dehydration)
   - Wind (pneumonia, pulmonary embolus)        • Wonder drugs (drug fever)

The most important initial step is to verify the actual temperature measurement for accuracy, followed by clinical assessment of the patient. Then the full fever work-up can proceed, if required.

10. **What are the advantages of fever?**

Fever enhances function of the immune system and is considered a host defense mechanism. Animal studies have shown higher survival rates in infected animals with fever compared with animals unable to increase temperature. Clinical studies in septic patients have yielded similar results in terms of higher survival rates. An exception to this is head injury, where benefit from the use of induced hypothermia has improved outcomes.

11. **What are the disadvantages of fever?**

Fever causes increases in oxygen consumption, heart rate, cardiac output, and elevation of serum catecholamine levels. Increased cardiovascular demands may be poorly tolerated by people with minimal cardiopulmonary reserve, such as those with heart failure or coronary artery disease.

12. **When should fever be treated?**

Treatment is indicated in critically ill patients with moderate-to-severe fevers and limited cardiopulmonary reserve. In sepsis, the results of treatment are difficult to interpret because thermoregulation may be altered. Of equal concern is the comfort of the patient. Antipyretics can cool the patient and provide mild analgesia.

13. **Are fever patterns meaningful?**

In the distant past, observation of fever patterns was a strategy for determining the cause. Certain infections regularly produce a particular fever pattern. This strategy, however, is helpful in only a few infectious diseases. Fevers may be viewed as acute, subacute, or chronic, with or without additional symptoms. For diagnostic purposes, febrile patients with localizing symptoms present few challenges. Fever patterns are of most help in diagnosing illnesses without localizing signs but are of limited value in hospital-acquired fevers.

14. **Which infectious diseases cause acute febrile illnesses without localizing signs?**

Typhoid fever, malaria, ehrlichiosis, roseola infantum, typhoidal tularemia, typhoidal Epstein-Barr virus, mononucleosis, miliary tuberculosis, early viral hepatitis, Rocky Mountain spotted fever, and some childhood rashes.

15. **What characteristics of fever can be observed?**
   - Magnitude        • Defervescence
   - Frequency        • Pulse/temperature relationships
   - Duration

16. **What information is provided by the magnitude of fever?**

The magnitude of the fever does not correlate with disease severity, but the peak of the elevation provides important information. Temperatures $> 41°C$ typically are not due to infectious causes.

17. **How is the frequency of fever described?**

The frequency of fever can be described as intermittent, sustained/continuous, or remittent. A double quotidian fever is the most specific pattern, associated with two fever spikes per day. Conditions that present with double quotidian fever include Still's disease, gonococcal endocarditis, and visceral leishmaniasis. Most infectious diseases have no specific fever pattern.

18. **What diagnostic clues are provided by duration and defervescence?**

The magnitude of acute infectious diseases improves or worsens within 2 weeks. If the fever lasts longer than 3 weeks it may be termed a prolonged fever. Fever of unknown origin (FUO) is defined by temperature ≥ 38.5°C for more than 3 weeks. Viral infections show a slow temperature decline, whereas bacterial infections show a prompt drop with appropriate treatment. Noninfectious fevers do not decrease without specific therapy. Steroids and antipyretics decrease temperature non-specifically. Occasionally, a febrile patient with viral pneumonia defervesces rapidly during the first 24–36 hours of treatment. Reappearance of fever suggests an infectious complication or drug fever. Reappearance after an initial response may be due to superinfection or antibiotic resistance.

### 19. Explain the significance of pulse/temperature relationships.

If the pulse is elevated out of proportion to the fever (relative tachycardia), the fever proba-bly is associated with a noninfectious cause or a toxin-mediated infection such as gas gangrene. If a hospitalized patient has fevers without associated tachycardia (relative bradycardia), the dif-ferential diagnosis can be narrowed to two causes: legionnaires' disease or drug fever.

### 20. What is the best way to monitor fever?

The most important part of temperature monitoring is to ensure that the reading is accurate and that each measurement is recorded, along with its site. Various body sites have different tem-peratures, so a consistent site of measurement is essential. Measurements at the bladder, rectum, right atrium, and tympanic membrane reflect higher temperatures because they are more central and reflect body systems that are highly vascular. Temperature is measured most accurately by an intravascular or bladder thermistor. Measurement by electronic probe in the mouth, rectum, or ex-ternal auditory canal is acceptable. Choosing the site of temperature measurement can be challeng-ing in some critically ill patients. An uncooperative, neutropenic, coagulopathic patient may best benefit by tympanic membrane temperature measurement. However, if the ear canal is obstructed (by wax, for example), the measurement will not be accurate. Axillary measurements should be used only if all other sites are not feasible; the probe should be placed over the brachial artery.

The measuring device should be properly calibrated, cleaned, and carefully maintained to prevent transmission of pathogens.

### 21. Describe the work-up for fever.

Once a fever is identified, the work-up is tailored to causes that may be life-threatening and causes that the clinician reasonably suspects. The work-up includes evaluation of vital signs and hemodynamic parameters to determine the urgency of the problem. The maximal temperature suggests whether the fever has an infectious or noninfectious cause. The patient should be exam-ined thoroughly for localizing signs. A review of medications may identify a drug source. Withdrawal of certain drugs, such as alcohol, opiates, barbiturates, and benzodiazepines, is some-times associated with fevers. Information provided by a positive blood culture has important prognostic and therapeutic implications. Further work-up includes evaluation of possible local sources of infection and appropriate laboratory and diagnostic tests.

### 22. When are blood cultures indicated? How are they obtained?

A new-onset fever requires blood cultures when clinical evaluation strongly suggests an in-fectious cause. Blood cultures should be obtained as soon after the development of fever as pos-sible to enhance the possibility of recovering the pathogen in the blood culture. A second pair of cultures should be obtained within 24 hours, as this procedure is thought to increase the chance of recovering the pathogen due to the often intermittent release. The cultures should be obtained from two separate peripheral sticks after appropriate skin disinfection with povidone iodine. Allow the skin to dry for 2 minutes. Alcohol is an acceptable alternative. The injection port of the culture bottle should be wiped with alcohol, and at least 10–15 ml of blood should be added to the bottle. Hospital protocol may have more specific information. The bottle should be labeled with time, date, and site for interpreting the result.

### 23. What methods are used to reduce fever?

Fever can be reduced with pharmacologic agents, cooling measures, or both.

### 24. What drugs are known to reduce fever?

Fever is suppressed by the administration of antipyretic agents such as aspirin, acetaminophen, or nonsteroidal anti-inflammatory drugs (NSAIDs). Steroids also blunt the fever response but are not used as antipyretics because of adverse side effects, including immunosuppression. Antipyretic drugs work by inhibiting prostaglandin synthesis and reducing the hypothalamic set-point.

### 25. Which antipyretic should be used?

Antipyretics vary somewhat, but overall they are relatively safe. Acetaminophen is the preferred agent for patients with clotting disorders, gastric ulcers, or asthma and in young children. It has no anti-inflammatory action. Acetaminophen toxicity is associated with renal and liver damage. The oral route is preferred in children because the rectal route is associated with erratic absorption. Route of administration in critically ill adults requires closer study. Aspirin has anti-inflammatory effects but is more toxic than acetaminophen. It is associated with hepatic, renal, and gastrointestinal toxicity and, in children, with Reye's syndrome. Aspirin also causes alterations in bleeding time.

### 26. What cooling methods are used?

Cooling is achieved by the use of physical and environmental measures. Specific methods include cooling blankets, ice packs, tepid water baths, alcohol sponges, decreased ambient air temperature, and removal of blankets. Nurses are often the decision-makers for initiating cooling measures, but research support for their use is limited.

### 27. Which cooling method is preferred?

The literature provides little information about the best cooling measures, how aggressively to cool, and when to cool the febrile critically ill patient. Two studies have examined the effects of physical cooling on metabolic and cardiovascular responses in critically ill adults. Currently, because of study limitation, treatment of febrile patients to improve hemodynamic values and decrease metabolic rate cannot be recommended. How quickly a patient can be cooled is not defined, but rapid cooling causes skin vasoconstriction and may induce shivering, which decreases heat loss. Patients should be allowed to determine the amount of clothing and blankets. The removal of blankets can increase discomfort, and the rate of fever rise is not significantly influenced. Convective cooling blankets (use of blowing cold air) have not been evaluated in a randomized clinical trial of critically ill patients.

### 28. What is the most important indication for use of cooling methods?

Hyperthermia, which results from inadequate peripheral heat dissipation, results in extremely high temperatures. The patient can experience delirium, seizures, and circulatory collapse. Cooling measures should be instituted immediately.

### 29. What is drug fever?

Drug fever is a febrile response to the drug without cutaneous changes. It is estimated to affect approximately 10% of hospitalized patients. Drug fever can result in prolonged hospitalization and unnecessary drug administration and lab testing. Early recognition can prevent complications and discomfort.

### 30. How are drug fevers classified?

Drug fevers are divided into five categories: (1) altered thermoregulatory mechanisms, (2) drug administration-related, (3) pharmacologic action of the drug, (4) idiosyncratic reactions, and (5) hypersensitivity reaction. The administration of Synthroid alters thermoregulatory mechanisms by increasing metabolic rate and heat production. Fevers related to drug administration are caused by contamination or irritation at the site of administration, as with IV infusions of cephalothin.

Sometimes the pharmacologic effect of a drug can cause fever. Chemotherapeutic drugs can cause fever related to the substances released from the damaged malignant cells. Malignant hyperthermia is an idiosyncratic reaction to inhaled anesthetic agents (halothane and isoflurane).

Neuroleptic medications such as haloperidol and chlorpromazine can cause hyperthermia as part of neuroleptic malignant syndrome. The most common cause of drug fever is a hypersensitivity response. If a rash is present, the diagnosis is obvious, but the rash is seen only in a minority of cases. Antigen-antibody complexes are formed and can stimulate release of endogenous pyrogens.

### 31. What are the clinical clues to drug fever?

Clinical features of a drug fever include an inappropriately well appearance, relative brady-cardia, high fevers, and, in some cases, a generalized maculopapular rash. The rash may be seen on the soles and palms and may be pruritic. The fever can occur anytime after the offending drug is given, but frequently occurs 1–2 weeks after initiation. The white blood cell count demon-strates leukocytosis with a left shift, and sedimentation rate is elevated. Eosinophils are typically present, but eosinophilia is uncommon.

### 32. Which drugs are associated with fever?

| MORE COMMON | | LESS COMMON | |
|---|---|---|---|
| Atropine | Cephalosporins | Allopurinol | Nifedipine |
| Amphotericin B | Phenytoin | Azathioprine | NSAIDs |
| Asparaginase | Procainamide | Cimetidine | Metoclopramide |
| Barbiturates | Quinidine | Hydralazine | Corticosteroids |
| Bleomycin | Salicylates | Iodides | Aminoglycosides |
| Methyldopa | Sulfonamides | Isoniazid | Macrolides |
| Penicillins | Interferon | Rifampin | Tetracyclines |
| | | Streptokinase | Clindamycin |
| | | Imipenem | Chloramphenicol |
| | | Vancomycin | Vitamin preparations |

### 33. What special considerations apply to fever in elderly patients?

Fever in the elderly is defined as persistent elevation of temperature, regardless of measure-ment technique: oral temperatures $\geq 37.2°C$ on repeated measurements or rectal temperatures $\geq 37.2°C$ on repeated measurements.

Fever in elderly patients requires a thorough investigation. The threshold for suspicion of in-fection is lower in mildly febrile elderly patients. Atypical presentation of infection is common. A significant proportion (20–30%) of older persons with serious infections present with an absent or blunted fever response, which may delay treatment and negatively influence outcomes. Mortality and morbidity rates for many infections are several-fold higher in the elderly.

Thermoregulation in the elderly is not well understood, but aging is thought to alter endoge-nous pyrogens, such as interleukin-1, interleukin-6 and tumor necrosis factor; to diminish sensi-tivity of the hypothalamus to endogenous pyrogens; and to impair the body's ability to produce and conserve body heat.

### 34. How can nurses offer support to patients with fever?

Fevers can cause discomfort, malaise, irritability, and fatigue. The use of analgesics and anti-pyretics can relieve such symptoms. Shivering is a particularly uncomfortable experience and can lead to or aggravate hemodynamic instability. The use of opioids or benzodiazepines may be in-dicated for comfort and for ensuring normal vital signs. Close attention to the skin is also needed, especially in patients who are febrile for prolonged periods (as with severe illness). The nurse can assess environmental causes of temperature variation such as air conditioning, heat losses from surgery, mattresses and/or beds, lights, cardiopulmonary bypass, peritoneal lavage, dialysis, res-piratory gases from a ventilator, and continuous renal replacement therapies. Critical care nurses should realize that mild-to-moderate fevers are beneficial and often better left untreated. When the decision not to treat a fever is made, the family should be reassured and informed of the ben-efits of fever.

BIBLIOGRAPHY

1. Cunha BA: Fever in the critical care unit. Crit Care Clin 14:1–14, 1998.
2. Cunha BA: Fever of unknown origin. Infect Dis Clin North Am 10:111–127, 1996.
3. Cunha BA: Treatment of fever. Infect Dis Clin North Am 10:33–44, 1996.
4. Henker R: Evidence-based practice: Fever-related interventions. Am J Crit Care 8:481–489, 1999.
5. Henker R: Use of blood cultures in critically ill patients. Crit Care Nurs 20:45–50, 2000.
6. Johnson DH, Cunha BA: Drug fever. Infect Dis Clin North Am 10:85–91, 1996.
7. Kluger MJ, Kozak W, Conn C, et al: The adaptive value of fever. Infect Dis Clin North Am 10:1–19, 1996.
8. Norman DC, Yoshikawa TT: Fever in the elderly. Infect Dis Clin North Am 10:93–99, 1996.
9. O'Grady NP, Barie PS, Bartlett J, et al:Practice parameters for evaluationg new fever in critically ill adult patients. Crit Care Med 26:392–408, 1998.
10. Rowsey PJ: Pathophysiology of fever. Part 1: The role of cytokines. Dimens Crit Care Nurs 16:202–207, 1997.
11. Rowsey PJ: Pathophysiology of fever. Part 2: Relooking at cooling interventions. Dimens Crit Care Nurs 16:251–256, 1997.

# 38. SEPSIS AND SYSTEMIC INFLAMMATORY RESPONSE SYNDROME

*Hildy Schell*, RN, MS, CCRN

## 1. What is systemic inflammatory response syndrome?

Systemic inflammatory response syndrome (SIRS) is a group of clinical signs and symptoms that result from a variety of acute injuries or illnesses. Causes of SIRS include trauma, burns, pancreatitis, infection, and drugs. The injury or infection stimulates inflammation throughout the body. The inflammatory response includes vasodilation, increased capillary permeability, microvascular clotting, and elevated temperature. SIRS presents clinically as fever or hypothermia, tachycardia, tachypnea, and/or leukocytosis or leukopenia. These early signs are followed by clinical manifestations of altered organ perfusion (e.g., altered mental status, hypoxemia, oliguria, mottled skin). When SIRS is caused by an infection, it is called sepsis.

## 2. What is sepsis?

Sepsis is the systemic inflammatory response to an infection. Sepsis is not synonymous with systemic infection. Sepsis is diagnosed in patients with clinical evidence of infection plus tachypnea, tachycardia, and fever (or hypothermia). The infection can be bacterial, viral, fungal, or protozoal/parasitic. Clinical evidence of infection can be described as a positive culture and/or a white blood count (WBC) count > 12,000 cells/mm$^3$, < 4,000 cells/mm$^3$, or > 10% band forms. Viral infections typically present with low WBC counts.

## 3. How are the clinical presentations of sepsis defined?

The clinical presentations of sepsis are defined along a continuum of increasing severity:

**Sepsis:** clinical evidence of infection including heart rate > 90 beats/minutes, respiratory > 20 breaths/minute, or partial pressure of carbon dioxide in arterial blood (PaCO$_2$) < 32 mmHg and/or temperature > 38°C or < 36°C.

**Severe sepsis:** sepsis plus evidence of hypotension or altered organ perfusion (e.g., altered mental status, hypoxemia, oliguria, elevated serum lactate levels). Hypotension is defined as systemic blood pressure (SBP) < 90 mmHg or a decrease in SBP by > 40 mmHg from baseline.

**Septic shock:** severe sepsis plus persistent hypotension despite IV fluid and pharmacologic resuscitative efforts.

#### 4. What two factors determine the severity of septic shock?

The two factors that determine the severity of septic shock are (1) pathogen characteristics (virulence, cell wall toxin, and mediators produced) and (2) host characteristics (susceptibility and response).

#### 5. Who is at risk for sepsis?

1. Immunocompetent hosts with overwhelming infections caused by pathogens, such as *Streptococcus* species and certain unidentified viruses.

2. Immunocompromised hosts with infections caused by more common and typically less toxic organisms, such as *Staphylococcus aureus* and *Candida albicans*. Risk factors for immunocompromise are age, malnutrition, chronic illnesses (e.g, diabetes, renal failure, liver failure, lupus erythematosus, HIV), trauma, pregnancy, radiation, splenectomy, and medications (e.g., immunosuppressive drugs, steroids, chemotherapy).

3. Critical care patients are at additional risk for developing infections and sepsis because of (1) the increased number of invasive lines, drains, and tubes; (2) the frequency of invasive procedures; and (3) the increased number and long duration of antibiotic use.

#### 6. What forms of hemodynamic monitoring are used in patients with septic shock?

Patients with septic shock require continuous electrocardiographic (ECG) monitoring, monitoring of arterial oxygen saturation, and invasive blood pressure monitoring. They may require invasive central venous or pulmonary artery catheterization for further assessment of cardiac function and fluid status.

#### 7. How does septic shock affect heart rate?

Tachycardia occurs as a response to fever and as a compensatory response for the low systemic vascular resistance (SVR) and preload seen in septic shock.

#### 8. Blood pressure?

Hypotension is related to low SVR, low intravascular volume, and/or inadequate ejection fraction. The degree of diastolic hypotension correlates with the low SVR.

#### 9. Cardiac filling pressures?

Cardiac filling pressures (preload), including central venous pressure and pulmonary capillary wedge pressure, are low prior to IV fluid resuscitation because of vasodilation, peripheral vascular shunt formation, and the increased third spacing of intravascular fluid secondary to severe capillary leak.

#### 10. Cardiac output?

Cardiac output (CO) is typically elevated to compensate for low systemic vascular resistance and increased metabolic needs related to sepsis. Some patients with septic shock present with low CO and biventricular hypokinesis on echocardiogram. This low CO state is thought to be caused by the cytokine, myocardial depressant factor, which is released during sepsis. This type of cardiac dysfunction is completely reversible and usually lasts 2–4 days.

#### 11. Systemic vascular resistance?

SVR is low because of vasodilation and increased peripheral vascular shunt formation caused by the cytokine and inflammatory response.

#### 12. Tissue oxygenation?

Mixed venous oxygen saturation ($SvO_2$) and the difference in arterial and venous oxygen content ($AVDO_2$) provide information about tissue oxygenation. In sepsis, $SvO_2$ is high and $AVDO_2$ is low because the oxygen content returning to the right side of the heart is high as a result of (1) the high CO that allows little time for oxygen diffusion at the tissue level and (2) the alteration in oxygen utilization by the tissues in sepsis.

**13. What compensatory mechanism mediates the metabolic changes associated with sepsis and SIRS?**

The compensatory mechanism for increased metabolic needs with sepsis or SIRS is mediated by the sympathetic nervous system (SNS). The SNS increases output of catecholamines (epinephrine and norepinephrine), cortisol, and glucagon. The results are increased CO, increased oxygen consumption, and hyperglycemia.

**14. How do sepsis and SIRS affect carbohydrate stores and metabolic rate?**

Carbohydrate stores (glycogen) typically are depleted within 12 hours, leading to protein and fat store breakdown as the primary and secondary sources of fuel. Hypermetabolism, an increase in the body's resting energy expenditure (REE), manifests as increased oxygen consumption and carbon dioxide production. The REE can increase up to 200% in patients with sepsis or SIRS.

**15. What is catabolism? How can it be minimized?**

Catabolism is the loss of lean body (muscle) mass as a result of proteolysis in sepsis and SIRS. The degree of catabolism is evidenced by the severity of the negative nitrogen balance study. The detrimental effects of hypercatabolism and multiple organ dysfunction syndrome (MODS) occur over time if sepsis is not adequately treated. Clinical manifestations include loss of lean body/muscle mass and severe weakness. Early nutrition intervention with enteral feeds, unless contraindicated, helps to minimize the complications of hypercatabolism and promotes healing.

**16. What is the primary goal in treatment of sepsis? How is it accomplished?**

The primary goal is to identify the source of infection. Obtaining blood, urine, sputum, cerebrospinal fluid, and/or other suspected body fluids or tissues for Gram stain and culture before administration of antibiotics is essential. The identified source or potential sources of infection should be removed as soon as possible. Antibiotics should be administered as soon as possible after cultures are obtained. Choice of antibiotics is based on the organisms typically found at the suspected sites as well as demographic data (e.g., residence in nursing home vs. recent travel in third-world country).

**17. What supportive therapies are used in the treatment of sepsis?**

Supportive therapies, including IV fluid resuscitation, vasopressors, inotropes, oxygen, and mechanical ventilation, should be instituted immediately. Adequate fluid resuscitation before adding or increasing vasopressor support helps to prevent potential complications. Fluid resuscitation with crystalloid and/or colloid fluids should be titrated to clinical end points of heart rate, mean arterial pressure (MAP), urine output, skin perfusion, and mental status. Blood products may be administered to keep the hemoglobin at 8–10 g/dl. Dopamine is the recommended first-line drug for increasing blood pressure after adequate fluid resuscitation. Norepinephrine and phenylephrine are alternative choices. Phenylephrine typically is used when tachyarrhythmias are present because, unlike dopamine and norepinephrine, it does not have positive chronotropic effects. Epinephrine is considered for use with refractory hypotension. Dobutamine is the first-line drug for inotropic support in patients with a low cardiac index ($<2.5$ L/minute/m$^2$). Dobutamine is usually used in conjunction with a vasopressor to maintain adequate MAP for organ perfusion.

**18. What other interventions are appropriate for patients with sepsis?**

Acid-base and electrolyte abnormalities should be monitored and treated as necessary. Interventions to prevent complications of immobility and altered tissue perfusion during septic shock include frequent repositioning, floating heels and pressure points off of pillows, passive range of motion to prevent joint stiffness, antithromboembolism therapies, and skin care (e.g., cleansing, moisturizers and/or moisture barriers). Early nutritional support, preferably enteral feedings, helps to minimize complications of hypermetabolism and catabolism.

**19. How is fever managed in patients with sepsis or SIRS?**

Patients with sepsis or SIRS can have intermittent or sustained fevers > 38.5°C for days. Elevated temperatures enhance the function of the cells of the immune system. Fever is a normal defense mechanism. Reducing fever should be a primary goal for patients at high risk for complications of fever, such as seizures or myocardial ischemia. Antipyretic medications (e.g., acetaminophen, ibuprofen) can be used around-the-clock. Cooling devices (e.g., blankets, ice packs, alcohol baths) have not been shown to be effective in reducing fever in patients with intact thermoregulation, although they can be used to promote patient comfort.

**20. What complications are associated with sepsis and SIRS?**

1. **Superinfections**, due most often to fungus (e.g., *Candida albicans*) or *Clostridium difficile*, are a complication of long-term or broad-spectrum antibiotic use in sepsis and SIRS. The normal flora of the skin, mucous membranes, and gastrointestinal tract provide a natural defense against toxic organisms. Antibiotics change the normal flora and allow growth of these pathogens.

2. **Disseminated intravascular coagulation** is stimulated by the cytokine and/or pathogen toxin injury to the vascular endothelium during sepsis.

3. **Profound weakness and limited mobility** are related primarily to the loss of muscle mass from catabolism and immobility during critical illness. Rehabilitation needs after leaving the ICU vary with the patient's age, comorbidities, complications, and degree of debilitation.

4. **MODS** results from hypoperfusion, perfusion abnormalities, and/or altered oxygen uptake by cells during sepsis and SIRS. MODS is considered a syndrome because the signs and symptoms are multiple and progressive. Organ systems are considered dysfunctional when they cannot maintain homeostasis or when they require supportive therapies to maintain homeostasis. The degree of organ dysfunction is a continuum that includes the possibility of return to normal function. The major organ systems affected in MODS are the pulmonary, renal, hepatic, cardiovascular, and central nervous systems.

**21. What kind of teaching is important for patients with sepsis and their families?**

Outlining the various interventions and explaining why they are necessary can be helpful to patients and families. They often want to know the normal timeframe for staying in the ICU. Because this is difficult to predict, reassure patients that they will stay in the ICU for close monitoring until they are stable and can be transferred safely to another level of care. Explaining that progress may take time and that "ups and downs" are expected in the usual trajectory may alleviate anxiety related to unrealistic expectations. Encourage and teach families to assist with providing direct care (e.g., bath, massage, range of motion exercises), as appropriate. These types of interventions promote understanding of the critical situation, encourage participation, and promote satisfaction for families and patients.

BIBLIOGRAPHY

1. Henker R: Evidence-based practice: Fever-related interventions. Am J Crit Care 8:481–487, 1999.
2. Members of the American College of Chest Physicians/Society of Critical Care Medicine Consensus Conference Committee: American College of Chest Physicians/Society of Critical Care Medicine Consensus Conference: Definitions for sepsis and organ failure and guidelines for the use of innovative therapies in sepsis. Crit Care Med 20:864–874, 1992.
3. Secor VH: Multiple organ dysfunction syndrome: Overview and conclusions. In Secor VH (ed): Multiple Organ Dysfunction and Failure, 2nd ed. St. Louis, Mosby, 1996, pp 402–423.
4. Shelton BK: Sepsis. Semin Oncol Nurs 15:209–221, 1999.
5. Sriskandan S, Cohen J: Gram-positive sepsis: Mechanisms and differences from gram-negative sepsis. Infect Dis Clin North Am 13:397–412, 1999.
6. Task Force of the American College of Critical Care Medicine, Society of Critical Care Medicine: Practice parameters for hemodynamic support of sepsis in adult patients in sepsis. Crit Care Med 27:639–660, 1999.

# 39. DISSEMINATED INTRAVASCULAR COAGULATION

*Carol Viele*, RN, MS

**1. What is disseminated intravascular coagulation?**

Disseminated intravascular coagulation (DIC) is generalized activation of the hemostatic system, which results in widespread fibrin formation followed by lysis within the vascular system. DIC can result in consumption of both platelets and clotting factors as well as microthrombus formation.

**2. What causes DIC?**

DIC does not occur in isolation; it is a symptom of an underlying disease. Many disease processes can cause DIC, which is the direct response to the presence of specific proteins or procoagulants. These agents, including tissue factor, tumor necrosis factor (TNF), and cell proteases, may be secreted by malignant cells.

**3. What causes DIC in critically ill patients?**

**Infection/sepsis:** bacterial, fungal, protozoal, and viral organisms.

**Trauma:** burns, "crush" injuries, snake bite.

**Obstetric complications:** abruptio placentae, placenta previa, amniotic fluid embolism, dead fetus, missed abortion, hydatidiform mole.

**Hematologic/immunologic disorders:** transfusion reactions, transplant rejection, anaphylaxis, autoimmune disorders, sickle cell crisis.

**Miscellaneous:** extracorporeal circulation, pulmonary or fat embolism, anoxia, acidosis, hyperthermia, hypothermia, hypovolemic or hemorrhagic shock, acute respiratory distress syndrome, sustained hypotension.

**4. What types of malignancies are associated with DIC?**

Both solid tumors and leukemia may cause DIC. Patients with mucin-secreting adenocarcinomas, prostatic carcinoma, and/or disseminated carcinomas are at highest risk. In addition, all leukemias may induce DIC. However, promyelocytic leukemia is associated almost universally with the development of some degree of DIC.

**5. What are the types of DIC?**

**Acute DIC** develops rapidly over a period of hours. The patient presents with sudden bleeding from multiple sites.

**Chronic DIC** is sometimes subclinical. It may develop over a period of months; eventually, however, it evolves into an acute DIC pattern of hemorrhage or thromboembolic episodes.

**6. What is the mechanism of clotting in DIC?**

Fibrin degradation products and D dimers are almost always abundant in DIC and frequently clump together. These fragments or clumps, particularly D dimers, competitively inhibit the formation and action of thrombin by binding to thrombin at its fibrinogen receptor site. These fragment complexes, if soluble, may deposit indiscriminately throughout the vasculature. Others bind abnormally to preexisting growing microthrombi, weakening clot structure.

**7. What is the mechanism of bleeding in DIC?**

Bleeding is due to failure of the clotting cascade, which results in systemic release of fibrinogen, fibrin degradation products, or D dimers. This release creates a host of circulatory disturbances, including the formation of small fragments that inhibit platelet function, large fragments that induce platelet clumping, and mixtures of soluble fragments that may increase capillary permeability. These disturbances may cause extravascular coagulation and interrupt endothelial activity. The result is significant bleeding throughout the vascular system.

### 8. What are the symptoms of DIC?

The most common sign of DIC is **bleeding**, usually manifested by ecchymosis, petechiae, and purpura. The patient usually presents with bleeding from multiple sites, including skin, nose, lungs, and central nervous system. The bleeding may range from continuous oozing of venipuncture sites, incisions, or wounds to uncontrollable hemorrhage that leads to shock and death unless intervention is swift and effective. Bleeding also may occur around tubes such as endotracheal, nasogastric, or Foley catheter. If DIC persists for more than a few hours, hemorrhages can be extensive and involve the pleura and pericardium. Patients may complain of dyspnea and chest pain.

**Neurologic alterations** may include headache, altered level of consciousness, irritability, restlessness, seizures, and coma.

**Cardiovascular changes** include tachycardia and ST-segment changes on the electrocardiogram (ECG).

**Renal symptoms** may include oliguria and hematuria.

### 9. What are the laboratory manifestations of DIC?

Platelet count, fibrin degradation products, prothrombin time (PT), activated partial thromboplastin time (aPTT), thrombin time (TT), and fibrinogen level are used to diagnose DIC. Patients with acute or chronic DIC show decreased platelet count, increased fibrin degradation products and D dimer assay, prolonged aPTT and PT, decreased fibrinogen level, decreased antithrombin III (ATIII) level, and prolonged TT.

*Laboratory Abnormalities*

| LABORATORY TEST | ABNORMALITY |
| --- | --- |
| Platelet count | Decreased |
| Fibrin degradation products | Increased |
| Prothrombin time | Prolonged |
| Activated partial thromboplastin time | Prolonged |
| Thrombin time | Prolonged |
| Fibrinogen | Decreased |
| Antithrombin III level | Decreased |
| D-dimer assay | Increased |

### 10. How is DIC diagnosed?

DIC is diagnosed on the basis of clinical presentation plus laboratory abnormalities. The aPTT is a less helpful test except in severe cases because it may be physiologically prolonged in children. Furthermore, it may be masked in adults by elevated factor VIII.

### 11. What is the goal of therapy?

The immediate goal of therapy is to stop the active bleeding and clotting. In addition, because DIC is not a single or specific disease but a syndrome, the underlying disease must be treated to resolve the problem.

### 12. How is DIC managed?

The overall management of DIC is controversial because of the lack of controlled studies of successful treatment interventions. However, the most important component in the management of DIC is to treat the underlying disorder. Management of DIC can be divided into two categories: use of blood component therapy and use of medications.

### 13. What blood components are used to treat DIC?

Platelet concentrates, cryoprecipitate, and fresh frozen plasma are frequently used in an attempt to control bleeding. Patients should be transfused only when the diagnosis is well established and clotting factors are depleted. The exception, of course, is the patient in a life-threatening situation that allows no time to establish diagnosis. Replacements for thrombocytopenia include 6–10 units of random donor platelets or a single unit of donor pheresed platelets. Hypofibrinogenemia (fibrinogen of < 100 mg/dl) may be treated with 8 units of cryoprecipitate. Each unit of cryoprecipitate contains 250 mg of fibrinogen. A prolonged PT due to factor deficiency may be corrected by administering two units of fresh frozen plasma. Depending on the severity of DIC, replacement therapy may need to be repeated every 8 hours, with adjustments for platelet count, PT, aPTT, fibrinogen level, and volume status. Replacements are discontinued when levels are normal or near normal. ATIII concentrate also has been used, either alone or in combination with heparin. No definitive studies show a decrease in the mortality rate with use of ATIII.

### 14. What medications are used to treat DIC?

Because patients with DIC have evidence of clotting in addition to bleeding, **heparin** may be used to prevent further clotting. It is indicated as a treatment for DIC in acute promyelocytic and acute monocytic leukemia during induction therapy. Heparin also is used to treat DIC-induced thromboembolic complications in large vessels and prior to surgery for metastatic carcinoma. **Fibrinolytic inhibitors** are used only in the setting of an undeniable threat to hemostasis, i.e., bleeding that does not respond to other measures.

### 15. What two fibrinolytic inhibitors are currently available?

Epsilon aminocaproic acid (EACA; Amicar) and tranexamic acid (Cyklokapron). EACA is a protease inhibitor that is uniquely reactive with plasminogen activators. It inhibits spontaneous fibrinolytic activity. A standard loading dose of 4 gm followed by 6–12 gm daily in divided doses provides sufficient plasma concentration to preserve the fibrin of a hemostatic vascular plug. The adverse effects are gastrointestinal disturbances, muscle necrosis, impotence, and the risk of creating clots in the urinary tract and bladder of patients with renal bleeding and hemorrhagic cystitis. Tranexamic acid is approximately 100 times more potent than EACA in inhibiting plasminogen activation. It has a greater specificity of action and fewer side effects. The current recommended dosage for managing systemic fibrinolysis is 30–50 mg/kg orally or 10 mg/kg intravenously every 12 hours. Tranexamic acid should be avoided with suspicion of renal bleeding or evidence of intravascular clotting to prevent cutting off the blood supply to the kidneys.

### 16. What nursing interventions are important in the general care of patients with DIC?

The nurse's role is to assess the patient for signs and symptoms of bleeding or thrombotic events. The nurse must use a thorough and organized approach, and physical assessment should be performed at least every 4 hours. Starting with the skin, the nurse inspects the patient from head to toe, including palms of the hands and soles of the feet, looking for petechiae or bruising. Particular attention should be paid to the sclera and buccal mucosa. The patient also should be queried about his or her vision. Blurred, cloudy, or diminished vision may indicate retinal hemorrhage and should be reported to the physician immediately. Inspect the oral cavity, evaluating for bleeding, ulcers, or hematomas. A mouth care regimen is imperative because oral cavity bleeding may be significant. Inspect both nares for signs of bleeding; epistaxis may be a significant source of blood loss. Proceed with your inspection to chest, back, abdomen, groin area, and lower extremities. Inspect pressure areas closely because patients may have petechiae, hematomas, and ecchymotic in these areas.

### 17. What nursing interventions are important in the intensive care unit (ICU)?

Patients in the ICU should be assessed for altered perfusion and decreased cardiac output. Assessment includes monitoring of vital signs, the 12-lead ECG, arterial blood gases, bowel sounds, urinary output, and mental status. Because the patient may be intubated and sedated, evaluation of mental status may be difficult. The cardiac evaluation should include an assessment for chest pain, dysrhythmias, murmurs, hypotension, tachycardia, or bradycardia. Pulmonary assessment includes identifying signs and symptoms of respiratory distress, dyspnea, tachypnea, or abnormal breath sounds. Because patients with DIC may develop diffuse alveolar hemorrhage, listening for rales, rhonchi, or areas of decreased breath sounds is important. It is also important to note any signs or symptoms of respiratory distress such as dyspnea, shortness of breath, nasal flaring, and increased respiratory rate.

**18. How does the presence of a central line affect nursing interventions in patients with DIC?**
In patients with a central line, bleeding from the site is common until the DIC is under control. Many leukemic patients with DIC require central line dressing changes every 2 hours because of bleeding. Pressure should be applied during each dressing change for a minimum of 5–10 minutes to reduce oozing. If pressure is not sufficient, Gelfoam sponges may be used at the exit site to enhance hemostasis. An alternative method is to apply topical thrombin to the Gelfoam sponges in an effort to control bleeding. Once the bleeding has stopped, the topical thrombin-soaked Gelfoam sponge should not be removed until it falls off; otherwise, the site may bleed again. The Gelfoam sponge will fall off when clotting conditions have returned to normal. Patients can lose units of blood from the central line site; up to 100 ml of blood may be contained within each hematoma. Inspection and assessment are key management methods.

**19. How is cardiac tamponade diagnosed and managed?**
In a few patients, cardiac tamponade may result from DIC and thrombocytopenia. This is an obvious medical emergency. Signs of tamponade may be acute in onset and include chest pain, shortness of breath, pulsus paradoxus, hypotension, and muffled heart sounds. Medical interventions should be initiated as appropriate.

**20. How should the abdomen be assessed?**
Patients with DIC may have symptoms of abdominal pain due to ischemic bowel. Abdominal examination should include listening for bowel sounds in all four quadrants; any areas with decreased or absent bowel sounds should be noted. Evaluation also should include palpation and observation of any acute peritoneal signs (e.g., rebound tenderness or a fluid wave related to bleeding in the abdominal cavity). The liver and spleen should be palpated and percussed to determine size and degree of tenderness. Any abnormal findings should be noted and reported to the physician. Urine and stool should be inspected for any sign of blood.

**21. What is the nurse's role in educating patient and family?**
Explain the syndrome, along with the expected treatment, whether it be blood components, heparin, and/or an antifibrinolytic agent. Patients and families are especially anxious because the patient looks very different from normal and bleeding is a scary symptom. Every effort should be made to explain the cause, treatment, side effects, and goals in the simplest way possible. Explanations should be repeated as often as necessary to reduce anxiety and increase patient/ family understanding. The more time the nurse can spend with the patient, the better. Many patients and family members ask how long the symptoms will last. Be honest, and tell them that it varies with each individual. The most important nursing intervention is to provide safe care during this highly stressful time.

**22. What is the prognosis of DIC?**
DIC and its underlying disorders contribute to a high mortality rate. Mortality correlates with the extent of organ or system involvement. It is also positively correlated with the degree of hemostatic failure and patient age. Mortality rates in various studies range from 42–86%, regardless of whether heparin is used.

### BIBLIOGRAPHY

1. Carey M, Rodgers G: Disseminated intravascular coagulation: Clinical and laboratory aspects. Am J Hematol 59:65–73, 1998.
2. Gobel B: Bleeding disorders. In Groenwald S, Frogge M, Goodman M, Yarbro C (eds) Cancer Nursing: Principles and Practice. Boston, Jones & Bartlett, 1993, pp 575–607.

3. Hathaway W, Goodnight S: Disorder of Hemostasis and Thrombosis: A Clinical Guide. New York, McGraw-Hill, 1993, pp 219–229.
4. Jandl J: Disseminated intravascular coagulation. In Jandl J (ed): Blood: Textbook of Hematology, 2nd ed. Boston, Little, Brown, 1996, pp 1440–1447.
5. Jones A: Hematological and immune disorders. In Hartshorn J, Sole M, Lamborn M (eds): Introduction to Critical Care Nursing. Philadelphia, W.B. Saunders, 1997, pp 376–400.
6. Kurtz A: Disseminated intravascular coagulation with leukemia patients. Canc Nurs 16:456–463, 1993.
7. Linker C: Blood. In Tiernery L Jr, McPhee S, Papadakis M (eds): Current Medical Diagnosis and Treatment. Norwalk, CT, Appleton & Lange, 1994, pp 415–466.
8. Schafer S: Oncologic complications. In Otto S (ed): Oncology Nursing, 2nd ed. St. Louis, Mosby, 1994, pp 376–440.
9. Seligsohn U: Disseminated intravascular coagulation. In Beutler E, Lichtman M, Coller B, Kipps T (eds): Hematology, 5th ed. New York, McGraw-Hill, 1995, pp 1497–1516.
10. Siegrist C, Jones J: Disseminated intravascular coagulopathy and nursing implications. Semin Oncol Nurs 1:237–243, 1985.

# 40. LEUKEMIAS AND BONE MARROW TRANSPLANTATION

*Mary Reid-Finlay, RN, MS, ACNP, CCRN, OCN, and Roberta Kaplow, RN, PhD, CCNS, CCRN*

### 1. What is leukemia?

Leukemia develops when immature or mature cells reproduce at an uncontrollable rate in the bone marrow. The cells begin to overpopulate the bone marrow and enter the bloodstream and lymphatic system. The cells then invade body organs and disrupt normal function. Eventually, the leukemic cells crowd out the healthy cells and prevent bone marrow from producing enough white blood cells (WBCs).

### 2. What are the types of leukemia?

The two types of leukemia are acute and chronic. They may involve two cell lines, lymphoid and myeloid. The lymphoid line produces lymphocytes, whereas the myeloid line produces monocytes and granulocytes, red blood cells, and platelets. Lymphocytic leukemia affects lymphocytes, and myelocytic (also known as myelogenous) leukemia involves monocytes and granulocytes. Either can occur in the acute form, which affects immature cells, or the chronic form, which involves cells at a more mature stage.

### 3. What are the acute leukemias?

With acute leukemia, WBCs do not develop into mature cells. The leukemias are differentiated according to the phase at which cell development ceases.

**Acute myelogenous leukemia** (AML; also known as acute myelocytic, myeloblastic, granulocytic, or nonlymphocytic leukemia) results in overproduction of abnormal, immature WBCs in the bone marrow. AML primarily involves the granulocytes, specifically the neutrophils.

**Acute monocytic leukemia** involves overproduction of monocytes.

**Acute promyelocytic leukemia** involves overproduction of promyelocytes (primitive granulocytes).

**Acute myelomonocytic leukemia** involves overproduction of monocytes and myelocytes (intermediate-stage monocytes).

**Acute lymphocytic leukemia** (ALL; also known as acute lymphatic, lymphoblastic, or lymphogenous leukemia) is characterized by production of immature lymphoid line cells.

## 4. What are the chronic leukemias?

In chronic leukemia, mature WBCs do not function normally.

**Chronic myelogenous leukemia** (CML; also known as chronic granulocytic, myelocytic, or myeloid leukemia) involves abnormal production of mature WBCs by the bone marrow, which results in an accumulation in the bone marrow and bloodstream. It also may involve production of granulocytes that grow and change in the myeloid line.

**Chronic lymphocytic leukemia** (CLL; also known as chronic lymphatic, lymphogenous, or lymphoid leukemia) involves overproduction of lymphocytes (B cells and T cells). It results in an abnormal accumulation of these cells in the bone marrow, blood, and lymph.

## 5. What is blast crisis?

Blast crisis occurs when peripheral blast counts are extremely elevated, resulting in leukostasis and impaired blood flow. The large and "sticky" blast cells occlude arterioles and capillaries. Blast crisis can occur in patients with acute and chronic leukemias. The blastic phase is one of three phases of CML; it is characterized by notable production of immature blast cells. Patients concomitantly develop progressive anemia and thrombocytopenia. During this phase, patients with CML resemble patients with acute leukemia. Cell development ceases at the blast (immature) phase rather than progressing to the mature granulocytic phase. The patient is immunocompromised because the large number of immature granulocytes are incapable of combating infection.

## 6. How do patients with blast crisis present?

The most common cause of admission to the intensive care unit (ICU) is sepsis or septic shock due to the inability of the body's defenses to combat infectious organisms. Altered perfusion related to blast crisis can present as headaches, altered mental status, or seizures related to increased intracranial pressure and/or cerebral infarcts. Dyspnea related to pulmonary emboli or infarcts may bring patients to the ICU. Patients also may present with joint pain and skin lesions due to excessive WBCs.

## 7. How is blast crisis treated?

Treatment of blast crisis includes administration of high-dose chemotherapy and corticosteroids to destroy the large number of abnormal cells. Leukapheresis may be performed to reduce circulating cells from the bloodstream. Radiation therapy may be used in the presence of related neurologic and pulmonary comorbidities. Patients in blast crisis also should receive chemotherapy prophylaxis for tumor lysis syndrome because of the large cell burden.

## 8. What is tumor lysis syndrome?

Tumor lysis syndrome (TLS) results when a large number of rapidly dividing cancer cells are killed (lysed) by antineoplastic therapy such as chemotherapy and/or radiation. TLS can result in potentially life threatening metabolic and electrolyte abnormalities. It usually occurs within the first 1–2 days of antineoplastic therapy but may occur within 7 days of treatment. It may last for up to 7 days after treatment has been completed.

## 9. What pathophysiologic changes occur with TLS?

Normal intracellular components include potassium, phosphorus, and nucleic acids. When tumor cells are killed, these contents are released into the bloodstream. Nucleic acids are converted to uric acid by the liver. Phosphorus binds with calcium. The end results are hyperkalemia, hyperphosphatemia, hyperuricemia, and hypocalcemia. Acute renal failure may result from the precipitation of uric acid or calcium and phosphorus.

## 10. Who is at risk for developing TLS?

TLS may occur in patients with rapidly growing tumor burden who receive antineoplastic therapy. The patients at greatest risk are those with bulky abdominal tumors. Specific tumors implicated in the development of TLS include Burkitt's lymphoma, chronic lymphocytic leukemia, chronic myelogenous leukemia, small cell lung carcinoma, breast cancer, and medulloblastoma.

Lymphomas and lymphoblastic leukemias have immature lymphoblasts that contain high phosphorus levels (4 times more phosphorus than mature lymphocytes). Hence, when the immature cells are lysed with antineoplastic therapy, hyperphosphatemia may result. TLS also has been reported in patients with rapidly growing ovarian cancer, metastatic melanoma, and metastatic gastrointestinal (GI) adenocarcinoma. Any patient with preexisting hyperuricemia, impaired renal function, dehydration, extensive lymph node involvement, multiple metastases, elevated WBC count, elevated levels of lactate dehydrogenase, lymphadenopathy, or splenomegaly are also at risk. Extensive cell death can occur after radiation therapy, placing patients at risk for TLS.

### 11. What are the signs and symptoms of TLS?

The manifestations of TLS depend on the degree of metabolic derangements. Patients with **hyperkalemia** may present with electrocardiographic (ECG) changes such as peaked T waves, flat P waves, wide QRS complexes, bradycardia, ventricular tachycardia, ventricular fibrillation, asystole, or pulseless electrical activity, depending on severity. Other signs and symptoms may include muscle weakness, twitching, tingling, or cramps. GI effects of hyperkalemia include increased bowel sounds, nausea, and diarrhea.

Patients with **hyperphosphatemia** present with renal impairment, such as azotemia, oliguria, or anuria. Other signs and symptoms include hypertension and edema.

Patients with **hyperuricemia** are lethargic and have renal impairment (decreased glomerular filtration rate [GFR]) similar to hyperphosphatemia as well as nausea and vomiting. The formation of uric acid crystals in the kidney can result in acute renal failure. Patients also may develop metabolic acidosis.

Clinical manifestations of **hypocalcemia** may include ECG changes such as prolonged QT interval, inverted T waves, ventricular dysrhythmias, heart block, or cardiac arrest. Neuromuscular symptoms include tetany, twitching, paraesthesias, and seizures. The primary GI symptom is diarrhea.

### 12. What measures are used to prevent TLS?

Preventative measures include identifying patients at risk for developing TLS and monitoring for electrolyte abnormalities. Prevention of hyperuricemia includes administration of allopurinol, which decreases uric acid levels by interfering with purine metabolism through inhibition of an enzyme (xanthine oxidase) that is essential for the conversion of nucleic acids to uric acid. Alkalinization of the urine with a sodium bicarbonate infusion is used to prevent renal damage and failure but has caused some controversy. Uric acid may crystallize in an acidic environment; hence, bicarbonate decreases the chance of renal obstruction. However, urinary alkalinization should be used cautiously because of the increased risk of precipitation in the kidneys from calcium-phosphorus binding and the risk of hypocalcemic-induced neuromuscular irritability.

### 13. How is TLS managed?

Goals of TLS therapy include maintenance of adequate fluid balance and adequate urinary output and prevention of life-threatening electrolyte abnormalities.

Patients should receive at least 3 liters of **hydration** daily. Aggressive intravenous hydration should begin 1–2 days before initiation of antineoplastic therapy and continue for a few days after treatment is completed.

Administration of **diuretics** or renal-dose dopamine helps to prevent fluid overload, electrolyte imbalance, and complications of uric acid build-up. Observation for hypokalemia and hypomagnesemia should accompany diuretic use. If fluid removal is not adequate with these measures, renal replacement therapies may be considered.

**Treatment of metabolic alterations** may include administration of calcium supplements and phosphate-binding antacids (e.g., Amphojel). Emergent treatment of life-threatening hyperkalemia may include administration of 50% dextrose in water (D50W) with insulin, sodium bicarbonate, or albuterol (Ventolin) or another pure beta stimulant. Each of these therapies temporarily shifts potassium back into the cell. Kayexalate and sorbitol should be administered to eliminate potassium from the body. If the patient has not developed any hyperkalemia-associated dysrhythmias, a dose of calcium chloride may be administered to protect the heart until potassium is removed from the body.

**Continuous renal replacement therapy** may be initiated to manage fluid overload, hyperuricemia, hyperphosphatemia, and metabolic acidosis related to TLS.

### 14. What nursing interventions are appropriate for patients with TLS?

Nursing management includes identifying patients at risk, initiating monitoring, and evaluating preventative and treatment modalities. Baseline renal function tests are performed in patients at risk before initiation of antineoplastic therapy. Patient and family education related to signs and symptoms of electrolyte abnormalities and renal insufficiency and the importance of prophylactic measures should be emphasized. Monitoring of renal and cardiac function, vital signs, fluid balance, and signs and symptoms of electrolyte and acid-base imbalances is essential. Monitoring of urine pH, which should be maintained at > 7, and maintaining urinary output of at least 3 L/day (or 150–200 ml/hr) are key nursing interventions. Monitor for early signs of a skin rash (associated with allopurinol), and treat with diphenhydramine and Sarna lotion if a rash is noted.

### 15. What is hemorrhagic cystitis?

Hemorrhagic cystitis is a bladder toxicity caused by cyclophosphamide (Cytoxan) and ifosfamide (Ifex) or radiation. Occasionally hemorrhagic cystitis is severe enough to warrant an ICU admission for monitoring and management. Cytoxan and Ifex are broken down by the liver into two compounds, phosphoamide mustard (active antineoplastic metabolite) and acrolein (inactive urinary metabolite). Acrolein binds to the mucous of the bladder, resulting in inflammation, erythema, ulceration, necrosis, and hemorrhage that lead to a reduction in bladder capacity and an increased risk for bladder cancer.

### 16. When does hemorrhagic cystitis present? How is it prevented?

Hemorrhagic cystitis may occur immediately or weeks after chemotherapy treatment. Once the chemotherapy is discontinued, the symptoms should subside. In some patients, however, cystitis may persist for weeks or months. Patients receiving Cytoxan may be premedicated with 2-mercaptoethane sulfonate sodium (MESNA) to prevent hemorrhagic cystitis. Aggressive prehydration with intravenous and oral fluids, diuretic use, and continuous bladder irrigations aid in diluting the metabolites in the urine.

### 17. What are the signs and symptoms of hemorrhagic cystitis?

Patients may present with one or more symptoms, depending on the extent of damage to the bladder. Symptoms include microscopic-to-gross hematuria, dysuria, increased frequency, blood clots, suprapubic discomfort, and frank hemorrhage.

### 18. How is hemorrhagic cystitis treated?

Once hemorrhagic cystitis has developed, the agent causing the cystitis should be eliminated or reduced in dosage. **Continuous bladder irrigation** with a three-way indwelling catheter infusing 1 L/hour of sterile water or saline solution helps to prevent clot formation. A decrease in flow from the catheter may indicate clot formation. Careful investigation is needed to rule out mechanical failure of the catheter vs. clot formation. Specific orders may be written to irrigate the catheter manually with sterile technique. If necessary, cystoscopy may be performed to cauterize bleeds and evacuate clots.

**Hyperbaric chambers** have been used in the treatment of radiation-induced hemorrhagic cystitis. Hyperbaric oxygen therapy has been shown to decrease bleeding.

**Prostaglandin E$_2$** may be used to treat hemorrhagic cystitis. It deactivates acrolein and is instilled directly into the bladder. The response to treatment may occur in 24 hours to 5 days. One of the side effects of prostaglandin E$_2$ is bladder spasm.

Hemorrhagic cystitis can be quite painful and may require **narcotics and antispasmodics**.

If hemorrhagic cystitis is refractory to conservative treatment, the patient may require instillation of **formalin** (1–4%) into the bladder via bladder irrigation. Formalin produces a protein precipitate when it comes in contact with the bleeding surface of the bladder. Because instillation of formalin is painful, the procedure usually is done in the operating room under general anesthesia. The patient is placed in the Trendelenburg position during the procedure to prevent ureteral reflux.

If all medical treatment fails, **suprapubic cystotomy** is indicated.

### 19. What nursing interventions are appropriate for patients with hemorrhagic cystitis?

Patients need frequent monitoring of serum electrolytes, blood urea nitrogen, and creatinine as well as urinalysis, and strict monitoring of intake and output. Monitor for bleeding (frequent assessment of vital signs and hemoglobin and hematocrit values), and assess for bladder distention and adequate urine output (at least 100 ml/hr). Diuresis may be required. Gentle irrigation of the urinary catheter using sterile technique may be done to prevent infection and further trauma. Pain management is essential because catheter manipulation as well as cystitis can cause discomfort.

### 20. Define bone marrow transplantation (BMT). What is its primary goal?

BMT is the intravenous infusion of pluripotent stem cells and progenitor cells. Its goal is to replace diseased marrow with healthy marrow. The diseased marrow may be related to a hematologic or nonhematologic malignant disorder.

### 21. What are the different types of BMT?

**Autologous transplant:** the patient receives his or her own bone marrow. The bone marrow is harvested, usually under general anesthesia in the operating room, when the patient is in remission. The posterior iliac crest and mediastinum are common sites of bone marrow aspiration. Multiple aspirations of bone marrow are collected, processed, cryopreserved, and then administered later when the patient needs the marrow.

**Allogeneic transplant:** the patient receives bone marrow from a related or unrelated donor with matching human leukocyte antigen (HLA) type. The procedure is the same as above.

**Peripheral blood stem cells transplant** (PBSCT): the patient receives an infusion of stem cells that have been harvested from peripheral blood. The donor (patient or related or unrelated donor) must receive hematopoietic growth factors to mobilize the progenitor cells. The procedure used to harvest stem cells, called apheresis, separates the stem cells out of the peripheral blood. It usually takes two or more apheresis sessions to collect the cells. Once the cells are collected, they are processed and administered when needed.

### 22. What complications are associated with BMT?

Patients receiving BMT may experience a myriad of complications, which can present during the conditioning regimen, during transplant, or days to years after transplant. These complications are related to treatment toxicities (e.g., radiation, high-dose chemotherapy drugs), the disease itself, and/or graft-vs.-host disease (GVHD). The following questions relate to complications that may be encountered in caring for BMT patients in the ICU.

### 23. What is mucositis?

Mucositis is inflammation and irritation of the mucosal layer. Oral, esophageal, gastric, or intestinal mucositis may occur after BMT as a result of high-dose chemotherapy (methotrexate), radiation, infection, and/or herpes simplex virus. The patient may present with mucositis of one or several GI locations.

### 24. How is mucositis managed?

Management of severe oral and/or esophageal mucositis includes maintaining an airway, preventing aspiration, pain management, frequent oral hygiene, nutritional support, symptom management and infection prophylaxis or treatment (i.e., antibacterial, antifungal, or antiviral agents). Management of gastric and intestinal mucositis includes monitoring of vital signs, intake and output, electrolytes, hematocrit, and hemoglobin; pain management, parenteral support; symptom management; and infection prophylaxis or treatment. Patients with severe cases may require intubation to maintain a patent airway, mechanical ventilation to provide adequate analgesic support, and blood product transfusions to treat blood loss from the irritated GI tract.

### 25. What are the causes of respiratory distress in BMT patients?

Common causes of respiratory insufficiency or failure include pneumonia, pulmonary fibrosis (due to radiation or GVHD), pulmonary hemorrhage, adult respiratory distress syndrome, atelectasis, bronchiolitis obliterans, and pulmonary embolism.

### 26. What is graft-vs.-host disease?

GVHD is an antigen-antibody reaction in which the allogeneic transplant (graft) recognizes the patient (host) as a foreign antigen and attacks. GVHD can affect any organ in the body (skin, lung, liver, kidney, GI tract).

### 27. What are the signs and symptoms of GVHD?

Clinical manifestations of GVHD affecting the skin are generalized redness, maculopapular rash, blisters and bullae, and finally desquamation. GVHD of the liver presents as jaundice, upper quadrant pain, hepatomegaly, and elevated liver function tests. GVHD of the GI tract presents as nausea, vomiting, anorexia, pain, and diarrhea. If the kidneys are affected, decreased urine output and increased levels of blood urea nitrogen and creatinine may be seen. GVHD of the lung presents as pulmonary edema, hypoxemia, and altered lung compliance. The alveolar parenchymal tissue is initially inflamed and then becomes fibrotic as it heals. The alveolar capillary membrane thickens because of the fibrotic tissue. As a result, diffusion of gases is not optimal. In addition, the distensibility of the lung is decreased and vital capacity is reduced.

### 28. How is GVHD diagnosed and treated?

The diagnosis of GVHD can be difficult and is confirmed by biopsy. Patients diagnosed with GVHD are immediately started on immunosuppressive therapy (e.g., cyclosporine, tacrolimus, and/or methotrexate). Management includes monitoring of vital signs, fluid balance, and laboratory results; parenteral support; pain management; and antimicrobial therapies to prevent infection due to impairment of mucosal integrity. Severe GVHD of the skin requires care that is similar to that of burn patients.

### 29. What is hepatic venoocclusive disease (VOD)?

Hepatic VOD is a complication of high-dose chemotherapy and high-dose radiation, which is used to precondition patients for BMT. VOD occurs in approximately 20% of BMT patients.

### 30. What is the mechanism of injury in hepatic VOD?

The mechanism of injury is not clear. According to one theory, injury is caused by cellular toxicity when the cells release tumor necrosis factor and coagulation is activated, resulting in endophlebitis, thrombus, and subsequent obstruction of the hepatic sinusoids and venules. VOD involves partial or complete occlusion of the terminal hepatic sinusoids and venules and sublobular veins, which results in hepatocyte necrosis.

### 31. What is the mortality rate of hepatic VOD?

Patients with chemotherapy-induced VOD have a 50% mortality rate.

### 32. What are the risk factors for developing VOD?

- History of hepatitis
- Age > 12 years
- Elevated levels of alanine aminotransferase (ALT) or aspartate aminotransferase (AST) before transplantation

• Unrelated allogeneic BMT
• Fever during preconditioning

Drugs associated with development of VOD include busulfan, amphotericin, and vancomycin. It is not clear whether the drugs or the infection that they treat is the predisposing factor.

### 33. How is VOD diagnosed?

Diagnosis of VOD is complex and difficult because of the multiple complications associated with BMT. An invasive diagnostic biopsy in pancytopenic BMT patients is not without risk of serious complication. Noninvasive procedures such as computed tomography scan, ultrasound, or Doppler studies can identify thrombus formation. Diagnosis may be made if the patient presents with two or more signs or symptoms within 2–3 weeks after transplantation. Signs and symptoms of VOD include edema, sudden weight gain (> 2% of body weight), jaundice, right upper quadrant abdominal pain (painful hepatomegaly), ascites, encephalopathy, and increased levels of serum bilirubin and ALT or AST. The onset of symptoms is usually within 1–2 weeks after transplantation.

### 34. What treatment is available for VOD?

Symptom management and supportive care are currently the only treatments for VOD. There is no known cure. Fluid management consists of sodium and water restriction, maintaining intravascular volume (e.g., hematocrit > 35%, administration of albumin), diuretics (e.g., spironolactone, furosemide), and low-dose dopamine for renal perfusion. Anticoagulation therapy (heparin) is usually standard to prevent further thrombus formation. Pain management is indicated for hepatomegaly. Meperidine is contraindicated because its metabolite, normeperidine, lowers the seizure threshold. Lactulose may be given prophylactically to minimize encephalopathic complications by decreasing the production of ammonia in the intestinal tract. Certain procedures, such as paracentesis to drain ascites fluid, chest tube insertion for pleural effusions, intubation for respiratory distress, and renal replacement therapy for associated renal failure, may be implemented to treat the sequelae of VOD.

### 35. What nursing interventions are appropriate for patients with VOD?

Nursing management includes frequent monitoring of serum electrolytes, liver function tests, fluid balance (intake and output, patient weight), vital signs, and abdominal girth (daily) as well as restriction of sodium intake. Patients receiving anticoagulation therapy should be placed on bleeding precautions and monitored closely. Nursing strategies include neurologic assessment (to evaluate any changes in mental status); pulmonary assessment (including breath sounds, and chest radiographs for pleural effusions); GI/urinary assessment (including management of abdominal girth and strict intake and output), nutritional assessments; and assessment for adequate pain control. The patient and family need education, reassurance, and emotional support during treatment and recovery.

### BIBLIOGRAPHY

1. Chernecky C, Berger B: Advanced and Critical Care Oncology Nursing: Managing Primary Complications. Philadelphia, W.B. Saunders, 1998.
2. Groenwald LS, Frogge MH, Goodman M, Yarbo CA (eds): Cancer Nursing: Principles and Practice, 4th ed. Boston, Jones & Bartlett, 1997.
3. Groenwald LS, Frogge MH, Goodman M, Yarbo CA: Clinical Guide to Cancer Nursing. Boston, Jones & Bartlett, 1998.
4. Shelton B: Oncology emergencies. In American Cancer Society: A Cancer Source for Nurses, 7th ed. Atlanta, American Cancer Society, 1997, pp 214–230.
5. Vujak D, Viele C, Caudell KA: Leukemia. Management strategies: The next generation. Onc Nurs Forum 23:478–486, 1996.

# 41. ONCOLOGIC EMERGENCIES

*Mary Reid-Finlay, RN, MS, ACNP, CCRN, OCN, and*
*Roberta Kaplow, RN, PhD, CCNS, CCRN*

### 1. Why do some oncology patients require intensive care?

Patients with cancer can develop serious complications related to the disease process, treatment modalities, or both. In caring for patients with oncologic emergencies and disorders, the goal is early recognition of the signs and symptoms and prompt treatment to prevent life-threatening complications.

### 2. What oncologic emergencies typically require intensive care?

* Spinal cord compression
* Superior vena cava syndrome
* Syndrome of inappropriate diuresis (SIAD)
* Cardiac tamponade
* Anaphylaxis
* Hypercalcemia
* Increased intracranial pressure (see Chapter 44)
* Sepsis (see Chapter 38)
* Disseminated intravascular coagulation (see Chapter 39)
* Adult respiratory distress syndrome (see Chapter 33)

### 3. What is spinal cord compression (SCC)?

SCC is caused by a tumor that exerts indirect or direct pressure on the spinal cord, affecting vascular supply. The decrease in blood flow to the spinal cord can result in infarct or vertebral collapse. Without early treatment, SCC can cause permanent damage to sensory or motor function that may lead to paresis or paralysis.

### 4. How is SCC classified?

* Intramedullary (within the spinal cord)
* Intradural (within the dura mater)
* Extramedullary (outside the spinal cord)
* Extradural (outside the dura mater)

SCC also can be due to direct extension of tumors within the epidural space through the intravertebral formations (rare: 1–3% of cases). Epidural tumors usually present in the later stages of metastatic disease.

### 5. Which patients are at high risk for developing SCC?

The incidence of SCC ranges from 5–10 % in patients with metastatic disease. The most common metastatic cancers causing extradural SCC are breast, prostate, lung, multiple myeloma, and lymphoma. Other cancers less commonly associated with SCC include melanoma, kidney cancer, gastrointestinal (GI) cancer, carcinomas, and sarcomas. Types of tumors that can cause SCC within the central nervous system are astrocytoma, ependymoma, hemangioblastoma, oligodendroglioma, and mixed glioma.

### 6. Do certain cancers metastasize to specific areas of the spine?

Yes. Patients with lung, breast, or prostate cancer, lymphoma, myeloma, or melanoma usually present with tumors in the thoracic area (70%). Tumors related to the lumbosacral area are usually lymphoma, melanoma, myeloma, or GI, kidney, prostate, breast, or lung cancers (20%).

Tumors related to the cervical area are usually breast, kidney, or lung cancer, lymphoma, melanoma, or myeloma (10%).

### 7. What are the early signs and symptoms of SCC?
The most common early complaint associated with the SCC is pain due to increased pressure in the epidural space. Ninety-five percent of patients complain of pain either in the cervical, thoracic, or lumbosacral areas weeks to months before other symptoms develop. The pain is located at the level of tumor involvement and often can be elicited by manual palpation. The patient with SCC also describes a localized or radicular, dull, and constant pain. The pain may become more severe when the patient coughs, bears weight, lies down, or performs a Valsalva maneuver.

### 8. What are the later signs and symptoms of SCC?
Later signs and symptoms include motor weakness, sensory deficits, and autonomic dysfunction. The patient with motor weakness may present with loss of muscle strength, changes in muscle tone, and motor deficits. Most patients have some type of motor weakness at diagnosis. Fifty percent of patients present with sensory and autonomic dysfunction. Sensory deficits may include numbness and paresthesia. Autonomic dysfunction involves impotency, urinary retention or incontinence, and constipation or diarrhea.

### 9. How is SCC diagnosed?
A thorough history, physical exam, and neurologic assessments evaluating pain and motor, sensory, and autonomic dysfunction provide valuable information. Spinal radiographs reveal erosion and lesions of the vertebral body and collapsed vertebral spaces. Magnetic resonance imaging (MRI) is commonly used in the diagnosis of SCC. It is a noninvasive procedure as well as sensitive and precise. MRI has replaced myelography, which is an invasive procedure involving injection of dye. A lumbar puncture may be performed for cytologic purposes.

### 10. What is the goal of treatment?
SCC is an emergency requiring early diagnosis and treatment to prevent further debilitating outcomes. Early treatment can prevent permanent damage such as paralysis, respiratory depression, and death. The goal for patients with SCC is to preserve existing neurologic function. The type and location of the tumor, onset of symptoms, and the patient's prognosis determine treatment.

### 11. What treatment modalities are available for SCC?
**Radiation treatments** are started immediately to prevent neurologic deficits. Research has shown that radiation is the best treatment; it is equivalent to surgery in terms of outcome and has lower morbidity rates. The radiation dose may range from 3000–4000 cGy over 2–4 weeks in fractionated doses. Pain may be relieved soon after treatments are started. Approximately 85% of patients with SCC report adequate pain relief. Approximately 50% of patients with neurologic deficits are stabilized.

**Steroids** are an accepted treatment for SCC and usually are used in conjunction with other modalities. The goal is to reduce the edema caused by compression. The many side effects include hyperglycemia, GI upset, electrolyte imbalances, bleeding, and psychosis.

**Surgical decompression** involves complete or partial removal of the tumor or laminectomy. It is performed in patients with radioresistant tumors or rapidly progressing neurologic deficit to prevent further deterioration.

### 12. What nursing interventions have high priority in patients with SCC?
The immediate goal is to stabilize the patient's condition, and the first step is to immobilize the patient to prevent further damage. Bedrest and logrolling are mandatory strategies. Once the patient is placed on bedrest, a prophylactic antiembolism regimen should be initiated, including sequential compression devices, antiembolism stockings, and/or subcutaneous heparin or low-molecular-weight heparin.

A complete pulmonary assessment is done to establish any deficits related to oxygenation and ventilation. Patients with a tumor in the cervical area (C4 and above) require emergency intubation to protect the airway. A manual resuscitator (bag-valve-mask), suction, and oxygen should be set up at the bedside and kept readily available.

The practitioner must perform a thorough neurologic assessment and be able to recognize the signs and symptoms of SCC so that the patient is diagnosed early. This assessment should focus on motor and sensory deficits and autonomic dysfunction. The initial assessment should be followed with assessments every 1–2 hours to monitor changes. A complete physical assessment, with assessment of pain, vital signs, and intake and output, is required.

### 13. Describe the management of pain due to SCC.

Pain is the most frequent complaint of SCC. Therefore, specific assessment tools should include a detailed description of the pain—onset, location, intensity, quality, duration, aggravating or alleviating effects, and rating on a scale of 0–10 (0 = no pain, 10 = worst pain possible). Pain management requires multiple interventions to relieve symptoms. Commonly used medications include steroids, nonsteroidal anti-inflammatory agents, opioids, antidepressants, and anticonvulsants. Nonpharmacologic approaches, in conjunction with pharmacologic agents, may help to provide comfort and optimize quality of life.

### 14. How are motor and sensory deficits managed?

If any motor deficits are noted, the patient may require assistance in turning to prevent pressure ulcers. Active or passive range-of-motion exercises should be incorporated once the patient is stabilized. Foot drop may be prevented with splints. A referral for physical therapy, occupational therapy, or rehabilitation may be necessary, depending on the degree of immobility. A patient may experience sensory deficits such as decreased sensation, paresthesias, numbness, tingling, hyperesthesias (unusual sensibility to sensory stimulation), or dysesthesias (sensation of pins and needles). Assessment of light touch, temperature, pinprick, or vibration can reveal sensory deficits. Patients with certain sensory deficits, such as loss of sensation in the lower extremity, are at risks for falls, self-injury, and alteration in skin integrity.

### 15. What does autonomic dysfunction involve? How is it managed?

Autonomic dysfunction involves the bladder and bowel and results in bladder retention or incontinence, constipation, or diarrhea. The nerves that control these functions have been altered by either sensation or complete dysfunction. Interventions such as intermittent bladder catheterization, retraining of the bladder, or bowel regimen may be required. Patients may present with a neurogenic bladder, in which obstruction is caused by interruption of the nerve supply. A loss in either voluntary or involuntary function of the bladder may occur. Patients with neurogenic bladders are at high risk for infection. Sexual dysfunction also needs to be assessed and may require referral to a counselor.

### 16. What is superior vena cava syndrome (SVCS)?

SVCS occurs when an intravascular clot, extrinsic compression, or tumor causes an obstruction that affects the SVC. Venous drainage above the obstruction in the upper thorax is impaired, causing impedance of venous return to the heart.

### 17. What causes SVCS?

The SVC is susceptible to obstruction because of its thin walls, low venous pressure, and anatomic location; it is surrounded by the lymph nodes, lungs, and major vascular structures. Tumors can easily penetrate the SVC directly or extrinsically. An intravascular clot can be formed by disruption of flow within the vessel by obstruction (tumor) or temporary or permanent indwelling catheters (e.g., central line, Silastic catheter, dialysis catheters).

### 18. What are the risk factors for SVCS?

Ninety-five percent of patients with SVCS have malignancies. The remaining 5% of cases are due to benign processes such as radiation fibrosis, infection, trauma, tension pneumothorax, mediastinal emphysema, sarcoidosis, aneurysm, arteriovenous fistula, pericarditis, and permanent or temporary catheters or devices (e.g., pacemakers).

### 19. What are the signs and symptoms of SVCS?

The onset of SVCS is rarely acute. Symptoms vary, depending on the extent of the obstruction. Usually symptoms progress slowly, and collateral circulation develops to compensate for the obstruction. Classic signs and symptoms include swelling or erythema in the face and/or neck; periorbital edema; jugular venous distention (JVD); swelling in the arms; and cyanosis. Other symptoms include dyspnea, tachycardia, dysphagia, tightness of the neck (Stokes' sign), hoarseness, stridor, epistaxis, chest pain, and hypotension. Headache, confusion, anxiety, changes in mental status, and blurred vision may be related to increased intracranial pressure.

### 20. How is SVCS diagnosed?

Tests that assist in the diagnosis of SVCS include chest radiograph, computed tomography (CT) scan, MRI, and contrast venography. These tests confirm the presence of any mass or obstruction adjacent to or within the SVC. If the malignancy is known, treatment may be started without a complete diagnostic work-up. If the diagnosis is unclear, confirmation is needed to treat SVCS unless the symptoms are life-threatening. Cytology testing is part of the diagnostic work-up and may include sputum cytology, thoracentesis, lymph node biopsy, CT-guided needle biopsy, mediastinoscopy, bronchoscopy, surgical biopsy, or thoracotomy.

### 21. What is the prognosis for SVCS?

The prognosis depends on the how rapidly the symptoms develop, histology and staging of the underlying malignancy, response to treatment, collateral circulation, and overall health status of the patient. If the cause of the SVCS is benign, the prognosis is excellent. If the cause of SVCS is metastatic disease, the median survival is 6–9 months after treatment.

### 22. How is SVCS most commonly treated?

The type of treatment depends on the history, location, and size of the tumor causing the obstruction. **Radiation** and **chemotherapy** are the two common treatments of choice. Lymphomas are radiosensitive, and relief can be attained within 3–4 days after treatment. The dosage of radiation depends on the histology of the tumor. If the patient presents with respiratory distress, immediate radiation is the treatment of choice. Chemotherapy can be used for chemosensitive tumors (e.g., small cell carcinoma, lymphoma). The decision to use combination chemotherapy depends on the histology of the disease.

### 23. What other treatments may be used?

If the cause of SVCS is related to thrombus, thrombolytic therapy is initiated. Depending on the extent of the thrombus, the catheter can be removed if the therapy is ineffective. Anticoagulation is used in conjunction with thrombolytics to prevent further development of thrombus. Surgical interventions, such as bypass, are rare. A combination of endovascular techniques (e.g., thrombolysis, angioplasty, stenting) may be used in conjunction with the above therapies. This approach has successfully relieved symptoms associated with SVCS. If the SVCS has affected the airway due to edema, steroids and diuretics are used.

### 24. What are the complications of SVCS?

Complications may be related to treatment:
- Bleeding due to thrombolytic or anticoagulation therapy, perforation, and hematoma from endovascular procedures
- Infection from endovascular procedures, steroids, chemotherapy, radiation, or any combination of these
- Pulmonary emboli due to thrombus formation
- Dehydration, electrolyte imbalances, hypotension, or any combination of these due to diuretics

### 25. What nursing interventions are appropriate for patients with SVCS?

Nurses caring for patients at high risk for developing SVCS should include the signs and symptoms of SVCS in **patient education** so that the patient can identify early symptoms and receive treatment. Early management of symptoms can prevent life-threatening complications such as airway obstruction, heart failure, and cerebral hypoxia.

**Baseline assessment of neurologic, pulmonary, and cardiovascular systems** is crucial to identify progression of symptoms. Respirations, pulses, blood pressure, and central venous pressure (CVP) should be assessed. Airway management includes reduction of edema with administration of diuretics and steroids, use of high Fowler's position (head of bed > 45–90° upright), oxygenation to maintain adequate pulse oximetry readings (> 95%), maintenance of oral airway, availability of suction at the bedside, and assessment of pattern and rate of respirations and breath sounds.

Patients with SVCS need **good skin care** because they are at risk for breakdown due to edema, radiation treatment, or both. Skin care involves elevation of upper extremities, keeping the skin clean and dry, especially where skin folds are present (e.g., underarms, breasts, and neck), and protecting the affected areas from trauma.

### 26. What are the components of the neurologic exam?

The neurologic exam should include assessment of mental status, level of consciousness, Glasgow Coma Scale, and neurovascular checks of the upper extremities. For management of increased intracranial pressure, refer to Chapter 44. For headache pain, medicate with analgesics as needed.

### 27. What are the components of the cardiovascular management?

Cardiovascular management includes maintenance of fluid and electrolyte balance and adequate cardiac output, assessment of pulses (including pulsus paradoxus), and monitoring of heart rate and rhythm. Strict intake and output should be maintained and recorded hourly to avoid alteration of fluid balance, which may exacerbate symptoms.

Intravenous access in the upper extremities should be avoided because of the high risk for thrombophlebitis. Blood pressure should be monitored through an arterial line to avoid use of a blood pressure cuff in the upper extremities. Inflation of the blood pressure cuff may cause more venous congestion in the affected area. If a blood pressure cuff is used, it should be placed on the lower extremities.

Bleeding precautions should be observed in patients receiving anticoagulation or thrombolytic therapy. Frequent monitoring of complete blood count, platelets, prothrombin time or international normalized ratio, and partial thromboplastin time are indicated. Patients typically present with anxiety, which may be related to respiratory distress, poor prognosis, or altered body image. Administration of sedatives that do not act on the central nervous system, a quiet, calm environment, emotional support, and reassurance that treatment will diminish the symptoms may decrease the level of anxiety.

### 28. What is the syndrome of inappropriate diuresis (SIAD)?

Antidiuretic hormone (ADH) regulates body fluid and sodium balance. Inappropriate levels of ADH lead to water intoxication and hyponatremia. SIAD, formerly known as the syndrome of inappropriate secretion of ADH, results from an excessive secretion of ADH. When ADH is secreted, water reabsorption in the distal tubules and collecting ducts of the kidneys is stimulated, leading to decreased urine excretion and concentrated urine. The plasma becomes more dilute, causing a lowering of plasma osmolality and dilutional serum sodium levels.

### 29. What causes SIAD?

SIAD is classified as an endocrine paraneoplastic syndrome. It is caused by the increased production of ADH by malignant cells. The extent of SIAD depends on the progression of the disease. Drugs that stimulate or potentiate the action of ADH have been associated with SIAD, including cyclophosphamide, vincristine, vinblastine, morphine, meperidine, barbiturates, tricyclic antidepressants, anesthetics, acetaminophen, chloralpamine, carbamazepine, and nicotine. Other factors that can increase production of ADH include infection, status asthmaticus, disorders of the central nervous system, endocrine disorders, surgery, severe pain, stress, nausea, positive pressure ventilation (PEEP), or any condition causing increased intrathoracic pressure or decreased venous return.

### 30. Which cancers are associated most commonly with SIAD?

The most common cancer associated with SIAD is small cell lung carcinoma. However, only 9–14% of patients develop SIAD. Other neoplastic etiologies include non–small cell lung cancer; carcinoid tumors; breast and brain tumors; squamous cell cancer of the head, neck, prostate, esophagus, pancreas, or colon; thymoma; and Hodgkin's and non-Hodgkin's lymphoma.

### 31. What are the signs and symptoms of SIAD?

Common signs include increased urinary sodium (> 20 mEq/L), increased urine osmolality (> 1000 mOsm/kg), serum hypoosmolality (< 275 mOsm/kg), and hyponatremia. Patients also may present with a wide range of symptoms, including fluid retention, weight gain, anorexia, nausea, vomiting, central nervous system manifestations (e.g., confusion, agitation, hallucinations), concentrated urine, and electrolyte imbalances. Such symptoms may be due to dilutional hypocalcemia, hyponatremia, and hypokalemia. The three categories of symptoms associated with SIAD are mild, moderate, and severe.

### 32. For which symptoms of SIAD should the patient be monitored?

**Mild** (serum sodium level = 125–135 mEq/L)
- Headache
- Lethargy
- Changes in behavior
- Ataxia
- Peripheral edema
- Muscle cramps
- Anorexia

**Moderate** (serum sodium level = 118–124 mEq/L)
- Irritability
- Disorientation
- Weakness
- Somnolence
- Hallucinations
- Tremors
- Nausea/vomiting
- Diarrhea
- Weight gain
- Oliguria

**Severe** (serum sodium level = 112–117 mEq/L)
- Obtundation
- Coma
- Seizures
- Inability to maintain airway and mobilize secretions
- Death

### 33. How is SIAD treated?

The treatment for SIAD includes management of the underlying problem and hyponatremia. In **less severe cases**, patients are placed on strict intake and output and maintained by fluid restrictions of 500–1000 ml/day to correct the hyponatremia.

Patients with **severe symptoms** require slow administration of hypertonic saline, diuretics, and electrolyte replacements. The serum sodium level should increase by only 1–2 mEq/hour to prevent complications of pulmonary edema, hypernatremia, changes in mental status, and/or seizures.

**Chronic SIAD** generally is treated with demeclocycline, an oral antibiotic that initiates diuresis by impairing the effect of ADH on the renal tubules. Side effects of demeclocycline include photosensitivity, nausea, and azotemia.

### 34. What nursing interventions are appropriate for patients with SIAD?

The nurse must monitor serum sodium, serum osmolality, and urine osmolality frequently, maintain strict intake and output (including insertion of a urinary catheter), and restrict fluids. Frequent neurologic assessments are necessary. Sudden changes in mental status may indicate worsening hyponatremia. In severe cases of hyponatremia, quick replacement of sodium also can cause changes in mental status and possible seizures. If the patient is confused, safety may be an issue. A calm environment, limited activity, and reorientation to person, place, and time are helpful.

If patients with SIAD complain of anorexia, nausea, or vomiting, a complete GI work-up may be required to investigate other possible causes. Patients with GI symptoms may need antiemetic medications. Educating the patient and family about symptoms is important to facilitate early assessment and treatment, which are essential for optimal patient outcome.

### 35. What patients are at risk for developing cardiac tamponade?

Malignancies are the most common cause of cardiac tamponade. Tumors usually associated with cardiac tamponade include lung, breast, lymphoma, and leukemia. When the tumor invades the pericardium or myocardium, venous and lymphatic drainage is obstructed. Patients who have received antineoplastic agents such as doxorubicin or daunorubicin are also at risk because of the cardiotoxic side effects. Postradiation pericarditis as well as compression of the pericardial sac from tumor (e.g., breast or lung cancer) also can cause tamponade.

### 36. What are the hemodynamic manifestations of cardiac tamponade?

The hemodynamic manifestations of cardiac tamponade depend on the amount of fluid in the pericardium, the rate of accumulation, and underlying cardiovascular function. Cardiovascular signs appear as fluid accumulation increases. An early sign is elevation in CVP; muffled heart sounds, decreased or absent apical pulse, and decreased cardiac output occur as fluid accumulates around the heart. If fluid accumulation is rapid, compensatory mechanisms do not have time to respond. The results are decreased stroke volume, hypotension, and tachycardia. The patient's stroke volume further diminishes, systemic vascular resistance increases, systolic blood pressure decreases, and diastolic blood pressure increases if treatment is not initiated. Blood pressure changes manifest as a narrowing of pulse pressure.

### 37. What other signs and symptoms are associated with cardiac tamponade?

If fluid accumulation is slow, patients may present with fatigue, shortness of breath, nausea, vomiting, diarrhea, hepatomegaly, and abdominal distention. When fluid accumulates quickly, tachypnea, dyspnea, orthopnea, and cyanosis develop concomitantly with hemodynamic compromise. Patients often have pulsus paradoxus, which is a decrease in systolic blood pressure of more than 10 mmHg during inspiration. Patients with tamponade may develop mental status changes as a result of decreased cerebral perfusion. A pericardial friction rub may be audible. Other manifestations may include anxiety, apprehension, agitation, hiccoughs, dysphagia, hoarseness, abdominal pain, low-grade fever, and peripheral edema. Prolonged hypotensive periods may result in oliguria or anuria related to altered renal perfusion.

### 38. How is cardiac tamponade diagnosed?

Several noninvasive and invasive diagnostic methods may be used to confirm the presence of cardiac tamponade. Echocardiography is the most sensitive and precise method. A chest radiograph may reveal an enlarged cardiac silhouette or "water-bottle heart," mediastinal widening, and cardiomegaly. A CT scan may reveal cardiac tamponade but does not provide data about cardiac performance. ECG changes in patients with cardiac tamponade are nonspecific but may include sinus tachycardia, presence of atrial or ventricular dysrhythmias, elevated ST segments, T-wave changes, low voltage QRS complexes, and electrical alternans. Pulmonary artery catheterization typically reveals equalization of right- and left-sided heart pressures, low cardiac output, increased systemic vascular resistance, and increased CVP, pulmonary artery pressure, and pulmonary artery wedge pressure. Because of the invasive nature and associated comorbidities, pulmonary artery catheterization is rarely used for the diagnosis of cardiac tamponade.

### 39. How is cardiac tamponade managed?

Before treatment of cardiac tamponade, **hemodynamic stability** should be attained by enhancing preload with aggressive fluid resuscitation using crystalloids or colloids. Cardiac performance can be enhanced with the titration of inotropic agents such as dopamine, norepinephrine, or dobutamine. Arterial vasodilators, such as nitroprusside, decrease systemic vascular resistance. Diuretics decrease preload and therefore should be avoided.

**Pericardiocentesis**, or aspiration of fluid from the pericardial space, is the most common effective approach. A large-bore needle is inserted under the xiphoid process and into the pericardial space. Fluid is gradually withdrawn with a syringe. Hemodynamic status usually improves at once, when as little as 50 ml of fluid is removed. Once the procedure is complete, a drainage catheter can be substituted for the needle and left in place until the output decreases to 50–100 ml over 24 hours.

### 40. How is the patient prepared for pericardiocentesis?
Preprocedure management of patients undergoing pericardiocentesis includes supportive therapy with oxygen, fluids, or inotropes, as clinically indicated. The patient should be prepared for possible sensations that may be experienced during the procedure, including the initial needle stick and burning during administration of the anesthetic, a pressure sensation during insertion of the needle, and some pain if the needle touches the pericardium.

### 41. Describe the nurse's role during pericardiocentesis.
The nurse's role includes obtaining intravenous access, positioning the patient in semi-Fowler's position, and administering sedation and analgesia as prescribed and indicated. The nurse assists the cardiologist by connecting the alligator clamp to the hub of the cardiac needle to provide an ECG trace in the V lead to guide needle placement into the pericardium, avoiding the myocardium. Nursing care during a pericardiocentesis includes frequent monitoring of vital signs, assessment of hemodynamic status, observing for dysrhythmias and other procedure-related complications, and monitoring the drainage that is aspirated.

### 42. Describe the nurse's role after pericardiocentesis.
Postprocedure care includes monitoring the patient's hemodynamic status and hourly intake and output, assessing for complications, and monitoring drainage if a catheter is left in place. Other nursing management includes providing emotional support; addressing psychosocial issues; educating the patient about signs and symptoms of fluid reaccumulation, the disease process, and treatment modalities; and stressing the importance of reporting significant signs of fluid reaccumulation.

### 43. How is reaccumulation of fluid prevented?
- A sclerosing agent, such as bleomycin, cisplatin, mitomycin C, doxycycline, minocycline, or fluorouracil, can be injected into the pericardial space via the pericardial catheter.
- Biologic response modifiers, such as interleukin-2, and radioisotopes also have been used.
- Systemic chemotherapy, external radiation, and hormonal therapy as treatments of the underlying malignancy have been effective in preventing recurrence.
- Pericardiotomy, or insertion of a balloon catheter into the pericardial sac through an incision of the pericardium, can be performed under local anesthesia at the bedside to promote drainage and prevent reaccumulation.

### 44. Define pericardial window and pericardiectomy.
A **pericardial window** is created by removal of a piece of pericardium. The procedure can be performed under general or local anesthesia in the operating room in patients who do not respond to other therapeutic interventions. Complications include infection, pneumothorax, pleural effusion, atelectasis, or pain.

**Pericardiectomy** is an excision of part or all of the pericardium and may be indicated for patients with pericarditis or with reoccurring cardiac tamponade. Complications include myocardial laceration, bleeding, scarring, and infection.

### 45. Which oncology patients are at risk for developing anaphylactic shock?
Anaphylactic shock in oncology patients has been associated with a number of antineoplastic agents. Patients are at higher risk for developing anaphylactic shock with intravenous (vs. oral) administration, drugs derived from bacteria (e.g., L-asparaginase), and repeated administration of

the agent. Anaphylactic shock is a life-threatening oncologic emergency. Respiratory and cardio-vascular complications have mortality rates of 70% and 24%, respectively. Prognosis is better for patients whose signs and symptoms are recognized and treated early.

### 46. When does anaphylaxis occur?

Anaphylaxis usually occurs within seconds to minutes after exposure to an allergen. The earlier the signs and symptoms appear, the more severe the reaction. A reaction may occur up to 1 hour after exposure to the antigen.

### 47. What are the signs and symptoms of anaphylactic shock?

The signs and symptoms are the result of the chemical mediators on the cardiopulmonary system. They include decreases in blood pressure, CVP, pulmonary artery occlusive pressure, and cardiac output as well as tachycardia due to preload reduction. Mental status changes range from a decrease in level of consciousness to coma. Patients experience dyspnea and prominent air hunger, hoarseness, stridor, and possibly complete airway obstruction due to laryngeal edema, laryngo-spasm, bronchoconstriction, and increased secretions. Urine output is decreased secondary to de-creased renal perfusion. Skin symptoms include itching and urticaria. Patients may have localized edema of the lips and tongue, pruritus, diaphoresis, or generalized erythema. Initially they may appear flushed but then develop pallor, cyanosis, or both. GI symptoms include nausea, vomiting, diarrhea, and abdominal pain. Patients also may experience a feeling of impending doom.

### 48. Describe the management of anaphylactic shock.

- In addition to maintaining a patent airway, the primary strategy is elimination of the causative agent.
- Endotracheal intubation, tracheotomy, or cricothyrotomy may be required to prevent as-phyxia due to laryngeal edema.
- Oxygen is administered to support delivery to tissues.
- Epinephrine is the initial drug of choice because of its rapid bronchodilator effects. The usual dose is 0.3 ml of 1:1000 via subcutaneous injection (if the patient is responsive) or 0.5–1 mg of 1:10,000 via slow intravenous injection (if the patient is not responsive). Absorption from the subcutaneous tissue is slow in the presence of hypotension. If the patient has a persis-tent airway obstruction, an epinephrine infusion at 2–4 µg/min may be required.
- Vigorous fluid resuscitation with isotonic solutions or colloids is required to correct fluid losses and restore hemodynamic stability.
- Administration of a vasopressor, such as dopamine or norepinephrine, may be indicated to treat hypotension while fluid resuscitation is in progress.
- Diphenhydramine, 25–50 mg, may alleviate urticaria.
- Aminophylline, 5–6-mg/kg bolus followed by an infusion of 0.6–1 mg/kg/min, occasion-ally is used if bronchospasm persists. Racemic epinephrine 2% also may be used to treat bronchospasm.
- Corticosteroids are administered to decrease bronchospasm and capillary permeability.
- Cardiac monitoring and frequent (every 5–15 min) monitoring of vital signs are required.

### 49. What is the nurse's role in management of patients with anaphylactic shock?

Nursing management includes identifying the patient at risk (e.g., patients with previous al-lergic reactions); premedicating the patient with hydrocortisone, diphenhydramine, or both; keeping emergency equipment and medications readily available; and instituting emergency measures if necessary. Patient education includes explaining the importance of reporting early signs and symptoms such as urticaria or erythema.

### 50. Define hypercalcemia of malignancy. What are the causes?

Hypercalcemia is defined as a serum calcium level greater than 10.5 mg/dl. Hypercalcemia of malignancy is most often caused by bone metastasis from squamous cell lung and breast cancer and kidney tumors. Other cancers, such as multiple myeloma, lymphoma, squamous cell cancer of the head and neck area, and bladder, esophageal, prostate, GI, ovarian, and thyroid cancers, also have been implicated. Bone metastasis causes bone destruction and release of calcium into the extracellular fluid. Antineoplastic therapies, such as estrogen, antiestrogen agents, and all-trans-retinoic acid, may intensify hypercalcemia. Other contributing factors include prolonged immobilization, increased secretion of parathyroid hormone by some squamous cell carcinomas, hyperparathyroidism, renal insufficiency, and dehydration. (See chapter 57.)

### 51. What is the treatment of hypercalcemia of malignancy?

The primary focus is treatment of the underlying malignancy. Tumor reduction or control is the only long-term effective measure to reverse hypercalcemia. Depending on the causative tumor, this goal can be accomplished with surgical resection, chemotherapy, radiation therapy, hormonal therapy, or any combination of the above. Emergent intervention must begin for patients who have a serum calcium level > 13 mg/dl or who present with signs and symptoms of hypercalcemia. Treatment includes vigorous rehydration, increasing renal calcium excretion, and decreasing bone resorption.

### 52. How is rehydration achieved?

Aggressive fluid resuscitation with 3–8 L of isotonic saline is needed to restore intravascular volume. Patients with serum calcium levels of 18–20 mg/dl are dehydrated as a result of nausea and vomiting and the kidney's inability to concentrate urine. Fluid also flushes out calcium and promotes urinary calcium excretion.

### 53. How is renal calcium excretion increased?

Furosemide produces sodium and calcium diuresis and prevents fluid overload and hypernatremia, but it should be administered only after volume expansion and rehydration have been achieved. Otherwise, furosemide may worsen the hypercalcemic state by promoting depletion of extracellular fluid and increased calcium reabsorption. Renal replacement therapies may need to be considered if serum calcium levels are severely elevated and cardiac or renal function is impaired. Bisphosphonates also are used.

### 54. How is bone resorption decreased?

When the patient is intravascularly depleted and renal function is normalized, antiresorptive therapy is used to decrease the rate of bone resorption and prevent worsening or recurrence of hypercalcemia. Therapeutic agents include calcitonin, plicamycin (mithramycin), etidronate, pamidronate, clodronate, alendronate, risendronate, tiludronate, YM175, and BM21.0955.

### 55. Describe the nursing management of patients with hypercalcemia of malignancy.

1. Identifying patients at risk and preventing serum calcium levels from becoming life-threatening are of paramount importance.

2. Cardiac status must be monitored because of aggressive volume resuscitation. Check for edema and shortness of breath, and evaluate breath sounds. Cardiac and hemodynamic monitoring is especially important in patients who have received cardiotoxic antineoplastic therapy (e.g., anthracyclines) because they are at risk for fluid overload. Ongoing observation for cardiac dysrhythmias (including tachycardia from dehydration) and ECG changes is essential.

3. Monitoring of serum chemistries, particularly potassium, magnesium, and phosphorus (given the potential electrolyte loss during therapy), and meticulous assessment of intake and output are essential.

4. Administration of furosemide after a normovolemic state has been achieved is controversial. Furosemide decreases calcium and sodium reabsorption. However, reabsorption of calcium will increase if the patient becomes intravascularly depleted as a result of the diuretic therapy.

5. Contributory factors to hypercalcemia of malignancy (e.g., immobility, dehydration) should be eliminated, as clinically indicated by the patient's medical condition.

6. Monitoring of renal and GI function can identify signs of dehydration and prompt appropriate interventions.

## BIBLIOGRAPHY

1. Chernecky C, Berger B: Advanced and Critical Care Oncology Nursing: Managing Primary Complications. Philadelphia, W.B. Saunders, 1998.
2. Gates R, Fink R (eds): Oncology Nursing Secrets. Philadelphia, Hanley & Belfus, 1997.
3. Clochesy JM, Breu C, Cardin S, et al: Critical Care Nursing, 2nd ed. Philadelphia, WB Saunders, 1996.
4. Groenwald LS, Frogge MH, Goodman M, Yarbo CA (eds): Cancer Nursing: Principles and Practice, 4th ed. Boston, Jones & Bartlett, 1997.
5. Groenwald LS, Frogge MH, Goodman, M Yarbo CA: Clinical Guide to Cancer Nursing. Boston, Jones & Bartlett, 1998.
6. Kaplow R: Cardiac tamponade. In Yarbro CA, Frogge MH, Goodman M, Groenwald LS (eds): Cancer Nursing: Principles and Practice, 5th ed. Boston, Jones & Bartlett, 2000, pp 857–868.
7. Miaskowski C, Gettrust K: Plans of care for specialty nursing. Oncology Nursing. Albany, NY, Delmar, 1995.
8. Shelton B: Oncology emergencies. In American Cancer Society: A Cancer Source for Nurses, 7th ed. Atlanta, American Cancer Society, 1997, pp 214–230.
9. Sorrell D, Mayo D: Superior vena cava syndrome. Clin J Oncol Nurs 2153–2154, 1998.
10. Tracey L, Kruger S: Leukemia. In Gates RA, Fink RM (eds): Oncology Nursing Secrets. Philadelphia, Hanley & Belfus, 1997, pp 96–107.

# 42. POSTOPERATIVE CARE OF LIVER, PANCREAS, AND RENAL TRANSPLANT PATIENTS

Hildy M. Schell, RN, MS, CCRN

### 1. What are the common indications for liver transplantation?

The most common indication for liver transplantation is end-stage liver disease (ESLD). The many causes of ESLD include hepatitis B and C, alcohol, primary sclerosing cholangitis, primary biliary cirrhosis, and metabolic disorders. Patients with ESLD awaiting transplantation typically receive maximal medical therapy for ascites, encephalopathy, gastrointestinal (GI) bleeding, and renal insufficiency. Acute or fulminant hepatic failure related to drug toxicity (e.g., acetaminophen), hepatitis A, autoimmune disorders, and mushroom poisoning is also an indication for transplantation.

### 2. Describe the status criteria for patients on a liver transplant waiting list.

The five categories on the liver transplant waiting list are based on the criteria of the United Network for Organ Sharing (UNOS):

**Status 1** is an adult patient in an intensive care unit (ICU) with fulminant hepatic failure, posttransplant hepatic artery thrombosis, or primary graft nonfunction. Such patients are expected to live less than 7 days without a transplant.

**Status 2A** is an adult patient with ESLD in an ICU who is expected to live less than 7 days without a transplant.

**Status 2B and 3** are patients with ESLD and significant complications. The severity of liver disease is scored by using the Child-Turcotte-Pugh system. They are not critically ill and may be in an acute care hospital or waiting at home.

**Status 7** is a temporary inactive status for patients with ESLD and a condition that renders them temporarily unsuitable for transplantation. The waiting time on a liver transplant list involves many variables and can last from days to months.

### 3. What is the surgical procedure for a liver transplant?

Depending on the surgical technique and procedure, liver transplants can take from 4–12 hours. Orthotopic liver transplants involve removing the recipient's native liver and placing the transplant in the same anatomic location. After removing the native liver, the vascular anastomoses (vena cava, portal vein, and hepatic artery) are completed. The biliary system is reconstructed by using a duct-to-duct anastomosis or a Roux-en-Y anastomosis to the jejunum. Drains placed around the liver that exit through the abdominal wall facilitate monitoring for bleeding and drainage of residual ascites. The resulting abdominal incision looks like the Mercedes symbol. Alternative procedures, such as living-related partial liver transplantation and use of split cadaver livers, are being done because of donor shortage and growing waiting lists. The recipients of these transplants are at higher risk for delayed graft function and bleeding complications.

### 4. What complications may occur during the postoperative period?

- Bleeding
- Hepatic artery thrombosis
- Bile duct leaks and strictures
- Renal insufficiency
- Infection
- Rejection
- Primary nonfunction of the graft

### 5. What are the most important monitoring considerations after liver transplant?

Because patients are at high risk for bleeding, it is important to monitor all intravenous line, drain, incision, and GI sites for bleeding. Hematocrit and hemoglobin, prothrombin time (PT), partial thromboplastin time (PTT), and platelet count should be monitored frequently and assessed in relation to the blood products administered. Some patients receive fresh frozen plasma (FFP) infusions at 50–300 ml/hr until the PT and international normalized ration (INR) are within an acceptable range and there is no indication of bleeding. Hemodynamics are monitored closely for signs of hypovolemia, hypervolemia, sepsis, and cardiac dysfunction. Standard care also involves monitoring of airway and respiratory status, weaning from mechanical ventilation, and extubation. Mental status assessment provides information about liver and renal function (e.g., clearing encephalopathy) and potential neurologic complications such as seizures or stroke. Laboratory monitoring of electrolytes, renal values, liver function tests, and arterial blood gases is essential for early detection of potential complications. Thorough assessment for signs of infection and use of good handwashing and aseptic technique are mandatory.

### 6. What drugs are used to prevent potential complications?

Postoperative regimens vary by transplant program and institution. Antimicrobial agents are used prophylactically to prevent bacterial (gram-positive and gram-negative), viral (herpes simplex and cytomegalovirus), protozoal (*Pneumocystis carinii*), and mucocutaneous fungal (candidal) infections. Additional antiviral agents are given as prophylaxis against recurrent hepatitis B (lamivudine and hepatitis B immunoglobulin) or hepatitis C (ribavirin and interferon) for patients with a history of these infections. Aspirin is started when bleeding complications are ruled out to prevent vascular thromboses. A proton pump inhibitor is given as prophylaxis for GI bleeding. Diuretics and renal-dose dopamine may be used to facilitate fluid removal.

### 7. What is the indication for renal transplantation?

End-stage renal disease (ESRD) requiring renal replacement therapy. The leading causes of ESRD in the United States are diabetes, hypertension, and glomerulonephritis. Renal transplantation can provide an improved quality of life for patients by eliminating dialysis dependence, diet restrictions, and ESRD-associated medical conditions. After the first year, the medical costs for a patient with ESRD are less after transplant than before transplant.

### 8. Describe the surgical procedure for renal transplant.

The transplant is placed in the extraperitoneal space of the iliac fossa of the pelvis. The vascular anastomoses are the renal artery to the recipient's iliac artery and the renal vein to the recipient's iliac vein. The ureter is anastomosed to the recipient's bladder using a tunneling technique to prevent urine reflux into the transplanted kidney. The resulting incision is located on the right or left side of the lower quadrant of the abdomen. This surgical procedure typically takes 2–4 hours. The recipient's native kidneys are not removed unless they are infected or contribute to other complications (e.g., uncontrolled hypertension).

**9. When do renal transplant patients require ICU care?**

Renal transplant patients typically go to the postanesthesia care unit for a few hours before being admitted to an acute care unit. They may require ICU care for airway compromise, suspicion of a perioperative myocardial ischemia, or hemodynamic instability or for close observation for other potential complications.

**10. List the potential complications of renal transplant.**
- Iliac artery or vein thrombosis
- Acute tubular necrosis (ATN)/delayed graft function
- Ureteral obstruction
- Urine leak (bladder, ureter, renal calyx)
- Acute rejection
- Infection

**11. What are the most important monitoring considerations after renal transplant?**

Hemodynamic and fluid status monitoring are essential in the assessment of graft perfusion and other tissue perfusion. Monitoring of blood pressure and central venous pressure is standard. Hourly urine output is measured during the first 24–48 hours to monitor function of the transplant. Renal laboratory values (creatinine and blood urea nitrogen) and electrolytes are monitored routinely. Respiratory status is monitored closely because pulmonary edema may result from fluid overload in patients with delayed transplant function. Pain assessment and management for incisional pain and bladder spasms are routine. The incision should be assessed for bleeding, leaks, hematoma formation, and signs of infection. Pedal pulses and edema of the leg on the transplanted side should be assessed to identify signs of iliac arterial or venous thrombosis. If present, the arteriovenous fistula or graft for hemodialysis access should be assessed routinely for bruit and thrill because it may be needed if ATN is present.

**12. What is the indication for simultaneous pancreas-renal (SPR) transplantation?**

Type I diabetes with ESRD or renal insufficiency is the indication for SPR transplantation. The goal is euglycemia and decreased azotemia (uremia), which improve peripheral neuropathies and gastroparesis and stabilize retinopathies associated with diabetes. Quality of life improves for SPR transplant recipients.

**13. What surgical procedures are used for simultaneous SPR transplantation?**

The bladder drainage (BD) and enteric drainage (ED) procedures are most commonly used for SPR transplantation. It is important to understand the surgical procedures for SPR transplant because they change monitoring and management regimens. In both procedures the kidney is transplanted as above, except that it is placed in the intraperitoneal space. When the BD procedure is used, the pancreas and an adjacent segment of duodenum from the donor are placed in the iliac fossa opposite the kidney. The donor's superior mesenteric and splenic arteries are anastomosed, via an extension of the iliac artery, to the recipient's iliac artery. The donor portal vein is anastomosed to the recipient's iliac vein. The duodenal segment attached to the head of the pancreas is anastomosed to the recipient's bladder to allow drainage of exocrine fluids and enzymes.

The vascular anastomoses are the same for the ED procedure, but the duodenal segment with the pancreas is anastomosed to a segement of the recipient's small bowel to allow exocrine drainage into the GI tract for reabsorption. Knowing which procedure was used is important because urine amylase levels are monitored for patients with SPR-BD transplants to assess for pancreas rejection. In addition, patients undergoing SPR-BD transplant are at risk for metabolic acidosis and dehydration related to loss of exocrine fluid, which is rich in bicarbonate. Patients undergoing SPR-ED transplant are monitored closely for signs of peritonitis related to a leak from the anastomotic site of the GI tract.

**14. What are the potential postoperative complications of SPR transplantation?**
- Perioperative myocardial ischemia
- Dehydration and metabolic acidosis (BD)
- Bleeding (vascular anastomotic site)
- Bladder leak
- Thrombosis of pancreas or kidney
- Hematuria
- Reflux graft pancreatitis (BD)
- Urethritis
- Infection
- Rejection

**15. What are the most important monitoring considerations after SPR transplant?**

Cardiac assessment and electrocardiographic (ECG) monitoring are important for early detection of myocardial ischemia. Monitoring of hemodynamics and fluid status is essential for assessment of kidney rejection, pancreas and renal perfusion, bleeding, potential infection, and myocardial ischemia. Monitoring of arterial blood gases enhances assessment of oxygenation, ventilation, and acid–base status. Patients with SPR-BD typically have metabolic acidosis. Many patients compensate by increasing their respiratory rate and tidal volume. If they do not compensate, sodium bicarbonate may be added to the IV maintenance solution. The abdominal drains are monitored for increased output and signs of bleeding. The amylase levels in drainage fluid and serum are monitored for signs of pancreatitis (elevated trends). Urine amylase levels are monitored for elevating trends, which can indicate rejection, in patients with SPR-BD. Glucose monitoring is done every 2 hours in the immediate postoperative period. Transient hypoglycemia in the first 12 hours is related to a "surge" of insulin from the transplanted pancreas directly into the systemic circulation without passing through the hepatic circulation. It can be treated with glucose. Hyperglycemia rarely occurs. It is a late sign of rejection or graft thrombosis.

Urine output is monitored for volume and bleeding. Significant hematuria can require transfusions and typically is treated with a continuous bladder irrigation and possibly a cystoscopy intervention (laser ablation, cautery). The abdomen and incision should be assessed for signs of hematoma and urine leak. Pain assessment and management for incisional pain and bladder spasms are routine. Pedal pulses and edema in both legs should be assessed to identify signs of iliac arterial or venous thrombosis.

**16. What drugs are used to prevent potential complications?**

The pancreas is a highly vascular, low-flow organ. Aspirin and dipyridamole are used to prevent graft thrombosis. They are started when postoperative bleeding is ruled out. Albumin and mannitol are administered to prevent graft edema and promote diuresis. Renal dopamine may be used to increase renal blood flow. An $H_2$-blocker or proton pump inhibitor is given to decrease the risk of GI bleeding. Antimicrobial agents are given to prevent bacterial (gram-positive and gram-negative), viral (herpes simplex and cytomegalovirus), protozoal (*Pneumocystis carinii*), and mucocutaneous fungal (candidal) infections.

**17. How is acute rejection diagnosed?**

Acute rejection is an immune-mediated inflammatory process in which T lymphocytes and cytokines attack the transplanted organ. Acute rejection is detected by clinical signs and symptoms and confirmed by biopsy. Patients may present with lethargy, fever, and pain or tenderness over the graft. Signs and symptoms of decreased function of the transplant also may be present. A renal transplant patient may present with decreased urine output, weight gain (fluid retention), and a rise in serum creatinine. A patient with SPR transplant may present with elevated serum and/or urine amylase levels plus decreased urine output. A liver transplant patient may present with elevated serum liver function tests, fever, and/or right upper quadrant tenderness. Early detection, diagnosis, and intervention are key to successful treatment of acute rejection. Patient education related to monitoring for these signs and symptoms is essential prior to discharge.

**18. What is the typical immunosuppressive regimen for transplant patients?**
- Corticosteroids
- Mycophenolate mofetil or azathioprine
- Cyclosporine-A, tacrolimus, or sirolimus
- Polyclonal or monoclonal antibody

## 19. Why are corticosteroids used?

Corticosteroids are used to prevent and treat rejection. They inhibit production of inter-leukin-1 (IL-1) from macrophages, which are involved in the initiation of acute rejection. Methylprednisolone is given in the immediate postoperative period (2 mg/kg/day), and the dose is tapered over a few weeks to a maintenance dose of prednisone. High-dose methylprednisolone (20 mg/kg/day) is used for 2–3 days as first-line treatment for acute rejection.

## 20. What is the function of mycophenolate mofetil and azathioprine?

Either mycophenolate mofetil or azathioprine is used solely to prevent rejection. Both de-crease the availablility of T and B lymphocytes, which are the active cells during rejection. An important side effect that requires monitoring is leukopenia.

## 21. Why is cycloporine-A or tacrolimus used in the immunosuppressive regimen?

Cyclosporine-A and tacrolimus are used only to prevent rejection. Both inhibit production of interleukin-2 (IL-2) and other cytokines from T lymphocytes. This inhibition suppresses activa-tion and further proliferation of T lymphocytes. Both drugs can be administered orally or as an infusion. Monitoring for renal dysfunction, hypertension, neurotoxicity, and hyperglycemia (tacrolimus) is important in the postoperative period.

## 22. What is sirolimus?

Sirolimus is a new drug used to prevent rejection and can be used to treat resistant rejection. Sirolimus blocks T-lymphocyte activation and proliferation in response to IL-2. Sirolimus is cur-rently available only as an oral solution. Important side effects that require monitoring are leukopenia, thrombocytopenia, rash, and hypertension.

## 23. What is the function of polyclonal or monoclonal antibodies?

A polyclonal or monoclonal antibody may be used as part of an induction regimen in the postoperative period or as treatment for steroid-resistant acute rejection. Both bind and remove T lymphocytes from circulation and may cause a cytokine release syndrome (e.g., fever, chills, rigors). Antithymocyte globulin (Atgam or Thymoglobulin) is a polyclonal antibody derived from rabbit or horse serum. Muromonab-CD3 (OKT3) is a monoclonal antibody that blocks the func-tion of the CD3 molecule in the T-lymphocyte membrane. Both are IV preparations that require premedication with a corticosteroid, acetaminophen, and diphenhydramine to prevent and mini-mize side effects. It is essential to monitor for signs and symptoms of anaphylaxis, fever, rigors, hypotension, and respiratory distress. Daclizumab is a new monoclonal antibody that blocks IL-2 from binding to receptors. Used to prevent rejection, it is administered intravenously in the im-mediate postoperative period and then every 2 weeks since it has such a long half-life (20 days).

BIBLIOGRAPHY

1. Albee B, Beckman NJ, Schell HM: Patients with end-stage renal disease. In Clochesy JM, Breu C, Cardin S, et al (eds): Critical Care Nursing, 2nd ed. Philadelphia, W.B. Saunders, 1996, pp 949–966.
2. Bush WW: Overview of transplantation immunology and the pharmacotherapy of adult solid organ trans-plant recipients: Focus on immunosuppression. AACN Clin Issues 10:253–269, 1999.
3. Freise CE, Narumi S, Stock PG, Melzer JS: Simultaneous pancreas-kidney transplantation: An overview of indications, complications, and outcomes. West J Med 170:11–18, 1999.
4. Heyneman LE, Keogan MT, Tuttle-Newhall JE, et al: Pancreatic transplantation using portal venous and enteric drainage: The postoperative appearance of a new surgical procedure. J Comput Assist Tomogr 23:283–290, 1999.
5. Humar A, Payne WD, Sutherland DE, Matas AJ: Clinical determinants of multiple acute rejection episodes in kidney transplant recipients. Transplantation 69:2357–2360, 2000.
6. Penko ME, Tirbaso D: An overview of liver transplantation. AACN Clin Issues 10:176–184, 1999.
7. Tolkoff-Rubin NE, Rubin RH: Recent advances in the diagnosis and management of infection in the organ transplant recipient. Semin Nephrol 20:148–163, 2000.

# IV. Neurology

# 43. NEUROLOGIC ASSESSMENT

*Heidi D. Clay, RN, MS, CCNS*

**1. Why are changes in mental status particularly important in critically ill patients?**

Some changes in mental status have important localizing value because they suggest the presence of focal brain lesions in particular areas.

**2. What particular challenges do critically ill patients present?**

It is difficult to obtain accurate mental status assessments in patients who receive mechanical ventilation, analgesics, neuromuscular blocking agents, or physical and/or chemical restraints. Timing of the neurologic exam is crucial in critically ill patients. The best possible exam is elicited when the patient is not sedated, paralyzed, or under the influence of opioids. Other factors that may affect neurologic status, such as abnormal laboratory values, hypoxemia, and hypercapnia, should be noted and recorded at the time of examination.

**3. List the seven traits that should be examined during mental status assessment of critically ill patients.**

1. General behavior (cooperation)
2. Mood or emotional state
3. Language
4. Orientation
5. Memory
6. Content of thought
7. Ability to acquire and manipulate knowledge

**4. How is general behavior assessed?**

Observe the patient's behavior, mode of speech or communication, grooming, and degree of cooperation. Uncooperativeness may be due to disturbance of consciousness, confusion, suspicion, delusion, hallucination, aggressiveness, or violence. An apparent lack of communication may be due to dysphasia (impairment of speech resulting from a brain lesion).

**5. How is mood or emotional state assessed?**

Assess for anxiety, depression, apathy, fear, suspicion, irritability, or euphoria. An aggressive euphoria is commonly seen after severe head injuries. Excessive display of emotion, such as laughing or crying suddenly, uncontrollably, inappropriately, and with excessive grimacing, is typical of pseudobulbar palsy and usually is due to bilateral cerebrovascular disease or corticobulbar lesions. This response usually is triggered by mildly humorous or sad situations.

**6. What is witzelsucht?**

Witzelsucht refers to the behavior of treating the examination as a joke and may be exhibited by patients with frontal lobe disease.

**7. How is language assessed?**

Note fluency and effort of speech as well as appropriateness of word choice. Test the patient's ability to name simple objects (e.g., pen, pencil tip, tie, clock), color (point to various objects), and body parts. Note the ability of nonintubated patients to repeat simple words (e.g., dog) or phrases of varying complexity (no ifs, ands, or buts). Comprehension of spoken language can be assessed in patients who cannot speak by asking them to make a fist, to point to the place where you entered the room, or to nod yes or no in response to questions.

**8. What are the six common types of aphasia?**
1. **Global aphasia:** the patient exhibits nonfluent speech, shows no speech comprehension, and cannot repeat.
2. **Broca's aphasia** (expressive, motor): the patient is not fluent in speech and usually cannot write but comprehends speech well.
3. **Transcortical aphasia:** the patient repeats well and comprehends speech but may not be fluent if a motor deficit is present. A sensory deficit presents as fluent speech without comprehension.
4. **Wernicke's aphasia** (receptive, sensory): the patient is fluent but does not comprehend speech, cannot repeat, produces neologisms, is unaware of his disabilities or situation, and has poor reading and writing ability.
5. **Conduction aphasia:** the patient is fluent and comprehends speech but repeats poorly, especially short words and phrases.
6. **Amnesic aphasia:** the patient has difficulty in naming objects and using nouns and prepositions.

**9. How is orientation assessed?**
Observe the patient's orientation to person, place, time, and situation, and note any trends or sudden changes.

**10. How is memory assessed?**
Elicit details and dates of recent and remote events, including birth date, marriage date, and names and ages of children. Illness may trigger poor power of concentration, but loss of recent memory and ability to retain and recall is common in organic dementias, although distant memory often is preserved.

**11. How is content of thought assessed?**
Assess patients for obsessions, phobias, delusions, compulsions, recurrent dreams or nightmares, depersonalization, or hallucinations.

**12. What elements are important to assess the ability to acquire and manipulate knowledge?**
- **General information:** ask for names of prominent political figures and the capitals of countries and states. Adapt questions to the patient's background and level of education.
- **Similarities and differences:** ask the patient to compare wood and paper, dwarf and child, and lie and mistake.
- **Calculations:** have the patient count backward from 100 by 7s or calculate interest at 6% for 18 months.
- **Retention:** ask the patient to repeat digits in natural or reverse order. Adults typically retain seven forward digits and five backward.
- **Right-left orientation and finger recognition:** ask the patient to touch his or her right ear with the left thumb.
- **Judgment:** ask the patient for the symbolic or specific meaning of simple proverbs; for example, "People who live in glass houses should not throw stones." The examiner must try to use proverbs that are familiar to the patient and match his or her culture and background.
- **Memory and comprehension:** tell a short story and ask the patient to retell it in his or her own words.
- **Communication skills:** assess the three primary modes of communication input (audition, vision, and tactile sensation) and the three modes of communication output (speech, graphic skills [writing, drawing], and kinetic skills [gestures, facial expressions]).

**13. How are agitation and psychosis differentiated from alterations in mental status?**

Psychoses may be present in patients who lose communication skills. Patients with poor fluency due to precentral lesions often seem mute or withdrawn and occasionally exhibit rage or cry when unable to express themselves. Patients with increased fluency due to posteriorly located lesions may appear psychotic. They may not understand verbal instructions and may babble at length, simulating the tangential speech typical of schizophrenic or manic patients. The most helpful differential assessment is that psychotic patients never seem to be in the same world with the examiner. The patient with defective cortical communication, by contrast, usually shows eagerness to communicate by any modality and works with the interested examiner despite all obstacles.

**14. Identify the twelve cranial nerves (CNs) and their functions.**

| | |
|---|---|
| CN I | **Olfactory nerve**, which carries sensations of smell from the nasal mucosa to the olfactory bulb. |
| CN II | **Optic nerve**, which carries visual impulses from the retina to the optic chiasma, optic tract, and lateral geniculate body. It acts as the afferent pathway for the pupillary light reflex via fibers traveling to the superior colliculus of the mid-brain. |
| CN III | **Oculomotor nerve**, which controls eye movement, eyelids, pupillary constriction, and accommodation of the lens. Autonomic fibers running in relation both to this nerve and CNs IV-VI regulate pupillary muscles. |
| CN IV | **Trochlear nerve**, which controls superior oblique eye movements. |
| CN V | **Trigeminal nerve**, which carries all forms of sensation from the face, anterior part of the scalp, eye, and anterior two-thirds of the tongue; gives motor power to the muscles of mastication; and carries sensation from the teeth, gums, mucous membrane of the cheeks, nasal passages, sinuses, and much of the palate and nasopharynx. |
| CN VI | **Abducens nerve**, which controls lateral rectus eye movements. |
| CN VII | **Facial nerve**, which stimulates motor function of the facial muscles, resulting in movement and expression. |
| CN VIII | **Vestibulocochlear (auditory) nerve**, which carries impulses of sound from the hair cells of the organ of Corti to the pons and regulates vestibular function. The vestibular nerve travels to the vestibular nuclei in the medulla and connects with the cerebellum, oculomotor nuclei, nuclei of the upper cervical nerves, spinal cord, and temporal lobes. |
| CN IX | **Glossopharyngeal nerve**, which carries common sensation from the pharynx, tonsils, soft palate, and posterior one-third of the tongue. It also senses taste from the posterior one-third of the tongue and supplies motor function to the palatal and pharyngeal muscles. |
| CN X | **Vagus nerve**, which supplies motor innervation to the vocal cords. |
| CN XI | **Accessory nerve**, which supplies motor power to the upper trapezius and sternocleidomastoid muscles and influences posture and movement of the head and shoulder girdles. |
| CN XII | **Hypoglossal nerve**, which controls all movements of the tongue and certain movements of the hyoid bone and larynx. |

**15. How is the olfactory nerve assessed?**

Use familiar odors such as coffee, peppermint, or vanilla to test its function. Avoid irritants such as ammonia and vinegar. The patient must identify the substance with eyes shut and one nostril occluded. Olfaction should be tested in cases of head trauma, when pathology at the base of the skull is suspected, and in patients with abnormal mental status. Complete or unilateral anosmia in the absence of intranasal disorders can suggest, for example, compression of the olfactory tract by an overlying meningioma, deep frontal lobe glioma, or fracture of the anterior fossa of the skull. Bilateral anosmia may be caused by sinusitis, colds, and heavy smoking.

**16. How is the optic nerve assessed?**

CN II is tested to measure visual acuity, to assess visual fields, and to determine whether any defect is due to local ocular disease. In the intensive care unit (ICU), near vision can be tested with standard Jaegar Type cards, which are held 30 cm (14 inches) from the patient's eyes. For patients with severe defects, cruder tests may be used, such as the ability to count fingers, detect hand movements, and detect changes from dark to light. The visual fields can be roughly tested by confrontation, with the patient situated about 1 meter from the examiner at eye level. With the left eye covered, the patient is instructed to look at the examiner's left eye. The examiner slowly raises both hands upward from a position where they can barely be seen in the lower two quadrants, and the patient signals when the examiner's moving hands first become visible. The upper and lateral quadrants are tested in similar fashion.

**17. Describe the five types of visual field lesions and the defects with which they are associated.**

1. **Optic nerve lesions**, which cause unilateral visual loss.

2. **Chiasmatic lesions**, which typically cause bitemporal hemianopsia.

3. **Lesions from the chiasma to the occipital cortex**, which can produce homonymous hemianopsia. Optic tract lesions produce a contralateral homonymous hemianopsia without macular sparing and typical incongruous fields.

4. **Temporal lobe lesions**, which may involve the inferior retinal radiations that move far anteriorly into the temporal lobe and can cause superior contralateral quadrantopsia.

5. **Occipital lobe lesions**, which can produce contralateral homonymous hemianopsia with macular sparing.

**18. Why are the oculomotor, trochlear, and abducens nerves assessed together? How is the assessment done?**

These three cranial nerves are tested together because their actions are so closely linked. Examine the size and shape of each pupil. Assess reactions of both pupils to a bright light flashed into each eye in a darkened room. Note the changes in the stimulated pupil and in the contralateral pupil. To test the accommodation-convergence response, the examiner asks the patient to focus alternately on two objects, one distant and the other 15 cm (6 inches) from the patient's face. Assess for strabismus (squinting), nystagmus (constant, involuntary, cyclical movement of the eyeball), ptosis (drooping of the upper eyelid), exophthalmos (bulging eyes), and pupillary abnormalities.

**19. Describe assessment of the trigeminal nerve.**

Test the patient's ability to perceive a pinprick or the touch of cotton over all three divisions of the face and the anterior half of the scalp. Corneal sensation may be elicited by touching the cornea from the side with a wisp of cotton as the patient looks upward. Test motor function by palpating the contraction of the masseter and temporalis muscles while the patient simulates a biting movement of the jaw. Assess for alterations in sensation and motor weakness.

**20. How is the facial nerve assessed?**

Note facial expression, mobility, and symmetry. Assess zygomaticus function (voluntary movements of the lower facial musculature) by having the patient smile, whistle, bare the teeth, and pucker the lips. Test upper facial musculature by having the patient close the eyes or wrinkle the forehead. Taste sensation of the anterior two-thirds of the tongue may be assessed in alert patients with suspected facial nerve injury. Facial nerve tests assess the presence, location, and origin of facial muscle weakness and impairments of taste. Results can be graded with a numerical score from 1 (no impairment) to 6 (no facial movement, including lack of ocular muscle contractions with attempted eye closure).

**21. How are the two functions of the vestibulocochlear nerve assessed?**

Test the **ability to hear** by the patient's response to the examiner's voice in ordinary conversation or by rubbing the thumb and forefinger together a few centimeters from each ear. More formal assessment is done with a vibrating tuning fork.

The caloric test can be used to evaluate **vestibular nerve function**. First, examine the eardrum to confirm absence of perforation. To test the vertical canals, the patient is placed with head raised 30° and tilted slightly forward; to test the horizontal canals, the patient lies supine with the head tilted back at an angle of 60°. The examiner slowly and steadily irrigates one external auditory canal with cool (30°C) or warm (40°C) water. Normally, cool water in one ear produces nystagmus on the opposite side, whereas warm water produces nystagmus on the same side. A useful mnemonic is **COWS**: **C**ool = **O**pposite and **W**arm = **S**ame.

Irrigation is continued until the patient complains of nausea or dizziness or until nystagmus is detected (normally 20–30 seconds). The test is discontinued after 3 minutes if no reaction occurs. No response to stimulation suggests brainstem injury. These tests assess the presence and origin of deafness and disturbances of vestibular function.

### 22. Describe assessment of the glossopharyngeal nerve .

Touch sensation can be tested on the soft palate and pharynx. The pharyngeal response (gag reflex) is tested bilaterally by using a suction catheter or tongue blade.

### 23. How is dysfunction of the vagus nerve detected?

Assess for dysfunction by noting the patient's ability to drink water and eat solid food. Note pharyngeal wall contraction in testing the gag reflex. Note the character, volume, and sound of the patient's voice. In comatose or aphasic patients, the exam may be limited to the gag reflex.

### 24. How is the accessory nerve assessed?

Test for wasting and weakness of the upper trapezius and sternocleidomastoid muscles. If the head falls forward, suspect trapezius weakness. If the head falls backward, suspect sternocleidomastoid weakness. Instruct the patient to rotate the head against resistance applied to the side of the chin. This test assesses the function of the opposite sternocleidomastoid muscle. To test both sternocleidomastoid muscles together, have the patient flex the head forward against resistance placed under the chin. Trapezius muscle function may be tested by having the patient shrug a shoulder against resistance.

### 25. What does assessment of the hypoglossal nerve involve?

Inspect the tongue for wasting, weakness, and involuntary movement. Ask the patient to stick out the tongue to assess voluntary muscle control. Examine the tongue for atrophy and tremors when it is protruded and at rest. Note any deviation of the protruded tongue. Tongue deviation pulls toward the side of the lower motor neuron weakness and opposite the side of upper motor neuron weakness. In patients with facial paresis, the protruding tongue may appear to deviate to one side. However, if the tongue is straight, the median portion should be aligned with the tip of the nose and the tip of the chin.

### 26. What causes pupillary constriction?

Pupillary constriction (miosis) may indicate a hemorrhage or a lesion in the hypothalamus, brainstem, or lateral aspect of the spinal cord.

### 27. What causes pupillary dilation?

Pupillary dilation (mydriasis) results from paralysis of the parasympathetic fibers at their origin in the midbrain, during their course with CN III, or at the ciliary ganglion in the eye. Mydriasis usually is caused by lesions related to vascular accidents in the midbrain, tentorial herniation (due to cerebral space-occupying lesions), or aneurysms of the carotid artery. Drugs such as atropine also cause mydriasis. In addition, the pupil of a blind or nearly blind eye may be dilated.

### 28. What causes nonreactive pupils?

Pupils that do not react to light are associated with a break in the pathway for light reflex. The break may be due to a lesion in the afferent loop (retina, optic nerve, or chiasma) or efferent loop (parasympathetic supply from the mid-brain running with CN III). Bilateral failure to react, with intact vision, usually indicates a mid-brain lesion. If a unilateral lesion exists in the afferent loop, both pupils react when the normal side is stimulated. If the efferent loop is involved, the affected pupil is unable to react with both sides stimulated.

### 29. What are the important elements of a motor examination?
The examination of motor function involves assessment of muscle power, tone, and bulk; coordination and gait; and abnormal movement. Occasionally an electric and chemical test is included.

### 30. How do you test muscle power, tone, and bulk?
1. Have the patient carry out movements against resistance.
2. Passive movements may be tested to ascertain range of motion.
3. Assess muscle tone by palpation and passive movement of the extremity muscles and joints.
4. Note the following:
   • Degree of resistance to passive movement, which is described as increased (rigidity) or decreased (hypotonicity)
   • Tone alterations, including spasticity, cogwheel rigidity, spasms, contractures, and hypotonia
   • Abnormal voluntary and involuntary movements. Describe involuntary movements, including tremors, athetosis (slow, irregular, twisting, snakelike movements in the upper extremities), chorea (involuntary muscle twitching of the limbs or facial muscles), and tics (involuntary spasmodic contractions of the face, mouth, eyes, head, neck, or shoulder muscles).

### 31. How are coordination, gait, and equilibrium tested?
A simple walking test can assess posture, gait, coordinated automatic movements (swinging arms), and ability to walk a straight line and make rapid turns. Unfortunately this test rarely can be performed in the ICU. The finger-to-nose and finger-to-finger tests assess cerebellar function and sensory, motor, and visual systems. For the finger-to-nose test, instruct the patient to place the tip of a finger on the nose and then touch the examiner's finger (which is placed at arm's length) repeatedly and as rapidly as possible. For the finger-to-finger test, instruct the patient to approximate the tips of the index fingers after the arms have been extended forward.

### 32. Which five reflexes are commonly tested? How are they graded?
1. Biceps reflex        3. Knee reflex        5. Babinski reflex
2. Triceps reflex       4. Ankle reflex

The first four reflexes are graded from 0 to 4+; the normal value is 2+. Assess and compare bilateral reflexes, particularly asymmetries in briskness. For the Babinski reflex, toes upgoing indicates reflex is present and downgoing absent (normal response in adult).

### 33. Describe the test for each of the five reflexes.
**Biceps reflex.** The examiner places a thumb on the patient's biceps tendon while the patient's elbow is flexed at a right angle and then strikes the thumb. A normal response is a slight contraction of the biceps muscle.

**Triceps reflex.** With the patient's elbow supported in the examiner's hand, the triceps tendon is sharply percussed just above the olecranon. Normally, the triceps muscle contracts with extension of the forearm.

**Knee reflex.** Ideally, the patient is seated at the edge of the bed with the legs hanging loosely. If the patient is bedridden, the knees can be flexed and supported over the arm of the examiner with the heels resting lightly on the bed. The patellar tendon is located and tapped lightly with a percussion hammer or fingers. The force of tapping is increased until contraction of the quadriceps muscle and knee extension can be elicited.

**Ankle reflex.** The Achilles' tendon is struck with a percussion hammer. Normally, the foot jerks and moves downward.

**Babinski reflex.** It is elicited by stimulating the plantar surface of the foot with a blunt point directed from the heel toward the ball of the foot, stopping at the metatarsophalangeal joints. If the response is difficult to obtain, it may be elicited by stimulating the lateral aspect of the sole. The sign is obtained with less difficulty if the patient is in the recumbent position with the hips and knees in extension and may be reinforced by rotating the patient's head to the opposite side. It may be inhibited when the foot is cold and increased when the foot is warm. The Babinski reflex has been called the most important sign in clinical neurology. If definitely present, it is always indicative of organic disease.

### 34. What is the purpose of the "doll's eyes" test? How is it done?

The doll's eyes test (like the caloric test; see question 21) assesses brainstem function in comatose and unconscious patients. The oculocephalic reflex can be elicited by rapidly rotating the head from side to side or up and down. In comatose patients with an intact brainstem, the eyes move conjugately in the direction opposite that of head rotation. The eyes do not move at all or eye movement is disconjugate in patients with brainstem dysfunction.

### 35. What is clonus?

Clonus refers to spasmodic alteration of muscular contractions between antagonistic muscle groups. It is caused by a hyperactive stretch reflex from an upper motor neuron lesion. Usually, sustained pressure or stretch of one of the muscles inhibits the reflex. Clonus may be elicited in patients with exaggerated hyperreflexia but also may occur without active eliciting measures and without movement of the limb as a whole. It presents when the affected muscle is under tension and is stopped immediately by altering the position of the limb so that the muscle is relaxed.

### 36. Why are sensory examinations difficult in critical care patients?

Sensory examination is based on the patient's subjective responses. The patient should be well rested and in a cooperative frame of mind before the exam is performed. ICU patients commonly suffer from environmental sensory overload, lack of sleep or regular rest patterns, effects of multiple medications, effects of illness or injury, and emotional upset or confusion. Abnormalities, especially of minor degree, should be reassessed.

### 37. Which sensory tests can be performed in the ICU?

**Pain.** Test the patient's ability to perceive pinprick or deep pressure. If results are abnormal, note the topographic or dermatome pattern.

**Temperature.** Use a tube of warm water and a tube of cold water to check the patient's ability to detect and distinguish between the two.

**Touch.** Test the ability to perceive light stroking of the skin with cotton.

**Vibration.** The patient should be able to feel the buzz of a tuning fork (at a frequency of 128 Hz) applied to the bony prominences (e.g., malleoli, patellas).

**Position sense.** Instruct the patient to close the eyes and then determine the position of the toes and fingers in an upward, downward, or neutral position when they are grasped by the examiner.

**Stereognosis and graphesthesia.** Instruct the patient to identify a familiar object (coin, key, paperclip) that is placed in the palm of the hand without allowing the patient to see it. To test graphesthesia, write a word or draw a letter or number in the palm of the patient's hand and ask the patient to identify it.

**Topognosis.** The examiner ensures that the patient's eyes are closed and then touches the patient's body and instructs the patient to point to the spot touched or to state the location.

### 38. What is the Glasgow Coma Scale?

The Glasgow Coma Scale (GCS) is designed as a practical method of assessing changes in level of consciousness based on eye opening and verbal and motor responses. The total score is the sum of the scores assigned to each response. The lowest score is 3, and the highest score is 15. This scale has been used to determine patient outcome at 3, 6, and 12 months after brain injury.

*Glasgow Coma Scale*

| POINTS | BEST EYE OPENING | BEST VERBAL RESPONSE | BEST MOTOR RESPONSE |
|---|---|---|---|
| 6 | — | — | Obeys |
| 5 | — | Oriented | Localizes pain |
| 4 | Spontaneous | Confused | Withdraws to pain |
| 3 | To speech | Inappropriate | Flexion (decorticate) |
| 2 | To pain | Incomprehensible | Extension (decerebrate) |
| 1 | None | None | None |

### 39. When is the GCS useful in critical care?

The GCS provides a consistent standard of assessment for patients who have suffered neurologic injury. In an attempt to avoid errors that often result from imprecise use of language by medical and nursing staff, the GCS does not appraise the finer qualities of the neurologic system. Ongoing assessments should include many details about the neurologic exam in addition to what the GCS chart provides.

### 40. How should I focus assessment of the patient who has undergone craniotomy for lesions of the frontal lobe?

- Check for contralateral weakness and pronator drift.
- Assess for expressive aphasia; impaired thought, reasoning, or memory; emotional lability; and urinary frequency and urgency.
- Monitor for focal, motor, or grand mal seizures.

### 41. For lesions of the temporal lobe?

- Assess visual field loss, memory, receptive aphasia, and dysnomia.
- Monitor for seizure activity.

### 42. For lesions of the parietal lobe?

- Assess for sensory deficits (i.e., contralateral neglect; impaired joint position, vibration, and light touch sensations; visual field loss; receptive dysphasia).
- Monitor for sensory seizures.

### 43. For lesions of the occipital lobe?

- Assess for contralateral homonymous hemianopsia (consult with neuroophthalmologist) and visual hallucinations.
- Monitor for seizure activity.

### 44. For lesions of the cerebellum?

- Assess for decreased coordination, ataxia of ipsilateral limbs, and nystagmus.
- Watch for signs of increasing intracranial pressure, including headache, decreased mental status or agitation, and vomiting due to hydrocephalus.

### 45. For lesions of the brainstem?

- Assess for cranial nerve palsies, sensory or motor impairment, and vomiting.
- Observe for ataxia.
- Be wary of sudden death due to brainstem herniation.

### 46. How is the level of the vertebral column involved in spinal cord injury (SCI) determined?

The signs of a lesion of the sensory pathways are extraordinarily constant, with only a slight range. The intensity of sensory abnormality, however, may range from total loss to slight reduction or even hypersensitivity. In the latter cases, experience is needed to judge the significance of any abnormality. The dermatome chart most easily and explicitly outlines zones of the body that correspond to level of SCI (see figures on following page).

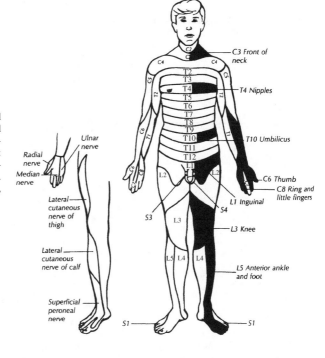

Front view of areas innervated by peripheral nerves *(left)* and dermatomes innervated by posterior roots *(right)*. (From Bates B: A Guide to Physical Examination and History Taking, 6th ed. Philadelphia, Lippincott, 1995, p 502, with permission.)

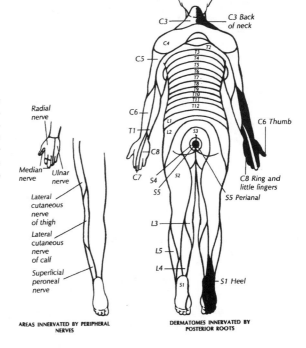

Rear view of areas innervated by peripheral nerves *(left)* and dermatomes innervated by posterior roots *(right)*. (From Bates B: A Guide to Physical Examination and History Taking, 6th ed. Philadelphia, Lippincott, 1995, p 503, with permission.)

AREAS INNERVATED BY PERIPHERAL NERVES

DERMATOMES INNERVATED BY POSTERIOR ROOTS

### BIBLIOGRAPHY

1. Barrows H: Guide To Neurologic Assessment. Philadelphia, Lippincott, 1980.
2. Bates B: A Guide To Physical Examination and History Taking, 6th ed. Philadelphia, Lippincott, 1995.
3. Collins R: Illustrated Manual of Neurologic Diagnosis. Philadelphia, Lippincott, 1982.
4. Conn P: Neuroscience in Medicine. Philadelphia, Lippincott, 1995.
5. De Jong R: Case taking and the neurologic examination. In DeJong RN (ed): The Neurologic Examination, 3rd ed. New York, Harper & Row, 1967, pp 1–61.
6. Lipson J, Dibble S, Minarik P: Culture and Nursing Care: A Pocket Guide. San Francisco, UCSF Nursing Press, 1996.
7. Johnson J, Blitzer A, Ossoff R, Thomas J (eds): American Academy of Otolaryngology–Head and Neck Surgery, Instructional Courses, vol. 3. Philadelphia, Lippincott, 1998.
8. Spillane J: Bickerstaff's Neurological Examination in Clinical Practice, 6th ed. London, Blackwell Science, 1996.
9. Waxman S: Correlative Neuroanatomy, 23rd ed. Stamford, CT, Appleton & Lange, 1996.

# 44. INVASIVE NEUROLOGIC MONITORING

*Lori Kennedy Madden*, RN, MS, ACNP

### 1. What patients may require invasive neurologic monitoring?

Any patient at risk for neurologic compromise or deterioration may require monitoring. Generally, this includes any patient with a Glasgow Coma Scale score of 8 or less and/or abnormalities on computed tomography (CT) head scan. Obvious candidates are patients with head injury, stroke, or brain lesion. Other patients, such as those with hepatic encephalopathy, are monitored for various neurologic complications related to their primary disease state.

### 2. What is the most common type of neurologic monitor in the intensive care unit (ICU)?

The most frequently used device is the intracranial pressure (ICP) monitor. However, the most common and least expensive method of monitoring is the neurologic examination.

### 3. What is the Monro-Kellie doctrine?

The Monro-Kellie doctrine describes the balance among three main cranial contents: blood, brain tissue, and cerebrospinal fluid (CSF). Under normal circumstances, compensatory mechanisms maintain the balance of these three components. In some circumstances, such as hemorrhage and cerebral edema, the balance of the three components may be compromised. If the volume of any of the three components is elevated, the volumes of the other two may decrease. For example, with increased tissue volume, as in cerebral edema, CSF may shunt to the subarachnoid space in the cervical spinal cord, or blood volume may decrease. This compensation can occur only to a certain extent.

### 4. What is the normal value for ICP? What may be the consequences of elevated ICP?

ICP is related directly to the volume in the cranium. Normal ICP is 0–15 mmHg. Elevation above normal may cause a decrease in blood flow, resulting in ischemia or structural injury from compression or shear of brain tissue against the skull. In the event of ischemia, the systemic blood pressure may increase to compensate for the increased ICP to maintain perfusion to the brain.

### 5. What is the purpose of ICP monitoring?

ICP is monitored in patients suspected of having an elevated ICP that can be treated. Monitoring of ICP allows treatment of elevated ICP and prevention of secondary injuries (such as structural injuries from shear or diminished blood flow and ischemia) that may result if ICP is left untreated. Usually, the goal is to keep ICP < 20 or 25 mmHg. Evidence suggests that aggressive treatment of elevated ICP improves patient outcomes. However, the issue of whether to monitor ICP has not been studied for ethical reasons.

With cautious attention to ICP, nurses at the bedside can identify what interventions (such as endotracheal suctioning, patient positioning, physical therapy, or physical or verbal stimuli) may deleteriously elevate the patient's ICP. Identification of such factors can help the clinician in planning treatment and care.

### 6. What are the different types of ICP monitors?

The gold standard of ICP monitoring is ventriculostomy, which involves placement of a small catheter in one of the two lateral ventricles containing CSF. This catheter usually is attached to a fluid-filled transducer that is connected to a bedside monitor for pressure monitoring and waveform evaluation. Other devices for ICP monitoring are drains and/or sensors placed in the parenchymal, subdural, or epidural space.

### 7. How is a ventriculostomy performed? Describe its advantages and complications.

A small flexible tube is inserted into one of the lateral ventricles. Using a fluid-filled system, the ventriculostomy is connected via a transducer to a pressure monitor. Ventriculostomy allows both pressure monitoring and CSF drainage. CSF drainage may be of therapeutic (e.g., to decrease ICP) or diagnostic value (e.g., specimen sampling for glucose, protein, and culture). Complications related to the use of a ventriculostomy include an approximate 1–10% risk of infection (causing ventriculitis or meningitis) and a 1–2% risk of bleeding.

### 8. How is parenchymal monitoring done? Describe its advantages and complications.

Parenchymal ICP monitoring involves a fiberoptic or strain-gauge device placed within the brain tissue for pressure monitoring. It may be placed in patients in whom CSF sampling or drainage is unnecessary or in patients with significant coagulopathies. Complications still include infection and bleeding (2%), although the incidence is lower with these devices in comparison with the ventricular catheter. Dislodgement of the cable/fiberoptics has been reported at a rate of 4%.

### 9. How are subdural monitors used? Why are they used less commonly now than in the past?

Subdural drains or monitors are placed between the dura and subarachnoid space. Monitors placed are usually fluid-filled or fiberoptic. Unfortunately, the fluid-filled devices can collapse and impair the waveform. Monitors placed in the subdural space have a lower rate of infection compared with ventriculostomy, but because of problems associated with subdural catheters, monitoring at this site is less common than in the past.

### 10. Where are epidural monitors placed? Why are they rarely used?

Epidural monitors are placed between the skull and the dura and provide an indirect measurement of ICP. As a result, they are less accurate and thus rarely used.

### 11. What information does the ICP waveform provide?

The analysis of various ICP waveforms has provoked much discussion. Yet the importance of the waveform is clear, whether or not it is present. If a good waveform is present, the pressure reading displayed on the monitor is more reliable. If the waveform is dampened, it reflects a mean pressure that is reasonably, if not completely, accurate. An exception is the fluid-filled system (i.e., for ventriculostomy) in which a blood clot or brain tissue has blocked the tubing. In this situation, the reading may be inaccurate until the obstruction is cleared, according to the policies of your neurosurgical service or institution.

### 12. Discuss the basic principles of waveform analysis.

The real-time waveform appears slightly similar to a vascular pressure reading. It has 3–4 peaks. The first peak (P1), called the percussion wave, is attributed to transmitted arterial pressure.

Two or three smaller peaks (P2, P3, and P4) have been attributed to choroid plexus or venous pressure artifact. Usually, these peaks occur in a stairstep fashion. However, P2 may become prominent as compliance decreases and/or ICP increases. The separate peaks may be less distinct or unnoticeable if the waveform is dampened.

A waves (plateau waves) are visible on analysis of larger spans of time with elevation of ICP to 60 mmHg or more for 5–20 minutes. B waves appear as sharp rhythmic oscillations of pressure values every 30–120 seconds and are seen in relation to respiratory patterns such as Cheyne-Stokes breathing. They are thought to progress to A waves. C waves occur every 4–8 minutes and relate to changes in blood pressure. Their effect is unknown.

### 13. What other neurologic parameters may be monitored?

Most other parameters monitor some aspect of blood flow, oxygenation, or metabolism. Examples that require invasive monitoring include cerebral perfusion pressure, jugular bulb oxygenation, tissue oxygenation, and microdialysis. Noninvasive examples include transcranial Doppler (TCD) examination, electroencephalography (EEG), CT of the head, and magnetic resonance imaging (MRI) of the brain. The primary objective behind monitoring much of these data is to avoid cerebral ischemia.

### 14. Define cerebral ischemia. What causes it?

Ischemia is a mismatch between oxygen supply and demand. Cerebral ischemia is defined in the vulnerable brain as cerebral blood flow (CBF) < 20 ml/100 gm/min. The cerebral metabolic rate of oxygen utilization is not matched by the supply of oxygen delivered by the blood. Reversible cellular injury results when the tissue demand for oxygen exceeds the supply and when toxic metabolites accumulate. Ischemia results whenever CBF falls below the ischemic threshold for the affected tissue. Initially, flow reductions are met with increased oxygen extraction to preserve tissue function and maintain adequate cerebral metabolic function. However, when the ability to increase oxygen extraction is exceeded, ischemia occurs.

### 15. What are the normal values for CBF?

The total CBF is approximately 50–55 ml/100 gm of brain tissue per minute, or about 15–20% of resting cardiac output. Overall flow in gray matter is normally 3–4 times higher than overall flow in white matter. Overall CBF is relatively constant, whereas regional CBF fluctuates to meet the metabolic needs posed by local physiologic changes during the course of various activities.

### 16. How does mean arterial pressure affect CBF?

CBF usually remains constant despite a wide range of mean arterial pressure (MAP). But extremely wide variations in blood pressure can affect CBF. When MAP ranges between 50 and 160 mmHg, CBF varies no more than 1–2 ml/100 gm of brain tissue per minute. If the arterial pressure is allowed to fall below 50 mmHg, however, CBF begins to fall passively with blood pressure. Conversely, if systemic blood pressure rises above 160 mmHg, CBF increases. Under pathologic circumstances, the brain's ability to maintain a constant blood flow over a wide range of cerebral perfusion pressures (a form of autoregulation) may be lost. The degree of loss of autoregulation is often directly proportional to the severity of injury.

### 17. When should CBF be monitored?

Severe neurologic injury or illness often leads to derangement of the cerebral vasculature and CBF, leaving the brain at risk of ischemia. Therefore, monitoring of CBF in such patients is useful for understanding the pathophysiology and effects of therapy.

### 18. How is CBF monitored?

The measurement of CBF in humans was first achieved in the 1940s by Kety and Schmidt. CBF is most commonly monitored by injection or inhalation of xenon, followed by a radiologic study. CBF also can be measured with positron emission tomography (PET) and single-photon emission computed tomography (SPECT).

### 19. What is cerebral perfusion pressure?

Cerebral perfusion pressure (CPP) is a derived value, not an actual measured datapoint, that is used to estimate CBF. It is calculated by subtracting ICP from MAP: CPP = MAP – ICP. The target CPP varies among centers but most often is $\geq 60$ or 70 mmHg. Current management strategies are to keep CPP at approximately 70 mmHg, but this practice has not been proved to improve outcome. CPP values below 50 mmHg are deleterious.

### 20. Describe the importance of jugular venous saturation monitoring.

Jugular venous oxygen saturation ($SjvO_2$) measures the balance between cerebral oxygen delivery and cerebral oxygen consumption. It enables clinicians to monitor global oxygenation of a cerebral hemisphere. Abnormalities that increase oxygen consumption or decrease oxygen delivery can decrease $SjvO_2$. Critical $SjvO_2$ levels are identified as desaturations to < 50%; the normal range is 60–85%. The occurrence of one or more episodes of desaturation is strongly associated with a poor outcome. However, there is a high incidence of false desaturations related to mechanical and monitor problems rather than true ischemia. True desaturation episodes have been attributed to hyperventilation, insufficient CPP, and severe vasospasm. In many instances, the tailoring of ventilation or induced hypervolemia and hypertension have reversed these low flow states.

### 21. How is $SjvO_2$ monitored?

An oximetric catheter is placed in either jugular vein and directed cephalad (toward the head) to the jugular bulb (approximately at the foramen of Monro). A lateral cervical spine/skull radiograph is obtained after placement to confirm approximate catheter tip location. The monitor is calibrated to a blood sample drawn slowly through the catheter and sent to the blood gas laboratory. Oxygen saturation may then be monitored continuously at the bedside.

### 22. What is $AJDO_2$?

$AJDO_2$ is the cerebral arteriovenous oxygen difference and represents the relationship between the metabolic rate for oxygen ($CMRO_2$) and blood flow of the brain (CBF), as noted in the following formula:

$$AJDO_2 = CMRO_2/CBF$$

Normal cerebral $AJDO_2$ is 1.8–3.9 millimoles/minute or 4.5–8.5 ml/dl. Because $CMRO_2$ and CBF are not commonly monitored, the following equation is most often used:

$$AJDO_2 = (SaO_2 - SjvO_2) \times 1.34 \times hemoglobin$$

where $SaO_2$ = oxygen saturation in arterial blood.

### 23. How are $AJDO_2$ values interpreted?

An increase in $AJDO_2$ suggests that metabolic oxygen demands are higher than the amount of blood flowing through the brain; thus, the brain may be ischemic or hypoxic. In contrast, a low $AJDO_2$ suggests a state of luxury perfusion, with relatively more blood flow than is needed to support the metabolic needs of the brain. In patients with neurologic injury or illness, $AJDO_2$ levels become an indicator of the adequacy of CBF for supporting metabolism.

### 24. What are the disadvantages of $SjvO_2$ monitoring?

Complications related to monitoring $SjvO_2$ include infection (0–5%) and carotid artery puncture (3–4%). The most concerning complication is carotid artery puncture. Trouble-shooting the $SjvO_2$ monitor is the biggest hurdle at the bedside, because the incidence of artifact/false values is very high. The table below provides a guide to trouble-shooting an $SjvO_2$ monitor.

---

*Jugular Bulb Monitoring: What to Do If SjvO$_2$ Is <60% or > 85%*

---

1. Check for quality of light intensity signal. Good quality signal = a more reliable value.
2. If you have a good signal:
   (1) Obtain a venous blood gas to calibrate/confirm the monitor value if you did not check calibration with a venous blood gas during your shift. Checking should be done regularly, according to institutional policy.
   (2) Is the venous blood gas value within 4% of the monitor reading? If not, recalibrate the monitor.
   (3) Notify the physician, and in the meantime consider the causes noted below. Determine whether any has occurred and whether it can be corrected:
      • Values < 60% suggest that supply is less than demand and may be caused by:

      | | |
      |---|---|
      | Decreased CPP | Decreased PaO$_2$ |
      | Decreased blood pressure | Decreased pH |
      | Decreased PaCO$_2$ | Vasospasm |
      | Increased ICP | Anemia |
      | Increased metabolic activity (e.g., fever, seizures) | |

      • Values > 85% suggest that supply is greater than demand and may be caused by:
      Decreased metabolic activity (e.g., barbiturate coma, heavy sedation, hypothermia, infarct, brain death)
      Increased PaO$_2$ beyond tissue needs
3. Notify the physician for evaluation and/or repositioning of the catheter, if necessary.

---

CPP = cerebral perfusion pressure, PaCO$_2$ = partial pressure of carbon dioxide in arterial blood, ICP = intracranial pressure, PaO$_2$ = partial pressure of oxygen in arterial blood.

### 25. What other invasive monitoring devices may be used?
   • Continuous partial pressure of brain tissue oxygen (PtiO$_2$)
   • Microdialysis
   • Laser Doppler flowmetry (LDF)

### 26. What is PtiO$_2$? How is it interpreted?
PtiO$_2$ is related to regional cerebral oxygenation. In contrast to SjvO$_2$ monitoring, PtiO$_2$ monitoring provides only local tissue oxygenation proximal to the probe. The threshold of ischemia in monitoring brain PtiO$_2$ has been identified as 10 mmHg. Early occurrence of PtiO$_2$ values below 10 mmHg indicates a poor prognosis. To recognize most accurately critical episodes of hypoxia or ischemia, PtiO$_2$ monitoring of cerebral oxygenation should be done in nonlesioned brain tissue that is vulnerable to ischemia.

### 27. How is cerebral microdialysis interpreted?
Cerebral microdialysate concentrations of several compounds provide interesting information about ischemia. Brain function and tissue integrity are highly dependent on continuous oxygen supply and clearance of carbon dioxide. Aerobic metabolism is the major energy source for normal brain. However, during hypoxia and ischemia, lactate accumulation may be seen, indicating anaerobic glycolysis after brain injury or illness. The strongest biochemical indicators of cerebral anoxia are elevations in the lactate-to-glucose ratio and in the concentrations of lactate and the excitatory amino acids glutamate and aspartate. Brain pH is inversely related to carbon dioxide levels in the brain. Poor outcomes are identified in patients with lower brain glucose levels and higher brain lactate levels.

### 28. How is LDF used?
LDF can assess a small volume of brain tissue, providing focal area monitoring. Local CBF is different from regional or global CBF. Small movement of the probe can cause significant changes in the absolute value of LDF. Artifact can result from a change in hemoglobin, strong external light presence, or change in probe contact with the cortex. These problems can be relieved by choosing a 15-minute interval of monitoring. CBF changes are detectable with LDF monitoring.

Because LDF changes occur linearly with changes in local CBF, LDF may be a good assessment of autoregulation.

**29. What noninvasive methods are available for neurologic monitoring?**
- CT head scan
- Brain MRI
- Angiography
- Transcranial Doppler (TCD)
- Nuclear medicine CBF study
- Xenon-enhanced CT scan
- EEG/computer-interpreted spectral analysis (CSA)
- Near-infrared spectroscopy (NIRS)
- PET
- SPECT
- Evoked potentials (EPs)

**30. When are CT head scans used?**
The CT head scan is frequently used to evaluate gross structural problems, skull fractures, and presence of blood. Patients are transported out of the ICU to the radiology department unless a portable CT scanner is available.

**31. When is brain MRI used?**
Brain MRI provides structural images with great detail. Because it employs a magnet, MRI should not be used in patients with implanted ferrous devices (e.g., some pacemakers, some aneurysm clips). It is particularly useful for patients with stroke or tumor. Patients are transported out of the ICU to the radiology department.

**32. What is the purpose of angiography?**
Angiography provides imaging of vascular structures. Patients must be able to tolerate injection of contrast dye (i.e., no allergy to iodine). Patients are transported out of the ICU to the interventional radiology suite.

**33. How is transcranial Doppler performed? What information does it provide?**
TCD is done at the patient's bedside. An ultrasound probe is held on the skin at various areas of the skull through "acoustic windows" of the relatively thin temporal bone, the foramen magnum, the orbit, under the mandible, or through a burr hole site.

TCD provides information about velocity of blood flow (cm/sec) in the major cerebral vessels. Depending on the ultrasound machine, vessel structures can be viewed and/or velocities can be measured (with a waveform somewhat similar to an arterial line tracing). Based on the location at which the probe is positioned, the direction in which the probe is pointed, the depth of the insonation, and the direction of flow, the clinician can identify what blood vessel is being monitored. Normal values are established in the literature. Elevated values have been confirmed via angiography to reveal vessel stenosis and vasospasm. TCD is commonly used to evaluate patients for vasospasm after aneurysmal subarachnoid hemorrhage. It also is used for emboli monitoring and as an adjunct in identifying the absence of blood flow in brain death.

**34. Describe the nuclear medicine CBF study.**
The nuclear medicine CBF study is based on the nitrous oxide technique of measuring blood flow, as described by Kety and Schmidt. After xenon injection or inhalation, 5–8 extracranial detectors serially measure changes in the concentration of xenon in the brain. This test is portable but both time-consuming and expensive.

**35. How are xenon-enhanced CT scans obtained?**
Stable xenon gas is administered after a conventional CT scan is obtained. Then a varying number of enhanced scans are obtained at 30-second intervals.

**36. How are EEG and computer-interpreted spectral analysis used?**
EEG closely correlates with rates of cerebral metabolism and is sensitive to both hypoxia and ischemia. EEG is the best method for detecting and localizing seizure activity. CSA breaks

raw EEG signal down into component frequencies and displays the contribution of each frequency to the total signal.

### 37. What information does NIRS provide? Why is its use limited?

NIRS provides an assessment of regional brain hemoglobin oxygen saturation by measuring the differential absorption of near-infrared light. The signal changes as quickly as EEG in response to progressive cerebral hypoxia. NIRS measures saturation in a local field (including arteries, capillaries, and mostly veins), then uses an algorithm to calculate the saturation in the area of cerebral saturation ($CSfO_2$). It use is limited because it provides a very small sampling volume and there is no consensus about its indications or normal values.

### 38. How is PET performed? What are its disadvantages?

Molecules labeled with radioactive isotopes are located within the brain and recorded by radiation-sensitive detectors outside the head. Compounds, such as oxygen and glucose, can be labeled to study different pathways of brain activity. PET can provide simultaneous measurements of regional CBF, metabolism, and biochemistry. PET scanning is time-consuming and expensive, costing thousands of dollars per session.

### 39. How is SPECT performed? What are its disadvantages?

Lipophilic radiolucent agents that emit single photons are injected intravenously and trapped in the brain in proportion to regional perfusion. It is not quantitative and cannot be repeated at frequent intervals.

### 40. When are evoked potentials used?

EPs provide information about cortical activity and neurologic function despite the presence of metabolic insults and medication effects. Many have used bilateral medial nerve sensory EPs to assess prognosis in comatose patients.

### 41. What other types of monitoring in the ICU benefit neurologic patients?

- Blood pressure monitoring (invasively via arterial catheter or noninvasively with an inflatable cuff) provides essential data related to cerebral perfusion.
- Cardiac telemetry
- Respiratory monitoring (e.g., rate, pattern)
- End-tidal carbon dioxide ($EtCO_2$) evaluates ventilatory function. Values are approximately 20% less than measured arterial carbon dioxide. Trending of carbon dioxide levels alerts the nurse to significant increases or decreases, both of which affect cerebral perfusion.
- Pulse oximetry ($SpO_2$) reflects but does not directly correlate with specific aspects of arterial oxygenation. Alterations in $SpO_2$ may affect oxygen delivery.
- Central venous pressure (CVP) monitoring helps to assess fluid volume status. Absolute numbers are less significant than monitoring of trends and responses to therapy.
- Pulmonary artery (PA) catheters allow measurement of PA wedge pressure. Although full of risk, they provide valuable information about volume status and cardiac function and are particularly useful in patients with a significant cardiac history.
- Oxygen saturation in venous blood ($SvO_2$) provides information about systemic oxygenation. $SVO_2$ values can be trended or used to determine prognosis.
- Temperature. Hyperthermia increases the metabolic activity of the brain, which subsequently increases CBF. Hyperthermia also increases ICP by elevating the brain's metabolic rate 7% for every Fahrenheit degree increase in body temperature above 100°.

### 42. What is the function of cardiac telemetry?

Variations in electrocardiographic (ECG) waveforms have been noted in patients with various neurologic disorders, particularly subarachnoid hemorrhage. Furthermore, responses to pathologic events are demonstrated by the development of bradycardia (e.g., Cushing's triad or spinal shock). ECG abnormalities should not be dismissed as secondary to neurologic disease without further cardiac investigation (i.e., to rule out cardiac ischemia or infarct).

### 43. Why is respiratory monitoring important?

Respiratory monitoring is important in neurologic patients in the ICU, because variations in rate and pattern may be suggestive of changes in neurologic status. Patients with elevated ICP may hyperventilate in an effort to decrease the elevation. Variations in hyperventilatory and hypoventilatory states are signs of neurologic dysfunction. Cheyne-Stokes breathing manifests as a crescendo-decrescendo respiratory rate, followed by a pause in respiration. Hyperventilation usually is a response to hypoxemia, metabolic acidosis, aspiration, or pulmonary edema. True central hyperventilation most often results from dysfunction in the pons. Cluster breathing involves periods of rapid irregular breathing followed by apnea and may seem similar to Cheyne-Stokes patterns. It may be a sign of lower pons or upper medulla dysfunction.

### BIBLIOGRAPHY

1. Coplin WM, O'Keefe GE, Grady MS, et al: Accuracy of continuous jugular bulb oximetry in the intensive care unit. Neurosurgery 42: 533–539, 1998.
2. Germon K: Intracranial pressure monitoring in the 1990s. Crit Care Nurs Q 17:21–32, 1994.
3. Ingvar DH, Lassen NA: Regional cerebral blood flow. Acta Neurol Scand 41(Suppl 14), 1965.
4. Kety SS, Schmidt CF: The determination of cerebral blood flow in man by the use of nitrous oxide in low concentrations. Am J Physiol 143:53, 1945.
5. Kiening KL, Unterberg AW, Bardt TF, et al: Monitoring of cerebral oxygenation in patients with severe head injuries: Brain tissue PO2 versus jugular vein oxygen saturation. J Neurosurg 85:751–757, 1996.
6. Lam JMK, Hsiang JNK, Poon WS: Monitoring of autoregulation using laser Doppler flowmetry in patients with head injury. J Neurosurg 86:438–445, 1997.
7. Lassen NA: Cerebral blood flow and oxygen consumption in man. Physiol Rev 39:183– 238, 1959.
8. Luerssen TG: Fiberoptic intraparenchymal pressure monitoring for the measurement of intracranial pressure in children. In Marlin AE (ed): Concepts in Pediatric Neurosurgery vol. 10. Geneva, Basel & Karger, 1990, pp 204–213.
9. Marshall LF, Bruce DA, Bruno L, et al: Role of intracranial pressure monitoring and barbiturate therapy in malignant intracranial hypertension. Case report. J Neurosurg 47:481–484, 1977.
10. Marx RB: Factors affecting intracranial pressure: A descriptive study. J Neurosurg Nurs 17: 89–94, 1985.
11. McCormick PW, Stewart M, Goetting MG, et al: Regional cerebrovascular oxygen saturation measured by optical spectroscopy in humans. Stroke 22:596–602, 1991.
12. Narayan RK, Kishore PR, Becker DP, et al: Intracranial pressure: To monitor or not to monitor? A review of our experience with severe head injury. J Neurosurg 56:650–659, 1982.
13. Robertson CS, Gopinath SP, Goodman JC, et al: SjvO2 monitoring in head-injured patients. J Neurotrauma 12:891–896, 1995.
14. Schneider GH, von Helden A, Lanksch WR, et al: Continuous monitoring of jugular bulb oxygen saturation in comatose patients—therapeutic implications. Acta Neurochirurg 134:71–75, 1995.
15. Schroeder ML, Muizelaar JP, Kuta AJ, et al: Thresholds for cerebral ischemia after severe head injury: relationship with late CT findings and outcome. J Neurotrauma 13:17–23, 1996.
16. Simon RH: Management of critical head injuries. Emerg Care Q 1:40–147, 1985.
17. Smith RW, Alksne JF: Infections complicating the use of external ventriculostomy. J Neurosurg 44:567–570, 1976.
18. Stuart GG, Merry GS, Smith JA, et al: Severe head injury managed without intracranial pressure monitoring. J Neurosurg 59:601–605, 1983.
19. Valadka AB, Goodman JC, Gopinath SP, et al: Comparison of brain tissue oxygen tension to microdialysis-based measures of cerebral ischemia in fatally head-injured humans. J Neurotrauma 15:509–519, 1998.
20. van den Brink WA, van Santbrink H, Avezaat CJ, et al: Monitoring brain oxygen tension in severe head injury: The Rotterdam experience. Acta Neurochir Suppl 71:190–194, 1998.
21. van Santbrink H, Maas AI, Avezaat CJ: Continuous monitoring of partial pressure of brain tissue oxygen in patients with severe head injury. Neurosurgery 38:21–31, 1996.
22. Zauner A, Doppenberg E, Woodward JJ, et al: Multiparametric continuous monitoring of brain metabolism and substrate delivery in neurosurgical patients. Neurol Res 19: 265–273, 1997.

# 45. STROKE MONITORING AND MANAGEMENT

*Nancy Ann Rudisill, RN, MSN, and Lori Kennedy Madden, RN, MS, ACNP*

### 1. What is stroke?

Stroke is defined as an acute neurologic deficit that persists more than 24 hours and is due to a reduction or loss of blood supply to an area of the brain. Stroke is not a specific disease but a syndrome with several subtypes and many potential causes. Specific neurologic deficits vary depending on the location, extent of the damage, and cause.

### 2. What is the ischemic cascade?

The ischemic cascade is a complex process at the cellular level. With the onset of cerebral ischemia, energy sources (oxygen and glucose) are depleted, and a cascade of biochemical events ensues. The two significant events are the excessive release of the excitatory amino acid glutamate from nerve terminals and influx of calcium into cells as the final common pathway to cell death.

### 3. What progress has been made in understanding the pathophysiology of acute ischemic stroke?

The timing of the various processes of the ischemic cascade and the potential time windows for different interventions are better understood. Furthermore, the importance of maintaining cerebral perfusion and optimizing systemic physiologic and biochemical factors to prevent neurologic deterioration is increasingly appreciated. Numerous antithrombotic and neuroprotective drugs have been evaluated in clinical trials. Although none has shown unequivocal benefits on its own, prospects for successful intervention are promising. Examples include different combinations of therapies targeted at various points of the ischemic cascade and different pathophysiologic stroke types. As a result of these potentially complex treatment regimens, patient care may be extremely challenging to health care professionals in the future.

### 4. What are the two basic types of stroke?

Strokes are usually classified, according to their etiologic basis, as either ischemic (83%) or hemorrhagic (17%).

### 5. What are the causes of stroke?

| HEMORRHAGIC STROKE | ISCHEMIC STROKE |
| --- | --- |
| Intracerebral hemorrhage | Large artery atherosclerosis |
| Subarachnoid hemorrhage | (embolus/thrombus) |
| | Cardioembolism |
| | Small vessel occlusion (lacuna) |
| | Nonatherosclerotic vasculopathies |
| | Hypercoagulable states |

### 6. How are ischemic strokes classified?

Ischemic strokes are classified as thrombotic or embolic. They are caused by blood clots that form in the brain vasculature (thrombus) and blood clots or pieces of atherosclerotic plaque or other material that travel to the brain from another location (embolus). Thrombotic stroke, the most common type, is usually associated with atherosclerotic narrowing of the arterial lumen, which eventually interferes with the blood supply nourishing the affected portion of the brain.

Embolic strokes often result from a cardiogenic embolism in patients with heart disease; however, they can originate anywhere. Patients with atrial fibrillation (Afib) are five times more likely to develop embolic stroke than patients without Afib.

**7. How are hemorrhagic strokes classified?**

Hemorrhagic stroke is classified according to the area of the brain in which the hemorrhage has occurred. Intracerebral hemorrhage (ICH) usually refers to cases of parenchymal hematoma not associated with trauma. Chronic hypertension is the most common cause of spontaneous ICH (60% of cases with hemorrhage) Subarachnoid hemorrhage (SAH) usually is associated with a ruptured cerebral aneurysm or ruptured arteriovenous malformation (AVM), accounting for approximately 25% of patients with hemorrhage. Other causes of hemorrhagic stroke include cerebral amyloidosis (in elderly patients), bleeding disorders, neoplasm, infection, trauma, reperfusion abnormalities, and drug abuse.

**8. What are the most common symptoms of stroke?**

- Sudden numbness or weakness of face, arm or leg, especially on one side of the body
- Sudden confusion, trouble with speaking or understanding
- Sudden trouble with vision in one or both eyes
- Sudden trouble with walking, dizziness, loss of balance or coordination
- Sudden severe headache with no known cause

Other important but less common symptoms include sudden nausea, fever, and vomiting, distinguished from viral illness by speed of onset (minutes or hours vs. several days), and brief loss of consciousness or period of decreased consciousness (fainting, confusion, convulsions, or coma).

**9. How is the diagnosis of stroke made?**

Stroke is diagnosed primarily on the bases of clinical presentation and neuroradiologic studies. A noncontrast computerized tomography (CT) scan of the head is currently the most important emergency diagnostic test in patients presenting with clinical manifestations of stroke. It is an invaluable means of distinguishing between hemorrhage and infarction. A head CT scan is by no means the only neuroradiologic examination performed in patients with cerebrovascular disease; it may be replaced or complemented by MRI. CT, however, is safe, noninvasive, and, in some instances, concludes the neurologic work-up. CT studies occasionally are complemented with dynamic CT and xenon enhancement to monitor the pathophysiologic changes of cerebrovascular occlusive disease.

**10. What findings may be seen on the head CT scan? How do they affect immediate response?**

CT scan results determine immediate treatment, as outlined below.

1. **Cerebral infarction:** if the patient meets all inclusion criteria and has no exclusion criteria, consider immediate treatement with tissue plasminogen activator (tPA; see question 21).

2. **SAH:** assess Hunt and Hess grade (see question 16) and Fisher grade (see question 17), obtain neurosurgery consult and urgent four-vessel cerebral angiogram, and provide supportive medical and nursing care.

3. **ICH:** assess Glasgow Coma Scale score (see question 14), obtain neurosurgery or neurology consult, determine cause of hemorrhage, and provide supportive medical and nursing care.

4. **Nonstroke lesion:** distinguish between encephalitis or intracranial mass (tumor, abscess, AVM, subdural hematoma, or epidural hematoma).

5. **Normal CT scan:** consider the following:
   - Seizure, migraine, hypoglycemia
   - Lumbar puncture for red blood cells, xanthochromia, white blood cells, protein, glucose, serology, and cultures (possible causes: SAH, meningitis, or encephalitis)
   - If history, exam, CT, and lab values are most consistent with cerebral ischemia and the patient meets all inclusion criteria and has no exclusion criteria, consider administering

tPA (see question 21); if the patient is not eligible for tPA, consider other acute therapy and provide supportive management.

## 11. What other studies may be done initially?

The aim of auxiliary tests in patients with acute stroke is to identify severity and subtype, to support treatment strategies, to identify additional risks, to give baseline information for follow-up studies, and to identify potential problems that may require intensive care. Examples include:

- Electrocardiography (ECG)
- Chest radiograph
- Blood tests (complete blood count, glucose, urea, electrolytes, coagulation)
- Urinalysis with microscopy to evaluate for hematuria (suggestive of a bleeding disorder or renal cardioembolism)
- Arterial blood gas or oximetry in comatose patients and patients with hypoxia or respiratory compromise
- Lumbar puncture (when stroke is suspected and the head CT scan is "normal," a lumbar puncture is sometimes done to confirm SAH)
- Transcranial Doppler

## 12. What historical data should be obtained?

- When did symptoms first occur?
- Was trauma involved?
- Did a seizure occur at the onset of symptoms?
- What medications is the patient taking? Warfarin?
- Does the patient have symptoms suggestive of myocardial infarction?
- Does the patient have symptoms suggestive of ICH?
- What is the patient's weight?

## 13. What scoring systems are used for patients with acute stroke?

Many scoring systems are used in patients with an altered level of consciousness. More important than the type of scale is the consistency with which its used. The most common assessment scales include the Glasgow Coma Scale (GCS), NIH Stroke Scale, Fisher grade, and Hunt and Hess score.

## 14. How do I figure out an accurate GCS score?

The GCS was developed originally for head-injured patients and is of limited use in patients with cerebral infarction, unless the presentation is complicated by massive edema and depressed level of consciousness (see Chapter 43).

## 15. What is the NIH Stroke Scale?

The National Institutes of Health Stroke Scale (NIHSS) allows health care professionals to document and communicate the severity of neurologic insult according to a standardized "severity of illness" scale. Moreover, it permits clinicians to compare the status of the patient by performing repeat evaluations to measure either improvement or worsening of clinical condition. It is most useful in patients with a focal neurologic deficit. The scores range from 0 (normal) to 42 (coma). In clinical trials, the scale has correlated with ICH complications and other outcome measures. Knowledge of the NIH Stroke Scale score before the administration of thrombolytic therapy is an important factor in discussing risks and benefits with the patient and family.

## 16. What is the Hunt and Hess Scale? When is it used?

The classification of SAH traditionally has been based on the patient's clinical neurologic status. The Hunt and Hess Scale is used to grade the clinical severity of SAH. Clinical grade correlates with neurologic outcome and risk of rebleeding and vasospasm.

*Hunt and Hess Scale*

| GRADE | CLINICAL CONDITION |
|-------|--------------------|
| I | Asymptomatic or mild headache and slight nuchal rigidity |
| II | Cranial nerve palsy, nuchal rigidity, and moderate-to-severe headache |
| III | Drowsy, confused, or mild focal deficit (e.g., hemiparesis, hemianesthesia) |
| IV | Stupor, moderate-to-severe hemiparesis, early decerebrate rigidity |
| V | Comatose and decerebrate rigidity |

### 17. What does the Fisher grade mean in patients with SAH?

Fisher and colleagues correlated the location and thickness of subarachnoid blood on CT scan with clinical outcome and likelihood of developing vasospasm. The Fisher CT grade is commonly used with the Hunt and Hess grade to gauge the severity of SAH.

*Fisher Grade in Subarachnoid Hemorrhage*

| GRADE | CT FINDING OF SAH |
|-------|-------------------|
| I | None |
| II | Diffuse, thin layer |
| III | Localized clot or thick layer |
| IV | Intracerebral or intraventricular blood |

### 18. What is the differential diagnosis of stroke?

- Seizures
- Hypoglycemia
- Hyperglycemia
- Hyponatremia
- Subdural hematoma
- Tumor
- Migraine
- Infections
- Drug overdose
- Hypertensive encephalopathy

Urgent identification of these conditions is particularly important if thrombolytic therapy is considered.

### 19. What medications are commonly used in stroke? Explain the action of each.

**Thrombolytics.** Thrombolytic (fibrinolytic) drugs help to reestablish cerebral circulation by dissolving (lysing) clots that obstruct blood flow. Most thrombolytics are plasminogen activators that stimulate factors in the blood, which ultimately break up the blood clot. To be effective, thrombolytic therapy should be administered as quickly as possible.

**Heparin.** Although studies are ongoing, the efficacy of heparin in acute ischemic stroke is not well-established. Nonetheless, anticoagulation with heparin is sometimes used in an effort to prevent or limit the progression of stroke in patients with atherothrombotic infarction. Heparin also is used to prevent recurrent embolism in patients with cardioembolic stroke. Heparin is contraindicated for 24 hours after intravenous tPA therapy. Antithrombotic agents used in acute ischemic stroke now include low-molecular-weight (LMW) heparins and heparinoids. Initial studies suggest that LMW heparins reduce disability and death even 6 months after stroke. Low-dose heparin and LMW heparins or heparinoids are strongly recommended for prophylaxis against deep venous thrombosis in immobilized patients after acute ischemic stroke.

**Neuroprotective agents.** Because ischemia is clearly a process and not an instantaneous event, it is possible to intervene and improve clinical outcome. Neuroprotective drugs minimize the effects of the ischemic cascade. Although no neuroprotective agents are yet available commercially, several different types are in clinical trials, including glutamate antagonists, calcium antagonists, opiate antagonists, and antioxidants.

**20. How do I manage the patient's blood pressure?**

Acute stroke produces an increase in blood pressure (BP) in approximately 80% of patients. Regardless of the treatment for stroke, BP should be monitored frequently. Control of BP is especially important in the setting of thrombolytic therapy, because elevated BP is associated with an increased risk of ICH. Minimal or moderate elevations in BP do not require urgent pharmacologic treatment, because BP usually declines spontaneously over time. As a guideline, antihypertensives are not required unless the mean arterial pressure is > 130 mmHg or systolic BP is > 230 mmHg. Systolic BP of 180–230 mmHg or diastolic BP of 105–120 mmHg may be treated with a beta blocker such as labetalol hydrochloride. If adequate reductions in BP are not achieved, intravenous sodium nitroprusside may be infused, starting at a dose of 0.5 µg/kg/min.

It is important not to overdo it! Rapid reduction of BP is not necessary and may cause a decrease in cerebral perfusion. No clinical evidence shows that lowering BP during a stroke is beneficial. This finding may surprise many clinicians, who draw on their experience with acute myocardial infarction (AMI). In AMI, lowering of BP reduces ischemia by reducing cardiac work. That benefit, however, does not apply to the brain. In fact, perfusion may be better when BP is high because vascular autoregulation is impaired in the ischemic brain. Therefore, a reduction to systolic BP of 200–220 mmHg and diastolic BP of 100–120 mmHg is probably adequate.

## MANAGEMENT AND TREATMENT OF ISCHEMIC STROKE

**21. What is tissue plasminogen activator?**

Tissue plaminogen activator (tPA) is an enzyme, found naturally in the body, that converts (or activates) plasminogen to plasmin, which dissolves blood clots. Intravenous tPA is now an approved treatment for patients who present within 3 hours of an ischemic stroke.

**22. What clinical research has been done on tPA therapy?**

In 1995 the results of the NINDS tPA Stroke Trial were published, and in the following year the Food and Drug Administration (FDA) approved recombinant tPA for treatment of acute ischemic stroke patients. The NINDS tPA trial showed a 30–50% relative (12% absolute) increase in favorable outcome (minimal or no disability) at 3 months for patients who received tPA. Unlike other thrombolytic trials, there was no difference in mortality rate between patients receiving tPA and patients receiving placebo (39% vs. 34%, respectively). Symptomatic hemorrhage occurred in 6.4% of patients receiving tPA and 0.6% of those receiving placebo. There was also a strong trend toward improvement in neurologic scores within the first 24 hours. Scores on the NIH Stroke Scale were significantly better at 24 hours in treated patients.

**23. Does tPA therapy require consent?**

Thrombolysis with tPA is not an experimental therapy; it is an approved treatment for stroke. Nevertheless, informed consent should be obtained from patients or their family if possible, just as for any procedure with significant risk. The potential benefits and risks should be thoroughly disclosed.

**24. When should I use tPA?**

Patients with sudden onset and persistent focal neurologic deficit should be considered for tPA therapy. Persistent symptoms after 1 hour have an 85% risk of stroke, with only a 15% chance of full recovery. Patients whose symptoms are rapidly resolving are most likely having a transient ischemic attack (TIA) and should not receive tPA.

*Eligibility Criteria for tPA Therapy*

- Age 18 or older
- Measurable neurological deficit
- CT does not show hemorrhage or nonstroke cause of deficit
- Time of onset within 3 hours of treatment

### 25. What are the absolute contraindications to tPA therapy?

- Isolated, mild deficits (NIH Stroke Scale score = 1or less)
- Neurologic signs that are improving rapidly (suggesting TIA)
- Seizure at the onset of stroke
- Symptoms suggesting SAH, even with normal CT
- Symptoms suggesting toxic/metabolic encephalopathy
- Blood glucose < 50 mg/dl or > 400 mg/dl
- Another stroke, intracranial surgery, or serious head trauma within past 3 months
- Current use of anticoagulants or international normalized ratio (INR) > 1.7
- Administration of heparin within 48 hours and prolonged PTT
- Platelet count < 100,000 µl
- Pretreatment systolic BP > 185 mmHg, diastolic BP > 110 mmHg, or aggressive treatment to bring BP below these limits
- Known intracranial neoplasm, AVM, or aneurysm
- Prior intracranial hemorrhage at any time

### 26. In which patients should tPA therapy be used with caution?

Give tPA with caution in patients with the following:
- Severe stroke (NIH Stroke Scale score over 22)
- CT evidence of large middle cerebral artery (MCA) infarction (sulcal effacement or blurring of gray-white junction in more than one third of MCA territory)

### 27. How do I administer thrombolytic drugs?

The recommended dose of tPA for stroke is 0.9 mg/kg, to a maximum of 90 mg. Ten percent of the dose is given as an initial IV bolus, and the remainder is infused over 60 minutes. Administer the entire drug solution using a normal saline flush at the end of the infusion. If the patient's condition worsens at any time during drug administration, the infusion should be stopped immediately until further assessment and head CT scan are completed.

The dose used for stroke is lower than the dose for myocardial infarction. No thrombolytic agent other than tPA is currently recommended. Patients already taking aspirin are not excluded from thrombolysis, but the guidelines warn against giving any other antithrombotic or antiplatelet agent, such as heparin, warfarin, aspirin, or ticlopidine, within the first 24 hours after treatment.

### 28. What are the essential components of nursing care when thrombolytics are administered?

During the first 24 hours, vital signs, neurologic status, and bleeding should be assessed frequently; continuous ECG monitoring is also essential. The patient-to-nurse ratio should be no more than 2:1 during this time.

### 29. Describe the assessment of neurologic status and vital signs.

Frequent monitoring of neurologic function after brain infarction is necessary but may be perplexing because of the variety of assessment tools currently in use. More important than the choice of scale is a uniform method of documentation of clinical neurologic status.

The NIH Stroke Scale is the tool of choice because it was designed specifically to assess stroke deficit. A complete baseline assessment should be obtained before drug administration. After drug administration, an abbreviated NIH Stroke Scale should be performed; vital signs should be assessed at 15-minute intervals for the first 2 hours, every half hour for the next 6 hours, then hourly until 24 hours after treatment.

### 30. What are the requirements for cardiac monitoring?

Cardiac arrhythmias are common in patients who have suffered a stroke. In addition, a significant percentage of elderly stroke patients may have low cardiac output at the time of the bleed. Pulmonary artery pressure monitoring may become necessary if aggressive BP manipulation or fluid management is anticipated. The cardiac examination includes assessment for tachypnea, tachycardia, jugular venous distention, and peripheral edema. If any symptoms or signs suggest the possibility of heart failure, a chest radiograph should be obtained.

**31. Describe the bleeding assessment.**
The primary complication from t-PA administration is intracranial hemorrhage (ICH). A patient who deteriorates neurologically after thrombolytic treatment is having an ICH until proved otherwise. The most common signs and symptoms of ICH are decreased level of consciousness, changes in motor examination, new headache, and increases in BP. Coagulation studies and CT scan of the head should be initiated immediately and tPA infusion stopped.

**32. What other nursing care issues should be considered?**
• Early mobilization
• Measures to prevent the subacute complications of stroke (aspiration, malnutrition, pneumonia, deep vein thrombosis, pulmonary embolism, decubitus ulcers, contractures, and joint abnormalities).
• Prophylactic administration of heparin or LMW heparins or heparinoids to prevent deep vein thrombosis is strongly recommended for immobilized patients. Intermittent external compression stockings are recommended for patients who cannot receive antithrombotic drugs.

## MANAGEMENT AND TREATMENT OF HEMORRHAGIC STROKE

**33. What causes spontaneous hemorrhagic stroke?**
1. **Arterial hypertension** is the presumed cause of spontaneous ICH in about 70% of patients presenting with hemorrhage.
2. **SAH** is caused most often by the rupture of an intracranial aneurysm and is associated with considerable morbidity and mortality. The International Cooperative Study on the Timing of Aneurysm Surgery reported a mortality and morbidity rate of 42% in 3521 patients admitted to neurosurgical services. Surgical clipping of the offending aneurysm is the therapy of choice for patients who survive to reach the hospital. Approximately 10% of all strokes in the United States per year are new cases of aneurysmal SAH.
3. The most frequent complication of **AVMs** is hemorrhage. AVMs characteristically rupture during the second to fourth decade of life, whereas hypertensive ICH usually occurs in an older population.
4. **Coagulopathic ICH** is usually secondary to underlying systemic disease or anticoagulation therapy and accounts for nearly 10% of ICH. Systemic diseases such as renal and hepatic failure, thrombocytopeni,a and leukemia produce coagulopathic states that can lead to spontaneous ICH.
5. **Drugs** appear to induce ICH through coagulopathy, hypersensitive vasculitis, or acute hypertension. The use of addictive drugs, especially cocaine and amphetamines, is a major cause of ICH in young adults.
6. **Other causes:** brain tumor, infection, dural fistula, venous sinus thrombosis, amyloid angiopathy.

**34. What are primary goals of emergency management of patients with ICH?**
The primary goals are to prevent subsequent damage from rebleed, edema, or hypoxia and to identify the cause, site and extent of the hemorrhage. In contrast to patients with ischemic stroke, who usually have a stable airway, many patients may arrive in the hospital already intubated and ventilated. Abnormalities in electrolytes and coagulation studies must be identified and corrected. An intravenous catheter is inserted for drug and fluid administration. In some centers, IV phenytoin is administered for seizure prophylaxis. Mannitol generally is given if the patient is stuporous or comatose. Patients who present with a moderate-to-large ICH, severe neurologic deficits, depressed level of consciousness, significant hypertension, or serious concomitant illnesses must be admitted to a critical care unit.

### 35. How is blood pressure controlled in patients with ICH?

BP reduction should be gradual and controlled. Acute normalization of blood pressure can be dangerous for several reasons. It may reduce local cerebral perfusion pressure (CPP) and cerebral blood flow (CBF) to ischemic levels, and in chronically hypertensive patients it may shift the autoregulatory curve to higher pressures. BP treatment must be tailored to the needs of the individual patient. As a guide, for patients with a history of significant hypertension, the MAP should be maintained initially in the range of 120 mmHg. Formerly nonhypertensive patients should have an MAP < 110 mmHg.

### 36. Describe the treatment of coagulopathies.

Coagulopathies must be reversed as soon as possible. Patients who are taking IV heparin should receive 1 mg protamine per 100 U of heparin. If the patient recently received a thrombolytic and is deteriorating, 5 gm of epsilon-aminocaproic acid (EACA) over 15–30 minutes and 10–15 bags of cryoprecipitate are often recommended. Warfarin should be reversed with vitamin K, three doses of 10 mg IV, and fresh frozen plasma to normalize PT. Factor IX concentrate can be used in addition to vitamin K (minimal dose = 50 U/kg). Patients with a platelet disorder due to leukemia or aplastic anemia should receive a platelet transfusion. If the patient is not actively bleeding, it does not make sense to use substances such as EACA, which may have a negative effect. As with BP control, the aggressiveness of therapy must be considered carefully.

### 37. How is increased intracranial pressure treated?

At what level ICP should be treated is a controversial issue. Current practice in most institutions is to maintain the ICP below 20 mmHg, using the following consecutive treatment regimen:

- Cerebrospinal fluid drainage through the ventriculostomy/ICP catheter
- Sedation with morphine sulfate or propofol
- Mannitol administration
- Paralysis with vecuronium or pancuronium
- Hyperventilation
- Induced coma with pentobarbital or etomidate
- Hemicraniectomy

### 38. How is cerebral perfusion maintained?

Most of the measures used to control ICP diminish CBF despite the fact that the most important determinant of neurologic recovery is maintenance of CBF. CPP is often used to titrate treatment and is calculated as follows: MAP – ICP = CPP. According to current thought, the CPP should be maintained around 70 mmHg (even if ICP cannot be kept below 20 mmHg). CPPs below 50 are associated with cerebral ischemia and poor outcome. CPP can be maintained by raising the MAP with ample fluids, colloids, or blood products and inducing arterial hypertension with phenylephrine. As with any other therapy, overly aggressive management can have deleterious effects and should be avoided.

### 39. What method is used for seizure control?

Anticonvulsants are frequently administered to patients who have had a seizure and patients with lobar or superficial subcortical bleeding. Phenytoin is the preferred agent with a loading dose of 15–18 mg/kg over 30–60 minutes and maintenance of 300 mg/day.

### 40. Why are ventricular catheters placed in patients with ICH?

Patients with ICH are at risk for chronic hydrocephalus. Ventricular catheters often are placed both for ICP monitoring and ventricular drainage. Persistent hydrocephalus can be treated surgically with a ventriculoperitoneal or lumboperitoneal shunt.

### 41. When is surgical management appropriate for ICH?

Size and location of the hemorrhage are used to predict the utility of surgical intervention. Operative evacuation of the hemorrhage may be beneficial or life-saving in patients with large hypertensive ganglionic hemorrhage or cerebellar hemorrhage, but this approach remains controversial. Surgery offers little benefit to patients presenting with a large hypertensive hemorrhage into the brainstem or thalamus.

**42. Describe the surgical management of aneurysmal hemorrhage.**

The essential, curative procedure for a ruptured cerebral aneurysm is direct clipping of the neck of the aneurysm. Surgery is considered high risk; morbidity and mortality rates are significant, even for unruptured aneurysms. Current practice is to clip the offending aneursym within 2–3 days after the bleed. This time frame generally provides the safest window before recurrent hemorrhage or vasospasm.

**43. What is vasospasm in patients with aneurysmal SAH?**

Cerebral vasospasm is the main reason for secondary deterioration after 4–7 days in both operated and nonoperated patients with SAH. Arterial narrowing develops in approximately 40–70% of patients, causing a delayed ischemic deficit in 20–30%. It is the leading cause of mortality and morbidity in patients who survive the initial hemorrhage.

**44. How is vasospasm managed?**

**Transcranial Doppler (TCD) ultrasonography** is a noninvasive alternative to cerebral angiography. It allows monitoring of changes in the cerebral circulation under both normal and pathologic conditions. TCD monitoring often is done on a routine basis after aneurysmal SAH and reliably detects cerebral vasospasm. In patients with vasospasm, TCD measurements often are used as a guide to therapy.

**Nimodipine** is the only medication shown to prevent vasospasm and improve patient outcome after aneurysmal SAH. Its use has become standard practice. In the United States, it is approved only for oral administration, whereas in Europe IV administration is sometimes used. The usual oral dose is 60 mg every 4 hr or 30 mg every 2 hr. Because of its vasodilator effect, BP should be carefully monitored.

**Hypertensive-hypervolemic hemodilution** (HHH) is achieved by increasing cardiac output and BP with aggressive intravascular volume loading and vasopressure medications. Fluid loading usually leads to hemodilution, which, if carried too far, reduces the relative content of blood cells and may lead to ischemia. Therefore, hematocrit values below 30% should be avoided. Vasoactive drugs are added to raise arterial pressure if intravascular volume expansion alone is inadequate. PA and/or CVP monitoring is helpful. HHH therapy should be individualized because successful treatment of ischemic deficits often occurs with hypervolemia and hypertension without hemodilution. Extreme caution should be exercised in caring for elderly patients or patients with a significant cardiac history.

**Transluminal balloon angioplasty** (TBA) of the major affected intracerebral arteries has led to successful resolution of medically refractory, angiographically demonstrated vasospasm and reversal of delayed neurologic deficit. The effect of TBA on the spastic arterial wall and the mechanism by which it results in long-lasting cerebral arterial dilation remain unclear. Patients must be moved out of the ICU to the radiology suite at a time when intensive monitoring and treatment are most critical. Ongoing studies are testing the concept of prophylactic TBA in patients at high risk for vasospasm. Prophylactic TBA usually is done immediately after surgical clipping while the patient is still under the influence of anesthetics. Although unproven, it is a promising therapy.

## BIBLIOGRAPHY

1. Braimah J, Kongable G, Rapp K, et al: Nursing care of acute stroke patients after receiving rt-PA therapy. J Neurosci Nurs 29(6):373–383, 1997.
2. Broderick J, Brott T, Barsan W, et al: Blood pressure during the first minutes of focal cerebral ischemia. Ann Emerg Med 22:1438–1443, 1993.
3. Davis S, Donnan G, Grotta J, et al: Interventional Therapy in Acute Stroke. London, Blackwell Science, 1998, pp 155–249.
4. Duldner JE, Emerman CL: Stroke: Comprehensive guidelines for clinical assessment and emergency management. Part II. Emerg Med Rep 18(21): 215–217, 1997.

5. Kassell NF, Torner JC, Haley EC: The international cooperative study on the timing of aneurysm surgery. Part I: Overall management results. J. Neurosurg 73:18–36, 1990.
6. Kay R, Wong K, Yu Y, et al: Low-molecular-weight heparin for the treatment of acute stroke. N Engl J Med 333:1588–1593, 1995.
7. Lappin R: Thrombolysis for stroke: A user's guide. Emerg Med 31(9):54–64, 1999.
8. Muizelaar JP, Peterson P: Current management strategies for traumatic brain and spinal cord injuries. In Peterson P, Phillis J (eds): Novel Therapies for CNS Injuries: Rationales and Results. New York, CRC Press, 1996, pp 62–63.
9. Peterson P, Guyot A, Zafonte R: Traumatic brain injury: Epidemiology, pathophysiology, and classification. In Peterson P, Phillis J (eds): Novel Therapies for CNS Injuries: Rationales and Results. New York, CRC Press, 1996, pp 5–7.
10. Rogers SJ, Sherman DG: Pathophysiology and treatment of acute ischemic stroke. Clin Pharmacol 12:359–376, 1993.

# 46. SEIZURE ASSESSMENT AND MANAGEMENT

*Mariann M. Ward, RN, MS, ANP*

## 1. What is a seizure?

A seizure is a discrete event, characterized by an excessive and synchronous discharge of cerebral neurons with associated sensory, motor, and/or behavioral changes. It is a symptom rather than a diagnosis of brain dysfunction.

## 2. How common are seizures?

Seizures are common and may present in a variety of clinical settings. Although the incidence and prevalence of seizure activity are influenced by various factors, approximately 1 in 11 persons will experience a seizure sometime in their lifetime. The incidence is highest during early childhood and late adulthood.

## 3. Are seizures and epilepsy the same thing?

No. A **seizure** is usually a self-limited event. If the underlying cause provoking disturbance in cerebral function (e.g., alcohol withdrawal, severe hyponatremia) can be identified and corrected, seizure activity is likely to stop. Long-term treatment with antiepileptic drugs (AEDs) is not required. **Epilepsy** refers to a group of chronic neurologic disorders characterized by recurrent (2 or more), unprovoked seizure activity of cerebral origin. Patients with epilepsy usually require long-term treatment with AEDs to achieve seizure control.

## 4. How are seizures classified?

Seizures are classified according to criteria established by the International League Against Epilepsy (ILAE).

### International Classification of Epileptic Seizures

I. **Partial seizures** (initial clinical and EEG findings demonstrate focal origin)
   1. Simple partial (no impairment of consciousness)
      • Focal motor activity
      • Somatosensory or special sensory symptoms
      • Autonomic symptoms
      • Psychic symptoms
   2. Complex partial (impairment of consciousness)
      • Simple partial onset followed by impairment of consciousness
      • Impairment of consciousness at onset
   3. Partial seizures evolving into a secondarily generalized seizure

*Table continued on following page*

*International Classification of Epileptic Seizures (Continued)*

II. **Generalized seizures** (clinical and EEG changes demonstrate bihemispheric involvement from onset)
   1. Absence              4. Tonic
   2. Myoclonic        5. Tonic-clonic (grand mal)
   3. Clonic              6. Atonic (akinetic/drop attacks)

III. **Unclassified seizures** (includes all seizures that cannot be classified because of inadequate or incomplete data and some that defy classification into a specific seizure type as defined above)

EEG = electroencephalography.
Adapted from the Commission on Classification and Terminology of the International League Against Epilepsy:Proposal for revised clinical and electroencephalographic classification of epileptic seizures. Epilepsia 22:489–501, 1981.

### 5. Is seizure classification important?

Yes. Accurate classification provides the cornerstone of seizure management from the initial diagnostic evaluation to decision-making about further evaluations and treatment.

### 6. What are common manifestations of seizure activity?

There are many different manifestations of seizure activity, depending on where in the brain the abnormal neuronal activity originates and to what areas, if any, it spreads. For example, simple partial seizures may manifest as an aura, a change in somatosensory, autonomic, or psychic phenomena often described by patients as a warning sign that a seizure is imminent. Depending on what part of the brain is affected, patients may describe an odd odor, unpleasant taste, sensory hallucination, feeling of intense fear, déjà vu, flushing, epigastric rising, flashing lights, or brief speech arrest. If motor cortex is involved, patients may experience unilateral, involuntary motor movements such as facial twitching, posturing of extremities, or tonic-clonic movements, but consciousness remains intact.

### 7. How do complex partial seizures often manifest?

Complex partial seizures may or may not begin as simple partial seizure but always involve impairment of consciousness. The patient may appear momentarily dazed or confused. Accompanying motor activity is usually minimal and often takes the form of various automatisms, such as lip smacking, chewing, and picking or fumbling movements of the hands. Dystonic posturing of extremities usually occurs on the side contralateral to the seizure focus. The postictal phase often is characterized by confusion; its duration is variable.

### 8. Describe the common manifestations of generalized seizures.

Generalized seizures demonstrate bihemispheric involvement from the onset and are characterized by impairment of consciousness (except for single myoclonic jerks). Motor manifestations depend on the amount of cortex affected. Absence (petit mal) seizures are an example of a generalized seizure type characterized by brief impairments of consciousness (a few seconds) without loss of postural tone or postictal confusion. Initially these spells often are thought to be simple "staring spells" and are not recognized as seizure activity.

### 9. Describe tonic-clonic convulsions.

A tonic-clonic convulsion is another type of generalized seizure and is what most people think of when they hear the word "seizure." This ictal event, often referred to as a grand mal seizure, classically begins with a loud cry, followed by tonic contraction of all extremities. Accompanying symptoms include respiratory impairment, pooling of secretions, cyanosis, pupillary dilation, and an increase in heart rate and blood pressure. Then the seizure evolves into the clonic phase, characterized by bilateral jerking movements of extremities. The severity decreases gradually as the periods of relaxation increase and the convulsion ends. The duration of the convulsion is usually less than 1–2 minutes, but the postictal phase is characterized by confusion and exhaustion that can last minutes to hours before full consciousness is regained.

## 10. What are the common causes of seizures other than epilepsy?

In addition to the causes listed in the table below, numerous medications and illicit drugs have the potential to cause seizures. Examples include high-dose penicillins, isoniazid, quinolones, meperidine, antipsychotics, barbiturate and benzodiazepine withdrawal, amphetamines, cocaine, and phencyclidine. Keep in mind that contributing factors and specific causes are often age-dependent.

*Causes of Seizures*

| | |
|---|---|
| Neonates (< 1 mo) | Perinatal hypoxia and ischemia |
| | Intracranial hemorrhage and trauma |
| | Acute CNS infection (bacterial and viral meningitis) |
| | Metabolic disturbances (hypoglycemia, hypocalcemia, hypomagnesemia, pyridoxine deficiency) |
| | Drug withdrawal |
| | Developmental disorders (acquired and genetic) |
| | Genetic disorders |
| Infants and children (>1 mo and < 12 yr) | Febrile seizures |
| | Genetic disorders (metabolic, degenerative, primary epilepsy syndromes) |
| | CNS infection |
| | Developmental disorders (acquired and genetic) |
| | Trauma |
| | Idiopathic |
| Adolescents (12–18 yr) | Trauma |
| | Genetic disorders |
| | Infection |
| | Brain tumor |
| | Illicit drug use |
| | Idiopathic |
| Young Adults (18–35 yr) | Trauma |
| | Alcohol withdrawal |
| | Illicit drug use |
| | Brain tumor |
| | Idiopathic |
| Older adults (>35 yr) | Cerebrovascular disease |
| | Brain tumor |
| | Alcohol withdrawal |
| | Metabolic disorders (uremia, hepatic failure, electrolyte abnormalities, and hypoglycemia) |
| | Alzheimer's disease and other degenerative CNS diseases |
| | Idiopathic |

CNS = central nervous system.
From Lowenstein DH: Seizures and epilepsy. In Fauci AS, et al (eds): Harrison's Textbook of Medicine, 14th ed. New York, McGraw-Hill, 1998, p 2316, with permission.

## 11. What are the common metabolic causes of seizures?

**Hyponatremia.** Seizures usually do not occur until serum sodium levels fall below 120 mEq/L. Convulsions are seen more frequently in patients experiencing acute onset of hyponatremia (< 12 hr).

**Hypoglycemia.** Seizures may occur when blood glucose levels fall below 40 mg/dl but respond well to treatment with glucose. Hypoglycemic seizures usually are generalized convulsions.

**Hyperglycemia.** Seizures also may result from elevated blood glucose levels (usually 600–800 mg/dl), although the range is quite broad. These seizures have predominantly focal features.

**Alcohol withdrawal.** Seizures usually occur in adults who have been alcoholics for several years, most of whom drink daily. Seizures are typically brief generalized tonic-clonic convulsions, the majority of which occur within 48 hours after cessation of alcohol consumption.

**12. What is the first priority when a patient has a seizure?**

The first priority is to ensure patient safety and maintain the airway. Never force anything into a patient's mouth. Prevent the patient from injuring himself or herself. Do not, however, forcefully restrain a patient unless he or she is at risk of inflicting significant self-injury. Pad the side rails, and maintain aspiration precautions by flattening the head of the bed and rolling the patient onto the side to promote drainage of secretions. Keep in mind that seizures rarely last more than 1–2 minutes. If the seizure activity does not stop, call for help (see question 30).

**13. What other nursing interventions are appropriate?**

Stay with the patient throughout the seizure until the patient returns to his or her cognitive baseline. Although the seizure itself may be brief, the postictal phase can last from minutes to hours, especially in the setting of a convulsion. However, if the patient fails to return to baseline in a sufficient amount of time, further investigation is warranted.

As potentially the only witness to the seizure, the nurse can play a key role in the patient's medical evaluation and management by providing an accurate and thorough assessment of the seizure event from beginning to end and documenting accordingly. Record not only your observations but also ask what the patient recalls once he or she has recovered.

**14. What should the nursing assessment and documentation include?**

- Precipitating events
- Occurrence of an aura
- Area of the body in which seizure activity was first observed
- Progression and duration of seizure activity
- Whether the patient was able to speak or follow commands during the seizure
- Head or eye deviation, posturing of extremities
- Whether the patient sustained injury during the seizure, including tongue or lip biting and falls
- Behavioral changes before and after the seizure
- Incontinence
- Evidence of a transient focal weakness after the seizure (Todd's paresis)
- Aphasia
- Preictal or postictal headache

**15. What other conditions can mimic seizure activity?**

The most common condition that causes episodic or recurrent paroxysmal events that can be commonly confused with seizure activity is syncope. Other conditions include migraine, transient ischemic attacks, narcolepsy, movements disorders (e.g., dystonias and tics), psychogenic seizures, panic attacks, and metabolic disturbances.

**16. How do you approach the work-up of new-onset seizures?**

Critically ill patients may experience a seizure in the ICU for various reasons. The first task is to determine whether the event was indeed a seizure. This goal is best achieved by thorough history taking. Obtain an accurate and detailed description of the event, interviewing both the patient, if he or she is able to participate, and witnesses to the event. Has the patient had seizures before? Is he or she taking any medications for seizures? Does the patient have a history of head trauma? If so, was the trauma associated with a loss of consciousness? Once the event has been determined to be a seizure, further investigation is focused on establishing etiology.

**17. What should you look for in the physical examination?**

Look for obvious signs of trauma, metabolic disturbances, infection, or systemic illness. A detailed neurologic examination should include assessment of mental status, including memory and language function; visual fields; sensory or motor deficits (symmetric vs. asymmetric findings); and coordination. Repeating the examination throughout the day is both necessary and helpful in differentiating postictal effects from static deficits.

### 18. What lab tests should be performed?

All patients should have routine lab tests, including complete blood count, electrolytes, calcium, magnesium, phosphate, blood urea nitrogen, creatinine, liver function studies, and glucose. Check AED levels if applicable. Additional tests based on clinical suspicion may include toxicology screen and blood cultures.

### 19. When is lumbar puncture indicated?

Lumbar puncture is indicated for all patients in whom meningitis or encephalitis is suspected. Lumbar puncture is also mandatory for patients with human immunodeficiency virus (HIV) infection.

### 20. What imaging studies are helpful?

Patients who have an unprovoked seizure should undergo a brain imaging study to look for underlying structural lesions (e.g., tumor, vascular malformation, abscess) that may be responsible for seizure activity. Magnetic resonance imaging (MRI) is the scan of choice because it is more sensitive than computed tomography (CT) in identifying most causative lesions. The exception is acute hemorrhage, in which case CT is superior. The newer functional brain imaging studies, positron emission tomography (PET) and single-photon emission tomography (SPECT), are not indicated in the initial evaluation.

### 21. What is the role of electroencephalography (EEG)?

An EEG measures the electrical activity of cortical surface neurons. It is a useful tool in detecting epileptiform activity, identifying an area of focal electrocerebral abnormality, and classifying seizure types. A normal EEG, however, does not exclude the possibility of seizure occurrence or recurrence. EEGs often are performed between seizures and may or may not reveal epileptiform activity. The significance of the EEG results should be determined in consultation with the neurologist interpreting the study.

### 22. How are seizures treated?

The first goal of treatment is to correct the underlying cause, if possible. Whether or not to treat a first isolated seizure of unknown etiology remains controversial. For patients likely to have recurrent seizures because the cause cannot be quickly or adequately reversed and for patients carrying the diagnosis of epilepsy, AEDs are the mainstay of treatment. The particular AED is chosen according to specific seizure type and side-effect profile. Complete seizure control with one AED (monotherapy) without untoward side effects is the goal.

### 23. List the common antiepileptic medications and their dosing regimens.

*Oral Antiepileptic Medications*

| GENERIC NAME | TRADE NAME | STRENGTH AVAILABLE* (mg) | TYPICAL ADULT STARTING DOSE† | TYPICAL INCREMENT AND RATE OF ASCENSION‡ |
|---|---|---|---|---|
| Carbamazepine | Tegretol | 100, 200 | 200 mg twice daily | 200 mg/wk (taken 3 or 4 times/day) |
| | Tegretol-XR | 100, 200, 400 | 200 mg twice daily | 200 mg/wk (taken twice daily |
| | Carbatrol | 200, 300 | 200 mg twice daily | 200 mg/wk (taken twice daily) |
| Ethosuximide | Zarontin | 250 | 250 mg daily to 250 mg twice daily | 250 mg/wk |

*Table continued on following page*

*Oral Antiepileptic Medications (Continued)*

| GENERIC NAME | TRADE NAME | STRENGTH AVAILABLE* (mg) | TYPICAL ADULT STARTING DOSE[†] | TYPICAL INCREMENT AND RATE OF ASCENSION[‡] |
|---|---|---|---|---|
| Felbamate | Felbatol | 400, 600 | 400 mg 3 times daily | 400–600 mg/wk |
| Gabapentin | Neurontin | 100, 300, 400 | 300 mg daily to 3 times day | 300 mg/wk |
| Lamotrigine | Lamictal | 25, 100, 150, 200 | 25 mg every other day (with valproate) to 25 mg twice daily (with carbamazepine, phenobarbital, or phenytoin) | 25 mg/2 wk |
| Phenobarbital | | 15, 30, 60, 100 | 100 mg/day | 15–30 mg/wk |
| Phenytoin | Dilantin | 30, 50, 100 | 300 mg/day | 25–30 mg/wk |
| Tiagabine | Gabitril | 4, 12, 16, 20 | 4 mg/day | 4 mg/wk (taken 2–4 times/day) |
| Topiramate | Topamax | 25, 100, 200 | 25 mg twice daily | 50 mg/wk |
| Valproate | Depakote | 125, 250, 500 | 250 mg 3 times/day | 250 mg/wk |

* Strengths listed are for tablet or capsule formulations of brand-name agents.

† Initiation doses for some agents vary, depending on concomitant medications, body weight, age of patient, and other factors. Consult prescribing information for each drug. Doses are for nonurgent initiation of medication; clinical circumstances may necessitate increased doses and accelerated titration. See prescribing information for pediatric doses, which are based on body weight and often must be administered more frequently than in adults.

‡ Rate of ascension may need modification, depending on seizure frequency and occurrence of adverse effects. Note that phenytoin may be increased in 25-mg increments by using a halved 50-mg Dilantin Infatab tablet or in 30-mg increments by using a 30-mg Dilantin Kapseal capsule.

Adapted from Marks WJ Jr, Garcia PA: Management of seizures and epilepsy. Am Fam Physician 57:1589–1600, 1998.

## 24. List the common side effects of oral AEDs.

*Common Side Effects of Oral Antiepileptic Drugs*

| DRUG | MOST COMMON DOSE-RELATED ADVERSE EFFECTS | NON–DOSE-RELATED AND IDIOSYNCRATIC REACTIONS |
|---|---|---|
| Carbamazepine | Dizziness, somnolence, ataxia, nausea, vomiting, diplopia, blurred vision | Hyponatremia, rash, Stevens-Johnson syndrome, leukopenia, aplastic anemia, agranulocytosis, transaminitis, hepatic failure |
| Ethosuximide | Anorexia, nausea, vomiting, drowsiness, headache, dizziness | Rash, Stevens-Johnson syndrome, hemopoietic complications |
| Felbamate | Anorexia, vomiting, insomnia, nausea, headache, dizziness | Aplastic anemia, hepatic failure |
| Gabapentin | Somnolence, dizziness, ataxia, fatigue | Weight gain, behavior changes, peripheral edema |
| Lamotrigine | Dizziness, ataxia, somnolence, headache, diplopia, blurred vision, nausea, vomiting, rash | Rash, Stevens-Johnson syndrome, transaminitis |
| Phenobarbital | Somnolence, cognitive and behavior effects | Rash, Stevens-Johnson syndrome, hemopoietic complications, transaminitis, hepatic failure |

*Table continued on following page*

*Common Side Effects of Oral Antiepileptic Drugs (Continued)*

| DRUG | MOST COMMON DOSE-RELATED ADVERSE EFFECTS | NON–DOSE-RELATED AND IDIOSYNCRATIC REACTIONS |
|---|---|---|
| Phenytoin | Ataxia, diplopia, nystagmus, slurred speech, confusion | Rash, Stevens-Johnson syndrome, hemopoietic complications, gingival hyperplasia, coarsening of facial features, transaminitis, hepatic failure |
| Tiagabine | Dizziness, nervousness, asthenia, confusion, tremor | Not established |
| Topiramate | Somnolence, dizziness, ataxia, slurred speech, psychomotor slowing, cognitive problems | Anemia, acne, alopecia, weight loss, transaminitis, nephrolithiasis |
| Valproate | Nausea, vomiting, tremor, thrombocytopenia | Weight gain, hair changes/loss, transaminitis, hepatic failure, rash, Stevens-Johnson syndrome |

Adapted from Marks WJ Jr, Garcia PA: Management of seizures and epilepsy. Am Fam Physician 57:1589–1600, 1998.

### 25. Define status epilepticus.

The Commission on Classification and Terminology of the ILAT defines status epilepticus as a condition that occurs "whenever a seizure persists for a sufficient length of time or is repeated frequently enough that recovery between attacks does not occur." Although this definition does not specify a length of time in which seizure activity must occur and continues to be a subject of debate, many clinicians agree that treatment should be initiated for continuous seizure activity lasting beyond 10 minutes.

### 26. Why is status epilepticus considered a medical emergency?

Status epilepticus is a medical emergency because prolonged, uncontrolled seizure activity can result in cardiorespiratory dysfunction, hyperthermia, and metabolic derangements that may lead to irreversible brain injury.

### 27. What are the most common causes of status epilepticus?

The most common causes of status epilepticus are AED withdrawal or AED noncompliance in patients with known seizure disorders. Other causes include acute metabolic disturbances (e.g., electrolyte abnormalities, sepsis, renal failure), central nervous system infection, stroke, tumor, head trauma, hypoxia, alcohol withdrawal, and medically refractory epilepsy.

### 28. How does status epilepticus present?

Status epilepticus may present with convulsive or nonconvulsive seizure activity. The most common presentation, generalized convulsive seizure activity, is associated with high morbidity and mortality rates. Nonconvulsive status epilepticus may present subtly, with little or no motor activity and perhaps with mild impairment of consciousness. Careful observation and sometimes EEG are required to detect its presence. Nonconvulsive status epilepticus also may present with continuous simple partial seizures, including epilepsia partialis continua (continuous clonic focal motor activity).

### 29. What are the initial steps in managing a patient in status epilepticus in the ICU setting?

Establish and maintain the airway, and provide adequate ventilation. Monitor vital signs, including pulse oximetry and continuous ECG monitoring. Establish and maintain intravenous access. Perform rapid blood glucose assay to assess for hypoglycemia (a treatable cause or early sequela of status epilepticus). If the patient is hypoglycemic, administer glucose in the form of 50 ml of 50% dextrose (adult dosage) intravenously. Glucose should be preceded by thiamine, 100 mg IV, to prevent Wernicke's encephalopathy when alcohol withdrawal is the underlying cause. Perform a brief physical and neurologic examination, and attempt to establish the cause. Draw blood for laboratory evaluations to determine specific causes. Start AED therapy without delay.

### 30. What is the treatment for status epilepticus?

Treatment is designed to control seizures quickly and aggressively. Lorazepam, 0.1mg/kg IV, followed by phenytoin, 20mg/kg IV (adult dosages), is currently preferred by many neurologists for the initial pharmacologic treatment of status epilepticus. Lorazepam rapidly arrests the seizure, but it does not provide adequate long-term protection against recurrence. It may cause respiratory depression, hypotension, and impairment of consciousness. The addition of phenytoin, while its onset of action is slower, provides prolonged seizure protection after the initial convulsions have stopped.

Every hospital should have a treatment protocol for status epilepticus and physicians and nurses should be ready to implement it as needed. The figure below summarizes the AED protocol for status epilepticus that is currently used at the University of California, San Francisco Hospital and Medical Center.

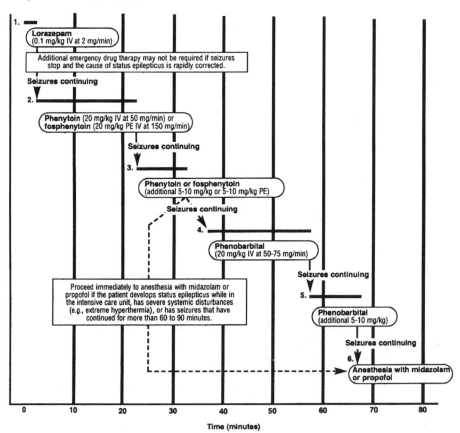

Antiepileptic drug therapy protocol for status epilepticus. IV = intravenous, PE = phenytoin equivalents. The horizontal bars indicate the approximate duration of drug infusions. (From Lowenstein DH, Alldredge BK: Status epilepticus. New Engl J Med 338:970–976, 1998, with permission. Copyright © 1998 Massachusetts Medial Society. All rights reserved.)

**31. What factors should be considered to ensure the safe administration of phenytoin and fosphenytoin in the treatment of status epilepticus?**

**Phenytoin** should be administered intravenously using a filter and mixed only with normal saline to avoid precipitation. The IV infusion rate should not exceed 50 mg/min to avoid significant hypotension and cardiac arrhythmias. Cardiac monitoring is required. Vital signs and neurological status should be assessed. Evaluate the IV site for patency, irritation, and extravasation.

**Fosphenytoin** is a water-soluble prodrug of phenytoin that may be used instead of phenytoin in the treatment of status epilepticus. Fosphenytoin dosages are expressed as phenytoin equivalents (PE). The main advantage of fosphenytoin is its ease in IV administration. It can be delivered in 5% dextrose in water or normal saline, does not require a filter, and is reported to have fewer infusion-site reactions than phenytoin. The maximal rate of infusion is 150 mg PE/min. Cardiac monitoring is required.

### BIBLIOGRAPHY

1. Commission on Classification and Terminology of the International League Against Epilepsy: Proposal for revised clinical and electroencephalographic classification of epileptic seizures. Epilepsia 22:489–501, 1981.
2. Engel J: Seizures and Epilepsy. Philadelphia, F.A. Davis, 1989.
3. Lowenstein DH: Seizures and epilepsy. In Fauci AS, et al (eds): Harrison's Principles of Internal Medicine, 14th ed. New York, McGraw-Hill, 1998, pp 2311–2325.
4. Lowenstein DH, Alldredge BK: Status epilepticus. N Engl J Med 338:970–976, 1998.
5. Marks WJ, Garcia PA: Management of seizures and epilepsy. Am Fam Physician 57:1589–1600, 1998.
6. Messing RO, Simon RP: Seizures as a manifestation of systemic disease. Neurol Clin 4:563–584, 1986.
7. Scheuer ML, Pedley TA: The evaluation and treatment of seizures. N Engl J Med 323:1468–1474, 1990.
8. Treatment of convulsive status epilepticus: Recommendations of the Epilepsy Foundation of America's Working Group on Status Epilepticus. JAMA 270:854–859, 1993.
9. Wyllie E (ed): The Treatment of Epilepsy, 2nd ed. Baltimore, Williams & Wilkins, 1997.

# 47. NEUROMUSCULAR DISORDERS: GUILLAIN-BARRE SYNDROME AND MYASTHENIA GRAVIS

*Siobhan* M. *Geary,* RN, MS

## GUILLAIN-BARRE SYNDROME

**1. What is Guillain-Barré syndrome (GBS)?**

GBS is an acute or subacute demyelinating polyneuropathy that affects primarily the motor component of the peripheral nerves (both cranial and spinal nerves). It is a self-limited disease that affects all ages and is thought to have an autoimmune cause.

**2. What factors predispose patients to develop GBS?**

Approximately 50–60% of patients with GBS have suffered a recent (within 1–3 weeks) respiratory or gastrointestinal infection caused by various pathogens (e.g., viruses or bacteria). In addition, 15% of patients have received a recent vaccination.

**3. Describe the pathophysiology of GBS.**

An immune-mediated response leads to destruction of the myelin sheath surrounding the axons of cranial and spinal nerves. Inflammation and edema of the cranial and spinal nerves also occur. The result is a loss of myelin and loss of the nerve's ability to transmit impulses, leading to a lack of motor movement. Remyelination occurs slowly.

## 4. What are the clinical manifestations of GBS?

GBS is characterized by areflexia and motor weakness. The initial clinical symptoms of GBS are usually paresthesias in the distal extremities, along with pain or stiffness in the proximal limbs, followed by a progressive weakness of the limbs, trunk, and cranial muscles. The weakness commonly begins in the legs, is symmetrical, and spreads in an ascending manner. As the disease progresses, the respiratory muscles often are involved. Other patterns of disease progression have been noted (e.g., descending GBS, pure motor GBS, and the Miller-Fisher variant of GBS), but they are not common. Other manifestations of GBS include autonomic dysfunction (blood pressure changes, dysrhythmias, ileus, urinary retention), fluid and electrolyte imbalances, sleep dysfunction, and pain.

## 5. What are the phases of GBS?

**Acute phase** (1–3 weeks): from the onset of the first symptom until the point of maximal deficit.

**Plateau phase** (days to weeks): little change in the neurologic exam.

**Recovery phase** (weeks to months): recovery of function as remyelination of damaged nerves occurs.

## 6. How is GBS diagnosed?

The diagnosis of GBS is made on clinical grounds, based on the acute onset of rapid and progressive weakness of both arms and legs, accompanied by areflexia. The diagnosis is supported by nerve conduction studies and electromyelograms showing evidence of a demyelinating polyneuropathy early in the course of the disease. Analysis of cerebrospinal fluid usually shows increased protein (about 7 days after onset of symptoms) without evidence of significant inflammatory cellular response. History of a recent infection supports the diagnosis.

## 7. Which patients with GBS require observation in the intensive care unit (ICU)?

ICU observation is required for patients with respiratory failure (due to weakness of the respiratory muscles) and/or patients with significant hemodynamic instability and cardiac disturbances (due to autonomic dysfunction). Patients with lower cranial nerve deficits affecting the ability to swallow and to protect the airway also may need ICU observation.

## 8. How is respiratory function monitored in patients with GBS?

Respiratory function is monitored at the bedside by measurements of vital capacity and maximal inspiratory and expiratory pressures. As vital capacity decreases, the patient's cough becomes weaker, and the patient may become dyspneic. Arterial blood gas (ABG) results are not a good measure of pulmonary function because they remain normal until respiratory weakness is severe. Patients are usually intubated when the vital capacity is less than 12–15 ml/kg of body weight, when maximal inspiratory pressure is less than –20 to –30 cm $H_2O$, when cranial nerve deficits are so severe that the patient cannot protect the airway, or when partial pressure of carbon dioxide rises and pH levels fall (respiratory acidosis). If the motor weakness progresses rapidly, early intubation may be considered.

## 9. How is GBS treated?

GBS is treated by either plasma exchange or high-dose intravenous immunoglobulin (IVIG). IVIG is easier to administer and costs less than plasma exchange; its use in the past was limited because its efficacy had not been determined. Recent studies have shown that the two therapies are equally effective in decreasing the number of days on a ventilator and the length of time until the patient can walk. Plasma exchange (removing 50 ml/kg of plasma on alternating days and replacing it with 5% albumin) should begin within 2 weeks of onset of disease to achieve maximal effectiveness.

## 10. What is the prognosis for GBS?

Prognosis for GBS is very good. Approximately 80–90% of patients recover with little or no neurologic sequelae. Mortality rates can be as high as 5–8%, with patients dying from the secondary effects of GBS. Mortality rates are higher among the elderly.

**11. What are the essential components of the nursing assessment for patients with GBS?**
- Neurologic function: monitor for increasing weakness, dysesthesias, and sensory changes.
- Respiratory function: monitor bedside pulmonary function tests; assess for accessory muscle use, dyspnea, signs and symptoms of pneumonia, weakening cough, hypoxemia, and ability to clear secretions and manage the airway
- Autonomic dysfunction: monitor for hypertension, orthostatic hypotension, electrocardiographic changes, cardiac dysrhythmias, abnormal hemodynamic responses to drugs, urinary retention, pupillary changes, sweating abnormalities, and gastrointestinal dysfunction.
- Pain: assess level of pain and patient's response to analgesics.
- Lab tests: assess electrolytes, ABGs.

**12. List important nursing interventions for the patient with GBS.**
- Aggressive pulmonary toilet
- Prophylaxis against deep venous thrombosis (DVT) (e.g., sequential compression devices, anticoagulants)
- Frequent turning and meticulous skin care
- Pain management and psychosocial support
- Communication strategies
- Maintenance of adequate nutrition
- Bowel and bladder care (try to prevent vagal stimulation by avoiding straining)
- Range-of-motion exercises, foot and hand splints

## MYASTHENIA GRAVIS

**13. What is myasthenia gravis (MG)?**
MG is a chronic, autoimmune disease of the neuromuscular junction characterized by muscle fatigue and weakness with repetitive activity. There are two peak incidences for the disease, depending on gender. The peak incidence for women is in the third decade; the female-to-male incidence is 4:1 before the age of 30. The peak incidence for men is in the fifth and sixth decades when the female-to-male ratio is 1:1.

**14. What are the two forms of MG?**
1. Generalized form (more common): involvement of any skeletal muscle.
2. Ocular form: involvement only of extraocular muscles.

**15. What other conditions are associated with MG?**
Patients with MG often have disorders of the thymus. Approximately 60% of patients have thymic hyperplasia, and another 10–15% have a thymoma. In addition, various autoimmune disorders are associated with MG.

**16. Describe the pathophysiology of MG.**
At the neuromuscular junction, acetylcholine (ACh) is released from the nerve ending after depolarization. It binds to the acetylcholine receptor (AChR) on the motor nerve to cause opening of the ion channel, which eventually leads to muscle fiber contraction. In MG, circulating antibodies to AChRs affect the transmission of nerve impulses at the neuromuscular junction by decreasing the number of receptor sites. Action potentials may not be generated, leading to decreased strength of the muscle contraction and muscle weakness.

**17. What are the clinical manifestations of MG?**
The onset of MG is usually gradual, and the course is variable, with periods of remission and exacerbation. MG is characterized by fatiguing weakness of striated muscle, and it has a predilection for extraocular and bulbar muscles. The patient often describes difficulty in sustaining muscle activity, which improves with rest.

**18. How is MG diagnosed?**

A strong suspicion of MG is based on the clinical findings described above. Confirmation is based on results of tests evaluating nerve and muscle function. For example, patients may be evaluated for signs and symptoms of improvement after the administration of edrophonium (Tensilon), a short-acting inhibitor of acetylcholinesterase, the enzyme that breaks down ACh. Patients also may be monitored for a progressive decrease in action potentials after repetitive electrical stimulation of a motor nerve. In addition, the presence of serum antibodies to AChR helps to confirm the diagnosis; they are present in 90% of patients with generalized MG.

**19. How is MG treated?**

1. Acetylcholinesterase inhibitors (e.g., pyridostigmine), which enhance the neuromuscular transmission of an impulse by preventing the degradation of ACh by acetyl cholinesterase
2. Long-term immunosuppression (e.g., prednisone, azathioprine, cyclosporine, cyclophosphamide)
3. Short-term immunomodulation (plasma exchange or IVIG)
4. Thymectomy

**20. What are the two most serious conditions associated with MG?**

Two conditions associated with MG can cause rapidly progressive weakness and respiratory failure. **Myasthenic crisis** is a severe worsening of MG. **Cholinergic crisis** is related to an overdose of acetylcholinesterase inhibitors and results in severe weakness due to continuous depolarization of the postsynaptic membrane, effectively creating a neuromuscular blockade. Cholinergic crisis usually is accompanied by excessive salivation, cramps, diarrhea, and blurred vision, and patients often have a history of an increase in pyridostigmine use. A test dose of edrophonium (Tensilon), a cholinesterase inhibitor, usually can differentiate the two conditions, but it may cause respiratory failure in cholinergic crisis. For this reason, emergency airway equipment should be available.

**21. Which patients with MG require ICU observation?**

Patients in a myasthenic crisis or cholinergic crisis should be monitored in the ICU, as should patients with respiratory muscle weakness, declining respiratory function, or difficulty in swallowing.

**22. What is the best way to assess respiratory function in patients with MG?**

Respiratory function is assessed using bedside pulmonary testing of vital capacity, maximal inspiratory flow, and maximal expiratory flow. The patient also should be assessed for signs and symptoms of respiratory difficulty.

**23. What conditions or agents can exacerbate MG?**

Infections, fever, stress, childbirth, surgery, and a number of medications (e.g., certain antibiotics, beta blockers, quinidine, certain antidepressants and anticonvulsants, procainamide).

**24. What specific nursing interventions are required for patients with MG?**

- Monitor respiratory function and perform respiratory toilet. Pay attention to the patient's ability to manage secretions.
- Perform neurologic assessment frequently, including cranial nerve assessment.
- Allow the patient to rest as much as possible. Always allow rest if you notice increased muscle weakness (e.g., new speech slurring, increased eye turning).
- Assess response to medications and monitor for side effects.
- Treat fevers and infections aggressively.
- Provide DVT prophylaxis.
- Monitor nutritional status.
- Provide family and patient support and communication strategies. Be aware that patients often know more about MG than you do.

## BIBLIOGRAPHY

1. Hickey JV (ed): The Clinical Practice of Neurological and Neurosurgical Nursing, 4th ed. Philadelphia, Lippincott-Raven, 1997.
2. Hund EF, Borel CO, Cornblath DR, et al: Intensive management and treatment of severe Guillain-Barré syndrome. Crit Care Med 21:433–446, 1993.
3. Kelly BJ: Landy-Guillain-Barré syndrome. In Parsons PE, Wiener-Kronish JP (eds): Critical Care Secrets, 2nd ed. Philadelphia, Hanley & Belfus, 1998, pp 340–342.
4. Kelly BJ: Myasthenia gravis. In Parsons PE, Wiener-Kronish JP (eds): Critical Care Secrets, 2nd ed. Philadelphia, Hanley & Belfus, 1998, pp 343–345.
5. Kernich CA, Kaminski HJ: Myasthenia gravis: Pathophysiology, diagnosis and collaborative care. J Neurosci Nurs 27:207–215, 1995.
6. Massey JM: Treatment of acquired myasthenia gravis. Neurology 48(Suppl 5):S46–S51, 1997.
7. Plasma Exchange/Sandoglobulin GBS Trial Group: Randomized trial of plasma exchange, intravenous immunoglobulin, and combined treatments in Guillain-Barré syndrome. Lancet 349:225–230, 1997.

# V. Gastroenterology and Renal Disease

# 48. NUTRITION ASSESSMENT AND CARE

*Colleen O'Leary-Kelley, RN, MS, CNSN*

### 1. What is the purpose of nutrition assessment?

A nutrition assessment is a comprehensive approach to determine nutritional status. It identifies patients who are undernourished or overnourished or at risk for developing malnutrition. After nutritional status is established, individual energy and protein requirements can be determined. Patients who are not expected to consume adequate nutrition may be started on enteral or parenteral nutrition support. Monitoring the efficacy of nutritional support is an additional goal of nutrition assessment.

### 2. What are the components of a nutrition assessment?

A nutrition assessment includes a complete history and physical examination, anthropometric measures, and biochemical tests. The history includes information about medical, social, and diet history. Signs of malnutrition and nutrient deficiencies are assessed during the physical examination. Body weight is the most commonly used anthropometric measure in hospitalized patients. Weight may be a less sensitive nutritional measure in patients with excessive fluid shifts after resuscitation. However, if hydration status is considered and weights are followed serially, they provide valuable information about changes in lean body mass.

### 3. Which lab tests are commonly used in nutritional assessment?

Common lab tests include albumin, prealbumin, transferrin, and retinol-binding protein. These visceral proteins are formed in the liver and correlate with body protein and energy status. Changes in levels of visceral proteins can be used collectively to determine nutritional status. They are influenced by nonnutritional factors such as intracellular fluid shifts and illness severity. As a result, no single test is used exclusively as a gold standard in nutritional assessment.

### 4. What is nitrogen balance?

Nitrogen balance is the difference between the amount of nitrogen ingested and the amount of nitrogen excreted. It is used to determine the adequacy of protein intake and is calculated as follows:

$$\text{Nitrogen balance} = [\text{protein intake (gm)}/6.25] - [\text{24-hour UUN (gm)} + 4]$$

where UUN = urinary urea nitrogen. One gram of nitrogen is equivalent to 6.25 gm of protein. Intake is calculated as the total amount of protein ingested divided by 6.25. Output is measured as the 24-hour total urinary nitrogen or urinary urea nitrogen plus a factor of 4 to account for nonurinary losses.

### 5. When are patients considered malnourished?

Patients are malnourished if intake is inadequate for more than 7 days or unintentional weight loss is more than 10% of usual weight. Patients with 85–90% of ideal body weight are considered mildly malnourished; with 75–84%, moderately malnourished; and with < 74%, severely malnourished. Patients with > 120% ideal body weight are considered overweight.

### 6. What complications are associated with malnutrition?

Malnourished patients have increased morbidity and mortality compared with adequately nourished patients. Malnutrition is related to wound infections, increased length of stay, delayed wound healing, and compromised immune function. Weaning from mechanical ventilation also may be delayed in malnourished patients.

### 7. How is the starvation of critical illness different from simple starvation?
Simple starvation is characterized by hypometabolism, which limits the loss of body protein as an energy source. The body adapts to starvation by gradually decreasing the need for glucose and begins to utilize fat and ketones for energy. Endogenous fat is the primary energy source. Hypermetabolism and catabolism leading to rapid loss of lean muscle mass characterize the stressed starvation associated with critical illness. Energy sources are derived from the break-down of endogenous protein and fat. The table below shows the differences between unstressed starvation and stress metabolism during critical illness:

*Comparison of Unstressed Starvation and Stress Metabolism*

|  | UNSTRESSED STARVATION | STRESS METABOLISM |
|---|---|---|
| Purpose | Conserve energy, preserve visceral proteins, and maintain vital organ function based on substrate demand and availability | Dynamic, changing process associated with marked alterations in metabolism that are difficult to suppress |
| Adaptive mechanisms | ↓ Resting metabolic rate<br>↓ Glucose utilization by CNS<br>Carbohydrates: gradual ↓ hepatic gluconeogenesis<br>Fat: ↑ utilization of fatty acids and ketones from fat catabolism<br>Protein: gradual ↓ urinary nitrogen excretion | ↑ Metabolic rate<br>↓ ↑ Body temperature<br>↑ Secretion of catecholamines, cortisol, and glucagon<br>↓ Serum insulin levels (in proportion to available glucose)<br>Carbohydrates: ↑ serum lactate and pyruvate levels, ↑ gluconeogenesis<br>Fat: ↑ serum free fatty acid levels<br>Protein: ↑ protein catabolism, ↑ urinary nitrogen excretion |
| Energy source | Glycogen stores depleted in first 6–12 hr<br>Fat: primary fuel | Amino acids: primary fuel<br>Fats: secondary fuel |

↓ = decreased, ↑ = increased, CNS = central nervous system.
From Leupold-DiCicco C, Monturo CA: Stress states: Trauma, burns, and sepsis. In Nutrition Support Nursing, Core Curriculum, 3rd ed. Silver Spring, MD, Aspen, 1996, pp 17–22, with permission.

### 8. What equations are used to determine energy requirements in critically ill patients?
One method of determining energy requirements is to provide 25–35 kcal for each kilogram of body weight. The **Harris-Benedict equation** also is used to estimate energy requirements:
Men: 66.47 + [13.75 × weight in kg] + [5.0 × height in cm] – [6.76 × age in yr]
Women: 655.1 + [9.56 × weight in kg] + [1.85 × height in cm] – [4.68 × age in yr]

Although used frequently, these equations are not accurate measures in critically ill patients. In an effort to increase accuracy, stress factors can be applied to the Harris-Benedict equation to account for disease and injury. The factors range from 1.2 for minor stress to 2.1 for severe stress. Use of the Harris-Benedict equation plus stress factors is associated with estimates in excess of actual energy requirements.

### 9. What is indirect calorimetry?
Indirect calorimetry is another method used to determine resting energy expenditure and energy requirements in critically ill patients. It can be performed using the gas exchange or Fick method.

### 10. Explain the gas exchange method of indirect calorimetry.
The gas exchange method of indirect calorimetry measures oxygen consumption ($VO_2$) and carbon dioxide production ($VCO_2$) to calculate resting energy expenditure through a series of equations. The measured resting energy expenditure can be used to determine energy needs.

Indirect calorimetry also can be used to calculate respiratory quotient (RQ), which is the ratio of $VCO_2$ to $VO_2$. RQ reflects the percent of fat and carbohydrate utilized by the body. Indirect calorimetry by gas exchange methods can be performed in both spontaneously breathing and mechanically ventilated patients using a device called an indirect calorimeter or metabolic cart.

## 11. What is the Fick method of indirect calorimetry?

The Fick method requires measurements using a pulmonary artery catheter and mixed venous blood samples to determine oxygen content and energy expenditure. The Fick method provides a reasonable estimate of energy requirements.

## 12. What are the clinical goals of nutrition support during critical illness?

Nutrition support includes enteral or parenteral formulas provided to patients who are unable to consume regular oral intake. The primary goal during critical illness is maintenance of nitrogen balance or minimization of additional nitrogen loss and nutrient deficiencies.

## 13. What are the recommended energy and protein requirements during critical illness?

*Metabolic Needs of Critically Ill Patients*

| COMPONENT | MODERATE STRESS | SEVERE STRESS |
| --- | --- | --- |
| Calories | Calculated REE | Calculated REE × 1.5 |
| Protein | 0.8–1.5 gm/kg/day | 1.5–2.5 gm/kg/day |
| Lipids | 20–30% of total calories (at least 2–6%; no more than 60%) | 20–30% of total calories (at least 2–6%; no more than 60%) |
| Nonprotein calorie-to-nitrogen ratio | 125–150:1 | 100:1 |
| Vitamins | RDA for water-soluble; 2–5 times RDA vitamin C; vitamin K weekly | 2 times RDA for water-soluble; 5–10 times RDA vitamin C; vitamin K weekly |
| Minerals | Twice weekly renal, magnesium, phosphorus, and calcium profiles | Daily renal and magnesium, biweekly phosphorus and calcium profiles; give zinc and copper empirically |

RDA = recommended daily allowance, REE = resting energy expenditure.
From Berry SM, Bower RH: Nutrition in critical illness and sepsis. In Torosian MH (ed): Nutrition for the Hospitalized Patient. New York, Marcel Dekker, 1995, p 382, with permission.

## 14. What are the advantages of enteral compared with parenteral nutrition support?

Enteral nutrition is the preferred route and is considered more physiologic than parenteral nutrition. It promotes gut motility and maintenance of intestinal barrier function. It may prevent translocation of bacteria from the gut, although this advantage has not been firmly established in human research. Enteral nutrition is less expensive and has fewer infectious and metabolic complications than parenteral nutrition.

## 15. When is enteral nutrition contraindicated?

Enteral nutrition should not be given in patients with intestinal obstruction or perforation, severe peritonitis, intractable vomiting, paralytic ileus, or severe diarrhea. Other contraindications include severe pancreatitis, enterocutaneous fistulas, gastrointestinal ischemia, and hemodynamic instability. The absence of bowel sounds is not a contraindication to enteral nutrition. Enteral feedings may be administered safely and absorbed into the duodenum or jejunum even when bowel sounds are not present.

## 16. What are the signs and symptoms of enteral feeding intolerance?

Manifestations of feeding intolerance include abdominal distention, nausea, vomiting, severe diarrhea, and abdominal discomfort.

**17. How can nurses reduce the risk of pulmonary aspiration in patients receiving enteral nutrition support?**

Pulmonary aspiration can be reduced or prevented by careful monitoring for signs of feeding intolerance. The head of the bed should be elevated to 30–45° during feeding. Postpyloric feeding with small-bore feeding tubes should be used when possible. Residuals should be checked every 4–6 hours initially, and feedings should be withheld for 1 hour with residuals > 150–200 ml. However, gastric residual amounts vary, depending on the rate of infusion. Prokinetic agents can be administered to promote gastric emptying. For patients with artificial airways, excessive secretions in the oropharynx should be suctioned frequently, and airway intracuff pressures should be maintained at 25 cmH$_2$O. Blue dye has been added to detect enteral formula in the airway. Glucose strips also have been used to detect the presence of formula in airway secretions. These practices do not differentiate oropharyngeal aspiration from aspiration of gastric feeding. Neither method is routine practice. Prevention of aspiration is preferred to detection after the fact.

**18. What is refeeding syndrome?**

Refeeding syndrome is defined as the metabolic complications that occur in malnourished patients who receive nutrition support after significant weight loss. Initiation of refeeding leads to a rapid change from catabolism to anabolism. Glucose becomes the primary fuel and insulin levels rise, promoting the shift of minerals and electrolytes into the cell. Rapid repletion with either enteral or parenteral nutrition promotes this intracellular shift, leading to depletion of serum levels of phosphorus, potassium, magnesium, and calcium. Patients may experience generalized muscle weakness, tetany, dysrhythmias, seizures, fluid retention, hemolytic anemia, and death due to cardiac or pulmonary failure. Clinicians must be aware of refeeding syndrome in patients who are at risk.

**19. How is refeeding syndrome prevented?**

1. Increase nutritional goals slowly during the first week.
2. Monitor and replace electrolytes aggressively.
3. Provide supplemental vitamins, especially thiamine.
4. Monitor closely for fluid overload and signs of congestive heart failure.

**20. What complications can develop in critically ill patients as a result of overfeeding?**

Overfeeding occurs when substrate is given in excess of requirements. It can stress the organ function of critically ill patients and potentially lead to serious complications. The complications associated with overfeeding include azotemia, hepatic steatosis, hypercapnia, hyperglycemia, hypertriglyceridemia, metabolic acidosis, and refeeding syndrome.

### BIBLIOGRAPHY

1. American Society for Parenteral and Enteral Nutrition Board of Directors: Guidelines for the use of parenteral and enteral nutrition in adult and pediatric patients. J Parent Ent Nutr 17(Suppl 4):5SA–11SA, 17SA, 1993.
2. Barton RG: Nutrition support in critical illness. Nutr Clin Pract 9:127–139, 1994.
3. Berry SM, Bower RH: Nutrition in critical illness and sepsis. In Torosian MH (ed): Nutrition for the Hospitalized Patient. New York, Marcel Dekker, 1995, p 382.
4. Brooks MJ, Melnik G: The refeeding syndrome: An approach to understanding its complications and preventing its occurrence. Pharmacotherapy 15:713–726, 1995.
5. Elpern EH: Pulmonary aspiration in hospitalized adults. Nutr Clin Pract 12:5–13, 1997.
6. Klein CJ, Stanek GS, Wiles CE: Overfeeding macronutrients to critically ill adults: Metabolic complications. J Am Diet Assoc 98:795–806, 1998.
7. Leupold-DiCicco C, Monturo CA: Stress states: Trauma, burns and sepsis. In Nutrition Support Nursing, Core Curriculum, 3rd ed. Silver Spring, MD, Aspen, 1996, pp 17–22.
8. McClave SA, Snider HL: Use of indirect calorimetry in clinical nutrition. Nutr Clin Pract 7:207–221, 1992.
9. Posa PJ: Nutritional support of the critically ill patient: Bedside strategies for successful patient outcomes. Crit Care Nurs Q 16:61–79, 1994.
10. Trujillo EB, Robinson MK, Jacobs DO: Nutritional assessment in the critically ill. Crit Care Nurse 19:67–78, 1999.

# 49.  DIARRHEA

*Colleen O'Leary-Kelley*, RN, MS, CNSN

### 1. What is the definition of diarrhea?

No single definition has been established for diarrhea. Current definitions include various stool frequencies, volumes, and weights. Diarrhea may be defined simply as several loose stools per day or, more specifically, as 500 ml of watery stool per day for two consecutive days. Regardless of how diarrhea is defined, the causes should be investigated and treated promptly to minimize complications. Complications include fluid, electrolyte, and nutrient losses and perianal skin breakdown, particularly for patients with limited mobility. The lack of a standard definition accounts for the wide range in reported incidence (32–62% in critically ill patients).

### 2. What are the most common causes of diarrhea?

Many factors associated with critical illness play a role in the etiology of diarrhea. The most common causes include antibiotics, enteric pathogens, and other medications, especially those containing sorbitol. The catabolic response and lack of nutrition associated with critical illness lead to atrophy of intestinal mucosa and reduced intestinal absorptive capacity. These conditions may subsequently cause diarrhea when enteral nutrition is initiated. Fecal impaction and bowel ischemia also may cause diarrhea.

### 3. What treatments are used to control diarrhea?

Initial treatment includes maintaining adequate hydration and limiting additional fluid and electrolyte losses. The rate of enteral infusion may be reduced, or the formula may be changed to a soluble fiber-containing formula. Gastric feeding is associated with diarrhea more often than intestinal feeding. Changing to duodenal feeding may decrease or eliminate diarrhea. An important aspect of treatment involves investigating the causative factors. Medications that promote diarrhea should be changed or discontinued. If diarrhea continues after enteric pathogens have been ruled out, antimotility drugs may be used. Pectin and banana flakes also have been used to decrease liquid stool and increase fecal mass.

### 4. How is low serum albumin related to diarrhea?

Hypoalbuminemia has been associated with the development of diarrhea, although a direct cause and effect relationship has not been established. Theoretically, a low serum albumin decreases intravascular oncotic pressure and impairs intestinal absorption, promoting formation of high volumes of liquid stool. Hypoalbuminemia may be more a sign of disease severity than a causative factor for diarrhea in critically ill patients.

### 5. What is *Clostridium difficile*?

*C. difficile* is an enteric pathogen that is a leading cause of diarrhea in hospitalized patients. *C. difficile* infection generally presents as colitis with moderate-to-profuse amounts of diarrhea. Patients taking antibiotics or with a recent history of antibiotic therapy are at particular risk. *C. difficile* infection is diagnosed by a positive toxin assay. Drugs that decrease gastric motility are contraindicated until infection is ruled out. The standard treatment for *C. difficile* infection is oral vancomycin in divided daily doses.

### 6. How can critical care nurses manage patients with diarrhea?

The first nursing priority is to determine the cause of diarrhea. Prevention of dehydration, electrolyte imbalance, skin breakdown and wound infection is also an essential aspect of care.

Emotional support and reassurance are needed during prolonged periods of diarrhea. Suggested interventions for the prevention and treatment of diarrhea are presented in the figure below.

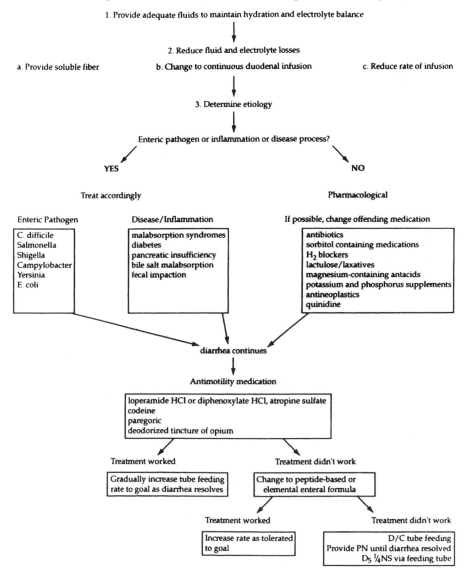

Treatment of diarrhea in tube-fed patients. (Reproduced with permission from the American Society for Parenteral and Enteral Nutrition (ASPEN) from Fuhrman MP: Diarrhea and tube feeding. Nutr Clin Pract 14:83–84, 1999.)

### 7. What methods are used to prevent and treat excoriation in patients with diarrhea?

Diarrheal stool contains digestive enzymes that cause local irritation, especially in patients with frequent loose stools. Keeping the skin clean and minimizing skin contact with stool are key principles of prevention and treatment. The skin should be cleaned gently with water and a pH-balanced agent, then gently dried. An ointment specially formulated to provide a barrier against moisture should be applied. For patients with large volumes of liquid stool, fecal incontinence devices may be applied directly to clean, dry skin or a barrier film surrounding the perianal area. The incontinence device can be attached to a gravity drainage bag to contain the liquid stool. For skin that is severely excoriated, gentle cleansing and application of ointment are recommended after each stool.

### BIBLIOGRAPHY

1. Bowling TE, Silk DBA: Diarrhea and enteral nutrition. In Rombeau JL, Rolandelli RH (eds): Clinical Nutrition: Enteral and Tube Feeding, 3rd ed. Philadelphia, W. B. Saunders, 1997, pp 540–553.
2. Emery EA, Ahmad S, Koethe JD, et al: Banana flakes control diarrhea in enterally fed patients. Nutr Clin Pract 12:72–75, 1997.
3. Fuhrman MP: Diarrhea and tube feeding. Nutr Clin Pract 14:83–84, 1999.
4. Ringel AF, Jameson GL, Foster ES: Diarrhea in the intensive care patient. Crit Care Clin 11:465–477, 1995.

# 50. FEEDING TUBES: PLACEMENT AND CARE

*Lisa Day, RN, PhD*

### 1. How is a feeding tube placed into the stomach?

The following technique is recommended in most basic nursing textbooks:

1. Sit the patient up in bed, and measure the tube from nose to ear and from ear to xyphoid process.

2. Flush about 5 ml of water through the tube to loosen the guidewire, and make sure that the guidewire pulls out easily.

3. Lubricate the end of the tube.

4. Begin by aiming for the back of the nostril with the patient's neck extended. Twirl the tube around if resistance is met at the nasopharyngeal junction.

5. As the tube advances down the back of the throat, the patient may begin to gag. At this point, flex the head forward and ask the patient to swallow as you gently float the tube down the esophagus and into the stomach.

6. It may be necessary to use a moist swab or, if the patient can tolerate it, ice chips to assist with swallowing.

### 2. What problems may be encountered in placing a feeding tube in the stomach?

Many ICU patients are not able to sit up in bed or swallow. Often they are endotracheally intubated and/or under the influence of neuromuscular blocking agents, sedatives, and narcotics. Under these circumstances the chance of placing a feeding tube into the lung is greatly increased. Furthermore, many physicians request postpyloric feeding tube placement to decrease the risk of aspiration. Given these circumstances, the technique for placing a nasogastric or nasoduodenal feeding tube must be modified.

### 3. Describe the modified technique for placing a feeding tube in the stomach.

The following is an adaptation of Ugo's technique for placing a small-bore feeding tube with a weighted tip in the stomach:

1. Measure the tube for the stomach and lubricate.

2. Position the patient supine with the head flexed forward and the head of the bed elevated as much as the patient will tolerate. Flexing the head decreases the chance of passing the tube into the trachea.

3. Advance the tube slowly as far as the stomach. Slow movement decreases the chance of kinking or knotting the tube.

If placement of the tube into the stomach is the goal, you can stop at this point.

### 4. What technique is used for placing the tube into the small bowel?

Small bowel placement also can be done at the bedside with the following technique:

1. Obtain a physician's order, and administer intravenously 20 mg metoclopramide hydrochloride (Reglan).

2. Thirty minutes after administrasiton of metoclopramide, follow the steps for placing the tube into the stomach (see question 3).

3. Once the tube is in the stomach, pump at least 150 ml of air through the tube. This technique distends the stomach and helps to move the tube through the pyloric sphincter.

4. Turn the patient onto his or her right side with the side as perpendicular to the bed as possible.

5. Try to get the patient as far onto the side as possible, using pillows or rolled-up blankets as props. The right side-lying position helps to move the tube by gravity.

6. Once the patient is positioned onto his or her side, attach a 60 ml syringe full of air to the feeding tube.

7. Begin advancing the tube slowly while injecting 10–20 ml of air with each small push.

8. If you are unable to inject air, the tube is kinked. Pull it back until air goes in easily, then start your advance over.

9. Go slow, about an inch with each advance, all the while injecting air.

10. Once you have about 3–4 inches of tube left, remove the guidewire and secure the tube to the patient's cheek or nose.

11. Confirm the position of the tube (see discussion in questions 6–12).

### 5. What are the major complications of feeding tube placement?

The two most dangerous complications are inadvertent placement of the tube into the trachea or lung and placement of the tube with the tip pointing back into the esophagus, which increases the risk of aspiration of stomach contents into the trachea. These complications can occur whenever a tube is placed blindly (i.e., without use of direct flouroscopy).

### 6. What is the most reliable way to confirm feeding tube position after blind placement? What are its disadvantages?

The most reliable way to confirm feeding tube position is by taking an abdominal flat-plate radiograph, which should be read by an experienced radiologist.

### 7. What are disadvantages of radiographic confirmation of feeding tube position?

All enteral medications and nutrition should be withheld until a radiographic report confirms that the tip of the tube is in the stomach or small bowel and not in the esophagus or lung. This approach can delay proper treatment of the patient; in addition, it is expensive and exposes the patient to radiation. Nonetheless, it may be the safest method for critically ill patients because it is the only sure way to determine in what part of the gastrointestinal tract the tube ends: esophagus, stomach, or small bowel.

### 8. What other technqiues are used to confirm feeding tube position?

The search for a reliable, inexpensive, and quick way to confirm tube position has led to the proposal of two promising methods. The second most reliable method is to test the pH of tube aspirate. The least reliable method is to auscultate the abdomen while injecting air through the tube.

### 9. How is pH testing used to confirm feeding tube position?

The pH of stomach fluid is lower than the pH of fluid from the lung. A pH < 5 indicates that the tube is in the stomach. This method has been successful even for patients taking hydrogen-receptor blockers for stress ulcer prevention (a common strategy in the intensive care unit [ICU]).

**10. What is a major disadvantage of pH testing?**

Unfortunately, pH testing is not a reliable way to distinguish between lung placement and small bowel placement because the pH of fluid from the small bowel is much less acidic than stomach fluid and therefore similar to lung fluid.

**11. How can this disadvantage be circumvented?**

Check the pH of the aspirate while the tube is still in the stomach, before advancing it into the intestine. A low pH at this point confirms placement in the gastrointestinal rather than the respiratory tract, and the tube can be safely advanced from the stomach.

Another suggestion is to test the pepsin and trypsin content of the aspirate. Lung fluid contains neither of these digestive enzymes, whereas pepsin (but not trypsin) is present in stomach fluid and trypsin (but not pepsin) is present in small bowel fluid. Measurement of enzyme levels as an adjunct to pH may be a good way to determine whether the feeding tube is in the lung, stomach, or small bowel. However, there is no easy bedside method for measuring enzyme levels, and the laboratory tests are not commonly done in hospitals.

**12. What is the role of auscultation in confirming tube position?**

An ICU nurse should *not* rely on auscultation alone to confirm feeding tube position. Skilled clinicians have been unable to distinguish the sound of air injected through a feeding tube into the stomach from the sound of air injected into the esophagus or lung. In the past, nurses relied on auscultation combined with observation of the patient's tolerance for the tube, based on the rationale that if the tube is in the lung, the patient will express some discomfort or acute respiratory distress. The auscultation and observation method for determining feeding tube position has come into disfavor in most ICUs. Because feeding tubes are small, patients sometimes tolerate lung misplacement without apparent discomfort, especially patients with decreased gag and cough reflexes. Given the fact that many ICU patients are sedated and/or under the influence of neuromuscular blocking agents, a misplaced tube may not be detected by this method until the patient has suffered extreme consequences.

**13. How can the nurse prevent a feeding tube from clogging?**

Most feeding tube occlusions occur when the tube is not flushed properly or when medications are administered through the tube improperly. Make sure that tablet forms of medications are crushed completely to a powder and thoroughly dissolved in warm water or normal saline. The solution must be sediment-free.

Following a standard plan for feeding tube maintenance also helps to prevent clogs, but many recommendations are not realistic for critically ill patients. For example, one plan suggests flushing the tube with 50–100 ml of water every 4 hours, before and after administering medications of any kind through the tube, after aspirating for residual volumes, and whenever tube feeding is stopped. This approach may prevent the tube from clogging, but it also may provide too much fluid in the form of free water to a patient with fluid overload or an electrolyte imbalance. If extra fluid is a concern, this plan can be adapted to use less fluid, but it is not clear how much is enough. If the patient's sodium is low, normal saline can be substituted for water.

**14. What should the nurse do if the feeding tube clogs?**

A clogged feeding tube can be reopened using carbonated cola, a solution of meat tenderizer, or a pancreatic enzyme solution. Meat tenderizer can be mixed with water to form a liquid solution but should not be used in patients who are allergic to papaya. Similarly, pancrealipase can be dissolved in water. First aspirate as much liquid as possible from the clogged tube. Flush at least 5 ml of declogging solution into the tube and clamp it. After 15 minutes, try to flush water or normal saline through the tube. If the tube is still clogged, take it out and replace it. Do *not* reinsert the guidewire to open a clogged tube.

## BIBLIOGRAPHY

1. Metheny N, McSweeney M, Wehrle MA, Wiersema L: Effectiveness of the auscultatory method in predicting feeding tube location. Nurs Res 39:262–267, 1990.
2. Metheny N, Reed L, Wiersema L, et al: Effectiveness of pH measurement in predicting feeding tube placement: An update. Nurs Res 42:324–331, 1993.
3. Metheny N, Stewart BJ, Smith L, et al: pH and concentrations of pepsin and trypsin in feeding tube aspirates as predictors of tube placement. J Parent Ent Nutr 21:279–285, 1997.
4. Metheny N, Wehrle MA, Wiersema L, Clark J: Testing feeding tube placement: Ausculataiton vs. pH method. Am J Nurs 98:37–43, 1998.
5. Ugo PJ, Mohler PA, Wilson GL: Bedside postpyloric placement of weighted feeding tubes. Nutr Clin Pract 7:284–287, 1992.
6. Webber-Jones J, Sweeney K, Winterbottom A, et al: How to declog a feeding tube. Nursing 92 22:62–64, 1992.

# 51. ACUTE PANCREATITIS

*KellyJane Harris*, RN, MS, CNS, CEN, CCRN

### 1. Describe the normal structure, location, and function of the pancreas.

The pancreas is located behind the stomach. The head of the pancreas sits in the concavity of the duodenum and is connected to the duodenum by one or two ducts. The tail lies against the spleen. The inferior vena cava, aorta, and hepatic artery are located near the head of the pancreas. It is structurally similar to the salivary glands, made up of small clusters of glandular epithelial cells. Pancreatic juice leaves the pancreas by way of the main pancreatic duct in the head of the pancreas. This duct joins with the common bile duct from the liver and gallbladder to become the common channel, which is surrounded by the sphincter of Oddi. The common channel enters the duodenum in a small raised area know as the ampulla of Vater.

The pancreas has **exocrine** and **endocrine** functions. The exocrine function is the release of enzymes: trypsin, lipase, and amylase. The acinar cells secrete these enzymes, which flow through the pancreatic duct to the duodenum. Trypsin breaks down proteins into amino acids. Lipase breaks down fat into fatty acids and phospholipids. Amylase breaks down carbohydrates into disaccharides and trisaccharides. Elastase is activated by trypsin and causes the dissolution of elastic fibers of blood vessels and ducts. The endocrine function is controlled by the islets of Langerhans. Alpha cells secrete glucagon, and beta cells secrete insulin.

### 2. What causes the inflammation of acute pancreatitis?

Acute inflammation of the pancreas results when the normally inactive enzymes in the pancreas are activated before secretion into the pancreatic duct. This process is usually associated with an obstruction, toxin, or trauma and leads to autodigestion. Damage to the cells results in release of more enzymes, which compounds the damage. Cytokine release leads to the **systemic inflammatory response syndrome** (SIRS).

Mild cases lead to interstitial edema of the pancreas and do not present with organ dysfunction. Severe acute pancreatitis may cause hemorrhage and necrosis. Approximately 80% of patients have **interstitial pancreatitis**; the remainder have the more severe form of **necrotizing pancreatitis**. Acute pancreatitis usually does not lead to chronic pancreatitis, but patients with chronic pancreatitis can have acute flare-ups.

### 3. What causes acute pancreatitis?

Alcohol abuse and biliary tract disease are the most common causes of acute pancreatitis (80%). Alcohol triggers excessive hydrochloric acid production in the gastrointestinal tract, which can cause spasm and inflammation at the sphincter of Oddi and obstruct the flow of enzymes. In biliary tract disease, duodenal contents back up into the pancreatic duct through the weakened sphincter, activating pancreatic enzymes. In elderly patients, gallstones are the primary cause because they obstruct normal enzyme flow. Other causes include blunt trauma, hyperparathyroidism, hypercalcemia, peptic ulcer disease, invasive procedures of the pancreas (e.g., endoscopic retrograde cholangiopancreatography [ERCP]), and medications (e.g., salicylates, corticosteroids, thiazides, propofol, pentamidine, sulfonamides, azathioprine, tetracycline, anticholinesterases, valproic acid, diuretics).

### 4. What are the signs and symptoms of acute pancreatitis?

The most common sign of acute pancreatitis is sudden onset of sharp abdominal pain, which may radiate to the back. It has been described as deep, visceral, and knife-like. Other signs and symptoms include nausea, vomiting, bloating, fever, tachycardia, dyspnea, hypotension, restlessness, and confusion. If the abdominal vasculature becomes involved, peritonitis or hemorrhage may result.

### 5. What is the significance of Ranson's criteria in patients with pancreatitis?

Ranson's criteria predict the severity of acute pancreatitis. Patients with fewer than three criteria have a predicted mortality rate of 1%. When three or four criteria are present, the mortality rate increases to 15–20%; when five or six criteria are present, it increases to 40%; and when more than six criteria are present, the mortality rate is higher than 50%. Ranson's criteria are based on the following data.

**On admission**
Age > 55 years
White blood cell (WBC) count > 16,000 cell/mm$^3$
Serum glucose > 200 mg/dl
Lactate dehydrogenase (LDH) > 350 IU/L
Aspartate aminotransferase (AST) > 250 U/L
**24–48 hours later**
10% decrease in hematocrit
Increase > 5 mg/dl in blood urea nitrogen
Serum calcium < 8 mg/dl
Base deficit > 4 mEq/L
Partial pressure of oxygen in arterial blood (PaO$_2$) < 60 mmHg
Estimated fluid sequestration > 6 L

### 6. What are Grey-Turner spots and Cullen's sign?

Grey-Turner spots (also known as Turner's sign) are bluish discolorations of the left flank. Cullen's sign is bluish discoloration of the periumbilical area. These signs may be seen in severe hemorrhagic pancreatitis and represent the presence of peritoneal fluid, which is blood-stained. They are seen in less than 3% of patients with acute pancreatitis.

### 7. What laboratory tests help to diagnose acute pancreatitis?

Serum levels of amylase and lipase are the hallmark tests for acute pancreatitis. The normal **serum amylase** level is 35–115 U/L. In acute pancreatitis, amylase levels may be higher than 300 U/L. In patients with gallstone pancreatitis, amylase values may be higher than 1000 IU/L. The amylase level usually rises within 12 hours after onset of symptoms, peaks within 20–30 hours, and returns to normal within 3–5 days. **Serum lipase** is more specific to acute pancreatitis. Normal values are 32–80 U/L. Lipase rises after 24 hours of illness. Because they may remain elevated for up to 14 days, serum lipase levels help to make a late diagnosis. Amylase and lipase values do not correlate with the severity of the pancreatitis.

WBC count increases in 80% of patients with pancreatitis in response to the inflammatory process. Serum glucose increases in severe cases because of the damage to pancreatic beta cells.

This damage impairs carbohydrate metabolism and may lead to diabetes mellitus. LDH and AST may be increased in the presence of alcoholic liver disease and acute pancreatitis associated with cholelithiasis. Serum calcium is decreased in severe disease as a result of hypoalbuminemia and altered fat metabolism because calcium binds to both proteins and free fatty acids.

### 8. What imaging modalities help to diagnose acute pancreatitis?

Computed tomography (CT) of the abdomen shows pancreatic fluid collections, abscesses, and necrosis. Plain films visualize perforated viscera and calcification in the pancreas as well as lower lobe pneumonia. The "sentinel loop" of small intestine with paralytic ileus may be visualized in the left upper quadrant of the abdomen. Ultrasound is used to visualize gallstones, dilation of the common bile duct, and ascites. ERCP usually is not done to diagnose acute pancreatitis, but it is used to locate and remove gallstones from the common bile duct in patients with pancreatitis due to gallstones.

### 9. What are the potential complications of acute pancreatitis?
- Hypovolemic shock
- Pancreatic fistula
- Pancreatic pseudocysts
- Pancreatic abscess
- Primary infections
- Secondary infections
- Pulmonary complications
- Disseminated intravascular coagulation

### 10. What causes hypovolemic shock? How is it managed?

Hypovolemic shock is caused by large fluid shifts from the intravascular space to the peritoneal and interstitial spaces. Up to 6 liters of fluid can be lost in the first 48 hours. Vomiting, diarrhea, nasogastric suction, and hemorrhage may contribute to the fluid loss. Hypoalbuminemia due to protein losses and nutritional problems may lead to third spacing of fluids and edema formation. Shock can cause hypoperfusion of the organs and lead to multiple organ dysfunction syndrome (MODS).

Aggressive fluid replacement is the initial therapy. If a patient does not respond to fluid therapy and is hemodynamically unstable, a pulmonary artery catheter may be placed to assess hemodynamic patterns and evaluate the effectiveness of interventions.

### 11. What is a pancreatic fistula? How is it managed?

A pancreatic fistula is an abnormal passage of pancreatic juice through a pancreatic ductal disruption that exits the pancreatic parenchyma. Fistulas can enter the peritoneal or retroperitoneal cavities or remain totally within the capsule of the pancreas. They are treated by endoscopic drainage or drainage through percutaneous, transenteric, or transpapillary catheters. After 4–8 weeks, when the inflammatory process has subsided, the portion of the pancreas containing the site of ductal disruption may be resected.

### 12. What are pancreatic pseudocysts? How are they managed?

Pancreatic pseudocysts are collections of pancreatic juices enclosed by a wall of fibrous granulation tissue. The wall lacks an epithelial lining and, therefore, is not a true cyst. Pseudocysts usually take about 4 weeks to form from pancreatic fluid collections. They usually remain sterile. If they become infected, they are treated as pancreatic abscesses. About 25–50% of pseudocysts resolve spontaneously if they remain sterile. Interventional radiologic catheter drainage of pseudocysts is avoided to prevent the possible introduction of a secondary infection. Operative intervention is avoided until after the pseudocyst is mature (e.g., after approximately 6 weeks) when a wall of granulated tissue is available for anastomosis.

### 13. What is a pancreatic abscess? How is it managed?

A pancreatic abscess is composed of pus with little or no necrosis. The abscess may erode through the retroperitoneum into the bowel, pleural space, mediastinum, or pelvis. Such erosion can lead to sepsis and death if left untreated. The development of pancreatic abscesses results in a doubling of the mortality rate. They are treated similarly to infected necrosis of the pancreas—with drainage and/or debridement.

### 14. In what setting do most primary infections occur? How are they treated?

Most primary infections occur in the presence of necrotizing pancreatitis. A patient with sterile pancreatic necrosis may wait up to 4 weeks to have a necrosectomy, when demarcation is evident for debridement. A necrosectomy is done if clinical evidence indicates that the necrosis is infected or if CT-guided aspiration reveals infected pancreatic or peripancreatic tissue. Open-packing or closed lavage drainage may be used in the operating room after a necrosectomy. Large volume irrigation or irrigation with sodium oxychlorosene also may be used. Usually 2–4 Davol drains are placed, although suction is not used longer than 5 days because of potential damage to surrounding tissues. A CT scan or an interventional radiologic procedure is done after a necrosectomy to visualize any remaining areas of necrosis or fluid collections. A percutaneous catheter can be placed to drain remaining fluid collections.

### 15. What causes secondary infections? How are they treated?

Translocation of bacteria from the colon is the leading cause of secondary infection in patients with necrotizing pancreatitis. The use of an antibiotic that is effective against enteric bacteria and that penetrates pancreatic tissue is more successful than the use of broad-spectrum antibiotics.

### 16. What pulmonary complications may result from acute pancreatitis? How are they managed?

Pulmonary complications range from hypoxemia to acute respiratory distress syndrome (ARDS). Pancreatic enzymes released into the circulation damage pulmonary vasculature and stimulate inflammation, which causes intrapulmonary shunt and hypoxemia. Exudate crosses the diaphragm and enters the pleural space via lymphatic channels, causing pleural effusions. Pulmonary compliance is decreased by pain, pleural effusions, abdominal distention, ileus, and a subdiaphragmatic inflammatory process. Fifty to seventy percent of patients with severe acute pancreatitis develop major respiratory complications. Most patients require oxygen therapy, and patients with severe acute pancreatitis may require mechanical ventilation with positive end expiratory pressure (PEEP).

### 17. What causes disseminated intravascular coagulation (DIC)?

DIC is caused by pancreatic inflammation, which prevents absorption of vitamin K from the gastrointestinal tract. Vitamin K deficiency inhibits coagulation of blood.

### 18. What nursing assessments and interventions are appropriate for patients with acute pancreatitis?

1. Assess level of consciousness. Monitor for confusion and hallucinations caused by electrolyte abnormalities or medications.

2. Pulmonary assessment includes listening to lung sounds and monitoring pulse oximetry ($SpO_2$). Bronchial breath sounds can indicate pleural effusion. Atelectasis and pneumonia can develop from hypoventilation associated with abdominal pain, immobility, and ascites. Decreased breath sounds and hypoxemia accompany atelectasis or pneumonia. Tachypnea can be caused by pain, anxiety, and increased metabolic demands related to SIRS. Frequent turning and repositioning may improve ventilation/perfusion mismatch. Encouragement of incentive spirometry and deep breathing can promote lung expansion and decrease atelectasis.

3. Monitor for cardiac and hemodynamic instability. Assess heart rate, blood pressure, peripheral pulses, capillary refill, and skin signs. If a patient becomes hemodynamically unstable, a pulmonary artery catheter may be placed. The nurse then can monitor central venous pressure, pulmonary arterial wedge pressure, and cardiac output.

4. Provide pain relief. Edema of the pancreas, obstruction of the biliary tree, and release of pancreatic enzymes into the pancreas and surrounding tissues cause pain. Historically, meperidine

was the drug of choice because it was thought not to cause spasm of the sphincter of Oddi. Now its use is controversial because it can induce seizures in patients with renal insufficiency. A long-acting somatostatic analog, such as ocreotide, may be effective in relieving pain that is unrelieved by opioids. Monitor the intensity of pain on a scale of 0–10 before and after pain medication is given to evaluate its effectiveness.

5. Assess fluid status. Hypovolemia induces the release of renin, angiotensin, and aldosterone, which leads to constriction of blood vessels and retention of sodium and water. The posterior pituitary gland also responds to the hypovolemia by releasing antidiuretic hormone, which also leads to retention of sodium and water. Therefore, it is important to monitor for edema and third-spaced fluid. In addition, assess for signs of hemorrhage. Grey-Turner spots and Cullen's sign indicate hemorrhagic pancreatitis. Monitor hematocrit and hemoglobin. Intake and output measures should be done every 2 hours while the patient is compromised or more frequently if indicated.

6. Assess blood sugar levels frequently to monitor for transient hyperglycemia. Monitor serum electrolytes to ensure replacement therapy is instituted when appropriate.

7. Assess skin integrity, which may be impaired by prolonged bed rest. Change patient position frequently, and assess dependent areas for signs of redness and irritation. Monitor for bruising caused by altered coagulation.

8. Treat nausea and vomiting, which are common complications caused by hypermotility or paralytic ileus secondary to altered blood flow. Most patients have a nasogastric tube to decrease the abdominal distention caused by paralytic ileus. Inspect the abdomen for distention, auscultate for bowel sounds, and palpate for ascites. Measure abdominal girth. Monitor nasogastric output for volume, pH, and characteristics. Monitor stools for malabsorption. Foul-smelling, fatty stools result from the pancreatic insufficiency and decreased lipase release from damaged pancreatic tissue.

9. Assess urine output hourly. It should be greater than 30 ml/hr. If the patient is not fully fluid-resuscitated, hypovolemia may lead to renal hypoperfusion and acute renal failure.

10. Assess all drains and invasive catheter sites for redness, drainage, and warmth. Maintain strict aseptic technique when caring for invasive catheters, drains, or wounds. Obtain cultures if signs or symptoms of infection are present.

11. Assess nutritional effectiveness by monitoring daily weight and tolerance of enteric feeding and total parenteral nutrition (TPN). Collaborate with the multidisciplinary team, including physician and dietitian, to determine the best nutritional regimen for the patient.

12. Assess the patient's knowledge and coping skills as well as the readiness of patient and family for receiving pertinent information. Assess social support, and give psychological support as needed. Refer to social services or support groups such as Alcoholics Anonymous if the patient has alcohol-induced pancreatitis.

### 19. Why are patients with acute pancreatitis at risk for developing acute respiratory distress syndrome (ARDS)?

The release of enzymes during acute pancreatitis causes damage to alveoli and pulmonary vasculature. Phospholipids hydrolyze surfactant in the alveoli. Levels of circulating free fatty acids (FFAs) are elevated by increased fat metabolism due to activation of lipase. FFAs damage the pulmonary capillary membrane, and noncardiogenic pulmonary edema develops. The criteria for ARDS are refractory hypoxemia ($PaO_2/FiO_2$ ratio $< 200$), bilateral infiltrates on chest radiograph, and no evidence of left-sided cardiac dysfunction.

### 20. What electrolyte disturbances are common in patients with acute pancreatitis?

Hypokalemia may be evidenced by hypotension, muscle weakness, apathy, confusion, paralytic ileus, and cardiac arrhythmias. It may be caused by fluid losses or nasogastric suction. Potassium should be replaced to a level above 3.5 mEq/L. The signs and symptoms of hypomagnesemia are hypotension, tachycardia, confusion, tremors, twitching, tetany, and hallucinations. When assessing for hypocalcemia, check for Chvostek's sign (facial twitching on tapping of the parotid gland), Trousseau's sign (carpopedal spasm on application of blood pressure cuff or tourniquet on the upper arm), and prolonged QT on the electrogram. Hypoalbuminemia deficiencies are common during the acute phase because of fluid shifts and excessive fluid replacement volume.

## 21. Describe the nutritional needs of patients with pancreatitis.

Patients with acute pancreatitis may develop severe nutritional problems related to hypermetabolism and catabolism. Nausea, vomiting, and anorexia lead to decreased food intake. Patients typically must avoid oral ingestion during the acute phase of the disease to reduce pancreatic enzyme release. A nasogastric tube may be placed to decompress the stomach if a paralytic ileus develops or to prevent aspiration of gastric contents in severe cases.

Alcoholic patients may have baseline malnutrition. Patients have greater caloric needs during acute pancreatitis because of increased metabolic demands caused by cytokine release and the neuroendocrine response to injury. Patients typically receive TPN or enteral feedings if oral intake is delayed more than 7 days. Lipids should be included in TPN unless the triglyceride levels are elevated above 500 mg/dl. When oral feeding is resumed, a low-fat, low-protein, high-carbohydrate diet may be started. Stool is usually monitored for fecal fat. Occasionally patients require pancreatic enzyme replacements to aid digestion.

## BIBLIOGRAPHY

1. Ambrose MS, Dreher HM: Pancreatitis: Managing a flare-up. Nursing 4:33–39, 1996.
2. Banks PA: Practice guidelines in acute pancreatitis. Am J Gastroenterol 3:377–386, 1997.
3. Batterden RA: Interventions for clients with problems of the gallbladder and pancreas. In Ignataviticus DD, Mishler MA, Workman ML (eds): Medical-Surgical Nursing: A Nursing Process Approach, 2nd ed. Philadelphia, W.B. Saunders, 1995, pp 1714–1723.
4. Bradley EL: Pancreatic abscess. In Cameron JL (ed): Current Surgical Therapy, 6th ed. St. Louis, Mosby, 1998, pp 502–506.
5. Coyne PJ: Assessing and treating the pain of pancreatitis. Am J Nurs 11:14–15, 1998.
6. Franklin CM, Darovic GO, Dan BB: Monitoring the patient in shock. In Darovic GO (ed): Hemodynamic Monitoring: Invasive and Noninvasive Application, 2nd ed. Philadelphia, W.B. Saunders, 1995, pp 463–478.
7. Goodley CD, Rattner DW: Pancreatic pseudocyst. In Cameron JL (ed): Current Surgical Therapy, 6th ed. St. Louis, Mosby, 1998, pp 507–509.
8. Mayer KL, Ho HS, Frey CF: Acute pancreatitis. In Cameron JL (ed): Current Surgical Therapy, 6th ed. St. Louis, Mosby, 1998, pp 487–493.
9. Meissner JE: Caring for patients with pancreatitis. Nursing 10:50–51, 1997.
10. Moss M, Goodman PL, Heinig M, et al: Establishing the relative accuracy of three new definitions of the adult respiratory distress syndrome. Crit Care Med 25:1538–1544, 1995.
11. Noone J: Acute pancreatitis: An Orem approach to nursing assessment and care. Crit Care Nurs 8:27–35, 1995.
12. Ruth-Sahd LA: Acute pancreatitis. Am J Nurs 6:38–39, 1996.
13. Smolen D: Structure and function of the liver, biliary tract, and exocrine pancreas. In Black JM, Matassarin-Jacobs E (eds): Medical-Surgical Nursing: Clinical Management for Continuity of Care, 5th ed. Philadelphia, W.B. Saunders, 1997, pp 1921–1929.
14. Traverso LW, Newman RM, Kozarek RA: Pancreatic ductal disruptions leading to pancreatic fistula, pancreatic ascites or pleural effusion. In Cameron JL (ed): Current Surgical Therapy, 6th ed. St. Louis, Mosby, 1998, pp 510–514.

# 52. LIVER DYSFUNCTION AND FAILURE

*Margaret M. Sullivan, RN*

### 1. How are liver dysfunction and failure classified?

Liver dysfunction is categorized as either acute or chronic. **Acute liver failure** is a sudden, severe impairment of hepatocyte function resulting in jaundice followed by encephalopathy in the absence of prior liver disease. Acute liver failure is divided into two categories: **fulminant hepatic failure** (FHF) and **subfulminant hepatic failure**. In FHF, hepatic encephalopathy develops within 8 weeks of onset of illness. In Sub-FHF, hepatic encephalopathy develops within 8 weeks to 6 months after the onset of illness.

**Chronic liver failure** is a result of ongoing hepatic inflammation and necrosis over 6 months or longer with persistent or intermittent elevation of alanine aminotranferase (ALT) levels. It is subdivided into **chronic persistent hepatitis** (CPH), **chronic lobular hepatitis** (CLH), and **chronic active hepatitis** (CAH). Since CPH and CLH do not progress to cirrhosis, this chapter discusses CAH as it relates to chronic liver failure.

### 2. What causes fulminant and subfulminant hepatic failure?

The most common causes are viral hepatitis A or B and acetaminophen toxicity. Other causes include autoimmune hepatitis, cytomegalovirus, herpes simplex virus, Wilson's disease, venoocclusive disease, orthoptic liver transplant with nonfunction of the primary graft, acute fatty liver of pregnancy, and ischemic injuries related to cardiogenic or hypovolemic shock, chronic right heart failure, and, in some cases, heat stroke. In Northern California the *Amanita phalloides* mushroom is a somewhat frequent cause of FHF during the rainy winter months. Both experienced and novice mushroom pickers have succumbed to FHF after ingesting *Amanita phalloides*.

### 3. What causes chronic liver failure?

The most common causes are viral hepatitis B, C, and D and alcoholic liver disease. Other causes include nonalcoholic fatty liver, hemochromatosis (iron overload), Wilson's disease (copper deposition), primary biliary cirrhosis, autoimmune chronic active hepatitis, primary sclerosing cholangitis, Budd-Chiari syndrome, and congestive heart failure. Some of these diseases are asymptomatic for many years, and the diagnosis is not made until liver function deteriorates to end-stage failure.

### 4. How is liver failure and dysfunction diagnosed?

Liver dysfunction is diagnosed by assessing liver function and coagulation tests along with clinical assessment. Test results vary and help to differentiate between FHF and chronic liver failure. Liver function tests evaluate hepatic cell integrity as well as excretory and synthetic function. (See table on pages 286–287 for interpretation of liver function tests.)

### 5. What are the complications of fulminant hepatic failure?

The patient with FHF may have some or all of the following complications: altered mental status, cerebral edema, coagulopathy, acute renal failure, sepsis, hemodynamic abnormalities, and metabolic disorders. Many of the complications of liver failure are directly related to abnormal function of the liver.

### 6. How do complications of chronic liver failure differ from those of FHF?

In chronic liver failure, complications typically occur at end stages of the disease. The same complications as FHF may occur, with the exception of cerebral edema. Other complications related to end-stage liver cirrhosis are portal hypertension, which causes ascites and varices; spontaneous bacterial peritonitis; and hepatorenal syndrome.

*Interpretation of Liver Function Tests*

**Cellular Integrity**

| TRANSAMINASES (INTRACELLULAR ENZYMES) | NORMAL (0–50 U/L) | MILD ELEVATION (50–400 U/L) | MODERATE ELEVATION (400–2000 U/L) | HIGH ELEVATION (2000–10,000 U/L) |
|---|---|---|---|---|
| Cellular injury causes release into serum<br>Alanine aminotransferase (ALT; relatively liver-specific)<br>12–59 U/L<br><br>Aspartate aminotransferase (AST; found in multiple organs; elevated in myocardial infarction, rhabdomyolysis; for liver injury, useful when interpreted with ALT)<br>16–41 U/L | Cirrhosis<br>Hemochromatosis<br>Alcoholic hepatitis | Drug-induced hepatic injury<br>Total parenteral nutrition<br>Autoimmune hepatitis<br>Intrahepatic tumor<br>Extrahepatic obstruction<br>Budd-Chiari syndrome<br>Venoocclusive disease<br>Congestive heart failure | Toxins<br>Ischemia<br>Acute biliary obstruction | Fulminant hepatic failure<br>Acetaminophen toxicity<br>Shock liver<br>Mushroom toxicity |

**Protein Synthesis**

| | | | | |
|---|---|---|---|---|
| Prothrombin time (PT): 11–14.5 seconds<br>International normalized ratio (INR): 0.8–1.2 | Short half-life of prothrombin makes PT a sensitive indicator for liver function | Elevation may be due to:<br>1. Inadequate supply of vitamin K<br>2. Liver parenchymal disease | To correct treat with vitamin K and/or fresh frozen plasma:<br>If PT decreases but does not correct: chronic hepatocellular disease, cirrhosis<br>In FHF, if PT is unresponsive to treatment, prognosis is poor | |
| Albumin<br>3.4–4.7 g/dl | Neither sensitive nor specific for liver disease; half-life: 15–20 days | Level reflects:<br>• Rate of synthesis<br>• Degradation rate | Useful in measuring progression of longstanding disease | |

**Excretory Values**

| MEASUREMENT | NORMAL | MILD ELEVATION | MODERATE ELEVATION | HIGH ELEVATION |
|---|---|---|---|---|
| Total bilirubin-<br><br>Conjugated and unconjugated bilirubin | 0.3–1.3 mg/dl<br><br>Hepatitis: chronic, auto-immune, viral | 1.4–4 mg/dl<br><br>Decompensated chronic liver disease<br>Early acute hepatitis<br>TPN<br>Biliary obstruction | 4–10 mg/dl<br><br>Acute hepatitis<br>Primary biliary cirrhosis<br>Primary sclerosing cholangitis | 10–50 mg/dl<br><br>End-stage liver disease<br>Hepatic sickle crisis<br>Acute hepatitis |
| Direct bilirubin<br><br>Unconjugated; does not cause rubinbilirubinuria | 0.1–0.3 mg/dl | 0.3–4 mg/dl<br><br>Hemolysis<br>Rifampin<br>Gilbert syndrome | 4–10 mg/dl<br><br>Hemolysis | > 10 mg/dl<br><br>Hepatic sickle crisis |
| Alkaline phosphatase (present in bile)<br><br>Present in bile canaliculi of hepatocytes; increased production by hepatocytes in biliary obstruction | 29–111 U/L<br><br>Chronic viral/autoimmune liver disease | 200–700 U/L<br><br>Primary biliary cirrhosis, cholangitis<br>Intrahepatic tumor<br>Extrahepatic obstruction | | > 700 U/L<br><br>Primary biliary cirrhosis<br>Primary sclerosing cholangitis<br>Sarcoidosis<br>Hepatic lymphoma |
| Gamma-glutamyl transpeptidase<br><br>Enzyme assists the transfer of amino acids across the cell membrane.<br>Highly concentrated in biliary ducts and canaliculi<br>More sensitive to biliary obstruction than alkaline phosphatase | 7–71 U/L<br><br>Genetic hemochromatosis<br>Cirrhosis | 250–500 U/L<br><br>Acute and chronic alcohol ingestion<br>Drugs<br>Chronic viral or auto-immune liver disease | 500–1000 U/L<br><br>Primary biliary cirrhosis, cholangitis<br>Intrahepatic tumor<br>Extrahepatic obstruction<br>Alcoholic hepatitis | > 1000 U/L<br><br>Primary biliary cirrhosis<br>Primary sclerosing cholangitis<br>Sarcoidosis<br>Hepatic lymphoma<br>Candidiasis |

### 7. What causes altered mental status in liver failure and dysfunction?

Altered mental status in patients with liver dysfunction may be caused by a number of conditions, including sepsis, uremia, intracranial hemorrhage, cerebral edema and increased intracranial pressure (ICP), hypoglycemia, hypercapnia, and drug intoxication. If these potential causes are ruled out, the likely cause is hepatic encephalopathy.

### 8. What causes hepatic encephalopathy?

Hepatic encephalopathy is a complex neuropsychiatric disorder related to metabolic abnormalities that occur only with significant liver dysfunction. The pathogenesis of hepatic encephalopathy is unclear, and no single cause has been found. Altered mental status may be related to decreased hepatic metabolism of nitrogenous waste byproducts and toxins from the blood and brain. The collateral vessels that develop because of portal hypertension shunt blood flow away from functioning cells in the liver. This shunting leads to an accumulation of substances such as ammonia, aromatic amines, and gamma aminobutyric acid, all of which have sedative properties and inhibit normal neurotransmission. Hepatic encephalopathy is exacerbated by ingestion of protein-rich food, gastrointestinal (GI) bleeding, infections, and severe fluid depletion related to overdiuresis. Although much attention is paid to monitoring ammonia levels, it is important to assess response to treatment with clinical evaluation of mental status.

### 9. How is encephalopathy graded?

There are two forms of encephalopathy in patients with liver dysfunction: subclinical and overt. In **subclinical encephalopathy**, which is identified by electrophysiologic and psychomotor tests, there is no change in level of consciousness. **Overt encephalopathy** is characterized as a change in mental status and/or movement disorders such as asterixis, hyperreflexia, muscle rigidity, extensor plantar response, parkinsonian features, and decerebrate posturing. Patients with FHF present with overt encephalopathy. Encephalopathy is graded from I to IV to assess the patient's mental state and neuromuscular response (see table below).

|  | MENTAL STATE | NEUROMUSCULAR RESPONSE |
|---|---|---|
| Grade I | Euphoria, mild confusion, slowness of mentation, slurred speech | Normal tone and reflexes, slight asterixis |
| Grade II | Accentuation of grade I, drowsy but speaking, inappropriate behavior | Asterixis easily elicited, reflexes brisk, muscle tone increased |
| Grade III | Sleeps most of time but arousable, incoherent or no speech, marked confusion | Asterixis if cooperative, upgoing extensor plantar clonus, localized flexion response to pain |
| Grade IVA | Responds to painful stimuli | Asterixis usually absent, sustained clonus, decerebrate posturing to pain |
| Grade IVB | No response to painful stimuli | No response |

### 10. What medications are used to treat encephalopathy?

Treatment is aimed at reducing ammonia toxicity. Lactulose, a disaccharide combination of lactose and galactose, draws ammonia from the blood into the bowel to be excreted in stool. Aminoglycoside antibiotics, such as neomycin, are used to inhibit ammonia-forming bacteria in the gastrointestinal tract. Short-term enteral antibiotics, in conjunction with lactulose, usually are administered in the inpatient setting. Patients should be monitored for nephrotoxicity and ototoxicity. Lactulose generally is not used for patients with FHF.

Patients with grade IV encephalopathy related to cerebral edema should be treated as any patient with increased ICP. Hyperventilation, osmotic diuresis, and drug-induced coma to reduce cerebral metabolism are common therapeutic interventions.

**11. What nursing interventions are important for patients with grade IV coma or cerebral edema?**

Cerebral edema occurs in 75% of patients with grade IV encephalopathy. A fiberoptic intracranial catheter is placed to monitor ICP and cerebral perfusion pressure (CPP). In caring for such patients, the following guidelines are important:

1. Monitor neurologic status every hour.

2. Keep CPP above 60 mmHg by optimizing perfusion with adequate intravascular volume. Vasopressors are titrated as needed to increase mean arterial pressure and perfusion to the brain.

3. Minimize any stimulation that may increase ICP.

4. Do endotracheal suctioning only when necessary.

5. Position the patient supine with the head of the bed elevated 10–30°.

6. Use towel rolls, sand bags, or IV bags to keep the head in neutral alignment and promote venous blood drainage from the brain.

7. Explain to family and friends at the bedside why it is important to minimize stimulation of the patient.

**12. What type of coagulopathy is associated with liver failure?**

Liver failure and dysfunction results in decreased synthesis of prothrombin, fibrinogen, and clotting factors V, VII, and X. As a result, prothrombin time is prolonged. Pancytopenia also results from hypersplenism due to hepatic congestion. Thrombocytopenia and poor platelet function are prevalent; 80% of patients have platelet counts below 100,000 cells/mm$^3$.

**13. When should a coagulopathy be treated or corrected?**

A coagulopathy is not treated unless active bleeding is present or an invasive procedure that may cause bleeding is scheduled. Patients with significant bleeding should receive platelets and fresh frozen plasma (FFP) along with red blood cells (packed RBCs or whole blood) to facilitate clotting and cessation of bleeding. FFP may be given as a bolus or as a continuous infusion. Patients are given subcutaneous vitamin K, which is essential to clotting. The most common sources of bleeding are the upper GI tract and nose. Patients also may have significant blood loss from oozing central IV sites. Use of Gelfoam soaked in a topical thrombin solution and a 2-lb weight source applied to the site can slow or stop the oozing.

**14. What is the typical hemodynamic profile of patients with liver dysfunction?**

Patients with acute and chronic liver dysfunction present with similar hemodynamic profiles. Typical hemodynamic values for patients with a PA catheter in place are high cardiac output (8–14 L/min) and low systemic vascular resistance (< 500 dynes/sec/cm$^5$). However, the mechanisms of this hyperdynamic response are different in acute and chronic liver failure.

Massive hepatic necrosis in FHF results in a shock-like state also known as systemic inflammatory response syndrome. Typical findings include peripheral vasodilation, low systemic vascular resistance (SVR), increased cardiac output, and elevated heart rate related to circulating inflammatory cytokines and the response of the sympathetic nervous system to injury. Such patients also may develop hypoxemia related to ventilation/perfusion mismatch and a pathologic supply dependency for oxygen consumption.

Patients with chronic liver dysfunction also have increased peripheral vasodilation, which leads to low blood pressure. The addition of portal hypertension results in increased blood flow through the splanchnic circulation and development of collateral vessels that increase circulating blood volume. This increased vascular capacitance related to collateral shunting contributes to low SVR, low blood pressure, and compensatory increase in cardiac output.

**15. What causes portal hypertension?**

Normal portal blood flow is 1–1.5 L/min with normal portal pressures of 5–10 mmHg. Portal hypertension (HTN) results from a back-up of blood flow related to obstruction in the liver. Portal pressure > 12 mmHg is diagnostic for portal HTN. The three classifications of portal HTN are based on the site of blood flow obstruction: (1) presinusoidal (e.g., portal or splenic vein thrombosis), (2) sinusoidal (e.g., cirrhosis or hepatic mass), and (3) postsinusoidal (e.g., Budd-Chiari and venoocclusive disease).

### 16. How do varices develop?

Increased resistance to portal blood flow results in the formation of portosystemic collateral vessels that divert blood flow to the systemic circulation by bypassing the liver. Varices are collateral vessels that form as a result of the increased resistance from portal HTN. They can form anywhere in the body but are seen primarily in the GI tract, especially the esophagus. They are diagnosed by direct visualization during endoscopy.

### 17. How are varices treated?

Therapies are aimed at preventing variceal bleeds. Nonselective beta blockers, such as nadolol or propranolol, reduce portal pressures and incidence of variceal bleeds in patients with liver failure. Bleeding varices can be banded or injected with a sclerosing agent under direct visualization by endoscopy. Placement of a transjugular intrahepatic portosystemic shunt in interventional radiology under fluoroscopic guidance is effective in decompressing varices by shunting portal blood flow to the systemic circulation.

### 18. How is variceal bleeding treated?

Patients with an active variceal bleed usually are treated with octreotide or vasopressin, both of which cause vasoconstriction of splanchnic circulation and reduce blood flow to the GI tract. They are started with an initial bolus followed by continuous IV infusion. Severe GI bleeds may require use of a Blakemore or Minnesota nasogastric tube. These tubes have esophageal and gastric balloons that can be inflated to tamponade bleeding sites and reduce blood flow to varices. Tension must be applied continuously to the tube to maintain pressure on the gastroesophageal junction, which reduces blood flow to the esophageal varices. Tubes typically are not used for longer than 24–48 hours to avoid complications of tissue necrosis, perforation, and airway compromise.

### 19. What factors contribute to the development of ascites?

- Increased hydrostatic pressure within the hepatic sinusoids, which forces the lymphatic drainage to weep across the liver capsule into the peritoneal cavity.
- Inadequate protein synthesis due to liver failure, which results in a decrease in osmotic pressure in the intravascular space.
- Movement of transudate fluid from the intravascular space into the peritoneal extravascular space as a result of the abnormal osmotic gradient. The resulting decrease in effective plasma volume stimulates aldosterone and antidiuretic hormone secretion, which leads to sodium and water retention by the kidneys.

### 20. Why are patients with liver failure at risk for acute renal dysfunction and failure?

Changes in the systemic circulation of patients with liver failure cause abnormal renal hemodynamics that alter renal perfusion. This disorder is called hepatorenal syndrome (HRS). Both renal blood flow and glomerular filtration rate are decreased. An overactive response from the renin-angiotensin-aldosterone system and the sympathetic nervous system results in excessive sodium reabsorption by the kidneys. Sodium retention results in an inability to excrete free water and leads to a dilutional hyponatremia. Such patients frequently have low serum sodium levels in the range of 115–130 mEq/L.

Multiple factors put these patients at risk for HRS and acute renal dysfunction or failure, including hypotension related to sepsis or bleeding; nephrotoxic agents such as aminoglycosides and IV contrast material; excessive diuretic therapy; and intravascular volume depletion.

### 21. What is the relationship between liver dysfunction and increased incidence of infection?

Liver dysfunction or failure impairs cell-mediated and humoral immunity, including neutrophil and Kupffer cell functions. Kupffer cells, which line the sinusoids of the liver, are macrophages that phagocytize 99% of intestinal bacteria that translocates into the portal circulation. Portosystemic shunting bypasses this immune function. Patients with FHF and high grades of coma have an 80% incidence of infection resulting from immobility, aspiration pneumonia, and increased numbers of invasive lines and procedures.

**22. What are the most common types of infection in patients with liver failure?**

Gram-positive bacterial and fungal infections. The gram-positive organisms are *Streptococcus* sp. and *Staphylococcus aureus*. Fungal infections usually are due to *Candida albicans*, although *Aspergillus* sp. has also been reported. The patient with chronic liver failure is at high risk for spontaneous bacterial peritonitis, in which the offending pathogens are usually *Eschericia coli, Klebsiella* sp., and *Streptococcus pneumoniae*.

**23. What are the signs and symptoms of spontaneous bacterial peritonitis?**

Patients may complain of abdominal pain and rebound tenderness with palpation. Fever and an increased white blood cell count also may be present. However, the patient may be asymptomatic with an increasing white blood cell count. Spontaneous bacterial peritonitis is diagnosed by a positive cell count and culture of ascites or peritoneal fluid obtained by paracentesis.

**24. What metabolic and electrolyte disorders are common in the patient with FHF?**

**Hypoglycemia** occurs in FHF and chronic liver disease as a result of increased circulating insulin and impairment of gluconeogenesis and glycogenolysis. Patients with FHF are at higher risk for hypoglycemia, but patients with chronic liver failure become more at risk as the disease progresses or with acute insults, such as infection or bleeding.

**Metabolic acidosis** is attributed to liver dysfunction and results from impaired lactate metabolism by the liver. It also is associated with tissue hypoxia and increased peripheral lactate production in patients with FHF.

Patients with central nervous system-induced hyperventilation, respiratory alkalosis, and resultant excretion of potassium in exchange for hydrogen ions develop **hypokalemia**. Other common electrolyte disturbances in FHF are **hypophosphatemia** and **hypomagnesemia**.

**25. What are the most important nursing interventions for patients with liver dysfunction?**

Critical care nurses play an important role in monitoring the subtle signs and symptoms that may lead to potential complications; instituting appropriate interventions; and providing education and comfort to patients and family during their stay in the intensive care unit:

1. Neurologic assessments should be performed frequently in patients with chronic liver failure and at least every hour in patients with FHF.

2. Because patients frequently have altered mental status ranging from agitation and combativeness to coma, it is important to keep the environment safe for the patient and clinicians. In severely agitated patients, monitor mental status for further deterioration.

3. Avoid medications that may impair ability to assess neurologic status. Propofol may be used for sedation in intubated patients. Its short duration of action allows discontinuance of the infusion to assess level of consciousness at prescribed intervals.

4. Closely monitor the patient's ability to protect the airway, especially if the patient has altered mental status.

5. Encourage coughing and deep breathing, or use incentive spirometry in patients with ascites or pleural effusions to prevent atelectasis.

6. Patients should be weighed daily.

7. Fluid intake and urine output should be strictly recorded.

8. Because patients find it difficult to adhere to fluid restrictions, allow them to have input in developing a plan on how to distribute fluid throughout the day. This approach gives the patient some sense of control.

9. Check glucose at least daily. Patients with FHF should be checked at least every 4 hours; every 2 hours may be more appropriate in severe cases.

10. Include dextrose in the IV fluids of patients with FHF. At the first sign of hypoglycemia, start an infusion of 10% dextrose in water to maintain a steady serum glucose level.

11. Include patient and family education. Families of patients with severe grade III and IV encephalopathy are especially anxious. Explanations should be repeated frequently to ensure understanding and to decrease anxiety, which may be related to the option of liver transplantation. They are concerned about whether they will receive a transplant in time and about the surgical and recovery process.

### BIBLIOGRAPHY

1. Bihari D, Gimson A, Williams R: Cardiovascular, pulmonary and renal complications of fulminant hepatic failure. Semin Liver Dis 6:119–126, 1986.
2. Garcia G, Keeffe E: Handbook of Liver Disease. London, Churchill Livingstone, 1998.
3. Jalan R, Hayes PC: Hepatic encephalopathy and ascites. Lancet 350:1309–1316, 1997.
4. Lee W: Acute liver failure. N Engl J Med 329:1862–1870, 1993.
5. Neuschwander-Tetri BA: Common blood tests for liver disease. Postgrad Med 98:49–63, 1995.
6. Siconolfi LA: Clarifying the complexity of liver function tests. Nursing 95:39–44, 1995.
7. Strauss F, Hansen BA, Kirkegaard P, et al: Liver function, cerebral blood flow, autoregulation, and hepatic encephalopathy in fulminant hepatic failure. Hepatology 25:837–839, 1997.
8. Sussman NL, Lake JR: Treatment of hepatic failure–1996: Current concepts and progress toward liver dialysis. Am J Kidney Dis 27:605–617, 1996.
9. Williams JW, Simel DL: Does this patient have ascites? How to divine fluid in the abdomen. JAMA 267:2645–2649, 1992.

# 53. GASTROINTESTINAL BLEEDING

*Robin Marci*, RN, MS, CCRN

### 1. How is gastrointestinal bleeding categorized?

Bleeding can occur anywhere along the length of the gastrointestinal (GI) tract. The source of the bleeding is classified as upper GI if it occurs above the ligament of Treitz at the duodenal/jejunal junction and as lower GI if it occurs below the ligament of Treitz.

### 2. Which category more commonly requires admission to the intensive care unit (ICU)?

An upper GI bleed, because the extensive arterial blood supply near the stomach and esophagus may result in rapid loss of large amounts of blood, hypovolemia, and shock.

### 3. What are the most common causes of upper GI bleeding?

- Peptic ulcer disease
- Stress ulcers in critically ill patients
- Erosive gastritis and esophagitis
- Esophageal varices
- Mallory-Weiss tears
- Esophageal and gastric tumors
- Angiodysplasias
- Arteriovenous malformations in the GI tract

### 4. What are the risk factors for upper GI bleeding?

The patient who presents to the ICU with GI bleeding usually has one or more of the following contributory comorbidities: coronary artery disease, past myocardial infarction, renal failure, history of alcohol abuse or hepatitis leading to chronic liver damage, past history of radiation therapy, and arthritis or chronic pain conditions treated with nonsteroidal anti-inflammatory drugs (NSAIDs).

### 5. What are the causes of peptic ulcer disease?

*Helicobacter pylori* is a treatable cause of peptic ulcer disease. In addition, the increased use of aspirin and NSAIDs has contributed to the development of peptic ulcers. Other risk factors include cigarette smoking, alcohol use, history of radiation therapy, and family history and genetic predisposition (e.g., Zollinger-Ellison syndrome).

### 6. How do stress ulcers develop?

Stress ulcers in critically ill, burn, or trauma patients are thought to develop in the setting of ischemic cellular injury of the GI tract due to hypotension or sepsis. Ischemic injury leads to a breakdown of the defensive mucosal barrier and the development of bleeding.

### 7. What causes gastritis and esophagitis?

The diffuse bleeding that results from erosive gastritis can develop in patients who use aspirin or NSAIDs. Other contributing factors are smoking, excessive stress, and use of medications such as corticosteroids. Esophagitis and resultant bleeding are thought to be brought on by the irritation of gastric reflux into the esophagus.

### 8. What causes esophageal varices?

Esophageal varices can lead to catastrophic bleeding because of their proximity to arteries. Varices result from increased pressure due to portal hypertension. They typically present in patients with end-stage liver disease or cirrhosis.

### 9. What are Mallory-Weiss tears?

Mallory Weiss tears occur at the junction of the esophagus and stomach as the result of forceful vomiting or coughing. Risk factors include a history of alcohol abuse, binge drinking, or bulimia.

### 10. What are the presenting signs and symptoms of an upper GI bleed?

Signs and symptoms depend on the extent and rapidity of blood loss as well as the patient's functional and physical status before the bleed. Symptoms range from feelings of weakness and activity intolerance to hypovolemic shock and death. Estimation of the amount of blood loss, based on the patient's history and presentation, helps to guide treatment and management decisions.

*Assessment of the Extent of Blood Loss and Clinical Manifestations*

| CLASS | APPROXIMATE AMOUNT OF BLOOD LOSS (ml)* | % OF TOTAL BLOOD VOLUME LOST | CLINICAL MANIFESTATIONS |
|---|---|---|---|
| I | 500–750 | 10–15 | None |
| II | 700–1200 | 15–25 | 1. Anxiety, tachycardia, tachypnea<br>2. Orthostatic hypotension<br>3. Urine output normal |
| III | 1200–1500 | 25–35 | 1. Anxiety, tachycardia, tachypnea<br>2. Restlessness, agitation<br>3. Systolic BP 90–100 mmHg in recumbent position (orthostatic hypotension)<br>4. Reduced urine output |
| IV | 1500–2000 | 35–50 | 1. Anxiety, tachycardia, tachypnea<br>2. Systolic BP ~ 60 mmHg<br>3. Reduced tissue perfusion<br>  • Cerebral: confusion, restlessness<br>  • Renal: oliguria (< 30 ml/hr)<br>  • Skin: diaphoresis, cool, clammy, pallor<br>4. Hypovolemic, hemorrhagic shock state |

* All blood loss estimates are acute losses in 60–70-kg person.
From Kelton JG: Management of the bleeding patient. In Sibbald WJ (ed): Synopsis of Critical Care, 3rd ed. Baltimore, Williams & Wilkins, 1988, p 245, with permission.

### 11. How does the appearance of the lost blood suggest its source?

It is possible to make an educated guess about the source of the bleeding based on the appearance of the blood lost. Patients with an upper GI source often present with bright red blood in the nasogastric tube drainage or vomitus. If the blood has spent any length of time in the stomach, it may have a coffee grounds appearance. Patients with lower GI generally do not vomit blood but have blood in their stool, ranging from occult to burgundy melena. Patients with extensive upper GI bleeding have melena as the blood passes through the GI tract. A large upper GI bleed also may have bright red or burgundy melena.

### 12. Which laboratory tests are used to assess patients with GI bleeding?

**Hemoglobin** (Hgb) and **hematocrit** (Hct) are assessed to identify the extent of blood loss. These results, however, may not reflect the true picture if the patient is still bleeding. Initial values also may reflect the fact that the patient is dehydrated as well as anemic. A drop in hematocrit of up to 6 points after crystalloid replacement reflects correction of dehydration. Repeat or serial Hbg/Hcts are obtained to evaluate the effectiveness of therapy and to determine whether the patient is still bleeding.

A rise in **blood urea nitrogen** (BUN) can reflect the presence of blood in the GI tract. **Creatinine** is an important indicator of kidney function; evidence of kidney failure in patients with a GI bleed is of concern because of the fluid resuscitation often required. Other baseline tests include electrolytes, glucose, and calcium.

**Other laboratory tests** depend on the perceived cause of the bleeding and the patient's history. Electrolyte levels help assess hydration status. Liver function tests include aspartate aminotransferase (AST), alanine aminotransferase (ALT), and lactic dehydrogenase (LDH); amylase levels assess for pancreatic damage. Coagulation tests such as the prothrombin time (PT), partial thromboplastin time (PTT), and platelet counts are often monitored as well.

### 13. How are the source and cause of GI bleeding determined?

**Endoscopy** is the preferred diagnostic test to locate the source of bleeding in the GI tract. The examined area should be as empty as possible, which is often problematic in patients who are still bleeding or cannot tolerate the necessary bowel preparation.

**Radiologic studies**, such as barium enema or barium swallow, also may be done to determine bleeding sites, but not in acutely bleeding patients. They can identify obstructions and lesions in the gut wall. Computed tomography (CT) scans performed with contrast assist in identifying bleeding sites throughout the GI tract.

When the source of bleeding is not readily apparent with the above diagnostic studies, a **red blood cell (RBC) tag study** can be performed. The patient is injected with a radioactive isotope (technetium Tc99) and taken to the nuclear medicine department at intervals of 1, 4 and 24 hours for a scan to follow the tagged RBCs. The radiologist may be able to identify small sources of bleeding (0.1ml/min), especially in areas that cannot be visualized by endoscopy.

Facilities with **interventional radiology** departments use angiography for diagnostic testing and therapeutic procedures. Once the bleeding site is identified, it may be possible to embolize the site under fluoroscopy and stop the bleeding without surgical intervention.

### 14. What are the priorities in managing GI bleeding?

The ABCs should be addressed first: airway, breathing and circulation. The patient should be given oxygen therapy to maximize the oxygen-carrying capacity of the remaining RBCs. For airway protection, the physician may elect to intubate the patient who has an impaired level of consciousness and who is vomiting. The next priorities are shock management, fluid status, volume replacement, and identification and management of the cause of the bleeding. At least two large-bore (16- or 18-gauge ) intravenous (IV) lines should be in place. A nasogastric (NG) tube should be placed in vomiting patients to decompress and drain the stomach and to minimize vomiting. A Foley catheter should be placed to monitor urine output.

### 15. What are the goals of fluid replacement therapy?

The overall goals of fluid therapy are maintenance of adequate circulating volume, blood pressure, and urine output; correction of tachycardia; and return of Hbg and Hct to baseline or normal levels. Initially, the fluid of choice for IV replacement is often crystalloid, either lactated Ringer's or normal saline solution. Plans for blood product replacement are based on the patient's history and presenting symptoms. If vital signs have not improved after 2–3 L of crystalloid, blood products are considered. Options include transfusion of crossmatched packed RBCs or, in the face of massive bleeding, uncrossmatched packed cells or whole blood. The patient also may require transfusions of fresh frozen plasma or cryoprecipitate to correct coagulopathies. Platelets may be transfused to maintain the platelet count above 50,000 cells/mm$^3$.

### 16. Which medications are used to treat GI bleeding?

Various medications can be used to manage the patient with GI bleeding in the critical care setting. Their overall goals include decreasing gastric acidity, treating infection, and controlling bleeding.

### 17. How is gastric acidity reduced?

Because of the risk of stress ulcer development in critically ill patients, especially those with GI bleeding, medications that decrease gastric acidity are commonly used. They include histamine 2 antagonists, such as ranitidine and cimetidine, and often are given intravenously as an intermittent dose or continuous infusion. They can be combined with an antacid through the nasogastric tube for increased effectiveness. Sucralfate also decreases pH in the stomach and is effective in management of duodenal ulcers. In addition, it forms a protective barrier over the mucosa. Sucralfate should be given as a slurry through the nasogastric tube and flushed with plenty of water. Sucralfate and antacids should be given at least 30 minutes apart to avoid diminishing their effectiveness. The nurse should note whether the patient has underlying kidney disease before giving antacids because of the possible development of electrolyte imbalances such as hypermagnesemia and hypophosphatemia.

### 18. Describe the medical treatment of patients with peptic ulcer disease.

Patients with peptic ulcer disease as a result of *H. pylori* bacteria are managed with a combination of proton pump inhibitors, such as omeprazole, to block the formation of gastric acid and antibiotics, such as clarithromycin and amoxicillin, to eliminate the bacteria. Patients should be taught not to break or open the pills but to swallow them whole.

### 19. What agent helps to prevent GI bleeding in patients on prolonged NSAID therapy?

Misoprostol is a synthetic prostaglandin E$_1$ analog that helps to replace gastric prostaglandins that have been reduced by prolonged NSAID regimens. In addition, it decreases gastric acid secretion and decreases the risk of gastric ulcer development.

### 20. How are acute bleeding episodes managed medically?

Medications available to manage acute bleeding episodes include pitressin and somatostatin, both given as continuous infusions. Pitressin is a potent vasoconstrictor. It also acts on the kidney's distal tubules to increase water reabsorption, thereby increasing intravascular volume and blood pressure. It is effective in decreasing bleeding from the GI tract through its vasoconstricting properties. However, the vasoconstriction occurs throughout the body and can contribute to hypertension, myocardial ischemia, and development of chest pain in patients with coronary artery disease. Pitressin also may be given as a direct infusion into the arteries of the GI tract to cause vasoconstriction and thereby decrease bleeding.

### 21. What agents are used to treat esophageal varices?

Somatostatin and its synthetic analog, octreotide, decrease bleeding in patients with esophageal varices, but their mechanism of action is not well understood. They are thought to decrease splanchnic and hepatic blood flow and thereby decrease bleeding from the varices. Octreotide is given as a 50-µg IV bolus, followed by a continuous IV infusion of 50–150 µg/hour for up to 72 hours after a bleeding episode.

## 22. What are the alternatives to medical management of peptic ulcer disease?

Peptic ulcer management includes **gastric lavage** to empty the stomach of blood, decrease vomiting, and prepare the upper GI tract for endoscopic visualization. Endoscopy is the preferred method for diagnosing the cause of upper GI bleeding. Endoscopic treatments include **sclerotherapy**, in which the bleeding site is scarred by injecting a sclerosing agent to prevent further bleeding. Esophageal varices can be banded during endoscopy to stop bleeding. This procedure is commonly used to treat severe hemorrhoids. Surgical interventions include gastric resections, vagotomy to decrease stomach acid secretion, or oversewing of ulcers that fail medical or endoscopic therapy.

## 23. What are the alternatives to medical management of esophageal varices?

In addition to endoscopic methods of managing esophageal varices, **mechanical tamponade** with a Sengstaken-Blakemore tube or Minnesota tube may be required as palliative therapy for patients whose bleeding cannot be controlled by medications or sclerotherapy. For patients with portal hypertension and associated variceal bleeding that has not responded to medical or surgical management, **transjugular intrahepatic portosystemic shunt** (TIPS) is another option. This procedure, done under fluoroscopy in the interventional radiology department, creates a portosystemic shunt by inserting a stent between the hepatic and portal veins. Surgical shunts, such as a portacaval or splenorenal shunt, redirect blood flow and temporarily relieve variceal bleeding.

## 24. What are the alternatives to medical management of Mallory-Weiss tears and tumors?

Depending on the length and depth of a Mallory-Weiss tear, endoscopy with sclerotherapy may be a treatment option. If this option is not possible, **surgical intervention** may be required to repair the tear.

Tumors that result in bleeding in the GI tract often are discovered and biopsied by endoscopy. Esophageal tumors that bleed and do not respond to mechanical tamponade generally require surgical resection. **Electrocoagulation** via endoscopy also has been used for the emergent control of nonvariceal upper GI bleeding.

## 25. What are the key priorities in caring for patients with acute upper GI bleeding?

- For any patient in the critical care setting, ABCs are the key priority. Make sure that the patient has a patent airway, is breathing adequately, and has a perfusing pulse and blood pressure.
- The nurse must assess the extent of blood loss and correlate it with the patient's signs and symptoms.
- It is important to monitor physical assessment findings and hemodynamic status and to ensure that the trend in vital signs is in the desired direction.
- Patient safety should be maintained by securing a necessary airway and IV lines and preventing falls related to confusion or hypotension.
- Management of anxiety is also a priority. Few things are more frightening to patients (or nurses) than vomiting large amounts of bright red blood. The combination of a calm demeanor, even when you are most concerned, with technical competence goes a long way toward reassuring patients and family members.

## 26. What are the key assessment areas for patients with acute upper GI bleeding?

- Airway
- IV intake and urine output
- Trends in vital signs
- Skin
- Lab values
- Abdominal assessment
- Neurologic assessment
- Pain
- Nutrition

**27. What does airway assessment involve?**

Watch for the development of respiratory compromise related to blood loss, fluid replacement, and gastric tubes. The patient's airway should be protected at all times. Other components of respiratory assessment include evaluation of oxygen saturation, lung sounds, respiratory characteristics (rate, depth and quality), and ABG results.

**28. What should you look for in monitoring IV intake and urine output?**

The patient should have a urine output of at least 30 ml/hr as hypovolemia is corrected. Close tracking of IV intake assists the nurse in determining the patient's progress toward hemodynamic stability.

**29. What should you expect when monitoring trends in vital signs?**

Expect to see an increase in blood pressure, elimination of orthostatic changes, and correction of tachycardia as hypovolemia is corrected and blood loss is replaced. In response to blood replacement, the patient's hematocrit should rise 3% for each unit of packed cells given.

**30. What skin signs are important to assess?**

Temperature, color, moisture, and tenting should be assessed on an ongoing basis. In response to the correction of hypovolemia and anemia, the patient's skin should warm and become less pale, with a decrease in diaphoresis and tenting.

**31. Which lab values should be monitored?**

Serial hemoglobin and hematocrit values, electrolytes, platelets, and PT/PTT. Calcium levels should be monitored when multiple units of blood are administered because the citrate used to anticoagulate the blood chelates calcium and may necessitate calcium replacement.

**32. What should abdominal assessment include?**

Baseline and ongoing abdominal assessment includes inspection, auscultation, and palpation. Monitor for changes in bowel sounds, evidence of abdominal distention, and location of masses or areas of discomfort.

**33. What should neurologic assessment include?**

Baseline and ongoing neurologic assessments are vital. Possible causes of a decrease in level of consciousness include circulatory overload, progressive liver failure, and stroke. Any deterioration in neurologic status requires immediate assessment and evaluation by the physician.

**34. How is pain managed?**

Using a standard pain measurement scale that the patient can understand and evaluating the patient's level of discomfort and response to pain relief measures are important components of pain management. Measures such as positioning, temperature adjustment, and mouth/nares care provide comfort to the patient. Often combined with discomfort is the stress of anxiety (see question 25). Reassurance and presence of the staff combined with anxiolytics such as midazolam or lorazepam help to decrease the patient's anxiety level.

**35. Why is nutritional assessment important?**

Assessment of nutritional risk factors should be part of the admission assessment, and referral to the dietitian for a complete nutritional evaluation should be done as early as possible. Nutritional repletion assists in the healing process as well as decreases the likelihood of developing an infection during hospitalization. Early nutritional evaluation and intervention are particularly important if the bleeding is related to a chronic condition (e.g., cirrhosis) that has interfered with the patient's nutritional intake on a long-term basis or if the patient is functionally impaired for other reasons.

**36. What are the arguments for and against the use of gastric lavage?**

Much controversy surrounds gastric lavage. Opponents believe that the installation of fluid into the stomach may dislodge any clot that has developed and lead to further bleeding. Advocates believe that it is important to clear the stomach of blood in order to locate the source of bleeding and to decrease the chances of vomiting and aspiration.

**37. Which is better for gastric lavage—room-temperature or iced saline?**

When lavage is performed, either normal saline solution or tap water at room temperature is preferred. Research demonstrates that the initial vasoconstriction caused by iced saline is followed by rebound vasodilation, which often results in more bleeding. It is not necessary to use saline exclusively; concerns about electrolyte loss with use of tap water have not been supported in clinical practice.

**38. Why is odor a concern in patients with GI bleeding? How is it managed?**

Blood that has been broken down by the GI tract has a strong and pervasive odor that affects both patients and staff. It does not help to attempt to mask the odor with another smell, such as peppermint oil or room freshener spray. In addition, opening windows is not an option in most critical care units. Successful interventions include wall- or counter-mounted charcoal air filters and odor-eliminating nonaerosol sprays. The door to the patient's room should be kept closed, as appropriate. The use of a negative airflow room does not eliminate the odor but decreases the airflow from the patient's room into the ICU. It is helpful to work with housekeeping and materials management departments to find new products on the market.

**39. What are the teaching priorities for discharge of patients with GI bleeding?**

Developing a discharge teaching plan for the patient with GI bleeding is an individualized process that depends on the cause of the bleeding as well as lifestyle factors. Most patients need to be educated about **lifestyle changes** such as avoidance of alcohol and cigarettes as well as the consequences if they do not make such changes. Patients also must be given resources to assist compliance. Although such decisions must be made by the patient, nurses can assist them in making an informed choice.

The patient probably will be discharged with **prescribed medications** to correct and prevent the recurrence of bleeding. They need education about the purpose, dosage, schedule, and possible side effects. Simple written instructions in addition to verbal instructions help patients to retain important information. Including significant others in the teaching plan is desirable whenever possible. Patients also need to be informed about **over-the-counter medications** that may cause further bleeding, such as aspirin or NSAIDs, and taught how to read labels carefully, because it may not be obvious which products contain these medications.

All patients and their significant others need education and written instructions describing **signs and symptoms that should be reported to their physician**. Any further evidence of bleeding, obvious melena, weakness, shortness of breath, or activity intolerance should be reported immediately. Patients must understand that blood transfusion reactions can be delayed and that they need to watch for signs and symptoms, such as jaundice, darkening of urine, or clay colored stools, that should be reported to their physician immediately.

## BIBLIOGRAPHY

1. Bouley G, Grimshaw K, Lindewall-Matto D, Kiernan L, et al: Transjugular intrahepatic portosystemic shunt: An alternative. Crit Care Nurse 16(1):23–29, 1996.
2. Cole L: Nursing management of the patient with acute upper gastrointestinal bleeding. In Ruppert SD, Kernicki JG, Dolan JT (eds). Dolan's Critical Care Nursing, 2nd ed. Philadelphia, F.A. Davis, 1996, pp 804–819.
3. Doyle RM, Johnson, PH (eds): Nursing 2000 Drug Handbook, 20th ed. Springhouse, PA, Springhouse Publishing, 1999.
4. Driscoll CJ: Acute gastrointestinal bleeding. In Bucher L, Melander S (eds): Critical Care Nursing. Philadelphia, W.B. Saunders, 1999, pp 725–744.

5. Friedman LS (ed): Gastrointestinal bleeding I. Gastrointest Clin North Am 22:717–887, 1993.
6. Kamen BJ: Combating upper GI bleeding. Nursing 99 32:1–6, 1999.
7. Smith SL: The gastrointestinal system. In Alspach JG (ed): AACN Core Curriculum for Critical Care Nursing, 5th ed. Philadelphia, W.B. Saunders, 1998, pp 647–714.
8. Zimmerman HM, Curfman K: Acute gastrointestinal bleeding. AACN Clin Issues 8:449–458, 1997.

# 54. ACUTE RENAL FAILURE

*Susan L. Robertson*, MS, RN, CNN

**1. What is acute renal failure?**

Acute renal failure (ARF) is defined as an acute deterioration in kidney function manifested as an inability to eliminate waste products and regulate fluid balance. Serum creatinine can increase by 25–50%. ARF occurs in 1–5% of hospitalized patients. Dialysis therapy may be necessary, depending on the severity of related clinical conditions. Unlike chronic renal failure, ARF is potentially reversible.

**2. How is ARF categorized?**

**Prerenal failure:** circumstances or conditions that decrease blood flow to the kidneys.

**Intrarenal failure:** conditions affecting internal structures of the kidney; most often, acute tubular necrosis (ATN).

**Postrenal failure:** conditions that obstruct urine outflow from the kidney.

**3. What are the potential causes of prerenal failure?**

1. Hypotension/hypoperfusion
   - Physiologic: gastrointestinal (GI) bleed, burns, cardiogenic shock, excessive sweating or diuresis, other GI losses, peritonitis, tumors
   - Mechanical: cardiac arrest and resuscitation, cardiac surgeries that require cross-clamping (decrease blood flow to renal arteries)
2. Change in peripheral vascular resistance: sepsis, antihypertensive drugs, drug overdose, anaphylactic reactions, neurogenic shock
3. Decreased cardiac output: myocardial infarction (MI), congestive heart failure (CHF), cardiac tamponade, dysrhythmias
4. Renal artery disorders: embolus or thrombus, stenosis, aneurysms, occlusions, trauma
5. Hepatorenal syndrome

**4. What are the potential causes of intrarenal failure?**

1. Ischemia: ATN, prolonged prerenal conditions
2. Nephrotoxic substances
   - Drugs: antineoplastics, anesthetics, antimicrobials, anti-inflammatory agents (steroids and nonsteroidals)
   - Contrast dye
   - Biologic: toxins, tumors, heme pigments (hemoglobin/myoglobin)
   - Environmental: pesticides, organic solvents, metals (lead, gold, mercury) plants and animals (e.g., mushrooms, snake venom)
3. Inflammatory processes: bacteria, viruses, toxemia related to pregnancy, trauma or radiation to kidneys, autoimmune hypersensitivity, tissue organ transplant rejection, obstruction (postrenal causes), intravascular hemolysis (transfusion reaction, disseminated intravascular coagulation [DIC])

4. Systemic and vascular disorders: renal vein thrombosis, nephrotic syndrome, malaria, multiple myeloma, sickle cell, diabetes, malignant hypertension, systemic lupus erythematosus
5. Pregnancy disorders: septic abortion, preeclampsia, abruptio placentae, intrauterine fetal death, idiopathic postpartum renal failure

## 5. What are the potential causes of postrenal failure?
1. Urinary tract obstruction: calculi (stones), strictures, tumors, blood clots, sloughed papillary tissue in ureters, surgical ligations, trauma, congenital abnormalities, foreign objects (plugged Foley catheter)
2. Enlarged prostate or benign prostatic hypertrophy (BPH)
3. Abdominal or pelvic tumors
4. Pregnancy
5. Neurogenic bladder secondary to spinal cord dysfunction or spinal cord injury
6. Drug-induced: ganglionic blocks, antihistamines

## 6. What are the most common causes of ARF?
Approximately 75% of all ARF cases are due to either prerenal disease (see question 3) or ATN. ATN develops when a toxic substance or ischemia damages the renal tubules.

## 7. Describe the typical presentation of ARF.
ARF typically presents as azotemia, or elevations in serum blood urea nitrogen (BUN) and creatinine (Cr). Acidosis, electrolyte imbalances (primarily hyperkalemia), and a change in urine output also may be observed. Alterations in urine output are defined as oliguria (< 400 ml/day) or nonoliguria (> 800 ml/day). Oliguric ARF has a poorer prognosis for renal recovery.

## 8. How is ARF diagnosed?
1. **History** helps to determine which events may have caused renal insult.
2. **Physical examination** includes assessment of edema (e.g. peripheral, sacral, facial, ascites), auscultation of lung sounds (rales), central venous congestion (jugular venous distention), and a review of patterns of weight losses or gains. These factors determine volume status as well as identify other systemic illnesses.
3. **Laboratory tests** that aid assessment include urinalysis (UA), urine electrolytes (potassium, sodium, chloride), fractional excretion of sodium (FeNa), and 24-hour urine collection to assess Cr clearance. A normal UA in patients with ARF suggests prerenal disease but also may be seen with obstruction, myeloma kidney, vascular disease (scleroderma), or, occasionally, ATN. Usual blood chemistries include electrolytes, BUN, Cr, osmolarity, and complete blood count (CBC).
4. **Imaging tests** include ultrasound to assess kidney size and structural abnormalities (cysts) and computerized tomography scans to identify lesions such as cancerous tumors or pheochromocytoma.

## 9. What is the significance of FeNa? How is it calculated?
FeNa assesses the percent of filtered sodium excreted in the urine and helps to assess renal tubular function. It is calculated with the following formula:

$$FeNa = \frac{UNa \times PCr}{UCr \times PNa} \times 100$$

where UNa = urinary sodium, PCr = plasma creatinine, UCr = urinary creatinine, and PNa = plasma sodium.

**10. Which urine tests are commonly performed in patients with ARF? How are they interpreted?**

| TEST | ABNORMAL FINDINGS | COMMENTS |
| --- | --- | --- |
| Urinalysis (detects presence of infection and severity of renal disease; white blood cell casts suggest intrarenal inflammation) | Red casts, dysphoric red cells, proteinuria, lipiduria | Diagnostic of glomerular disease or vasculitis |
| | Granular and epithelial cell casts | Brown/muddy casts strongly suggest ATN |
| | Hematuria and pyuria (with no variable casts) | May be seen in interstitial nephritis, glomerular disease, vasculitis, obstruction, renal infarction |
| | Eosinophilia | May be seen in interstitial nephritis, but absence does not exclude diagnosis |
| | Pyuria (alone) | Be sure that sample is free of vaginal secretions; indicative of urinary tract infection; sterile pyuria suggests tubulointestinal disease |
| Urine microbiology (presence of infectious organisms) | Identified organisms: colony counts 10,000–100,000 | Avoid contaminants; clean catch or sterile specimen from catheter |
| Urine electrolytes (to measure excretion of particular electrolytes in urine; sodium is important to evaluate renal abnormalities) | Normal sodium: 20–200 mEq/L<br>Normal potassium: 25–125 mEq/L<br>Normal chloride: 100–250 mEq/L<br>Normal calcium: 110–125 mEq/L<br>Normal phosphate: 1 gm/24 hr<br>Normal magnesium: 6–10 mEq/L | Urinary sodium < 20 mEq/L indicates volume depletion or decreased renal blood flow and suggests that renal tubules are intact and actively conserving sodium. High values (> 40 mEq/L) indicate that kidneys are losing ability to concentrate, as in acute and chronic renal failure |
| FeNa (assesses renal tubular function) | See question 9 | Usually < 1% in persons with normal renal function or prerenal disease; levels > 2% suggest ATN |
| 24 hour collections (protein/Cr clearance) | Normal protein = < 150 mg/day<br>Normal Cr clearance:<br>　Males: 120 + 25 ml/min<br>　Females: 95 + 20 ml/min | Collection must include all samples; restart if sample is lost or wasted during collection time; store sample in cool container (on ice) to prevent degradation<br>Cr clearance < 15 ml/min indicates chronic renal failure |

**11. Which are the risk factors for developing ARF?**
- Infections requiring treatment with nephrotoxic antibiotics
- Frequent bouts of hypotension
- Volume depletion (e.g., surgery patients, dehydrated elderly patients)
- Preexisting conditions that can cause renal insufficiency (e.g., MI, coronary artery disease, hypertension, diabetes, cirrhosis)

**12. Which electrolyte disorders are often seen in patients with ARF?**
- Increased·potassium
- Increased phosphate
- Increased magnesium
- Decreased calcium

### 13. What complications or life-threatening situations are associated with ARF?

- Pulmonary edema
- Hyperkalemia
- Anemia/bleeding

### 14. Describe the pathophysiology of pulmonary edema.

As glomerular filtration rate (GFR) falls below 4–5 ml/min, large amounts of water are retained in the blood; as intake exceeds output, volume overload occurs. Capillary hydrostatic pressure increases, and fluid moves from vascular space to interstitial spaces, resulting in tissue edema and third-spacing in the tissues. In addition, if albumin is low, plasma intravascular oncotic pressure decreases, and fluid moves from the vascular to the interstitial space.

### 15. How is pulmonary edema treated?

Treatment for pulmonary edema includes identifying causes of fluid imbalance, monitoring vital signs, maintaining strict and accurate intake and output, and removing excessive fluid. Diuretics are helpful if reserve kidney function is present, but often aggressive volume removal is necessary via renal replacement therapy.

### 16. What causes hyperkalemia?

High potassium, the most common electrolyte abnormality in ARF, is caused primarily by decreased GFR and, therefore, an inability to excrete potassium. Hyperkalemia can result from multiple blood transfusions, IV fluids or medications with potassium, excessive bleeding, cellular injury or catabolism, and metabolic acidosis. In patients with chronic renal failure, hyperkalemia often results from excessive ingestion of potassium-rich foods.

### 17. What are the signs and symptoms of hyperkalemia?

Signs and symptoms of hyperkalemia include peaked T waves on the ECG, GI disturbances due to alteration in gut motility, and muscular weakness.

| Potassium levels 6.0–7.0 | Potassium levels 8.0–9.0 |
| --- | --- |
| Tall, tented T waves | Widened QRS complex and loss of P wave (sine waves) |
| Prolonged PR interval | Slow rhythms (sinoatrial rhythms) |
| | Lower extremity muscle weakness |

### 18. How is hyperkalemia treated?

Treatment for hyperkalemia includes identifying and correcting the cause. Calcium gluconate, insulin, glucose, and occasionally bicarbonate can help to shift potassium back into the cells to stabilize cardiac rhythm. If the patient does not have significant ECG changes, a cation exchange agent (Kayexalate) can be used to eliminate potassium via the gut. However, the most effective treatment to remove potassium is hemodialysis.

### 19. What causes anemia and bleeding?

Frequent blood draws for lab tests, severe GI losses, depleted iron stores, and decreased production of erythropoietin contribute to anemia once the GFR falls below 20–30 ml/min. Blood loss related to anticoagulants (e.g., heparin) and frequent clotting during dialysis also contribute to anemia. Platelet function becomes abnormal in uremic patients and thus increases risk for bleeding.

### 20. What clinical conditions are associated with ARF?

- Uremic pericarditis
- Hepatorenal syndrome (HRS)
- Nephrotic syndrome

### 21. What causes uremic pericarditis?

Inflammation of the pericardial sac may be due to uremic toxins, infection, or immunologic factors. Uremic pericarditis often develops in patients with CRF who do not receive adequate dialysis.

### 22. What are the signs and symptoms of uremic pericarditis?

The classic clinical presentation includes fever, chest pain, and a friction rub audible at the left mid-to-left sternal border. The friction rub results from inflamed parietal and visceral layers of the pericardial sac. Usual ECG findings include ST-segment elevation with upward concavity, possible T-wave inversion after the acute phase, low-voltage QRS, and depressed PR segment in the limb leads and leads V2–V6. Arrhythmias associated with uremic pericarditis include atrial fibrillation and atrial flutter. Complications of uremic pericarditis include pericardial effusion and cardiac tamponade.

### 23. How is uremic pericarditis treated?

Treatment requires daily hemodialysis or continuous renal replacement therapy (CRRT) without anticoagulation (no heparin), medications (corticosteroids, nonsteroidal anti-inflammatory drugs) and, in severe cases of excessive fluid, pericardiocentesis or pericardial window.

### 24. What causes hepatorenal syndrome? What are the signs and symptoms?

HRS is a prerenal condition that may accompany cirrhosis. It is possibly related to altered distribution of extrarenal circulating volume and the resultant changes in renal hemodynamics. The typical patient has jaundice, hypoalbuminemia, splenomegaly, ascites, portal hypertension, oliguria, benign urinary sediment, low sodium excretion, and azotemia.

### 25. How is HRS diagnosed and treated? What is the prognosis?

HRS is a diagnosis of exclusion after other causes of ARF have been ruled out. Treatment includes maintenance of adequate fluid balance, prevention of hypotension and hypovolemia, avoidance of neomycin and other nephrotoxic drugs, and renal replacement therapy, if needed. HRS has a poor prognosis secondary to combined liver and renal failure. Of note, renal function may return after liver transplant. Kidneys can be transplanted from donors with HRS if they are histologically normal.

### 26. What causes nephrotic syndrome? What are the signs and symptoms?

Nephrotic syndrome often accompanies systemic lupus erythematosus, diabetes, Goodpasture syndrome, and amyloidosis. The glomerular basement membrane is damaged by immune complexes, nephrotoxic antibodies, or nonimmune mechanisms. Proteinuria commonly results from increased capillary permeability, low albumin, edema, hyperlipidemia (due to increased liver production of lipids or interference with peripheral or liver lipid utilization), and lipiduria.

### 27. How is nephrotic syndrome treated? What are the potential complications?

Treating nephrotic syndrome requires identification of the underlying cause. Potential complications include skin breakdown, infection, thrombosis, fluid imbalance, ARF, and nutritional problems.

### 28. Which therapies are used for ARF?

ARF is treated either medically or with renal replacement therapy (RRT). Medical management includes blood pressure support (e.g., vasoactive drugs such as dopamine, diuretics) and discontinuation of toxic agents. If a particular renal toxin is vital to the patient's treatment regimen, dosages are adjusted to account for the kidneys' limited ability to eliminate the drug. Dialytic therapy in the form of intermittent hemodialysis (IHD), peritoneal dialysis, or continuous renal replacement therapy (CRRT) assists the patient with fluid and electrolyte homeostasis.

### 29. What is intermittent hemodialysis?

IHD is a process in which solutes are cleared from the blood through diffusion across a semipermeable membrane. The blood compartment is separated from the dialysate compartment by the semipermeable membrane. The membrane and diffusion gradient created by the dialysate solution allows passage of some molecules (waste products) but restricts or prevents the passage of others. Depending on the blood circuit pressures and membrane characteristics, plasma water can move into the dialysate compartment and contribute to desired fluid removal. Potential complications of IHD include hypotension, dehydration, altered drug levels, anemia, circuit clotting, and vascular access infection.

### 30. What is pure ultrafiltration?

Pure ultrafiltration (PUF) is used when the primary goal is to remove fluid. Blood goes through the dialyzer (artificial kidney or filter), but no dialysate fluid is used. A small percentage of solute is removed through convection or "solute drag." PUF can be performed before dialysis, after dialysis, or independently. Desired weight loss and the time required to achieve the net loss are programmed into the machine. Because minimal solute exchange occurs, the patient often remains hemodynamically stable; thus, more fluid can be removed in less time.

### 31. What is the difference between CRRT and IHD?

CRRT is continuous therapy provided over 24 hours, whereas IHD is provided over 2–4 hours daily or on an as-needed basis. Blood flows are lower (100–150 ml/min) with CRRT than with IHD (250–450 ml/min). CRRT is provided solely in the critical care setting, whereas IHD can be done at the bedside in the ICU, on the medical ward, or in a specially designated acute dialysis unit. CRRT requires specialized critical care training and is labor-intensive due to the strict monitoring of the patient and the CRRT circuit. IHD and CRRT can remove large amounts of fluid via an extracorporeal circuit, but both require specialized training and education for nursing staff. Both therapies also can alter hemodynamics drastically and create electrolyte imbalances if not prescribed and managed appropriately.

### 32. Describe the roles of dialysis and critical care nurses during IHD.

Caring for critically ill patients during IHD is a collaborative process. The **dialysis nurse** performs the predialysis assessment, verifying with the bedside nurse what medications should be withheld (e.g., antihypertensives, antibiotics) and obtaining an accurate weight before initiating treatment. During IHD, the dialysis nurse monitors vital signs frequently, along with blood flow, ultrafiltration rates, vascular access, membrane pressures from the circuit, and amount of fluid removed.

The role of the **critical care nurse** includes patient assessment, hemodynamic monitoring, maintenance or alteration of medication schedules (depending on drug dialyzability), and maintenance of blood pressure by titration of vasoactive drugs during treatment. If blood products are ordered, the critical care nurse coordinates administration to coincide with IHD.

### 33. What parameters should be monitored in patients with ARF?

1. Urine output—quality as well as quantity. Because ARF occurs on a continuum and is reversible, careful trending of urine output serves as a measure of renal function and facilitates early intervention.

2. Hemodynamic parameters, including heart rate and rhythm, blood pressure, and filling pressures (central venous pressure, pulmonary capillary wedge pressure). Heart rate and rhythm may change as a result of electrolyte alterations.

3. Lab values for all electrolytes, BUN, Cr, hematocrit, platelet count, and arterial pH.

4. Drug levels (especially for antibiotics). Many drugs are cleared renally and/or nephrotoxic.

5. Volume overload (lung sounds, edema) and/or depletion (loss of turgor, thick sputum, hypotension) due to diuretics or RRT.

### 34. What other systems does ARF affect?

**Neurologic system.** An altered level of consciousness or encephalopathy can develop from uremic toxins and/or electrolyte imbalance. Seizures and altered muscular activity (asterixis) also may develop.

**Pulmonary system.** The lungs are at risk for pleural effusions and pulmonary edema secondary to changes in capillary permeability.

**Cardiovascular system.** The heart is at risk for abnormal rhythms secondary to electrolyte imbalances (hyperkalemia and hypocalcemia).

**GI system.** Carbohydrate metabolism is altered by elevated insulin levels, which are due to decreased insulin degradation by the kidneys. In addition, uremia can cause anorexia, nausea, vomiting, diarrhea, and intestinal irritation. Such alterations in the GI system can lead to malnutrition.

**Skin.** The skin is at an increased risk for breakdown due to changes in volume, especially when edema is present.

### 35. What other areas should the nurse monitor closely?

Whether the patient is on IHD or CRRT, the bedside nurse is responsible for maintaining vascular access and ensuring proper function and patency. Maintain patency by instilling the proper concentration and amount of anticoagulant in both ports of the catheter whenever it is not in use. Aseptic technique is important during catheter assessment. Assess the site for infection, and change dressings at regular intervals. Monitor for potential complications, including infection, air embolus, clotting of the limbs, and bleeding from the catheter.

### 36. How can the risk of ARF be minimized in critically ill patients?

1. Maintain adequate blood pressure, and prevent dehydration.

2. Maintain accurate records of intake and output trends to detect drops in urine output and/or fluid overload.

3. Identify patients at risk for ARF, and monitor baseline Cr and urine output.

4. Discontinue or adjust nephrotoxic agents to prevent further damage or other complications.

### 37. What other support can critical care nurses offer to patients with ARF?

As with all critical illnesses, psychosocial issues and difficulty in coping with illness are important concerns for the patient and all involved parties. The critical care nurse can educate patient and family about ARF and the particular therapies that are used. Listening, answering questions, and addressing concerns honestly help to reduce anxiety. Being the patient's advocate includes coordinating care and maintaining communication among the many services and team members involved with the patient's care.

### BIBLIOGRAPHY

1. Black R (ed): Rose and Black's Clinical Problems in Nephrology. Boston, Little, Brown, 1996.
2. Chertow G, Christiansen C, Cleary P, et al: Prognostic stratification in critically ill patients with acute renal failure requiring dialysis. Arch Intern Med 155:1503–1511, 1995.
3. Davda R, Guzman N: Acute renal failure: Prompt diagnosis is the key to effective management. Postgrad Med 96(5):89–101, 1994.
4. Daugirdas J, Ing T: Handbook of Dialysis, 2nd ed. Boston, Little, Brown, 1994.
5. Lancaster L (ed): Core Curriculum for Nephrology Nursing, 3rd ed. Pitman, NJ, Anthony J. Jannetti, 1995.
6. Parker J (ed): Contemporary Nephrology Nursing. Pitman, NJ, Anthony J. Jannetti, 1998.
7. Stark J: Dialysis choices: Turning the tide in acute renal failure. Nurs 97 Feb:41–46, 1997.

# 55. CONTINUOUS RENAL REPLACEMENT THERAPIES

Hildy M. *Schell*, RN, MS, CCRN

### 1. List the acronyms used in reference to continuous renal replacement therapies.

| | |
|---|---|
| CRRT | Continuous renal replacement therapy |
| SCUF | Slow continuous ultrafiltration |
| CAVH | Continuous arteriovenous hemofiltration |
| CVVH | Continuous venovenous hemofiltration |
| CAVHD | Continuous arteriovenous hemodialysis |
| CVVHD | Continuous venovenous hemodialysis |
| CAVHDF | Continuous arteriovenous hemodiafiltration |
| CVVHDF | Continuous venovenous hemodiafiltration. |

### 2. Define the following terms.

**Hemofiltration/ultrafiltration:** the process by which plasma water and solutes are separated from blood across a semipermeable membrane as a result of a transmembrane pressure gradient.

**Ultrafiltrate:** the plasma water and solutes removed from the blood during hemofiltration.

**Ultrafiltration rate** (UFR): the amount of ultrafiltrate produced per unit of time (ml/min or ml/hr).

**Effluent:** the output from the UF side of the circuit. It may be ultrafiltrate (CVVH) or ultrafiltrate plus dialysate (CVVHD and CVVHDF).

**Clearance:** the volume of plasma from which a substance is completely cleared per unit of time (ml/min).

**Dialysis:** the process by which solutes are separated from blood across a semipermeable membrane as a result of a diffusion gradient.

**Dialysate:** the synthetic solution administered into the ultrafiltration compartment of the hemofilter to create a diffusion gradient that facilitates solute clearance.

**Hemodiafiltration:** the process of concurrent dialysis and large-volume ultrafiltration using replacement fluid to maintain a prescribed fluid balance.

**Diafiltrate:** dialysate plus ultrafiltrate produced during hemodiafiltration.

**Hemofilter:** a blood filter separated into two compartments (blood and ultrafiltrate) by a semipermeable membrane.

**Replacement fluid:** the solution administered through the CRRT circuit to achieve high-volume UFRs and to maintain the fluid, electrolyte, and acid-base balance.

### 3. What are the traditional indications for CRRTs?

The indications for and prescription of renal replacement therapies for acute renal failure (ARF) have not been well established. The indications are extrapolated from guidelines used to prescribe intermittent hemodialysis (IHD) and plasma ultrafiltration for patients with end-stage renal disease (ESRD). Traditional indications for initiating renal replacement therapy for patients with ARF are as follows:

1. Symptomatic uremia (altered mental status, bleeding, pericarditis)
2. Acid-base disturbances (metabolic acidosis)
3. Electrolyte abnormalities (hyperkalemia, hyponatremia, hyperphosphatemia)
4. Severe fluid overload refractory to diuretics

CRRTs are indicated for patients with ARF who may not tolerate IHD due to hypotension, arrhythmias, and/or increased intracranial pressure.

### 4. What indications for CRRTs are still under evaluation?

1. Myoglobin removal in patients with rhabdomyolysis
2. Endotoxin and cytokine removal in patients with sepsis and systemic inflammatory response syndrome
3. Fluid and cytokine removal in patients with acute respiratory distress syndrome

CRRTs effectively remove myoglobin, which leads to ARF in patients with rhabdomyolysis. Myoglobin has a molecular weight of 17,000 daltons, which is too large to be cleared by traditional hemodialysis hemofilters. The clearance and adsorption of endotoxin, complement (C3a and C5a), and proinflammatory cytokines (tumor necrosis factor-alpha, interleukin (IL)-1, IL-6, IL-8, and IL-10) have been demonstrated in human studies, but clinical benefit and outcomes need further investigation.

### 5. How are the various types of CRRT differentiated?

The different types of CRRT are named and defined by the goal of therapy and the methods of operation. The CRRT system uses arterial and venous blood (AV) or venous blood alone (VV). Blood flow through the AV circuits is maintained by the mean arterial pressure generated by the patient's cardiac output. Because venous pressure is low, a blood pump is required to generate flow through the circuit for VV therapies. The primary goal of therapy may be (1) fluid removal via hemofiltration (H), (2) solute removal via dialysis (HD), or (3) large-volume hemofiltration plus dialysis via hemodiafiltration (HDF).

### 6. What is the goal of slow continuous ultrafiltration?

The goal of SCUF therapy is fluid management with low UFRs (120–500 ml/hr) in patients with refractory edema, with or without renal dysfunction. SCUF can have either arteriovenous or venovenous blood flow and does not require specific replacement fluid because of the low UF volumes.

### 7. What type of access is required for CRRTs?

The ideal access catheter is short and has a large bore to minimize resistance, yet is not large enough to compromise perfusion or venous return. The AV therapies require two large-bore, single-lumen catheters. Adults typically require 7- or 8-French arterial catheters and 7- to 12-French venous catheters. The catheter lengths vary from 10 to 20 cm, depending on the insertion site.

For VV therapies, a dual-lumen venous catheter may be placed, using one lumen for return blood flow. Two temporary or long-term, single-lumen, large-bore venous catheters also can be placed. The femoral artery is most commonly used for arterial access for AV therapies. Typical venous access sites for AV or VV therapies are the femoral, subclavian, or internal jugular vein. Increased intraabdominal pressure, changes in intrathoracic pressure, patient movement, catheter kinking, and clot in the catheter or in the vessel influence blood flow through the access catheters.

### 8. What two types of filters may be used in a CRRT system?

**Flat-plate filters** have a semipermeable membrane that lines 15 plates and is housed in a rectangular casing. The semipermeable membrane separates the filter into two compartments.

**Hollow-fiber filters** are used more commonly. They are composed of thousands of tiny cylindrical, straw-like hollow fibers enclosed in a cylindrical casing. The "straws" are the semipermeable membrane that separates the blood compartment (inside the straws) from the UF compartment (outside the straws).

Both filters have biocompatible membranes made from polysulfone or polyacrylonitrile materials. They clear solutes of low and mid-range molecular weight. The average surface area of adult hemofilters is 0.6 m². They do not stimulate leukotriene and complement activation, whereas the cellulose membranes previously used for IHD activated inflammatory mediators. Hemofilters have ports for blood inflow and outflow, dialysate infusion, and ultrafiltrate outflow.

### 9. What are the other components of the CCRT circuit?

The other components of the CRRT circuit include blood tubing, UF tubing and collection bag, dialysate infusion tubing, replacement fluid infusion tubing, and anticoagulation infusion port or tubing. The blood pumps used in VV therapies require a roller pump, an air detector, ability to transduce circuit pressures, and alarm systems.

**10. What is the mechanism for fluid removal in CRRTs?**

The transmembrane pressure gradient (TPG) in the hemofilter determines UF production or fluid removal. The TPG is the difference between the hydrostatic and oncotic pressures across the semipermeable membrane in the hemofilter. Positive (higher) hydrostatic pressure is generated by blood flow in the blood compartment, which forces fluid across the semipermeable membrane into the UF compartment. The hydrostatic pressure in the UF compartment is low; the pressure is regulated by the placement of the UF tubing and collection bag or by a pump that pulls fluid from the blood compartment. Oncotic pressure is created by the plasma proteins, which exert pressure to hold fluid in the blood compartment. The movement of plasma water and non–protein-bound solutes across the semipermeable membrane into the UF compartment occurs when the net hydrostatic pressure exceeds the oncotic pressure. In some systems the TPG is calculated by adding the pre- and post-filter pressures and subtracting the UF/effluent pressure.

**11. What factors influence blood flow through the hemofilter?**

1. Location and diameter of the access catheters
2. Length and diameter of the blood tubing
3. Blood viscosity and presence of clot in the circuit
4. Rate of blood flow

The rate of blood flow is determined by the patient's mean arterial pressure (MAP) in AV therapies. A minimum MAP of 60–70 mmHg is required for effective ultrafiltration in CAVH, CAVHD, and CAVHDF. The speed of the blood pump determines the rate of blood flow in VV therapies. Most of the pumps can be set to deliver blood flow rates up to 300 ml/min during CVVH, CVVHD, and CVVHDF. The rate of blood flow is the main determinant of fluid removal in CRRTs.

**12. What is the effect of negative hydrostatic pressure in the UF compartment?**

A negative hydrostatic pressure in the UF compartment has a significant effect on fluid removal. Placement of the UF collection bag below the level of the hemofilter creates a siphon effect, which increases the negative hydrostatic pressure and enhances fluid removal. Approximately 0.75 mmHg of negative pressure is generated for each centimeter that the UF collection bag is lowered. This fact is relevant for systems that do not use a UF pump. Most systems have a UF pump that regulates the negative hydrostatic pressure, thereby limiting or increasing the amount of UF removed each hour.

**13. What are the mechanisms for solute removal in CRRTs?**

The mechanisms for solute removal during CAVHD, CAVHDF, CVVHD, and CVVHDF include diffusion and convection. Approximately 80% of the total clearance of small solutes is due to diffusion and 20% is due to convection.

**Convection** is the transport of solutes in fluid ("solute drag") across a semipermeable membrane. Convective transport of solutes depends on the rate of UF and the surface area and permeability of the semipermeable membrane. Higher UF rates produce more convective clearance of solutes. Solute removal occurs during CAVH and CVVH therapies because of convection, although usually the primary goal of these therapies is fluid removal.

**Diffusion** is the movement of solutes across a semipermeable membrane from a compartment of higher concentration to one of lower concentration. Diffusion is affected by the concentration gradient, temperature, surface area, thickness, and charge of the semipermeable membrane as well as by the size and charge of the solute. Countercurrent dialysate is infused through the UF compartment of the hemofilter to create a diffusion gradient between the blood and the UF compartments. The countercurrent flow provides a fixed concentration gradient from the inlet to the outlet of the hemofilter.

#### 14. How is the dialysate infused? What is the standard dialysate flow rate?

A dialysate is used during CAVHD, CAVHDF, CVVHD, and CVVHDF to provide a diffusion gradient to enhance the removal of solutes. The dialysate is infused into the UF compartment via a port near the return end of the hemofilter to produce a flow in the opposite direction of the flow of blood. The standard dialysate flow rates used in CRRTs range from 1,000 to 2,500 ml/hour.

#### 15. What type of dialysate solutions are used?

Dialysate solutions can be purchased or custom-made to meet specific patient needs. In the past, peritoneal dialysis solutions were used as the dialysate in CRRT systems. The high dextrose concentrations in these solutions can diffuse into the blood compartment, resulting in significant hyperglycemia and increased calories. Commercially available, premixed dialysates for CRRTs are composed of sodium chloride (140 mEq/L), potassium chloride (2 mEq/L), calcium chloride (3.5 mEq/L), magnesium chloride (1.5 mEq/L), sodium lactate (30 mEq/L), and dextrose (100 mg/dl). The potassium concentration can be adjusted to meet the patient's needs. Recently, bicarbonate-based dialysates have become commercially available. The nurse must know the composition of the dialysate used during CRRT when evaluating solute removal and the patient's clinical condition.

#### 16. What is the role of replacement fluid?

Replacement fluid (RF) typically is used during CAVH, CAVHDF, CVVH, and CVVHDF to provide the intravascular volume necessary for high-volume ultrafiltration and electrolyte replacement. RF rates can range from 100–4,000 ml/hr depending on the patient's dialysis and acid-base needs.

#### 17. Describe the composition of replacement fluids.

The composition of solutions used for RF are determined by the electrolyte and acid-base needs of individual patients and/or by institutional practice guidelines. Most RF solutions contain electrolytes and/or bicarbonate, as indicated. RF may be infused before or after the hemofilter. When RF is infused before the hemofilter, it causes hemodilution, which may reduce the clotting of the hemofilter. A disadvantage of the prefilter technique is that electrolytes in the RF also are lost in the ultrafiltrate.

#### 18. Is anticoagulation required during CRRT?

CRRTs may be initiated and maintained without anticoagulation. Protein adsorption to the semipermeable membrane and clotting in the hemofilter occur over time and can affect clearance rates. Clotting may occur in the access catheter, hemofilter, or in the venous trap of the VV circuit. Anticoagulation may be used to prevent filter and circuit clotting and to maximize the clearance capacity of the hemofilter membrane. The anticoagulant is infused before the hemofilter with the goal of anticoagulating the circuit, not the patient. The risk-benefit ratio of anticoagulation needs to be addressed for each patient receiving CRRT. It is essential to determine whether prolonging the circuit life a few days or increasing the clearance margin outweighs the risk of bleeding.

#### 19. How is anticoagulation implemented?

Continuous infusions of low-dose heparin (100–600 U/hr) are typically used to anticoagulate CRRT circuits. Activated clotting times (ACTs) or partial thromboplastin times (PTTs) are monitored every 4–6 hours during continuous anticoagulation therapy. The heparin dose may be adjusted based on evidence of clotting in the hemofilter circuit or to meet a clotting time goal of 1.5–2 times normal. The blood sample for the PTT test may be obtained from the postfilter section of the circuit or from the patient. It is important to sample blood consistently from one site to interpret results accurately.

Some centers use regional trisodium citrate anticoagulation, which requires posthemofilter infusion of calcium to reverse the effects. Citrate anticoagulation requires adjusting the dialysate bicarbonate and sodium content as well as close monitoring of acid-base and electrolyte status.

### 20. What does the nurse need to know about drug dosing during CRRT?

Many variables influence drug removal and dosing during CRRT. Unfortunately, no comprehensive reference is available to identify which drugs need to be adjusted during CRRT. Therapy variables include the type of hemofilter membrane (large or small pores) and whether dialysis, hemofiltration, or hemodiafiltration is performed. The properties of the drug that affect removal include molecular weight, volume of distribution, sieving coefficient (SC), protein binding, elimination, and nonrenal clearance of the drug. Critically ill patients with ARF typically have altered volumes of distribution because of fluid overload and altered drug-clearance related to their disease state. Therapeutic drug level monitoring should be performed frequently during CRRT, if possible.

### 21. What is the sieving coefficient (SC)?

The SC is the ability of a drug to cross the hemofilter membrane. The SC can be calculated by dividing the drug concentration in the prefilter blood by the drug concentration in the UF. Drugs that freely move across the hemofilter membrane have an SC of 1. Drugs such as vancomycin, metronidazole, and amikacin have SCs > 0.80. The SC can determine CRRT clearance but does not account for clearance by the liver and kidney.

### 22. What are the potential complications of CRRTs?

1. Air embolization is a risk when extracorporeal circuits (especially blood pumps) are used, even though they have air detectors and alarm systems. The AV circuits do not have alarm systems. The circuits should be monitored frequently for movement of air or clot through the tubing.

2. Hemorrhage may be due to disruption of the arterial or venous access or anticoagulation.

3. Ischemia and injuries to vessels from large-bore arterial catheters may occur in patients undergoing AV therapies.

4. Normothermic patients may become hypothermic and febrile patients may become normothermic during CRRT because of the cooling of blood in the extracorporeal circuit. The blood tubing is exposed to room temperature, and/or the room temperature dialysate runs countercurrent to the patient's blood. The temperature of the blood is reduced through convective heat loss. Infusion of large volumes of room-temperature RF also reduces the temperature of the blood. Fluid warmers and air-warming blankets can be used if the patient's temperature drops below 36°.

5. Significant alterations in electrolyte and acid-base balance can be catastrophic if the patient's laboratory values are not monitored closely.

6. Miscalculations of intake, output, RF, or patient fluid removal rates can lead to significant fluid overload or depletion, resulting in pulmonary edema or hypotension, respectively.

7. Frequent filter or circuit clotting is considered a complication because it disrupts the effectiveness of the continuous therapy.

8. Other potential complications related to CRRTs are infection and hemofilter rupture.

### 23. What are the advantages of CRRTs?

CRRTs have many advantages over intermittent therapies. Critically ill patients may develop arrhythmias, increased intracranial pressure, and/or hemodynamic instability during intermittent therapies. These adverse effects may be related to the significant extracorporeal blood volume or rapid fluid, electrolyte, or osmolality shifts during a 2- to 4-hour therapy session. The slow and continuous fluid and solute removal during CRRT results in less hemodynamic instability and fewer acute changes in intracranial pressure.

Patients who require large volumes of intravenous fluids (parenteral nutrition and medications) and/or frequent blood product transfusions benefit from CRRTs because UFRs are continuously adjusted to maintain a prescribed fluid balance. Fluid restrictions, concentrating medications, and limiting nutritional support because of the risk of volume overload are not concerns during CRRT. The use of CRRTs during long surgical cases has facilitated fluid and anesthesia management during the perioperative period.

Renal recovery in critically ill patients receiving IHD for ARF may be prolonged by use of hypotension and vasopressors during therapy. In theory, CRRTs protect the kidneys from further ischemic injury and thereby enhance renal recovery because less hemodynamic instability occurs during continuous therapies. This theory is supported only by anecdotal clinical reports at this time.

### 24. What are the disadvantages of CRRTs?

The disadvantages of CRRTs relate to the intensive labor and competency requirements. Providing safe and effective CRRT requires extensive and ongoing training for nurses and physicians. The therapy is labor-intensive and requires a minimal staffing of 1 nurse to every patient. Another disadvantage is that the therapy needs to be discontinued for patient transport.

### 25. What are the major nursing responsibilities for CRRT management?

**Emergency management.** Understanding the CRRT circuit and its potential complications allows the nurse to prioritize actions during patient emergencies. The procedure for discontinuing fluid removal while continuing blood circulation can be implemented if the patient becomes hypotensive during CRRT. Emergent discontinuation should be performed if hypotension and/or arrest is not quickly reversed with resuscitative efforts or if a power failure occurs.

**Safety.** Protective devices (goggles, gloves, mask) should be worn to prevent splash and body fluid exposure.

**Circuit monitoring.** Assess the circuit and hemofilter for signs of clotting, filter rupture, and air. Monitor the circuit pressures and alarms, and troubleshoot as necessary.

**Patient monitoring and management.** Monitor fluid, hemodynamic, and metabolic status. Monitor for signs and symptoms of potential bleeding, alteration in perfusion, alteration in skin integrity, immobility, and infection. Provide education to family and patient about CRRT. Mix and administer appropriate RF, anticoagulant, and dialysate prescriptions. Perform calculations and document per procedure. Implement a plan for prevention of potential complications.

### BIBLIOGRAPHY

1. Bellomo R, Ronco C, Mehta RL: Nomenclature for continuous renal replacement therapies. Am J Kidney Dis 28:S2–S7, 1996.
2. Burrow-Hudson S: ANNA Standards and Guidelines for Clinical Practice for Nephrology Nursing, 5th ed. Pitman, NJ, ANNA, 1999.
3. Clark WR, Mueller BA, Kraus MA, et al: Solute control by extracorporeal therapies in acute renal failure. Am J Kidney Dis 28:S21–S27, 1996.
4. Kaplan AA: Continuous renal replacement therapies in the intensive care unit. J Intens Care Med 13:85–105, 1998.
5. Levraut J, Ciebiera J-P, Jambou P, et al: Effect of continuous venovenous hemofiltration with dialysis on lactate clearance in critically ill patients. Crit Care Med 25:58–62, 1997.
6. Palsson R, Niles JL: Regional citrate anticoagulation in continuous venovenous hemofiltration in critically ill patients with a high risk of bleeding. Kidney Int 55:1991–1997, 1999.
7. Politoski G, Mayers B, Day T, Swartz M: Continuous renal replacement therapy: A national perspective AACN/NKF. Crit Care Clin North Am 10:171–177, 1998.

# VI. Metabolic and Endocrine Disorders

## 56. DIABETIC KETOACIDOSIS AND HYPERGLYCEMIC HYPEROSMOLAR NONKETOTIC SYNDROME

*Dianne M. Schultz*, RN, BS, BSN

**1. What is diabetic ketoacidosis (DKA)?**

DKA is a life-threatening complication of diabetes mellitus (DM) due to severe alterations in the metabolism of carbohydrates, proteins, and lipids as a direct result of an absolute or relative insulin deficiency coupled with elevation of stress hormones. It is characterized by hyperglycemia, acidosis, and ketosis.

**2. Describe briefly the pathogenesis of DKA.**

Absolute or relative insulin deficiency creates an environment of hyperglycemia and acute intracellular starvation. As a compensatory response, the body releases glucagon, cortisol, catecholamines, and growth hormone. These counterregulatory hormones serve in various capacities to alter hepatic metabolism of carbohydrates, proteins, and fats in an effort to provide glucose for the cells. Unfortunately, the body does not recognize that the diabetic patient cannot provide the required insulin for utilization of this glucose. The result is a worsening of hyperglycemia secondary to glycogenolysis and gluconeogenesis. Metabolic acidosis develops from ketogenesis which produces acetone (nonacid ketone) and acetoacidic and β-hydroxybutyric acid (ketoacids).

**3. How does the renal response to hyperglycemia contribute to the pathogenesis of DKA?**

Hyperglycemia causes serum hyperosmolarity, which creates disturbances in fluid and electrolyte balances. Intracellular dehydration occurs as water is drawn from the cells down the osmotic gradient to the extracellular compartment. As the renal threshold for glucose is surpassed, glucosuria ensues, causing an osmotic diuresis with water losses exceeding electrolyte losses (hypotonic fluid losses). The resultant dehydration decreases glomerular filtration rate (GFR) and glucose excretion by the kidneys, worsening the hyperglycemic-hyperosmotic state.

**4. How does DKA affect the cardiovascular system?**

Decreased myocardial contractility and loss of arterial vascular tone due to acidosis, coupled with dehydration, can result in circulatory collapse. Decreased tissue perfusion and oxygen delivery can lead to a concomitant lactic acidosis. Hyperkalemia can develop as potassium exits cells with intracellular water and as intracellular potassium is exchanged for extracellular hydrogen, a normal compensatory response to acidosis. Hyperkalemia can cause serious life-threatening cardiac arrhythmias.

**5. What is hyperglycemic hyperosmolar nonketotic syndrome (HHNS)?**

Like DKA, HHNS is a complication of DM initiated by insulin deficiency. The pathophysiology of both conditions is similar, but the hyperglycemia, hyperosmolarity, and dehydration are of a greater magnitude in HHNS. In addition, ketoacidosis is not present. Most authorities regard the two syndromes on a continuum, with pure DKA at one end, pure HHNS at the other end, and a considerable amount of overlap in between. Thirty-three percent of patients present with features of both conditions. Various theories for the lack of ketoacidosis in pure HHNS have been presented, but the actual explanation remains elusive. Without the toxic affects of severe acidosis, the patient with HHNS tends to be less acutely ill initially. The more extended period before medical help is sought is believed to be responsible for the more profound hyperglycemia.

## 6. Does the development of DKA versus HHNS correlate with a specific type of DM?

DKA is more commonly associated with type I or insulin-dependent diabetes mellitus (IDDM) and HHNS with type 2 or non–insulin-dependent diabetes mellitus (NIDDM). However, both may occur in either type of diabetic and at any age. The average age of the patient with DKA is approximately 43 years, whereas with HHNS it is approximately 60 years.

## 7. What are the most common precipitating events of DKA and HHNS?

Anything that evokes a stress response can precipitate DKA and HHNS. Infection is the most common precipitator, especially pneumonia and urinary tract infections. Other causes include omission of or inadequate use of insulin in DKA, new onset of diabetes, and clinical conditions such as myocardial infraction, cerebrovascular accident, gastrointestinal bleed, trauma, surgery, and pancreatitis. Certain drugs such as phenytoin, thiazide diuretics, beta blockers and calcium channel blockers also can be responsible. In approximately 20% of patients an underlying etiology is not found, leading to the theory that emotional stress may be a factor as well.

## 8. How do the clinical manifestations of DKA compare with those of HHNS?

Presentation depends on how early medical help is sought, the nature of the precipitating event, fluid intake, and coexisting medical problems (see figure on following page). Tachycardia, orthostasis, hypotension, poor skin turgor, dry mucous membranes, and decreased or absent urinary output are common to both but usually more severe in HHNS because of the more extreme dehydration. Nausea, vomiting, and abdominal pain may be present in both and subside as the condition resolves. However, an intraabdominal process should be ruled out. If improvement with therapy is not noted, further investigation is needed.

Tachypnea and Kussmaul respirations, as the body attempts to compensate for ketoacidosis, and a fruity odor to the breath due to elevated levels of plasma acetone are characteristics of DKA only. The patient with HHNS may present with seizures, focal neurologic signs, and mental status changes ranging from confusion to frank coma. Often it is the altered mental status that causes the family to seek medical attention. DKA is associated with mild confusion to severe lethargy but rarely coma. Patients with DKA are more likely to be hypothermic than patients with HHNS. Hypothermia does not preclude infection. Neither condition induces fever; if fever is present, it most likely indicates an infection.

## 9. How do the more significant laboratory findings of DKA compare with those of HHNS?

| TEST | DKA | HHNS |
| --- | --- | --- |
| Glucose (mg/dl) | 300–800 (average: 500) | 600 to > 3000 (average: 1200) |
| Serum osmolarity (mOsm/L) | Variable (typically < 340) | 320 to > 460 |
| pH | < 7.3 (typically 6.8–7.2) | > 7.3 (lower with sepsis or other cause) |
| Bicarbonate (mEq/L) | < 15 (usually 5–10) | > 20 |
| Sodium (mEq/L) | Low to normal (total body depleted) | 124–140 (total body depleted) |
| Potassium (mEq/L) | 5–8 (total body depleted) | 4.5–5 (total body depleted) |
| Blood urea nitrogen (mg/dl) | 25–50 | > 50 (hemoconcentration) |
| Hematocrit (%) | Normal or elevated | Elevated (may be > 60%, hemoconcentration) |
| White blood cells (mm) | 15,000–40,000 (due to acidosis, stress hormones, and hemoconcentration) | 20,000 |
| Urine ketones | Present | Absent |
| Serum ketones | Present | Absent |

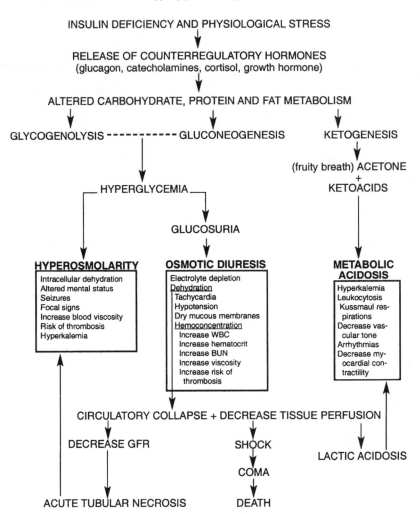

Pathophysiology and clinical presentation of diabetic ketoacidosis and HHNS.

## 10. Why is the serum sodium deceptively low relative to the degree of dehydration?

It reflects a dilutional effect from the intracellular water shifts into the extracellular space. A corrected sodium is obtained by adding 1.6–1.8 mEq/L of sodium to the serum value for each 100 mg/dl of glucose over 100. This relationship is not precise but is considered a reasonable approximation with all of the osmotic shifts taken into account.

## 11. Is there a correlation between the degree of hyperosmolarity and degree of altered mental status?

Yes. The correlation between serum osmolarity and mental status is strong. Coma in DKA and HHNS is seen only when the **effective** serum osmolarity exceeds 340 mOsm/L.

## 12. What is the difference between effective osmolarity and total serum osmolarity?

The effective osmolarity is considered a more meaningful measurement than total serum osmolarity. Because urea freely crosses cell membranes, it equilibrates between the intra- and extracellular compartments and therefore does not effectively contribute to the flow of water between the two areas. The formula for effective osmolarity leaves out the urea component:

$$2 \text{ (serum sodium)} + \text{glucose}/20$$

The formula for total serum osmolarity includes blood urea nitrogen (BUN):

$$2 \text{ (serum sodium)} + \text{glucose}/20 + \text{BUN}/2.8$$

This difference can be quite significant. For example, the patient with HHNS may present in a coma with Na = 140 mEq/L, glucose = 800 mg/dl, and BUN = 84 mg/dl. The total serum osmolarity is 350 mOsm/L, and coma may be attributed to the osmolarity. An effective osmolarity of only 320 mOsm/L indicates that the coma is due to some other cause. If the effective osmolarity is not calculated, diagnoses such as meningitis, which requires immediate antibiotic therapy, or cerebrovascular accident may be missed.

### 13.  What are the most important therapeutic interventions in DKA and HHNS?

1.  The first priority is to restore normal circulatory volume and tissue perfusion and to avoid cardiovascular collapse through **hydration**.

2.  **Insulin therapy** is essential to supply glucose to the cells. Insulin deficiency initiates the process and it will continue unrestrained until insulin is supplied. Until the cells receive glucose, normal patterns of nutrient utilization and termination of ketogenesis in DKA cannot occur.

3.  Despite normal or elevated potassium levels initially, total body depletion is marked, and with the initiation of therapy potassium levels fall precipitously. Timely **potassium replacement** is vital to prevent life-threatening hypokalemia and its potential to cause respiratory failure and cardiac arrest.

4.  **Identifying and treating the precipitating event** is essential for terminating the stress that led to the initial decompensation.

### 14.  What amount and type of fluid are recommended for hydration?

Restoration of fluid volume is initially aggressive and should be guided by clinical presentation, laboratory findings, age, and cardiac and renal status. Recommendations for amount, type, and rate of fluid replacement vary. Some clinicians argue for hypotonic saline initially in patients with HHNS, especially if the corrected serum sodium is > 140 mEq/L. Most advocate isotonic saline, 1–2 or more liters over the first few hours, to achieve hemodynamic stability and good urine output. Slower rates may be used for patients with preexisting cardiovascular disease or renal insufficiency. Subsequently, the fluid is changed to hypotonic saline to provide more free water because water was lost in excess of electrolytes during osmotic diuresis.

### 15.  At what rate should fluid volume be restored?

Some authorities recommend rapid restoration of euvolemia to decrease the risk of thromboembolic events, which is high in this patient population because of dehydration and hyperviscosity. Others suggest that half of the fluid deficit should be supplied over the first several hours, with the remainder supplied over a more prolonged period to avoid potential complications of fluid overload. Clearly, individualized management with ongoing reassessment is critical. New onset of respiratory distress, shortness of breath, and decreased oxygen saturation may be related to overzealous hydration, pulmonary embolus, or myocardial infarction.

### 16.  When are intravenous fluids with dextrose started?

When serum glucose falls to 250–300 mg/dl, a dextrose-containing solution is initiated, with continuation of insulin therapy. Many clinicians express concern that a decrease in glucose below this level during the first 24 hours of therapy predisposes to the development of cerebral edema. The evidence for this concern is conflicting and permits no definitive conclusions. A dextrose solution also supplies a steady source of cellular energy until the patient is adequately recovered to take oral fluids. Since insulin must be continued to correct the acidosis of DKA, which takes twice as long to correct as the hyperglycemia, a dextrose solution is essential to prevent hypoglycemia.

### 17.  When should insulin therapy be initiated?

The use of insulin before hydration has the potential for serious adverse affects. When insulin is provided, glucose begins to move into the cells, lowering serum osmolarity. As a result, the osmotic gradient changes, favoring the flow of water from the extracellular to the intracellular compartment and further depleting intravascular volume. Thus the already dehydrated hypotensive patient may be placed at serious risk for cardiovascular collapse and shock. In addition, a further increase in blood viscosity through hemoconcentration increases the risk of thrombosis. Therefore rehydration, at least 1 L during the first hour, should be started before initiation of insulin therapy.

### 18. What is the goal of insulin therapy?

The goal of insulin therapy is a gradual but steady decline in serum glucose to a target of 300 mg/dl at a rate not exceeding 75–100 mg/dl/hr. Faster rates of decline can result in undesirable fluid and electrolyte shifts and possibly increase the risk of cerebral edema associated with rapid correction of hyperosmolarity, according to some authorities.

### 19. How is this goal achieved?

Because insulin has a short half-life (about 7 minutes), the goal is best achieved through continuous insulin infusion, which provides a steady serum insulin level and thus a predictable decrease in glucose. The infusion usually is started at 5–10 U/hr and adjusted to provide the desired results. The infusion may be preceded with an insulin bolus. Lower doses may be needed in patients with type II diabetes, who secrete some endogenous insulin and may be sensitive to exogenous insulin. Most clinicians view the subcutaneous route of insulin administration as unacceptable because of poor cutaneous perfusion and erratic absorption. Because insulin adheres to infusion tubing, 50 ml of the insulin preparation should be flushed through the tubing to saturate the binding sites. This technique ensures that the calculated dose is the actual dose delivered to the patient.

### 20. Why do serum potassium levels fall with initiation of therapy?

With institution of hydration and insulin therapy, potassium levels fall rapidly for four reasons: dilution by IV fluid administration, increased urinary excretion as extracellular volume expansion augments urinary output, the movement of potassium into cells with insulin and glucose, and the exchange of potassium ions for cellular hydrogen ions as acidosis begins to correct. A corrected serum potassium value for the acidosis can be determined by subtracting 0.6 mEq from the serum potassium for each decrease in pH of 0.1 from a normal pH of 7.4. The nurse should anticipate and carefully monitor these shifts.

### 21. How should potassium replacement be managed?

Potassium may be required in the initial fluid replacement if the presenting serum potassium level is low or normal. Such patients are at highest risk for sudden hypokalemia, especially with institution of insulin therapy, which rapidly shifts potassium into cells. The nurse should check the most recent serum potassium level before initiating insulin orders. Otherwise, potassium replacement starts when serum potassium is ~ 5mEq/L and adequate urinary output has been established. In addition to following serum electrolytes every 1–2 hours initially, continuous ECG monitoring should be used adjunctively. Tall, peaked T waves can represent hyperkalemia, whereas flattened T waves and U waves represent hypokalemia.

### 22. Why are frequent neurologic assessments important?

Patients with DKA or HHNS must be monitored for two neurologic conditions:

1. **Vascular thrombosis,** which is a relatively frequent complication because of blood hyperviscosity, remains one of the primary causes of death. Any vessel may be involved (e.g., coronary, pulmonary, mesenteric, renal, limb vessels), but thrombosis is especially prevalent in cerebral vessels.

2. **Cerebral edema**, generally viewed as a complication of therapy, is relatively uncommon but carries a mortality rate of 90%. It develops during the first 24 hours of therapy, usually when the patient is showing signs of recovery. It is more frequent during the resolution of DKA than HHNS

and is seen more often in children than adults. The most plausible theory to date suggests that development of an unfavorable osmotic gradient causes a shift of extracellular water into the brain cells. No single factor appears to be the culprit; therefore, a gradual steady reduction of glucose, less aggressive replacement of water losses with hypotonic solution, and attention to adequate sodium replacement are recommended to minimize rapid decreases in serum osmolarity. Either failure to note steady improvement in neurologic status or observation of deterioration warrants immediate investigation and aggressive intervention. Warning signs and symptoms may include headache, increased confusion, bradycardia, and vomiting.

### 23. Should phenytoin be administered to patients with HHNS and seizure activity?

No. Phenytoin is generally ineffective in controlling the seizures, but of greater importance, it can precipitate HHNS in patients with type II diabetes by impairing endogenous release of insulin. Cases of phenytoin-induced HHNS also have been recorded in nondiabetic patients.

### 24. When should the transition from continuous IV insulin to subcutaneous insulin be made?

Intravenous insulin therapy is discontinued when the patient is awake, oriented, capable of eating, has no serum ketones, has a pH > 7.3, and has a serum bicarbonate level > 15–18 mEq/L.

### 25. How can a safe transition be achieved ?

Any sudden interruption in availability of insulin can result in a relapse of DKA within a few hours. Because the half-life of IV insulin is so short and the peak action of subcutaneous insulin is approximately 4 hours, the subcutaneous regimen must be initiated at least 1–2 hours before discontinuation of the insulin infusion. Unfortunately, the subcutaneous regimen often is written as part of the transfer orders from the critical care unit to the ward. Cases of relapse after patient transfer have been documented. Such relapses are not surprising because unplanned delays can occur in transferring patients and in implementation of transfer orders. The critical care nurse can ensure a safe transition with uninterrupted insulin therapy by obtaining orders to initiate the subcutaneous insulin regimen while preparing the patient for transfer and before discontinuing the insulin infusion.

## CONTROVERSIES

### 26. Should bicarbonate therapy be used for management of acidosis?

Many clinicians are opposed to bicarbonate therapy in the treatment of DKA because no evidence indicates that routine use of bicarbonate provides any therapeutic advantage or improved outcome. In addition, the many theoretical negative affects include worsening of cerebral and intracellular acidosis. Others believe that the adverse clinical consequences of severe acidosis outweigh such considerations. Most of the literature suggests the cautious approach of supplying small doses of bicarbonate when the pH is < 7.0 or serum bicarbonate is < 5 mEq/L with maximal respiratory compensation or if lung disease is present and the patient cannot compensate well. Small doses also are recommended for symptomatic patients with arrhythmias or persistent hypotension secondary to the negative inotropic affect of acidosis. Under these conditions doses to achieve but not exceed a pH of 7.1 are suggested.

### 27. Should phosphate be replaced in patients with hypophosphatemia?

Complications of hypophosphatemia, which include respiratory depression, decreased myocardial contractility, and decreased tissue oxygen delivery, are considered rare or at least clinically silent. No clinical benefit from routine phosphate replacement has been noted in the treatment of DKA or HHNS, but reports of hypocalemia with tetany as a result of phosphate replacement are numerous. Thus many clinicians oppose IV phosphate replacement. Others suggest small amounts of replacement if the serum phosphate falls below 1 mg/dl—the level at which the patient may become symptomatic. The adverse affects can be minimized through slow delivery at a rate not exceeding 3–4 mmol/hour.

## Appendix: Useful Formulas and Relationships

1. Effective osmolarity = 2 (serum sodium) + serum glucose/20

2. Relationship between pH and serum potassium: for each 0.1 change in pH there is an inverse change of 0.6 mEq/L in serum potassium.
   Example: initial laboratory findings: pH = 7.0 and potassium = 4.5 mEq/L
   pH corrected to 7.4 will cause a fall in potassium to 2.1 mEq/L

3. Serum sodium corrected for effect of hyperglycemia: there is approximately 1.6 mEq/L dilutional decrease in serum sodium for each 100 mg/dl of glucose over 100.
   Corrected serum sodium = $\dfrac{\text{(serum glucose} - 100)}{100} \times 1.6 + \text{serum sodium}$

4. Fluid volume deficit (FVD) in liters = patient's body weight (kg) × 0.6 $\dfrac{\text{(plasma Osm} - 280)}{280}$
   You need to know the patient's pre-illness weight.

5. Rate of intravenous phosphate replacement = 0.05 mmol/kg/hr

### BIBLIOGRAPHY

1. Cydulka R: Diabetes mellitus and disorders of glucose homeostasis. In Rosen P, Barkin R (eds): Emergency Medicine, 4th ed. St Louis, Mosby, 1998, pp 2456–2470.
2. Israel SR: Diabetic ketoacidosis. Emerg Med Clin North Am 7:859–869, 1989.
3. Karam JH: Pancreatic hormones and diabetes mellitus. In Greenspan FS, Strewler GJ (eds): Basic and Clinical Endocrinology, 5th ed. Stamford, CT, Appleton & Lange, 1997, pp 640–651.
4. Kitabchi AE, Wall BM: Diabetic ketoacidosis. Med Clin North Am 79:9–37, 1995.
5. Lorber D: Nonketotic hypertonicity in diabetes mellitus. Med Clin North Am 79:39–52, 1995.
6. Pope DW, Dansky D: Hyperosmolar hyperglycemic nonketotic coma. Emerg Med Clin North Am 7: 849–857, 1989.
7. Siperstein MD: Diabetic ketoacidosis and hyperosmolar coma. Endocrinol Metab Clin North Am 21:415–432, 1992.
8. Unger RH, Foster DW: Diabetes mellitus. In Wilson JD, Foster DW, Kronenberg HM, Larsen PR (eds): Textbook of Endocrinology, 9th ed. Philadelphia, W.B. Saunders, 1998, pp 1010–1039.

# 57. ELECTROLYTE DISTURBANCES

*Stacey A. Hallatt, RN, MS*

**1. List the major electrolytes and their normal values.**

*Major Electrolytes and Their Normal Values*

| ELECTROLYTE | EXTRACELLULAR (SERUM) | INTRACELLULAR |
|---|---|---|
| Sodium | 135–145 mEq/L | 10–20 mEq/L |
| Potassium | 3.5–5.0 mEq/L | 130–140 mEq/L |
| Calcium | 8.5–10.4 my/dl | |
| Ionized calcium | 1.0–1.3 mmol/L | |
| Magnesium | 1.5–2.5 mEq/L | 30–40 mEq/L |
| Phosphorus | 2.5–4.5 mg/dl | |
| Chloride | 95–105 mEq/L | |
| Albumin | 3.5–6.0 gm/dl | |
| Glucose | 90–120 mg/dl | |

**2. What is the normal osmolality of serum?**

290 mOsm/L.

**3. How is serum osmolality controlled?**

Osmolality is exquisitely controlled through the interactions of antidiuretic hormone (ADH) release and stimulation of thirst. ADH has two control systems:

1. **Osmoreceptors** are highly sensitive and stimulate the release of ADH in response to high osmolality.

2. **Volume and pressure receptors**, which are more potent, trigger the release of ADH in response to low intravascular volume.

## SODIUM IMBALANCES

**4. Define hyponatremia. What is its physiologic significance?**

Hyponatremia is defined as a sodium serum level < 130 mEq/L. Serum sodium level represents the osmolality of extracellular fluid. A low serum sodium, therefore, indicates a low serum osmolality.

**5. What causes hyponatremia?**

Hyponatremia results from either an excess of fluid (dilutional hyponatremia) or an excessive loss of sodium with free water replacement.

**6. With what conditions and interventions is hyponatremia often associated?**

- Administration of hypotonic intravenous (IV) fluids or irrigation fluids in response to volume loss in postoperative patients.
- Edematous or low cardiac output states: congestive heart failure (CHF), nephrotic syndrome, and cirrhosis of the liver cause the kidneys to retain abnormal amounts of sodium and water. ADH is released in response to a low effective circulatory volume.
- Diuretic therapy with sodium wasting-thiazide diuretics.
- Extensive fluid loss secondary to gastrointestinal (GI) loss, insensible loss, fistulas, drains, or burns with hypotonic fluid replacement.
- Syndrome of inappropriate ADH (SIADH): water retention is caused by the release of ADH. Several drugs, central nervous system (CNS) diseases, pulmonary diseases, neoplasms, and the postoperative state can result in increased ADH release.
- Medications: opiates, vincristine, tolbutamide, chlorpropamide, oxytocin, and desmopressin cause drug-induced SIADH.
- Late stage of advanced renal insufficiency: impaired glomerular filtration rate results in water retention.
- Alcoholism, especially heavy beer drinking, and ingestion of large amount of solute-poor fluid with diet lacking in protein.
- Endocrine disorders: hypothyroidism and adrenal insufficiency.

**7. What is the relationship between volume status and hyponatremia?**

Hyponatremia may exist in the presence of euvolemia, hypervolemia, and hypovolemia. It is important to evaluate relative changes in sodium and/or volume status.

In **euvolemic hyponatremia**, total sodium remains normal despite an increase in total body water (TBW). No edema is present. Euvolemic hyponatremia may be seen in postoperative patients receiving hypotonic fluids or in patients with SIADH.

In **hypovolemic hyponatremia**, the loss of sodium is greater than the loss of TBW, as seen in GI loss or burns. Hypovolemic hyponatremia also occurs with osmotic diuresis and nephropathies.

In **hypervolemic hyponatremia**, the increase in TBW exceeds the increase in sodium. This marked increase in extracellular fluid results in edema. CHF, cirrhosis, and renal insufficiency are associated with hypervolemic hyponatremia.

### 8. When does hypoosomolar hyponatremia occur?

When ADH is released appropriately to volume but inappropriately to osmolality.

### 9. Does hyponatremia always reflect true hypoosmolality?

No. Severe hyperglycemia, for example, causes a shift of water from the intracellular to the extracellular space in attempt to equalize osmolarity among compartments. This process results in transient hyponatremia. It should not be treated and will resolve as the hyperglycemia is corrected.

### 10. What are the most significant clinical manifestations of hyponatremia?

As fluid shifts from the extracellular to intracellular space in an attempt to establish osmolar equilibrium, cellular swelling results. Thus the clinical presentation of hyponatremia is related to cerebral edema. Symptoms include anorexia, nausea, vomiting, headache, confusion, lethargy, muscle cramps or twitching, and agitation. Severe cases may result in seizures or coma. The severity of symptoms is related to the degree of hyponatremia and the rapidity of onset (acute or chronic). Additional signs may relate to fluid status. A patient with hypovolemic hyponatremia may present with signs of dehydration: tachycardia, decreased urine output, hypotension, or orthostasis. A hypervolemic patient may present with pulmonary or peripheral edema, ascites, or S3 gallop.

### 11. What is the primary cause of morbidity and mortality in patients with acute hyponatremia?

Acute hyponatremia develops in 48 hours or less and is considered a medical emergency. The cerebral cells do not have time to compensate for the rapid influx of water. Brainstem herniation and death ensue as the midbrain is compressed within the confines of the skull.

### 12. Why must extreme caution be observed in correcting hyponatremia?

In chronic hyponatremia, the brain cells initiate a compensatory mechanism whereby solutes are extruded out of brain cells into the extracellular space. This mechanism balances the osmolarity among compartments and limits the influx of water, which can cause cerebral edema. If sodium is replaced rapidly, cell shrinkage results because the brain cells cannot reverse the process abruptly.

### 13. What is central pontine myelinolysis (CPM)? Describe the symptoms and treatment.

CPM is a poorly understood, yet serious condition that may result from rapid correction of hyponatremia. Symptoms include altered mental status, seizures, dysphagia, and quadriparesis. The goal of treatment is to prevent permanent neurologic injury. Sodium should be replaced to halt severe symptoms such as seizure activity, but at a rate not to exceed 12 mEq/L/day.

### 14. Describe the role of nursing in the treatment of hyponatremia.

Nursing plays a critical role in the documentation, assessment, and evaluation of fluid and electrolyte balance. Prescribed treatment is based on severity of symptoms, onset and cause of hyponatremia, and fluid status. Water restriction alone may be sufficient treatment in an euvolemic patient. Hypovolemic patients require volume replacement with normal saline. Hypervolemic patients require water restriction and normal saline. If symptoms are profound, hypertonic 3% saline may be administered over 1–2 hours for rapid sodium replacement of 4–6 mEq/L. The infusion should be stopped as soon as symptoms subside. Three percent saline is not used for normalizing sodium levels but to prevent cerebral damage. Monitor vital signs and electrolytes closely.

### 15. What is hypernatremia?

Like hyponatremia, hypernatremia is primarily a disturbance in water balance. It usually indicates dehydration rather than an increase in total body sodium. Hypernatremia is defined as serum sodium > 145 mEq/L.

### 16. What causes hypernatremia?

- Decreased thirst or inability to self-regulate fluid intake. Thirst is the primary stimulus to consume fluid in response to hyperosmolarity or hypovolemia. Primary hypodipsia is a problem with the thirst centers in the hypothalamus. The elderly have a blunted thirst response. Unresponsive or intubated patients are unable to rely on thirst to maintain fluid balance.

- Fluid loss: burns, fistulas, vomiting, diarrhea, osmotic diuresis, and insensible losses, including fever tachypnea and mechanical ventilation.
- Diabetes insipidus (DI). Central DI is associated with inadequate production of ADH, which is necessary for water conservation by the kidneys. Nephrotic DI is the inability of the kidneys to respond to ADH.
- Hypertonic fluids: tube feeding, parenteral fluid administration.
- Intrinsic renal disease: the kidneys are unable to filter and excrete sodium. The elderly have decreased renal concentrating ability.
- Rare causes of hypernatremia include Cushing's syndrome and primary hyperaldosteronism, which result in an increase in sodium and water retention.

### 17. Why are patients in the ICU at greater risk for developing hypernatremia?

1. Fluid restrictions are common in ICU patients, who may be unable to interpret or communicate thirst because of sedation, intubation, advanced age, or decreased level of consciousness.

2. ICU patients undergo aggressive diuresis for numerous disorders, such as pulmonary edema and congestive heart failure.

3. Postoperative patients are subject to losing volume through blood loss or drains without adequate replacement.

4. Febrile states often cause hypernatremia.

### 18. What is the role of the ICU nurse in the recognition of hypernatremia?

Hypernatremia is often iatrogenic. The ICU nurse must monitor closely and document fluid balance, observe for signs and symptoms of electrolyte abnormalities, and report changes to the physician. It is the nurse's responsibility to suggest clinical laboratory studies as indicated (i.e., electrolytes after significant diuresis) and to report the findings.

### 19. What are the clinical manifestations of hypernatremia?

Hypernatremia indicates a hyperosmolar state. In response to an elevation of extracellular electrolytes, cellular shrinking occurs as fluid shifts out of cells into the extracellular space. Such cellular changes are responsible for the clinical manifestations, which are primarily neurologic. The severity of symptoms correlates with the extent of serum hyperosmolarity. Initial symptoms, such as altered mental status, may be vague. Other symptoms include thirst , nausea and vomiting, irritability, disorientation, muscle twitching and hyperreflexia, lethargy, stupor, and coma. Although elevated sodium may exist in euvolemic and hypervolemic states, it is seen primarily with hypovolemia. Therefore, manifestations of hypovolemia may be noted, including hypotension, tachycardia, flushed skin, hyperventilation, and oliguria.

### 20. Why is it critical to begin treatment of hypernatremia immediately?

The mortality rate ranges from 40–60% in hospitalized patients with hypernatremia. Delays in treatment increase morbidity and mortality. The goal is to normalize the serum osmolarity to protect the brain. Neurologic outcome is highly dependent on the duration of hypernatremia and the rate at which it is corrected.

### 21. Should hypernatremia be corrected rapidly? Why or why not?

No. Although identification and initiation of treatment should begin without delay, the correction of hypernatremia should take place over 48–72 hours. The treatment is fluid repletion rather than sodium removal. Brain cells have adapted to the hyperosmolar state through the uptake of electrolytes and accumulation of organic osmolytes to retain cellular volume. Rapid water replacement can cause significant cerebral edema. The cells must be given adequate time to reverse the adaptive process.

### 22. Describe the treatment for hypernatremia.

Hypovolemic patients initially should receive normal saline to stabilize hemodynamics and perfusion. Then the water deficit should replaced slowly with hypotonic fluid or 5% dextrose in water

(D5W) to correct serum sodium at a rate not to exceed 2 mEq/L/hr. Hypervolemic patients are treated with a combination of diuretics and D5W. Dialysis may be necessary in patients with renal failure or dysfunction.

Antidiuretic replacement with 5–10 U of aqueous vasopressin is the initial treatment of choice for acute hypernatremia secondary to central DI. Desmopressin is the long-term treatment of choice in patients with central DI. It is given intranasally, typically at 10–20 μg once or twice daily. Electrolytes should be monitored frequently during therapy.

## POTASSIUM IMBALANCES

### 23. What causes hypokalemia?

Hypokalemia may result from inadequate potassium intake but more frequently results from potassium loss. Common causes of potassium loss include GI losses from vomiting, diarrhea, nasogastric suctioning, laxative abuse, or gastric and intestinal surgeries and renal loss with diuretic therapy, renal tubular acidosis, or hyperaldosteronism. Transcellular shifting of potassium in the presence of alkalosis may result in hypokalemia as potassium moves intracellularly in exchange for hydrogen ions. Additional causes of hypokalemia include hepatic disease, acute alcoholism, and medications such as insulin, steroids, aminoglycosides, angiotensin-converting enzyme (ACE) inhibitors, beta-adrenergic agonists, and diuretics.

### 24. What clinical findings may be seen in hypokalemia?

The clinical presentation of hypokalemia is vague and similar to hyperkalemia. It involves the GI, renal, musculoskeletal, cardiac, and nervous systems. The transcellular gradient of potassium is crucial in determining the cellular membrane potential. Changes in serum potassium significantly affect the cardiovascular system, neuromuscular system, and conduction of nerve impulses.

**Cardiovascular:** hypotension, arrhythmias (e.g., premature atrial and ventricular contractions), ventricular irritability, depressed ST segment, flattened T waves, prominent U waves, and cardiac arrest. Monitor for signs of digitalis toxicity because hypokalemia may potentiate digoxin effects.

**Neuromuscular:** muscle weakness or cramping, paresthesias, fasciculations and tetany, diminished tendon reflexes, and paralysis

**Neurologic:** depression, psychosis, delirium, and hallucinations.

**Respiratory:** shallow respirations that may result in respiratory failure.

**GI:** anorexia, nausea and vomiting, abdominal cramping, constipation, and ileus.

**Genitourinary:** polyuria or polydipsia.

### 25. How is potassium replaced?

**Oral replacement.** In mild or asymptomatic hypokalemia, the oral route is preferred because it is relatively safe and potassium is readily absorbed in the GI tract. Potassium chloride (KCl), the typically prescribed form, is available in liquid, powder, or tablets. Oral potassium may cause GI irritation; single doses should not exceed 40 mEq.

**Intravenous replacement.** Intravenous KCl may be administered for severe or symptomatic hypokalemia. It must be diluted and *never* given by IV push. It is toxic to peripheral veins; unfortunately, with a peripheral IV, potassium must be replaced slowly with substantial volume. Ten mEq KCl should be diluted in 100 ml and given over 1 hour; 20 mEq/ hr is acceptable when delivered through a central line.

### 26. What causes hyperkalemia?

• Renal failure: decreased glomerular filtration rate impairs potassium secretion in acute and chronic renal failure.

• Metabolic acidosis: hydrogen ions move intracellularly in exchange for potassium ions.

• Conditions that result in the cellular release of potassium, including rhabdomyolysis, sickle cell disease, tumor lysis syndrome, blood transfusions, burns, and crush injuries.

- Medications: beta blockers, ACE inhibitors, potassium-sparing diuretics (e.g., spironolactone), nonsteroidal anti-inflammatory drugs, cyclosporine, or excessive administration of oral or IV potassium.
- Hypoaldosteronism
- Insulin deficiency

### 27. Explain the relationship between hyperkalemia and acidosis.

In an attempt to normalize serum pH and maintain electroneutrality, hydrogen ions move into cells in exchange for potassium. This cellular redistribution results in a transient hyperkalemia that corrects itself as the acidosis resolves. Monitor arterial blood gas pH along with serum potassium to evaluate treatment.

### 28. What electrocardiographic (ECG) changes may occur with hyperkalemia?

The elevation of extracellular potassium changes the resting potential, thereby decreasing the automaticity and depolarization velocity of cardiac cells. A progression of conduction disturbances is associated with serum potassium levels. Life-threatening arrhythmias, however, may occur without warning.

### 29. List the progression of ECG changes.

- Tall peaked T waves
- Initial shortening of PR interval
- Widening of QRS complex with prolonged PR interval
- Widened, low-amplitude P waves
- QT prolongation
- ST elevation or depression
- P waves disappear
- Marked widening of QRS complex
- Increased risk of ventricular fibrillation or asystole

### 30. What clinical findings are associated with hyperkalemia?

Ninety-eight percent of potassium is located within cells; only 2% is found in the extracellular space. This distribution creates a significant transcellular gradient, which is responsible for establishing the cellular resting membrane potential. An increase in serum potassium reduces the membrane potential, slows the conduction velocity of the impulse, and inactivates the sodium channels. Consequently, cardiovascular and neuromuscular manifestations are the most common. Clinical findings include:

- **Cardiac:** bradycardia, pauses, ventricular arrhythmias, and cardiac arrest
- **Neuromuscular:** paresthesias, twitching, muscle weakness, diminished deep tendon reflexes, paralysis
- **Neurologic:** apathy, confusion
- **GI:** abdominal cramps, nausea, diarrhea

### 31. What are the goals of treatment?

Treatment of hyperkalemia is directed at protecting the myocardium, temporarily shifting extracellular potassium into cells, and promoting renal and intestinal excretion of excessive potassium.

### 32. What agents are used to treat hyperkalemia?

**Calcium chloride** (CaCl). In severe hyperkalemia with ECG changes, IV CaCl is given to stabilize the heart. Calcium antagonizes the effects of hyperkalemia, stabilizing the membrane potential and restoring membrane excitability. Calcium acts immediately, but it is a temporary measure with effects lasting approximately 30–60 minutes. A normal adult dose of CaCl is 5 ml of a 10% solution over 2 minutes. CaCl has three times as much calcium as calcium gluconate; 10 ml of 10% calcium gluconate may be administered over 2 minutes.

**Dextrose and insulin.** Also a temporary measure, administration of dextrose and insulin is directed toward shifting excessive potassium intracellularly. The standard dose is 50 ml of 50% dextrose (25 gm) by IV push, followed by 10 U of regular insulin by IV push. Onset of action is about 30 minutes, and the effects lasts for several hours. Serum potassium should drop by 1–2 mEq/L. The standard doses may be repeated.

**Sodium bicarbonate.** Acidosis may cause hyperkalemia through an exchange of hydrogen ions and potassium across the cell membrane. Sodium bicarbonate temporarily increases serum pH, thereby promoting movement of potassium into cells. Unfortunately, this measure, too, merely buys time (approximately 15–30 minutes). The usual adult dose is 1mEq/kg by IV push.

**Kayexalate.** This binding resin promotes the elimination of potassium. It may be given orally, mixed with sorbitol, or administered as a retention enema. Several doses may be necessary to lower potassium. One dose typically results in a 0.5–1.0 mEq/L decrease in serum potassium.

**Diuretics.** Diuretics such as lasix promote renal excretion of potassium. Patients with renal insufficiency may require higher doses. It is important to monitor volume status and to realize that diuresis is not a fast acting treatment.

### 33. When is dialysis necessary?

Dialysis may be necessary for potassium removal in severe symptomatic hyperkalemia or in patients with renal failure.

## CALCIUM IMBALANCES

### 34. How is calcium balance maintained?

Serum calcium is maintained within a normal range of 8.8–10.4 mg/dl through a complex feedback loop involving vitamin D, parathyroid hormone (PTH), and calcitonin. Vitamin D and PTH increase serum calcium levels by acting on bone, kidneys, and intestinal absorption; calcitonin increases calcium loss.

### 35. What causes hypocalcemia?

- Renal failure: the kidneys are unable to reabsorb calcium or to produce the hormone required to activate vitamin D, and hyperphosphatemia decreases calcium absorption.
- Hypoparathyroidism: most commonly secondary to surgical removal of the parathyroid glands, extensive neck surgery, and cancer. PTH promotes release of calcium from bones and promotes reabsorption by the kidneys.
- Malabsorption of vitamin D: vitamin D promotes calcium absorption and bone resorption.
- Hyperphosphatemia: excessive phosphorus binds with calcium to form salts that deposit in the tissue. It also inhibits calcium absorption in the gut.
- Alcoholism and malnutrition: poor absorption of calcium and inadequate intake.
- Hypomagnesemia: suppresses PTH secretion
- Transfusions of blood products with citrate (e.g. fresh frozen plasma): citrate binds with calcium.
- Antineoplastic drugs
- High calcitonin levels: enhance calcium excretion, decrease reabsorption, and decrease amount of calcium available from bone.
- Hypoalbuminemia: approximately 40% of calcium is bound to protein (mostly albumin). A decrease in albumin results in less bound calcium and a decrease in total serum calcium.

### 36. What laboratory tests are useful in diagnosing the cause of hypocalcemia?

- Serum calcium: normal range = 8.8–10.4 mg/dl.
- Ionized calcium: 50% of extracellular calcium is ionized. Ionized calcium is the calcium form, unbound to protein. Normal ionized calcium = 1.0–1.30 mmol/L.
- Albumin level: hypoalbuminemia is the most common cause of hypocalcemia.

**37. How is calcium corrected in hypoalbuminemic patients?**

Corrected calcium (mg/dl) = measured total Ca (mg/dl) + 0.8 [4.4 − serum albumin (gm/dl)], where 4.4 represents the average normal albumin level. In cases of hypocalcemia with low albumin levels, calcium should not be replaced if corrected calcium or ionized calcium levels are within the normal range.

**38. What are the clinical signs and symptoms of hypocalcemia?**

Calcium affects nerve transmission and muscle and cardiac function. Neuromuscular irritability is the predominant clinical manifestation of hypocalcemia.

- **Neuromuscular:** tetany, numbness, muscle spasms, positive Chvostek's sign (tapping the facial nerve about 2 cm anterior to the tragus of the ear results in twitching at the angle of the mouth, followed by the nose, eye, and facial muscles), positive Trousseau's sign (carpal spasm is noted on inflation of a blood pressure cuff above systolic pressure).
- **Neurologic:** irritability, confusion, hallucination, memory loss, anxiety, dementia, seizures.
- **Cardiac:** decreased myocardial contractility, CHF, hypotension, arrhythmias.
- **Pulmonary:** stridor, wheezing, bronchospasm secondary to smooth muscle contraction.
- **GI:** abdominal spasms, biliary and intestinal colic, dysphagia secondary to smooth muscle contraction.

**39. When should you administer calcium chloride? Calcium gluconate?**

**CaCl** is the drug of choice in life-threatening emergencies. It contains 272 mg of elemental calcium in 10 ml of solution, 3 times more than calcium gluconate. CaCl may be administered by slow IV push (100–300 mg) or as a continuous infusion, starting at 0.5 mg/kg/hr.

**Calcium gluconate** is the drug of choice in nonemergent situations. It contains 90 mg of elemental calcium in 10 ml of solution.

Both drugs carry the same list of indications and side effects. Either drug may be prescribed for treatment of magnesium toxicity, cardiac resuscitation, severe hyperkalemia, or hypocalcemia.

**40. What are the nursing implications for administering IV calcium?**

Precautions are the same for either form of calcium, but because CaCl is more potent than calcium gluconate, it must be administered with particular care. The nurse should do the following:

1. Carefully monitor vital signs and electrolytes throughout therapy.

2. Confirm patency of the IV catheter to avoid vein irritation or necrosis.

3. Monitor for side effects, including bradycardia, cardiac arrest, metallic or chalky taste, tingling sensation, and hot flashes. Signs of overdose include lethargy, nausea and vomiting, weakness, hypercalcemia, and sudden death.

4. In the event of hypercalcemia, sodium chloride and lasix may be given to promote renal excretion of calcium.

**41. What is the main contraindication to administering IV calcium?**

Digitalis is a relative contraindication to IV calcium because the combination may result in cardiac arrhythmias.

**42. What causes hypercalcemia?**

Hypercalcemia (serum calcium level > 10.5 mg/dl) results from increased absorption, reabsorption by the kidneys, or increased intake.

Two illnesses that commonly result in hypercalcemia are hyperparathyroidism and malignancies. **Hyperparathyroidism** leads to elevated levels of circulating PTH, which mediates an increase in renal reabsorption of calcium, stimulates bone release of calcium, and enhances intestinal absorption of calcium. The incidence of hyperparathyroidism is higher among women over 60 years of age. **Malignancy-associated hypercalcemia** may result from lung or breast cancer, which contributes to hypercalcemia through osteoclastic activity of the bone. Furthermore, a PTH related protein is produced in some malignant tissues. About 10–20% of cancer patients develop hypercalcemia during the course of their disease.

**Other causes** include excessive vitamin D and calcium supplementation in patients with renal failure, immobility, granulomatous disorders (e.g., sarcoidosis), metastasis to the bone from multiple myelomas or malignancies, drugs that result in an increase in PTH release (e.g., thiazide diuretics, lithium), milk-alkali syndrome, and hypervitaminosis A, which increases bone resorption.

### 43. What diagnostic tests are useful in diagnosing the cause of hypercalcemia?
- Serum PTH. The normal range is 2–6 mol/L. In the presence of hypercalcemia, PTH should be suppressed. If it is not suppressed, the diagnosis of hypoparathyroidism is supported.
- Parathyroid hormone-related peptide (PTHrP), which is responsible for malignancy related hypercalcemia.
- 1,25-Dihydroxyvitamin D is useful in the diagnosis of hypercalcemia secondary to sarcoidosis or other granulomatous disease.

Remember that alterations in serum protein alter the serum calcium level. Confirm hypercalcemia by correcting calcium for albumin level and checking the ionized calcium.

### 44. What are the clinical manifestations of hypercalcemia?
Signs and symptoms are often subtle and nonspecific; they progress with the severity of hypercalcemia.
- **Neurologic:** as the severity of hypercalcemia progresses, neurologic findings advance from subtle confusion and personality changes to lethargy, muscle weakness, hypotonicity, flaccidity, arthralgias, impaired memory, slurred speech, stupor, and coma.
- **Renal:** calcium calculi with associated thigh or flank pain, polyuria, polydipsia.
- **GI:** nausea and vomiting, anorexia, constipation.
- **Cardiac:** shortened QT interval, hypertension, bradycardia, arrhythmias.
- **Integumentary:** calcifications in the cornea and skin may result in severe itching.

### 45. How is hypercalcemia treated?
1. Fluid, fluid, fluid: encourage 3-4 L/day, unless contraindicated, to promote renal excretion of calcium
2. Hydrate with IV saline to expand extracellular volume, thus inducing calciuresis.
3. Do continuous cardiac and neurologic monitoring throughout therapy.
4. Discontinue calcium and/or vitamin D supplements.
5. Give loop diuretics concurrently with hydration to promote renal excretion and prevent volume overload.
6. Administer other drugs (see question 46) as appropriate.
7. Teach patients to avoid foods and liquids high in calcium, particularly dairy products.
8. Practice safety precautions; patients may be weak, confused, and disoriented.
9. Document! Strict documentation of fluid balance, system assessments, and electrolytes, including sodium, calcium, phosphate, and magnesium.

### 46. What other drugs may be used to treat hypercalcemia?
- Biphosphates inhibit osteoclastic activity. Pamidronate is the most potent and effective treatment for acute hypercalcemia. For severe hypercalcemia, a single 90-mg dose may be diluted in 500-1000 ml of normal saline and infused over 24 hours.
- Mithromycin inhibits RNA synthesis in osteoclasts. The typical dose is 25 µg/kg IV, given over 4–6 hours. Unfortunately, mithromycin has significant side effects and is contraindicated in patients with renal or hepatic dysfunction or coagulopathies.
- Calcitonin, 2–8 U/kg, may be given IV, subcutaneously, or intramuscularly every 6–12 hr. Calcitonin is a hormone that promotes calcium excretion and inhibits bone reabsorption.
- Gallium nitrate alters the structure of bone crystal to inhibit bone reabsorption. Renal insufficiency is a contraindication because gallium nitrate is nephrotoxic.
- IV phosphate lowers serum calcium through calcium-phosphate precipitation. Serious complications include acute renal failure, hypotension, and myocardial infarction.

**47. When is dialysis necessary?**

Dialysis is necessary in patients with renal failure.

## MAGNESIUM IMBALANCES

**48. How is magnesium balance regulated?**

Magnesium is absorbed by the intestines (ileum) and excreted and regulated by the kidneys. The normal serum magnesium level is 1.5–2.2 mEq/L.

**49. What are the common causes of low magnesium levels?**

1. **Alcoholism:** 30–80% of alcoholics have low magnesium levels related to poor diet and poor absorption.

2. **GI loss:** magnesium normally is absorbed in the small bowel. Malabsorption results from radiation to the bowel and bowel resection or bypass. Chronic diarrhea, inflammatory bowel disease, and laxative abuse may cause hypomagnesemia through lower GI secretions. Malnutrition is also a contributing factor in alcoholics and diabetics.

3. **Renal loss:** results from primary renal disorders such as acute renal necrosis, renal tubular acidosis, or postobstructive diuresis. Diuretic therapy, interstitial nephritis, and drugs such as cisplatin, amphotericin B, and tobramycin can cause increased magnesium excretion. Uncontrolled diabetes and alcoholism may result in magnesium loss through osmotic diuresis.

4. **Redistribution:** refeeding malnourished or alcoholic patients with high-protein, high-calorie supplements causes magnesium to shift into cells. Insulin also drives magnesium intracellularly. Hungry bone syndrome causes magnesium to shift into newly formed bone.

5. **Endocrine disorders:** renal wasting of magnesium may result from primary aldosteronism and hypoparathyroidism.

**50. How common is hypomagnesemia in ICU patents?**

About 50–60% of ICU patients develop hypomagnesemia.

**51. Describe the clinical presentation of hypomagnesemia.**

Hypomagnesemia manifests primarily in the neurologic, neuromuscular, GI, and cardiac systems. As in hypocalcemia, signs and symptoms may include positive Chvostek's and Trousseau's signs, muscle cramps, tremors, tetany, and hyperactive deep tendon reflexes. Monitor for central nervous system hyperexcitability (e.g., irritability, combativeness, psychosis). Further neurologic signs include confusion, memory loss, hallucinations, vertigo, ataxia, and seizures. Evaluate the ECG for ST segment depression, prominent U waves, loss of voltage, prolonged PR interval, widened QRS, and flat or depressed T waves. Monitor for arrhythmias such as premature ventricular contractions, supraventricular tachycardia, ventricular tachycardia (VT), and ventricular fibrillation (VF).

**52. Describe the role of nursing in magnesium replacement.**

1. Oral supplementation may be given for mild or chronic hypomagnesemia. Magnesium gluconate, oxide, and hydroxide are the oral forms. Diarrhea is the most common side effect.

2. For moderate-to-severe hypomagnesemia, 1–4 gm of 50% magnesium sulfate ($MgSO_4$), diluted in normal saline or D5W, may be administered intravenously over 30–60 minutes. Rapid administration may cause cardiac or respiratory arrest. Atrioventricular block is a contraindication.

3. Replace cautiously in patients with impaired renal function.

4. Monitor and take precautions for hypotension, respiratory depression, venous irritation, diminished deep tendon reflexes, and hypocalcemia.

5. Have IV calcium available to antagonize the effects of magnesium intoxication.

**53. What are the indications for emergent IV administration of magnesium sulfate?**

- Severe symptomatic hypomagnesemia: $MgSO_4$, 5 gm diluted in 1000 ml of solution may be infused over 3 hours.

- Preeclampsia: total dose of 8–15 gm of $MgSO_4$ may be required. Infusion rate is typically 1–2 gm/hr.
- Convulsive states: $MgSO_4$, 1–4 gm, may be necessary. Dose may not exceed 4 gm/ 250 ml D5W over 90 minutes.
- Torsades de pointes, recurrent or refractory VT or VF: $MgSO_4$, 1–2 gm diluted in 100 ml of solution, may be given over 1–2 minutes, followed by continuous infusion. Note that a side effect of ibutilide, a newer antiarrhythmic drug, is torsades de pointes. Check magnesium levels before initiating ibutilide, and have magnesium readily available.

## 54. For what other indications is IV $MgSO_4$ under investigation?

Investigational uses include reduction of incidence of myocardial infarction-related arrhythmias and adjunctive therapy in acute asthma.

## 55. What causes hypermagnesemia?

**Renal failure** is the most common cause of hypermagnesemia. Other causes include:
- Excessive intake from magnesium-containing antacids or laxatives
- Parenteral magnesium, infusions for the treatment of eclampsia, or other iatrogenic interventions
- Intracellular release of magnesium secondary to tumor lysis syndrome, rhabdomyolysis, or neoplasms with skeletal involvement
- Decreased GI elimination with increased absorption due to bowel obstruction, narcotics, or chronic constipation
- Diabetic ketoacidosis with decreased magnesium excretion secondary to extracellular volume contraction
- Hypoparathyroidism
- Adrenal insufficiency
- Lithium intoxication

## 56. List the progression of physical findings as the level of serum magnesium rises.

The clinical findings of hypermagnesemia reflect its sedative effect on the myoneural junction and muscle cell excitability. Generally, symptoms progress with the rise in magnesium levels as follows: skin flushing, nausea and vomiting, muscle weakness, lethargy, diminished deep tendon reflexes, hypotension, arrhythmias, intraventricular conduction delay, heart block, stupor, coma, ventilatory failure, asystole, and death.

## 57. How is severe hypermagnesemia treated?

- Intravenous fluids are administered to dilute extracellular magnesium concentration. Fluids, however, may be contraindicated in patients with poor renal function.
- Diuretics are given in conjunction with fluid to promote renal excretion of magnesium.
- Calcium is given for severe symptoms to antagonize directly the effects of magnesium. Heart block and respiratory depression should be reversed with 5–10 mEq (10–20 ml) of 10% calcium gluconate.
- Hemodialysis may be necessary for life-threatening symptoms in patients with renal failure.

## PHOSPHATE IMBALANCES

## 58. Define hypophosphatemia.

Normal serum phosphate levels range from 2.5–4.5 mg/dl in adults. Moderate hypophosphatemia is defined as 1–2 mg/dl and severe hypophosphatemia as < 1.0 mg/dl.

## 59. What causes hypophosphatemia?

**Increased urinary excretion:** hyperparathyroidism, osmotic diuresis, kidney transplants, renal tubular defects, malignancies, extracellular volume expansion.

**Decreased intestinal absorption or phosphate deficiency:** phosphate-binding antacids or sucralfate, vitamin D deficiency, chronic alcoholism, chronic diarrhea.

**Intracellular shift:** alkalosis, especially respiratory alkalosis, is the most common cause of hypophosphatemia. Glucose or carbohydrate administration, insulin, hyperalimentation, nutritional recovery, and refeeding syndrome drive phosphate into the cells. Cellular uptake of phosphate also is increased with rapidly growing malignancies and during recovery from severe burns as the body enters a catabolic state.

## 60. What are the clinical manifestations of hypophosphatemia?

Phosphate depletion compromises all systems; it is necessary for the integrity of cellular structure and provision of energy for cellular functions.

- **Neuromuscular:** skeletal and smooth muscle weakness, paresthesias, muscle tenderness, peripheral neuropathy.
- **Pulmonary:** respiratory depression.
- **Cardiac:** myocardial depression, hypotension, arrhythmias.
- **Neurologic:** altered level of consciousness, malaise, seizures, coma, peripheral nystagmus.
- **Hematologic:** hemolytic anemia, impaired oxygen release from red blood cells.

## 61. When is IV rather than oral phosphate therapy appropriate? How is it administered?

IV phosphate replacement should be reserved for severe or symptomatic hypophosphatemia. Recommended doses vary, but generally 8–15 mmol of potassium phosphate may be given slowly over 4–6 hours. The maximal infusion rate is 0.2 mmol/kg/hr. Depending on sodium and potassium levels, phosphate may be administered as potassium or sodium phosphate. Oral phosphorus may be used to treat mild-to-moderate asymptomatic hypophosphatemia.

## 62. What are the side effects of IV phosphate therapy?

Side effects include hyperphosphatemia, hyperkalemia or hypernatremia, hypocalcemia, and their associated manifestations. They can be minimized through slow infusion and close monitoring of electrolytes. IV phosphate replacements should be used cautiously in the presence of renal failure.

## 63. What causes hyperphosphatemia?

**Renal dysfunction or failure**, acute or chronic, is the most common cause of hyperphosphatemia. Other causes include:

- Extracellular shift of phosphorus, which may result from cellular injury, rhabdomyolysis, trauma, burns, cancer, chemotherapy, prolonged immobilization, severe hemolysis, infection, tumor lysis syndrome, or acidosis.
- Excessive intake or administration, which may result from transfusion of stored or outdated blood, IV phosphate, and use of phosphorous-containing laxatives or enemas.
- Hypoparathyroidism, which decreases renal excretion of phosphate.
- Hyperthyroidism, which increases phosphate reabsorption by the kidneys.

## 64. What risks are associated with hyperphosphatemia?

**Metastatic calcification** is the greatest cause of morbidity in prolonged hyperphosphatemia. Soft tissue calcification may affect the heart, lungs, blood vessels, kidneys, brain, eyes, and skin.

It is crucial to recall the inverse relationship between phosphorus and calcium. **Hypocalcemia** can cause elevated serum phosphorus levels. Neurologic findings include muscle spasms, circumoral paresthesias, tetany, positive Chvostek's and Trousseau's signs, altered mental status, delirium, confusion, and seizures. Cardiovascular manifestations include hypotension, heart failure, and prolonged QT interval on ECG.

## 65. What are the goals of treatment in patients with hyperphosphatemia?

Treatment is aimed at the underlying cause of hyperphosphatemia. Goals include reduction of serum phosphate and elevation of serum calcium.

### 66. What agents are used to treat hyperphosphatemia?

**Oral phosphate binders** lower serum phosphate by decreasing GI absorption. Calcium carbonate may be initiated at 1 gm orally 3 times/day with meals and slowly increased to a maximal dose of 3 gm 3 times/day. Aluminum is the most effective binder, but the risk of aluminum toxicity has limited its use, especially in patients with renal failure. The usual dose of aluminum hydroxide or carbonate is 1–2 600-mg tablets orally 3 times/day with meals.

**Diamox** may be given to promote renal excretion of phosphorus when the kidneys are functional.

**Calcium chloride or gluconate** may be given to replace calcium and to decrease phosphorous absorption. Refer to section on calcium for dosage and administrative guidelines.

### 67. What is the role of dialysis?

Continuous renal replacement therapies effectively remove phosphorous and may be necessary in patients with renal dysfunction or failure.

### BIBLIOGRAPHY

1. Arnold JL, Bibb J: Hypophosphatemia. www.emedicine.com/emerg/topic278.htm, 1998.
2. Beach C: Hypocalcemia. www.emedicine,com/emerg/topic271.htm, 1997.
3. Craig S: Hyponatremia. www.emedicine,com/emerg/topic275.htm, 1997.
4. Dittrich KL, Walls RM: Hyperkalemia: ECG manifestations and clinical considerations. J Emerg Med 65:449–455, 1986.
5. Fung J, DeBlieuz P: Hyperphoshatemia. www.emedicine.com/emerg/topic266.htm, 1998.
6. Gahart BL, Nazareno AR: Intravenous Medications, 16th ed. St. Louis, Mosby, 2000.
7. Healey PM, Jacobson EJ: Common Medical Diagnoses: An Algorithmic Approach, 2nd ed. Philadelphia, W.B. Saunders, 1994.
8. Hemphill R: Hypercalcemia. www.emedicine.com/emerg/topic260.htm, 1997.
9. Innerarity SA, Stark JL: Fluid and Electrolytes, 3rd ed. Springhouse, PA, Springhouse Corporation, 1997.
10. Kunis CL, Lownstein J: The emergency treatment of hyperkalemia. Med Clin North Am 65:165–176, 1981.
11. Palevsky PM: Hypernatremia. Semin Nephrol 18:20–30, 1998.
12. Perez N, Blumstein H: Hypermagnesemia. www.emedicine.com/emerg/topic262.htm, 1998.
13. Perez N, Blumstein H: Hypomagnesemia. www.emedicine,com/emerg/topic274.htm, 1998.
14. Preston RA: Acid-Base, Fluid, and Electrolytes Made Ridiculously Simple. Miami, MedMaster, 1997.
15. Spratto GR, Woods AL: Delmar's Nurse's Drug Reference. Albany, NY, Delmar Publishers, 1997.
16. Wilson M, Sinert R: Hypernatremia. www.emedicin.com/emerg/topic263.htm, 1998.
17. Zwanger M, Garth D: Hyperkalemia. www.emedicine.com/emerg/topc261.htm, 1998.
18. Zwanger M, Garth D: Hypokalemia. www.emedicine.com/emerg/topic273.htm, 1998.

# VII. Sedation and Pain Management

## 58. AGITATION AND DELIRIUM

*Margaret H. Doherty*, RN, MSN, CCRN

### 1. What is agitation?

Agitation is a syndrome of excessive nonpurposeful motor activity with internal tension. It can cause panic, excessive startle reflexes, and paranoia and usually is a behavior of delirium. In the intensive care unit (ICU), the patient may be pulling at tubes, hitting the staff, and moving all extremities in a restless manner.

### 2. What is delirium?

Delirium is an acute and reversible abnormal mental state characterized by disorientation, fear, misconception of sensory stimuli, hallucinations, and usually agitated behavior. The person perceives the environment as hostile and threatening. Although delirium can manifest as hypoactive behavior, 67% of delirious patients are hyperactive.

### 3. What is the difference between delirium and dementia?

Dementia is an irreversible organic state due to brain dysfunction and has a gradual onset. Both dementia and delirium cause disorientation, but dementia involves a more ordered thought process. Although agitation is present with both conditions, dementia involves ritualistic behaviors such as pacing. Both conditions have pathophysiologic etiologies.

### 4. What physiologic factors contribute to the development of delirium?

- Alterations in neurotransmitter levels (e.g., acetylcholine, dopamine, gamma aminobutyric acid, serotonin)
- Corticosteroids, catecholamines, and histamine, which affect arousal, attention, cortical function, and limbic activities
- Multiple pharmacologic interventions with adverse side effects (common in ICU patients)

### 5  What environmental factors contribute to the development of delirium?

Sensory overload, sleep deprivation, and perceptual alterations. In the ICU, equipment, alarms, and number of staff cause a high noise level that leads to sensory overload. Sleep deprivation may result from frequent nursing and medical interventions and excessive noise. Patients often are not allowed to sleep for 90-minute periods. Perceptual alterations are common in the elderly and may be complicated by pathologic conditions.

### 6. What is the most significant risk factor for delirium?

Advanced age. The incidence of delirium among elderly patients in the critical care setting is 10–15%. Organ dysfunction and increased sensitivity to the effects of drugs are contributing factors.

### 7. Who else is at risk for the development of delirium?

Critically ill patients are at risk because of their complex pathology, multiple interventions, pharmacologic management, and environmental factors. Patients with a history of drug abuse, multiorgan dysfunction, hemodynamic compromise, joint replacement surgery, cardiovascular surgery, traumatic brain injury, and shock are also at high risk.

**8. Describe the assessment of at-risk patients.**

An initial physical exam and history, including identification of risk factors and neurologic assessment, are mandatory. Ongoing assessment should include observation for early signs of agitation in high-risk patients (see question 11).

**9. What physiologic disorders commonly cause agitation and delirium?**

The most common cause is hypoxia, followed by electrolyte imbalances, hypo- or hyperglycemia, cerebral hypoperfusion, infection, myocardial ischemia, and pain. Cerebral hypoperfusion may be due to hypovolemia or hemodynamic instability. Acute infections in the elderly, such as urinary tract infections and pneumonia, may manifest as confusion and hallucinations.

**10. What drugs cause agitation and delirium?**

- Analgesics: opiates, salicylates, ibuprofen
- Antibiotics: aminoglycosides, ciprofloxacin, cephalosporins
- Anticholinergics: antihistamines, phenothiazines
- Antiepileptics: phenytoin, sodium valproate, primidone
- Antineoplastics: interleukin-2, cyclosporine
- Cardiovascular agents: angiotensin-converting enzyme inhibitors, lidocaine, quinidine, calcium channel blockers
- Diuretics: furosemide, hydrochlorothiazide
- $H_2$ blockers: cimetidine, ranitidine
- Sedative-hypnotics: benzodiazepines, propofol
- Sympathomimetics: cocaine, phenylephrine

Critically ill patients who require many of the above drugs must be monitored closely for early signs of agitation and delirium. Withdrawal from specific central nervous system drugs (e.g., alcohol, benzodiazepines, cocaine, heroin, opiates) also can cause an agitated delirium. A thorough drug history helps the critical care nurse anticipate, prevent, and manage such withdrawal.

**11. What are the early signs of agitation and delirium?**

- Slight restlessness
- Fearful look in the eyes
- Fingering of tubes or bedding
- Looking at the ceiling in a startled manner
- Anxiety
- Sudden increase in heart rate or blood pressure
- Sudden inability to follow simple commands
- Disorientation

**12. What are the advanced signs of delirium?**

- Sudden agitation
- Increased restlessness
- Sudden attempts to hit staff or get out of bed
- Sudden changes in vital signs

**13. How is length of stay affected by the presence of delirium?**

Length of stay often is prolonged because of possible adverse consequences. Premature self-extubation interferes with recovery, may cause myocardial ischemia and dysfunction, and may increase total body oxygen consumption and alter end-organ function. Research has shown that adequate management of agitation with an effective sedation protocol decreases length of ICU stay, length of hospital stay, time with mechanical ventilation, and time of agitation.

**14. What are the key nursing responsibilities in caring for agitated and delirious patients?**

1. In addition to thorough ongoing assessment, the nurse must consider patient safety. Prevention of agitation and delirium in high-risk populations is ideal.

2. Watch for early signs and treat the cause aggressively.

3. Allow at least 90 minutes of uninterrupted sleep during evening and night shifts.

4. Involve the family in patient orientation and hand-holding to decrease anxiety and fear.

5. Physically restrain the patient as little as possible. Physical restraint increases agitation and may be perceived as abuse by the agitated or delirious patient.

6. Monitor lab values for abnormalities and trends:

- Hemoglobin and hematocrit
- Arterial blood gases
- Pulse oximetry
- Electrolytes
- Glucose
- Blood urea nitrogen
- Creatinine
- Liver function studies
- Drug toxicity levels
- Albumin

7. Monitor level of consciousness (LOC) and watch for subtle changes in behavior and perception. LOC is the most sensitive indicator of alterations in neurologic, respiratory, and cardiovascular function.

8. Develop a goal of management with each patient that includes cooperation, comfort, and trust in the environment.

9. Administer sedatives as prescribed, and monitor for response and side effects (see Chapter 61).

## 15. Why should albumin levels be monitored?

Patients with low albumin levels are at risk for inadequate therapeutic levels of protein-bound central nervous system drugs. The incidence of adverse effects from such drugs is also increased.

## 16. What other management strategies should be addressed?

1. Attempt to correct abnormal lab values as soon as possible.
2. Maintain optimal oxygenation and adequate cerebral perfusion.
3. Individualize the sedation protocol to each patient's needs.
4. Frequent orientation by care providers is essential.
5. Do *not* tell critically ill patients with many tubes in various parts of the body to "relax."
6. Different types of music can be incorporated into patient care in the ICU.
7. Approach the patient with kindness and patience (especially important because perceptual alterations contribute to the development of delirium).

## 17. What is the role of physical restraint with limb ties, chest vests, or mittens?

Physical restraints are used when the patient is a danger to self or staff. They are part of many critical care protocols for ventilated patients. However, legal aspects must be considered to ensure patient safety, including appropriate use, frequent monitoring, reevaluation of need, skin and circulation monitoring, and repositioning.

## 18. What risks are associated with the use of physical restraints?

Patient safety is compromised because patients cannot protect themselves from harm. Risk of death is related to airway compromise or asphyxiation. Other risks include discomfort, altered perfusion, mistrust of staff and environment, fear, and increased agitation.

## 19. What are the key nursing responsibilities associated with the use of restraints?

1. The nurse must assess the need for restraints on an individual basis instead of restraining patients routinely.
2. The nurse should identify alternatives, such as asking family members to sit with the patient, adequate sedation, and frequent reorientation in a calm and caring manner.
3. The nurse must encourage a multidisciplinary approach that evaluates the cause of the agitation and develops a comprehensive plan to improve patient comfort and decrease the need for restraints.
4. The nurse must establish trust and rapport with patients so that they experience less anxiety and fear and are more cooperative with necessary care.

## 20. What risks are associated with self-extubation?

The patient may be unable to ventilate and oxygenate effectively. Another risk is the inability to reintubate, if necessary, because of airway edema or anatomic limitations. This problem, however, is uncommon. The mortality rate associated with early self-extubation is less than 1%.

### 21. What else should the nurse consider in patients who attempt self-extubation?

Often the patient is ready to be extubated and no longer requires mechanical ventilation. The staff must assess the readiness to be weaned from the ventilator and extubate as soon as possible to prevent the potential complications of self-extubation. In addition, the frequency of restlessness and agitation in patients who self-extubate indicates inadequate sedation or analgesia.

### 22. What kind of institutional approach facilitates management of delirium?

A systems approach using agitation and delirium as indicators can be evaluated with a quality improvement process. For example, the staff of an ICU can choose self-extubation as a quality indicator and monitor the incidence and timing of self-extubation, the patient's relationship with the staff, and use of medications. Such data can be compared with other ICUs, regionally or nationally, to develop a plan focused on decreasing the number of self-extubations and increasing patient comfort.

In addition, staff competency requirements related to sedative administration and implementation of a sedation protocol can improve outcomes of agitated patients. Staff competency includes both knowledge and skills. The nurse should be able to identify causes and symptoms of agitation and delirium; describe patient goals for therapy; evaluate use of pharmacologic and nonpharmacologic interventions; and use a sedation scale and sedation protocol appropriately. With nursing competency and a multidisciplinary systems approach, critically ill patients with agitation and delirium can receive safe and compassionate care.

### BIBLIOGRAPHY

1. Antoni-Jordi B, Perez M, Bak E, Mancebo J: A prospective study of unplanned endotracheal extubation in intensive care unit patients. Crit Care Med 26:1180–1186, 1989.
2. Brook AD, Aherns TS, Schaiff R, et al: Effect of a nursing-implemented sedation protocol on the duration of mechanical ventilation. Crit Care Med 27:2609–2615, 1999.
3. Doherty MH, Plowfield L, Ware C, West CM: Impact of critical illness on the patient and family. In Bucher L, Melander S (eds): Critical Care Nursing. Philadelphia,W.B. Saunders, 1999, pp 51–92.
4. Haskell RM, Frankel HL, Rotondo MF: Agitation. AACN Clin Issues 8:335–350, 1997.
5. Holland C, Cason CL, Prater LR: Patients' recollection of critical care. Dimens Crit Care Nurs 16:132–140, 1997.
6. Nion LC: Establishing alternatives to physical restraints in the acute care setting: A conceptual framework to assist nurses' decision making. AACN Clin Issues 7:591–602, 1996.
7. Simpson T, Rayshan E, Cameron C: Patients' perceptions of environmental factors that disturb sleep after cardiac surgery. Am J Crit Care 5:173–181, 1996.
8. Sullivan-Marx EM, Strumpf NE: Restraint-free care for acutely ill patients in the hospital. AACN Clin Issues 7:572–578, 1996.
9. Wunderluch RJ, Perry A, Lavin MA, Katz B: Patients' perceptions of uncertainty and stress during weaning from mechanical ventilation. Dimens Crit Care Nurs 18:2–10, 1999.

# 59. NEUROMUSCULAR BLOCKING AGENTS

Sandra Rowlee, MS, RN, CNS, ACNP-CS

### 1. What is a neuromuscular blocking agent (NMBA)?

Neuromuscular blocking agents (NMBAs) are drugs that cause complete relaxation of the skeletal muscle. They are structurally related to the neurotransmitter acetylcholine (ACh) and affect the performance of the neuromuscular junction.

### 2. Discuss briefly the history of NMBAs.

South American Indians first used the NMBA curare for hunting. The animals died by asphyxiation when paralyzed by arrows poisoned with curare. The first clinical use of curare was described in 1932, when neuromuscular blockade was given to control muscle spasms associated with tetanus. Ten years later, curare was given in the operating room to facilitate muscle relaxation and intubation.

### 3. Explain the physiology of the neuromuscular junction (NMJ).

An impulse or nerve stimulation travels down the axon to the NMJ, causing an influx of calcium ions into the axon terminal. It is here that choline from the cholinergic neurons is combined with acetate from the plasma to form ACh. After calcium generates the release of ACh from the presynaptic vesicles, the neurotransmitter traverses the synaptic cleft and binds to the receptor sites on the muscle cell membrane. Membrane permeability is increased, allowing a rapid exchange of sodium and potassium ions in the muscle fiber. Depolarization is initiated, causing an action potential that spreads through the muscle fibers and produces a muscle contraction. ACh is quickly inactivated by acetylcholinesterase, thus repolarizing the muscle fibers and restoring muscle permeability.

### 4. How are NMBAs classified?

The functional structure of ACh is duplicated in the chemical structure of NMBAs. NMBAs may be classified as either depolarizing or nondepolarizing agents. A **depolarizing agent** combines with the endplate receptors, resulting in persistent depolarization and skeletal paralysis because a depolarized membrane cannot respond to subsequent stimuli. Succinylcholine is the only clinically used depolarizing agent. Its primary use is to facilitate intubation.

**Nondepolarizing agents** compete with ACh to occupy the postsynaptic receptors, resulting in neuromuscular blockade. The level of skeletal paralysis increases in direct correlation to the number of receptor sites occupied by the agent. Nondepolarizing NMBAs may be further classified by duration as either short-, intermediate-, or long-acting.

### 5. List the common NMBAs, specifying their structure/class, onset and duration of action, and initial dose.

| AGENT | DURATION OF ACTION | STRUCTURE/CLASS | INITIAL DOSE (MG/KG) | ONSET (MIN) | CLINICAL DURATION OF ACTION (MIN) |
|---|---|---|---|---|---|
| Succinylcholine (ND) | Ultra short | Acetylcholine-like | 1.0–1.5 | 0.5–1.0 | 4–6 |
| Mivacurium (D) | Short | Benzylisoquinolinium ester | 0.15–0.25 | 1.5–3 | 12–20 |
| Atracurium (D) | Intermediate | Benzylisoquinolinium ester | 0.4–0.5 | 2–3 | 20–45 |
| Vecuronium (D) | Intermediate | Steroid-based compound | 0.08–0.10 | 2–3 | 20–35 |
| Rocuronium (D) | Intermediate | Steroid-based compound | 0.5–1.0 | 1.0–1.5 | 20–40 |
| Doxacurium (D) | Long | Benzylisoquinolinium ester | 0.025–0.08 | 5 | 55–160 |
| Pipecuronium (D) | Long | Steroid-based compound | 0.07–0.085 | 2.5–3 | 60–120 |
| Pancuronium (D) | Long | Steroid-based compound | 0.04–1.0 | 2–3 | 60–100 |

ND = Nondepolarizing; D = Depolarizing

### 6. What are the indications for use of NMBAs?

The most common indications for use of NMBAs in the critical care setting are to facilitate intubation and mechanical ventilation, to assist in controlling increased intracranial pressure, to eliminate shivering, to decrease oxygen consumption, to control agitation, and to facilitate diagnostic procedures and studies. Less frequent indications include supportive therapy for cardiovascular instability and tetanus.

Most recommendations for the use of NMBAs have been extrapolated from their use in patients undergoing surgical procedures or from experimental data in animal studies. Application of these recommendations to the hemodynamically unstable critically ill patient should be considered on a case-to-case basis.

### 7. What is the most common use of NMBAs? Which agents are used most frequently?

In 1992, Klessig and colleagues conducted a national survey on the practice patterns of anesthesiology intensivists using NMBAs. NMBAs were used most frequently to facilitate mechanical ventilation (89%), and vecuronium and pancuronium were the most frequently used agents. A survey completed by Hansen-Flaschen and colleagues in 1993 showed similar results.

### 8. What is the most prominent complication of NMBA use? Who is at risk?

Over the past 10 years, persistent or prolonged paralysis has become the most prominent complication of NMBA use. Patients at greatest risk include those with renal or hepatic dysfunction and those receiving concomitant aminoglycosides or steroids.

### 9. What other complications and side effects are associated with NMBAs?

1. Accidental disconnection from the ventilator, resulting in hypoxemia, hypercarbia, and death
2. Failure to cough, leading to retention of secretions and atelectasis
3. Autonomic and cardiovascular interactions
4. Muscle deconditioning
5. Skin breakdown
6. Leukocyte interactions
7. Prolonged muscle weakness and paralysis

### 10. Can the effects of NMBAs be reversed?

Reversal of neuromuscular blockade can be achieved in two ways: spontaneously, as the plasma concentration of the NMBA declines, or with the use of acetylcholinesterase inhibitors (only with nondepolarizing NMBAs). They bind to and inhibit acetylcholinesterase, the enzyme that degrades ACh, resulting in an increased amount of ACh in the synaptic cleft. The most common agents currently in use are neostigmine, pyridostigmine, and edrophonium. Unfortunately, the reversal agents are not effective if 100% of the ACh receptors are blocked, and they may even deepen the blockade.

### 11. What are the adverse effects of acetylcholinerase inhibitors?

Adverse effects of acetylcholinesterase inhibitors are common and may lead to dangerous complications in critically ill patients. Examples include bronchospasm, cardiac arrhythmias (including bradycardia, complete heart block, and cardiac arrest), increased pulmonary secretions, and gastrointestinal hypermotility.

### 12. What technique is used to monitor the depth of neuromuscular blockade?

For more than 20 years, nerve monitoring has been used in research and clinical practice. In the early 1960s, peripheral nerve monitoring was used to research the effects of myasthenia gravis. A few years later, anesthesiologists adopted this technique to guide drug therapy. Because serum drug levels are inaccurate and sensitivity to NMBAs varies, the depth of neuromuscular blockade must be monitored. In the ICU, the depth of blockade should be measured and recorded at least every 4 hours.

### 13. How is peripheral nerve monitoring done in the ICU?

**Clinical observation** focuses on muscle movements, such as the ability to open the eyes or breathe spontaneously. The most frequently used definitive measures are the head lift and hand grip. Five seconds or more for each of these measurements is considered a positive result.

The **peripheral nerve stimulator** (PNS) is an inexpensive, small, battery-operated device that generates an external electrical stimulus. Delivery of the stimulus to an isolated nerve elicits a chain of events resulting in neuromuscular transmission and muscle contraction. The electrical current is delivered through two electrodes, which are positioned over a superficial nerve. There are three types of electrodes: needle, ball, and pregelled (most common).

**14. What are the different modes of PNS?**

1. Single twitch uses one electrical impulse with a duration of 0.2–0.3 milliseconds (ms), causing a brief muscle contraction. This mode requires a control response and is not commonly used.

2. Posttetanic count (PTC) is a measurement of posttetanic facilitation after the delivery of rapid electrical impulses at 30, 50, or 100 Hz and is seen only in nondepolarizing blockade. Repeated use of PTC is painful and may harm the NMJ.

3. Double-burst stimulation (DBS) consists of two short bursts of 50 Hz separated by 750 ms. DBS also results in muscle contractions.

4. Train-of-four (TOF) is a series of 4 stimuli of 2 Hz delivered every 0.5 second(s). TOF results in 4 short muscle contractions.

**15. Which mode is used most commonly?**

TOF is the most convenient and commonly used method, but DBS may be more accurate.

**16. How are the results recorded?**

Depending on the mode used, the number of twitches observed and/or felt should be counted and evaluated in proportion to the number of twitches given by the PNS. When TOF is used, for example, the number of twitches demonstrated by the patient is recorded over the number 4 (i.e., 2/4).

**17. Which nerve should be used for PNS monitoring?**

No scientific evidence justifies the use of one particular nerve or monitoring technique. Several nerves have been suggested: ulnar, facial, posterior tibial, and peroneal. The ulnar nerve is the most frequently used site.

**18. How is the ulnar nerve used for PNS monitoring?**

The ulnar nerve evaluates the motor response of the adductor pollicis brevis muscle of the thumb. Electrodes are placed at the wrist, one at the head of the ulna and the other 3–4 cm away in a straight line.

**19. How is the facial nerve used for PNS monitoring?**

The facial nerve is stimulated at the temporal branch, which causes a contraction of the orbicularis oculi muscle toward the forehead. Electrodes are placed about 2 cm lateral to the outer canthus of the eye and proximal to the tragus of the ear. The facial nerve is more resistant to NMBAs than the ulnar nerve and may show more responses at the same level of blockade, leading to an underestimation of the level of neuromuscular blockade.

**20. How is the posterior tibial nerve used for PNS monitoring?**

The motor response of the posterior tibial nerve is similar to that of the ulnar nerve. Electrodes are placed behind the medial malleolus in the groove near the Achilles' tendon. Electrical stimulation results in plantar flexion of the great toe.

**21. How is the peroneal nerve used for PNS monitoring?**

In peroneal nerve stimulation, electrodes are placed posterior to the lateral malleolus and lateral to the neck of the fibula. Stimulation results in dorsiflexion of the foot. Few data are available about this nerve site.

**22. What are the protocols for NMBAs and PNS?**

Unfortunately, few protocols have been published. The primary goals of a protocol should be to standardize the care of patients receiving NMBAs and to prevent complications. A multidisciplinary approach is essential. A protocol should describe how to administer and monitor NMBAs and include safety measures and specific nursing interventions necessary for the best patient outcome.

## 23. What nursing interventions are important in patients treated with NMBAs?

1. Safety measures are a priority. A face mask and Ambu bag should be kept at the bedside. All equipment alarms should be on and audible.

2. When the patient is fed enterally, the head of the bed should remain elevated to prevent aspiration. If the bed needs to be put into a flat position, the feeding should be stopped. Gastric residuals should be checked regularly.

3. NMBAs provide no analgesic or sedative effects. Although the patient appears comatose, he or she may be awake and have the feeling of being buried alive. Administration of analgesia and sedation is mandatory, preferably by continuous infusion. Astute assessment skills will recognize an increase in heart rate or blood pressure as a sign of discomfort.

4. Reorient the patient frequently to time and place.

5. Give reassurance that close monitoring is consistent, and explain all procedures.

6. Place a sign at the bedside, explaining that the patient is able to hear but cannot physically respond.

7. Because NMBAs prevent the patient from blinking, corneal abrasions are a common side effect. Eyes should be lubricated frequently with artificial tears or gellike lubricants.

8. A neurologic assessment is virtually impossible except for pupillary function. The pupillary reflexes are controlled by smooth muscle and will not be affected by NMBAs. Pupil size and reactivity should be assessed and documented consistently.

9. Decrease the risk of skin breakdown by frequent repositioning and use of an air flotation mattress.

10. Passive range-of-motion exercises help to prevent joint stiffness and disuse atrophy of muscles.

11. Pad bony prominences.

## 24. How can the nurse offer support to family and loved ones during the use of NMBAs?

Observing a loved one under the influence of NMBAs is a scary and uncomfortable experience. Provide education. Explain the effects and reasons that NMBAs are used. Include the family in the care of the patient. For example, teach visitors the importance of range-of-motion exercises and how to do them. Encourage family and friends to talk to the patient. Provide an environment conducive to healing. Enlist the help of a social worker and/or chaplain if needed.

### BIBLIOGRAPHY

1. Dickens MD: Pharmacology of neuromuscular blockade: Interactions and implications for concurrent drug therapies. Crit Care Nurs Q 18:1–12, 1995.
2. Davidson JE: Neuromuscular blockade: Indications, peripheral nerve stimulation, and other concurrent interventions. New Horizons 2:75–84, 1994.
3. Dulin PG, Williams CJ: Monitoring and preventive care of the paralyzed patient in respiratory failure. Crit Care Clin 10:815–829, 1994.
4. Ford EV: Monitoring neuromuscular blockade in the adult ICU. Am J Crit Care 4:122–130, 1995.
5. Hoyt JW: Persistent paralysis in critically ill patients after the use of neuromuscular blocking agents. New Horizons 2:48–55, 1994.
6. Klessig HT, Geiger HJ, Murray MJ, Coursin DB: A national survey on the practice patterns of anesthesiologist intensivists in the use of muscle relaxants. Crit Care Med 20:1341–1345, 1992.
7. Miller JN: Comprehensive review: Neuromuscular blocking agents in critical care. Crit Care Nurse Q 18:60–73, 1995.
8. Prielipp RC, Coursin DB: Applied pharmacology of common neuromuscular blocking agents in critical care. New Horizons 2:34–47, 1994.
9. Rowlee SC: Monitoring neuromuscular blockade in the intensive care unit: The peripheral nerve stimulator. Heart Lung 28:352–364, 1999.
10. Susla GM: Neuromuscular blocking agents in critical care. Crit Care Nurs Clin 5:297–311, 1993.

# 60. PAIN MANAGEMENT

*Kathleen A. Puntillo, RN, DNSc, FAAN*

### 1. What is the significance of unrelieved pain to critically ill patients?

Nurses diagnose and treat pain to enhance patient comfort, to relieve suffering, and to prevent and limit tissue injury and its sequelae. Poorly controlled pain can stress the sympathetic nervous system (SNS), leaving vulnerable patients at risk of complications. It activates the metabolic stress response, which can result in hyperglycemia, lipolysis, muscle breakdown, and delayed wound healing. Pain can also produce anxiety, disturb sleep, and cause confusion, delirium, and paranoia. Any or all of these responses to unrelieved pain can prolong convalescence. Thus, pain is a significant stressor that needs the aggressive attention of critical care nurses.

### 2. Do definitions of pain provide direction to practice in a critical care setting?

Yes and no. The International Association for the Study of Pain (IASP) defines pain as "an unpleasant sensory and emotional experience associated with actual or potential tissue damage, or described in terms of such damage." This definition emphasizes that pain is multidimensional but that identifying the cause of pain is not a prerequisite to valdiation of the patient's self-report. McCaffery's definition of pain also provides great latitude for the patient: pain is "whatever the experiencing person says it is, existing whenever he says it does." However, the problem with both definitions, from a critical care perspective, is that many patients cannot verbalize their pain. Thus, clinicians must be aggressive in their approach to assessing pain.

### 3. How can we assess pain in critically ill patients?

Just do it! Use whatever means are appropriate for the individual patient. Clearly, the patient's self-report of the pain's intensity and location is ideal. Many ICU patients are capable of using pain scales, even if they are intubated. A form that includes a number of methods used by critical care nurses to assess pain can be laminated and placed at patients' bedsides. The 0–10 pain intensity scale and body outline diagram (see figure on following page) allow the patient to point to the appropriate number and body location of the pain.

### 4. What can be done if the patient is not able to communicate?

When the patient is not able to self-report, nurses must rely on other measures of pain. Systematic observation of behaviors and physiologic signs such as increased heart rate and blood pressure can increase the accuracy of the nurse's assessment. The other side of the bedside form provides a checklist, derived from research, that nurses can use to observe patients for pain (see figure on following page).

### 5. What caveats about pain assessment should the nurse keep in mind?

- Individual, cultural, and care-related differences can influence how patients behave in the presence of pain.
- Absence of pain behaviors does not mean absence of pain.
- Changes in physiologic parameters occur for many reasons; they are not always valid indicators of pain.
- Physiologic responses to pain become dampened over time and in the presence of certain drugs (e.g., beta blockers).
- Pain is known by the company it keeps. If there is any reason that pain may be present, health professionals should assume that the noncommunicative patient has pain.
- When in doubt and the patient is unable to communicate, assess possible sources of pain and treat accordingly.
- Use family and friends, who can provide information about a patient's pain history, during pain assessments.

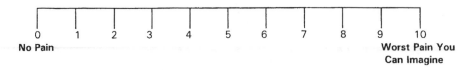

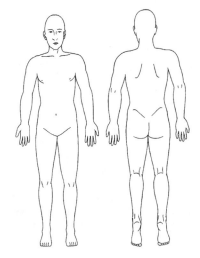

The 0–10 pain intensity scale *(above)* and body outline diagram *(left)* are important tools for the assessment of pain and should be kept at the patient's bedside.

**P**ain

**A**ssess

**I**ntervene

**N**ote (document assessment and response to intervention)

## Assess

| | |
|---|---|
| • Intensity ➜ | Use 0 - 10 scale <u>whenever possible</u> |
| • Location ➜ | Use Body Outline diagram if needed |
| • Behaviors ➜ | e.g.:<br>✓no movement<br>✓grimacing, frowning<br>✓restlessness<br>✓tense/stiffness<br>✓splinting |
| • Physiologic<br>  Signs ➜ | e.g.:<br>↑ HR<br>↑ BP or ↓ BP<br>↑ RR<br>Perspiration |

✱<u>Remember:  Absence of pain signs does not mean absence of pain</u>✱

**Intervene:**    Give analgesics as ordered and provide comfort measures.

**Note:**    <u>Document:</u> •   Initial assessment of pain<br>                              •   Interventions<br>                              •   Response to interventions

Pain asssessment reference. (From Analgesic, Sedation, NMBA Administration Reference card in Drip Chart Books and Pain Management in Adults. UCSF Nursing Policy and Procedure Manual, Vol. 1.)

**6. Why is it important to know the pain and analgesic history of a critically ill patient?**

The patient's pain and analgesic history can significantly influence the present pain experience and response to analgesic interventions. For example, a patient with cancer who has received long-term opioids at home is not "opioid-naive." ICU analgesic doses should be calculated to include at-home maintenance dose as well as the dose now needed for specific pain problems. Likewise, a patient with a history of chemical dependency who is admitted to ICU needs higher baseline doses for maintenance. A patient's pain history informs the nurse about ongoing problems, such as chronic back pain, that need to be taken into consideration as pharmacologic and nonpharmacologic analgesic interventions are planned.

**7. Can use of a physiologic framework of pain assist the critical care nurse in choosing pain management methods?**

A framework that depicts physiologic mechanisms of pain transmission and inhibition can assist the nurse in choosing and advocating for pain management methods that seem appropriate for a specific patient (see figure below). For example, nonsteroidal antiinflammatory drugs (NSAIDs) are effective at the source of tissue injury, as are cold and heat. Regional nerve blocks with anesthetic agents inhibit the transmission of pain across fibers that run from periphery to central nervous system (CNS). Spinal opioids provide a localized vs. systemic response and minimize untoward systemic effects. Intravenously (IV) administered opioids work systemically because of the multiple locations of opioid receptors. Nonpharmacologic interventions can augment the body's natural pain inhibition system. Through activation of pain inhibitory fibers that descend from the brain to spinal cord, ascending pain transmission is blocked. Distraction, patient control, information, and relaxation are believed to promote pain inhibition. The critical care nurse can refer to this physiologic framework and relate the patient's particular pain problem to possible interventions.

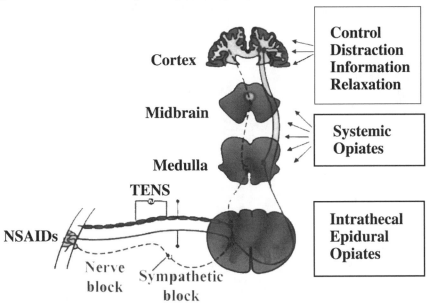

Pain therapies and proposed sites of action. (Modified from Fields HL, Levine JD: Pain: Mechanisms and management. West J Med 141:347–357, 1984.)

**8. What analgesics are used most frequently in critical care settings?**

Opioid analgesic therapy is the mainstay pharmacologic treatment modality for pain in critically ill patients. The table on the next page presents information about the systemic opioids most frequently used in critical care.

*Systemic Opioids for the Treatment of Acute Pain*

| DRUG | ADMINISTRATION ROUTE (MG/KG) | FRONT LOAD[1,2] (MG/KG) | MAINTENANCE DOSE[3] (MG/KG) | FREQUENCY[4] (HR) |
|---|---|---|---|---|
| Agonists | | | | |
| Codeine | PO | 1.5 | 0.75 | 3–4 |
| | SC, IM | 1.0 | 0.5 | 3–4 |
| Hydrocodone[5] (Vicodin) | PO | 0.15 | 0.07–0.15 | 4–6 |
| Oxycodone (Percodan) | PO | 0.15 | 0.07–0.15 | 3–4 |
| Morphine | PO | 0.5–1.0 | 0.5–1.0 | 4 |
| | Slow-release PO[6] | 1.0 | 1.0–2.0 | 12 |
| | SC, IM | 0.15 | 0.1–0.2 | 3–4 |
| | IV | 0.15 | 0.01–0.04/hr | Continuous |
| Hydromorphone (Dilaudid) | PO | 0.04–0.08 | 0.04–0.08 | 3 |
| | SC, IM | 0.02–0.04 | 0.03–0.06 | 3 |
| | IV | 0.02 | 0.01/hr | Continuous |
| Oxymorphone | SC, IM | 015 | 0.1–0.2 | 3–4 |
| Methadone | PO | 0.2–0.4 | 0.1–0.4 | * |
| | SC, IM | 0.15 | 0.1–0.2 | * |
| | IV | 0.15 | † | — |
| Levorphanol | PO | 0.02–0.04 | 0.02–0.04 | — |
| | SC, IM | 0.02 | 0.01 | — |
| | IV | 0.02 | † | — |
| Fentanyl | IV[7] | 0.0008–0.0016 | 0.0003–0.0016 hr | Continuous |
| | Transdermal | | | |
| Sufentanil | IV[7] | 0.0001–0.0003 | Not established | — |
| Alfentanil | IV[7] | 0.03–0.05 | 0.06–0.09/hr | Continuous |

[1] IV front loading dose should be titrated slowly to reduce risk of overdose.

[2] Except in pediatric patients, body weight is not an accurate predictor of effective opioid dose. Titration to desired effect for each patient is necessary.

[3] Maintenance dose usually is approximately one-half the effective loading dose.

[4] If pain breakthrough occurs before scheduled maintenance dose, give one additional maintenance dose and continue schedule

[5] Available only in combination with aspirin or acetaminophen in the U.S.

[6] Nearest dosage increment must be chosen; if tablets are broken, immediate release can occur.

[7] Short duration of action makes IV infusion only practical route of administration.

* Watch for accumulation, especially after 48 hours of administration.

† Long duration of action renders drug unsuitable for continuous infusion.

Modified from Brady LB, Edwards WT (eds): Management of Acute Pain: A Practical Guide. Seattle, IASP Press, 1992, pp 15–16.

## 9. How do you choose the appropriate mode and route of analgesic administration?

The enteral route is generally avoided in critically ill patients because absorption of drugs may be diminished. In considering the IV route, remember that a continuous infusion (vs. bolus doses) provides a steady plasma concentration and, ultimately, a better therapeutic window. Patient-controlled analgesia (PCA) should be considered for patients who are able to self-administer analgesic medications. This mode allows patients to feel more in control of their situation. The epidural route of administration offers many advantages. It can provide profound analgesia while minimizing adverse systemic effects from opioids. Numerous studies have documented better outcomes in patients receiving epidural analgesics vs. as-needed IV opioids. The epidural route should be considered as an option for patients without contraindications (e.g., coagulopathies, sepsis).

## 10. Why is dosing often complicated in critically ill patients?

Because of significant organ dysfunction and hemodynamic abnormalities in critically ill patients, the pharmacokinetics and pharmacodynamics of drugs show significant interindividual variation. A standard drug dose may be toxic for some patients, subtherapeutic for others, and completely effective for a few.

### 11. What key points should be kept in mind about morphine, fentanyl, and meperidine?

Morphine may stimulate histamine release from mast cells, causing allergic reactions and cardiovascular instability. Fentanyl does so to a lesser degree. Fentanyl metabolism is not significantly affected by renal disease, making it a good choice for long term use in patients with renal insufficiency. Morphine and meperidine have active metabolites and should be used cautiously in patients with renal disease. Use of meperidine is not recommended because accumulation of its active metabolite, normeperidine, can lead to central nervous system (CNS) hyperexcitability. Accumulation can cause seizures.

### 12. What is the role of ketorolac in the ICU?

Ketorolac (Toradol) is an NSAID that can be administered IV to substitute for or augment the effects of opioids. Its potency is comparable to various doses of morphine and meperidine. Ketorolac is contraindicated in the presence of bleeding, renal insufficiency, and active peptic ulcer disease. However, its use should be considered for certain ICU patients, especially if inflammation is a component of the patient's pain.

### 13. What is the role of regional nerve blocks in the ICU?

Some critically ill patients obtain considerable relief through the use of regional nerve blocks. Anesthetic agents such as bupivacaine injected into intracostal fibers or added to epidural opioid infusions block pain fiber transmission in the area of infusion. Intracostal blocks have been used with much success to relieve pain associated with blunt chest trauma or thoracic surgery.

### 14. Why are drug interactions of particular importance in critically ill patients?

Many drugs used for analgesia in the ICU are generally protein-bound and eliminated primarily by the liver. Thus they are susceptible to a variety of drug interactions that either decrease or increase their effectiveness and duration of action.

### 15. What other caveats about analgesics in the ICU should be kept in mind?

- Most of the analgesics used in the ICU may accumulate and have prolonged effects with extended drug administration.
- Opioids are not amnestic agents and, thus, should be used in combination with drugs that cause amnesia (e.g. midazolam) if amnesia is a treatment goal.
- Elderly patients are at higher risk for toxicity because they are more likely to exhibit decreased drug clearance and have concurrent risk factors. However, caution should be balanced with provision of effective pain management.
- When bolusing with opioids, know times to onset and peak effect as well as duration of effect of the specific opioid. Operating within the therapeutic window of an analgesic agent is essential.

### 16. Define opioid tolerance, dependence, and addiction. How common are they in the ICU?

**Tolerance** is a physiologic state in which increasingly greater amounts of opioids are needed to achieve a similar analgesic effect. **Physical dependence** is present if a withdrawal syndrome occurs when opioids are withheld. It, too, is a physiologic process that may be due to rebound of CNS noradrenergic activity depressed by chronic opioid use. **Addiction** is a psychological dependence on opioids evidenced by compulsive drug-seeking behavior. Addiction is often associated with physiologic dependence.

### 17. How common are tolerance, dependence, and addiction in the ICU?

Critical care patients who receive continuous opioid infusions for any length of time often exhibit tolerance and dependence, whereas addiction is extremely rare in patients who were opioid-naive prior to admission.

## 18. How is tolerance recognized and managed?

The first sign of tolerance may be a decrease in duration of effective analgesia. Tolerance can be delayed by combining opioids with nonopioids or switching to another type of opioid. With the latter strategy, one-half of the predicted equianalgesic dose should be selected as the starting dose, because there is not complete cross-tolerance among opioids.

## 19. What are the signs and symptoms of dependence? How are they managed?

Patients who have developed physical dependence from long-term opioid use are at risk of developing an abstinence syndrome (i.e., going into withdrawal) if the opioids are abruptly discontinued. Signs of the abstinence syndrome include anxiety, irritability, salivation, lacrimation, rhinorrhea, diaphoresis, piloerection, nausea, vomiting, abdominal cramps, and insomnia. To avoid the abstinence syndrome, opioids should be withdrawn slowly. A recommended weaning regimen is to administer one-half of the previous daily dose given every 6 hours for the first 2 days. Then reduce the dose by 25% every 2 days.

## 20. How are opioid-addicted patients managed?

Opioid-addicted patients admitted to the ICU have a physiologic need for continued opioid administration. This need should be managed pharmacologically so that patients receive the comfort that they deserve.

## 21. What is preemptive analgesia? Why is it important?

Once acute pain escalates and becomes established, it is more difficult to control—even with higher doses of analgesics. Preemptive analgesia is the administration of an analgesic before a noxious stimulus is rendered to prevent amplification and hyperexcitability of the CNS. It is postulated that hyperexcitability leads to CNS sensitization, which, in turn, can cause the development of persistent pain. Acute pain, most often experienced after tissue injury, is the highest risk factor for the development of a debilitating persistent pain syndrome. Most preemptive analgesia studies have been limited to surgical pain, and results are not yet well established. However, it is important for the critical care nurse to recognize the potential for long-term adverse consequences and the potential value of treating pain before it occurs.

## 22. What is the nurse's role in preemptive analgesia?

- Plan for the administration of analgesics before any potentially painful procedure.
- Be the patient's advocate when other health professionals plan to initiate painful procedures by insisting on prior administration of an analgesic.
- Attend to the analgesic's profile of action (i.e., time to peak effect and duration of effect) before and during a painful procedure so that its efficacy is optimal.

## 23. Why is procedural pain an important pain in the ICU?

Pain that accompanies diagnostic or treatment-related procedures can be both a physiologic and psychological stressor to patients. Indeed, thousands of painful procedures are performed every day in critical care settings. Even the frequently performed procedure of turning or being turned in bed is painful for many patients. In fact, in a large multisite study, turning was the most painful of six common procedures performed on hospitalized patients.

The frequency with which painful procedures are performed may serve as a barrier to adequate pain control because the procedure and accompanying pain become so commonplace to healthcare providers. However, procedural pain should not be minimized, and analgesia should never be withheld for a painful procedure unless immediate treatment of cardiorespiratory instability is required or a competent patient declines treatment.

## 24. What interventions may be used for procedural pain?

Selection of interventions should be individualized, and use of a combination of interventions should be considered. The table below summarizes common options.

*Interventions for Procedural Pain*

| INTERVENTION | MECHANISM OF ACTION | SPECIAL CONSIDERATIONS |
|---|---|---|
| IV administration of opioids | Promotes analgesia by mimicking endogenous opioid system | Fentanyl is a rapid-acting opioid; its rapid onset and short duration of action promote dose adjustment and make it highly suitable for pain management during procedures |
| IV administration of benzodiazepines (BZDs) | Sedative and amnesic properties augment analgesia | Should not be administered in place of analgesics<br>Midazolam is the most rapid-acting of commonly used BZDs; this factor promotes dose adjustment |
| IV administration of propofol | Ultra-short–acting anesthetic with amnestic, hypnotic, and anxiolytic properties | Can cause hypotension when administered rapidly and with bolus doses<br>Sedative effects are dose-dependent and short-lived, making it a suitable agent for procedures<br>Should be administered along with analgesics because it possesses no analgesic properties |
| IV admistration of ketamine | Dissociative anesthetic; causes individual to be separated from surroundings<br>Induces sedation, amnesia, and analgesia | Activates SNS; can be administered in patients with hypotension or respiratory depression<br>Structurally similar to phencyclidine (PCP), causing hallucinatory effects<br>Because unpleasant dreams and emergent delirium are common, should be used in conjunction with BZDs |
| Relaxation techniques, distraction (e.g., with music), information, visual imagery | Nonpharmacologic interventions thought to activate endogenous pain inhibitory systems | Should be used as adjuvants to pharmacologic agents<br>Provide patient with sense of control<br>Specific information about expected sensations can decrease pain intensity and distress<br>Some require prior training, which may preclude widespread use in ICU |

SNS = sympathetic nervous system.

## 25. Why is it important to have a systematic, standardized method of documenting pain, analgesic interventions, and patients' responses?

This information is as important to a patient's well-being as are other data collected and documented, considering the patient's physiologic and psychological vulnerability. Better pain management and decreased pain have resulted from systematic nursing documentation on pain assessment forms or bedside flow sheets. Documentation of degree of relief after an intervention communicates the effects of the interventions to other health care team members and provides guidance to subsequent treatment decisions.

### BIBLIOGRAPHY

1. Acute Pain Management Guidelines Panel: Acute pain management: Operative or medical procedures and trauma. Clinical Practice Guidelines (AHCPR Pub No 92-0032), Rockville, MD, 1992, US Department of Health Care Policy and Research.
2. American Pain Society. Principles of Analgesic Use in the Treatment of Acute Pain and Cancer Pain, 4th ed. Glenview, IL, American Pain Society, 1999.

3. Cammarano WB, Pittet J, Weitz S, et al: Acute withdrawal syndrome related to the administration of analgesic and sedative medications in adult intensive care unit patients. Crit Care Med 26:676–684, 1998.
4. International Association for Study of Pain: Pain terms: A list with definitions and notes on usage. Pain 6: 249–252, 1979.
5. McCaffery M: Nursing Management of the Patient with Pain. Philadelphia, J.B. Lippincott, 1979.
6. Puntillo KA, Casella V: Pain, analgesia, and sedation. In Kinney MR, Dunbar SB, Brooks-Brunn JA, et al (eds): AACN's Clinical Reference for Critical Care Nursing, 4th ed. St. Louis, Mosby, 1998.
7. Puntillo KA, White C, Morris A, et al: Patients' perceptions and responses to procedural pain: Results from Thunder Project ® II. [in review].
8. Stannard D, Puntillo K, Miaskowski C, et al: Clinical judgment and management of postoperative pain in critical care patients. Am J Crit Care 5:433–441, 1996.
9. Summer GJ, Puntillo KA: Management of surgical and procedural pain in a critical care setting. Crit Care Nurs Clin North Am [in review].

# 61. SEDATION

*Margaret H. Doherty, RN, MSN, CCRN*

### 1. What is sedation?

Sedation is the pharmacologic use of central nervous system (CNS) depressants to reduce fear, anxiety, and agitation.

### 2. How is the need for sedation determined?

The need for sedation is based on the underlying pathologic condition, the primary goals of treatment, the physiologic stress response to illness, and the presence of agitation and delirium. The many causes of fear, anxiety, and agitation in critically ill patients include underlying pathology and medical interventions. Agitated delirium impairs cellular metabolism, increases oxygen consumption, and threatens the success of necessary interventions, such as intravenous (IV) medications and mechanical ventilation.

### 3. What are the most common goals of sedation?

Compliance with therapy, patient comfort and safety, and conscious sedation during a specific procedure.

### 4. What are the major risks of using sedatives?

Adverse side effects and interference with assessment of changes in neurologic status.

### 5. Describe the nurse's role in assessing the need for sedation.

1. The nurse must consider the purpose and goal of sedation, which may vary with each patient (see question 3).

2. A careful history (e.g., drug use, alcohol abuse, chronic illness, normal coping behaviors) is necessary to determine the cause of agitation and to identify the most effective sedative for each patient.

3. The patient should be assessed for restlessness, agitation, hallucinations, acutely altered level of consciousness, and attempts at self-extubation, all of which may indicate the need for sedation.

### 6. What types of patients should be sedated?

An individualized approach to sedation is mandatory, but the following principles should be kept in mind:

1. Agitated patients with head injury should be sedated enough to reduce intracranial pressure but not to the point that it is impossible to assess neurologic status.

2. Research indicates that sedation decreases the severity of ischemia in agitated patients who have undergone open-heart surgery by deactivating the stress response.

3. In patients with an acute myocardial infarction, sedatives are used to relieve anxiety, opioids to relieve pain. Opioids also provide some central nervous depression and sedation.

4. Intubated patients should be sedated to decrease oxygen consumption and energy expenditure because agitation is a hypermetabolic state.

**7. Which class of agents is used for effective sedation in the intensive care unit (ICU)?**

Benzodiazepines increase the action of two inhibitory neurotransmitters, gamma aminobutyric acid (GABA) and glycine, and cause sedation, anxiolysis, decreased skeletal muscle contraction, and amnesia.

**8. Describe the use of specific benzodiazepines.**

**Midazolam** (Versed) is used to maintain compliance with therapy and for conscious sedation with specific procedures. It is highly lipophilic and absorbed rapidly into the brain and fat stores. It can be given by IV bolus, 1–4 mg, or infusion, 1–4 mg/hr. Possible side effects include respiratory depression, hypotension, and excessive sedation.

**Diazepam** (Valium) is another lipophilic benzodiazepine with a sudden onset of action. But it has a prolonged duration of action because of its active metabolite, dimethyl-diazepam, which prolongs the sedative effect up to 96 hours, especially in patients with decreased metabolism or severe liver disease. For this reason, it is not recommended in the critical care setting.

**Lorazepam** (Ativan) is highly effective with many patient populations. Because it is hydrophilic, it has a longer serum half-life. Lorazepam can be given IV, intramuscularly (IM), or sublingually (SL). The SL route is convenient when the patient has no IV access; the dose is the same as for the IV route (1–4 mg). Because it is metabolized in the liver by microsomal enzymes instead of conjugation, lorazepam does not have an altered effect or prolonged duration of action in patients with severe liver disease. It is the drug of choice for alcohol withdrawal protocols. Doses are quite variable and often need to be adjusted because of tolerance.

**9. What other sedatives are used?**

Propofol (Diprivan) and haloperidol (Haldol).

**10. Describe the appropriate use of propofol.**

Propofol is a short-acting sedative-hypnotic agent used for sedation and induction of general anesthesia. It has a rapid onset of action (30 seconds) and duration of 3–10 minutes because of its high lipophilicity. It must be given via IV infusion and is appropriate only when sedation is required for < 72 hours. Patients must be mechanically ventilated or have their airway continuously monitored. Infusion rates typically start at 5 μg/kg/min for at least 5 minutes. The rate can be increased in increments of 5–10 μg/kg/min every 5–10 minutes until the desired level of sedation is achieved. The sedative effect is enhanced when opioids are administered concomitantly for pain management. If a second CNS depressant is added, the dosage needs to be decreased to prevent adverse side effects such as oversedation. Propofol has no analgesic properties; analgesics should be given as needed or if painful procedures are anticipated.

**11. What contraindications and adverse side effects are associated with propofol?**

Contraindications include pregnancy and allergies to soy bean oil or egg lecithin. Possible adverse side effects include hypotension, reduced myocardial contractility, increased risk of infection due to the lack of an antimicrobial additive, hypertriglyceridemia related to lipid content, and loss of airway protective mechanisms.

**12. Describe the appropriate use of haloperidol.**

Haloperidol is an antipsychotic agent that stabilizes the neurotransmitter dopamine and improves cognitive function. Clinical research with agitated critically ill patients has demonstrated its synergistic effects with benzodiazepines, especially lorazepam. For example, a combination of lorazepam 1–4 mg IV, and haloperidol 1–4 mg IV, can be titrated to the desired effect in management of agitation.

### 13. What adverse effects are associated with haloperidol?
Possible adverse effects with short-term use of haloperidol include prolongation of the QT interval.

### 14. What factors help to choose the right sedative and right dose for an agitated patient?
- Underlying pathology
- Patient's age
- Cause of agitation
- Goal of sedation
- Length of required sedation
- Pharmacokinetics of the specific drug

The initial dose should be the lowest possible, with upward titration to the desired effect. The dose should be decreased when the patient is oversedated. With elderly patients, the general rule is to "start low and go slow."

### 15. How is level of sedation assessed?
The following scale may be included in the ICU 24-hour flow sheet to remind nurses to document level of consciousness (LOC) at frequent intervals; it also may be used in conjunction with pain management:

1 = awake, alert      4 = confused
2 = drowsy            5 = stuporous
3 = sleeping          6 = comatose

### 16. What is the Modified Ramsay Scale?
The Modified Ramsay Scale is another tool for assessing agitation and effectiveness of sedation. If the goal is level 3, for example, each nurse can medicate the patient with this goal in mind.

Level 1: anxious, agitated, or restless
Level 2: cooperative, oriented, and tranquil
Level 3: responsive only to commands
Level 4: responsive to gentle shaking
Level 5: responsive to noxious stimuli
Level 6: unresponsive to firm nail bed pressure or other noxious stimuli

### 17. What is a sedation protocol? What are its advantages?
A sedation protocol is a standardized plan of care that guides nurses in meeting the goal of sedation and effectively managing agitated delirium (see figure on following page). It provides useful information about which drug is indicated and which dosage is appropriate for a particular patient. It also emphasizes the importance of patient comfort as a quality issue. Research has shown that a nurse-driven sedation protocol reduces the length of ICU stay, hospital stay, time on the ventilator, and time of sedation.

### 18. What technique is recommended for sedative administration?
Therapeutic levels of the appropriate drug can be maintained with IV bolus or IV infusion. IV boluses must be diluted on an ml-per-ml basis and given over 10–60 seconds. This slower push allows the drug to bind to plasma proteins, especially albumin. The unbound portion binds to specific receptors, such as GABA/benzodiazepine receptors in the CNS. This technique minimizes adverse effects due to an excessive blood level of unbound drug.

### 19. How often should the patient be unsedated? Why?
The patient should be unsedated or "lightened up" once per shift or once daily to assess neurologic status and effectiveness of sedation. Specific techniques, included in the sedation protocol, allow the patient to be assessed neurologically without becoming severely agitated. An LOC scale should be used frequently with assessment of vital signs. The nurse must be vigilant during lightening-up periods and assess the risk-benefit ratio of less sedation. For example, a patient

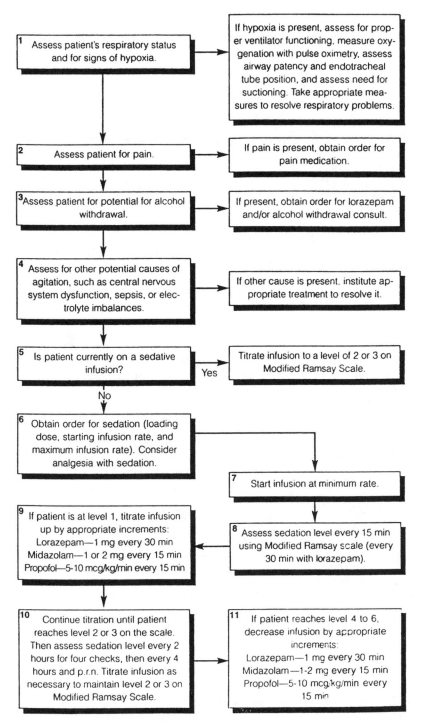

Protocol for sedating intubated patients who appear agitated. (Reprinted with permission of the author, Jan Powers, RN, MSN, CCRN.)

with traumatic brain injury must have neurologic assessments at frequent intervals. However, if he or she is agitated, intracranial pressure may increase and cause further damage. The goal in this setting is to maintain the ideal level of sedation with small changes in the sensorium. In general, a multidisciplinary approach provides the safest sedation and care.

## 20. What other nursing responsibilities help to ensure sedation?

1. The nurse must decrease stimuli, such as pain, fever, anxiety, fear, seizure activity, and hypovolemia, that may increase the stress response. A calm and caring approach is essential. Minimization of the stress response helps to decrease energy expenditure and oxygen consumption.

2. The patient must be monitored continuously to achieve the goals of therapy and to prevent complications. Attention must be paid to lab values, fluid status, organ perfusion, and oxygenation, all of which may affect sedation.

3. The nurse must be aware of high-risk patients, such as the elderly, who are sensitive to the effects of sedatives and may experience adverse side effects because of decreased liver metabolism and renal excretion.

## 21. Can patients develop tolerance to sedatives?

Yes. Over time the GABA receptors change shape and decrease in number so that more drug is needed to achieve the same effect. In this context, undersedation is likely. The nurse must monitor the level of sedation closely. In additions, patients receiving sedation for management of agitation should receive the minimal effective dose for the shortest period to prevent complications. If tolerance is present, a different type of benzodiazepine can be used.

## 22. What is conscious sedation?

Conscious sedation is a state in which the patient receives drugs with the intent of inducing a depressed level of consciousness so that a particular procedure can be performed. The patient retains the ability to maintain a patent airway and responds appropriately to verbal and tactile stimuli.

## 23. What are the key nursing responsibilities with conscious sedation?

Nursing priorities are based on the goals of patient safety and compliance during a procedure such as cardioversion or bronchoscopy. A thorough assessment that includes a health history, current pathology/diagnoses, vital signs, pulse oximetry, and estimation of hydration status must be done before the procedure. This assessment helps the nurse to identify patients at increased risk for complications (see question 24). Other nursing responsibilities include:

1. Obtaining IV access
2. Monitoring airway patency
3. Monitoring vital signs (heart rate, blood pressure, respiratory rate, and pulse oximetry)
4. Monitoring level of consciousness during the procedure
5. Ensuring availability of emergency equipment (e.g., suction and defibrillator) and medications (e.g., naloxone [Narcan], an opioid reversal agent, and flumazenil [Romazicon], a benzodiazepine reversal agent).
6. Ensuring ongoing and effective communication about the patient's condition with the physician during the procedure.

## 24. What factors place patients at increased risk for complications during conscious sedation?
- Noncompliance/lack of cooperation
- Extremes of age
- Severe underlying cardiac, pulmonary, hepatic, renal, or CNS disease
- Sleep apnea
- Pregnancy
- History of substance abuse

## 25. What drugs are used for conscious sedation?

The most commonly used sedatives are short-acting opioids such as fentanyl and short-acting benzodiazepines such as midazolam. If two agents are used, smaller doses of each drug may achieve adequate conscious sedation.

### 26. What are the nursing priorities after the procedure is completed?

Patient safety is the primary goal. Patients must be allowed to recover completely from the procedure and from the sedation. Careful monitoring is essential during the recovery period. Because sedatives can affect coordination for several hours, patients are instructed not to drive and must have an identified means of returning home. Discharge instructions should include pertinent information about safety issues and possible side effects.

### 27. How can competency related to sedation be ensured?

The nursing staff must work closely with pharmacists and physicians to develop sedation protocols and to identify education strategies related to sedation management. Knowledge of the causes of agitation and delirium is essential for nursing assessment. Minimizing agitation in the critical care setting is everyone's responsibility. The pharmacokinetics of each drug must be considered in choosing the best sedative for a particular patient. Nonpharmacologic interventions are important adjuncts that increase comfort, decrease anxiety and fear, and enhance the quality of patient care.

### BIBLIOGRAPHY

1. Davidson JE: Managing sedation in the intensive care unit: An advanced practice resource. Critical Care Nurse Educational Series, 1997, pp 1–10.
2. Hooper VD, George-Gay B: Sedation in the critically ill patient. Crit Care Nurs Clin North Am 9:395–409, 1997.
3. Kixmiller JM, Schick L: Conscious sedation in cardiovascular procedures. Crit Care Nurs Clin North Am 9:300–311, 1997.
4. Lilley LL, Aucker RS: Pharmacology and the Nursing Process, 2nd ed. Mosby, St. Louis, 1999.
5. Luer JM: Sedation and neuromuscular blockade in patients with acute respiratory failure. Aliso Viejo, CA, AACN Crit Care Publication: Care of the Mechanically Ventilated Patient Series, 1998, p 1027.
6. Mirski MA, Muffelman B, Ulatowski JA, Hanley DF: Sedation for the critically ill neurologic patient. Crit Care Med 23:2038–2053, 1995.
7. Powers J: A sedation protocol for preventing patient self-extubation. Dimens Crit Care Nurs 18:30–34, 1999.
8. Puntillo K, Casella V, Reid M: Opioid and benzodiazepine dependence: Application of theory to critical care practice. Heart Lung 26:317–324, 1997.
9. Shapiro BA, Warren J, Egol AB, et al: Practice parameters for intravenous analgesia and sedation for adult patients in the intensive care unit: An executive summary. Crit Care Med 23:1596–1600, 1995.
10. Shields RE: A comprehensive review of sedative and analgesic agents. Crit Care Nurs Clin North Am 9: 281–287, 1997.

# 62. EPIDURAL CATHETER MANAGEMENT

*Sheila Gleeson*, RN, BSN

### 1. What are epidural catheters? When are they used?

An epidural catheter is a thin plastic catheter that is placed into the epidural space between the dura mater and vertebral arch. Epidural catheters are inserted into either the thoracic or lumbar region of the spinal cord. Opioids and/or local anesthetics are administered through the catheter to provide analgesia and/or anesthesia during procedures, surgery, and the postoperative period.

### 2. Who benefits from epidural catheter analgesia?

Many different patient populations benefit from epidural analgesia. Surgical patients undergoing thoracic, major intraabdominal, peripheral vascular, orthopedic, gynecologic, and obstetric procedures are frequently managed intra- and postoperatively with epidural catheters. Patients with chronic pain, cancer, and trauma can achieve effective pain relief with a variety of drugs that are infused via epidural catheter.

### 3. What are the contraindications to epidural cathter placement?

Contraindications to epidural catheter placement include severe infections, sepsis, coagulopathies, increased intracranial pressure, various spinal problems, and patient refusal.

### 4. What are the advantages of epidural analgesia and anesthesia?

Infusion of medication specifically where the pain receptors are located in the spinal cord can inhibit neuronal firing. This proximity to pain receptors makes it possible to use 10 times less opioid than by the intravenous (IV) route.

### 5. What types of drugs are used?

Opioids and local anesthetics are frequently combined and infused in very low concentrations to achieve a powerful pain-mediating effect. Segmental anesthesia and continuous postoperative analgesia are achieved with continuous epidural infusions.

### 6. How do epidurally administered local anesthetics work?

Local anesthetics bind nerve roots that enter and exit the spinal cord. By using low concentrations of anesthetics, sensory pathways are blocked while motor fibers remain intact. Ropivacaine and bupivacaine are used most often because they allow better sensory block. Local anesthetics act synergistically with opioids and have a dose-sparing effect. The benefits of using the two agents together are that lower doses of opioids provide effective pain relief and the incidence of side effects is reduced.

### 7. How do epidural opioids work?

Opioids work by moving across the dura mater into the spinal cord, where they bind to opiate receptors and reduce presynaptic neurotransmitter release. Morphine, fentanyl, and hydromorphone are commonly used for epidural analgesia. It is essential to use preservative-free morphine and fentanyl to avoid potential neurotoxicity and spinal cord injury. Morphine and fentanyl have different drug solubility characteristics that influence volume of distribution, onset, duration of action, and side effects. Hydrophilic opioids cross the dura mater slowly, stay in the cerebrospinal fluid (CSF) longer, and have a slower onset of action. Lipophilic opioids cross the dura mater easily and rapidly and have a shorter duration of action.

### 8. Summarize the pharmacologic characteristics of the epidural opioids.

| DRUG | SOLUBILITY | ONSET | DURATION |
|------|------------|-------|----------|
| Fentanyl | Lipophilic | Rapid: 10–30 min | Short: 2–5 hr |
| Morphine | Hydrophilic | Slow: 60–120 min | Long: 8–22 hr |
| Hydromorphone | Lipophilic and hydrophylic | Intermediate: 30–45 min | Intermediate: 5–8 hr |

### 9. What risks are associated with combining opioids and local anesthetics?

Local anesthetics may cause hypotension and motor weakness. The dose of opioid and local anesthetic must be titrated carefully to minimize these risks. If the infusion rate is increased to treat pain, the anesthetic dose also is increased. The concentrations and/or ratios of the two agents can be adjusted to minimize the risks of hypotension and excessive motor weakness.

### 10. What nursing interventions are important when epidural pain management is initiated?

1. Emergency supplies and equipment should be accessible on units where patients with epidural catheters are managed. This includes an oxygen set-up, self-inflating resuscitation bag, and naloxone (reversal agent).

2. Patients should be educated about pain assessment with the 0–10 intensity scale (0 = no pain, 10 = worst pain) and potential side effects (e.g., tingling or numbness of fingers or mouth from local anesthesia) before initiation of epidural therapy.

3. Review the epidural prescription for appropriateness of medications and dosages.

4. The infusion pump should be set to administer only 2 hours of medication.

5. Aspirate the epidural catheter before connecting the infusion tubing to confirm placement.

6. Free flowing CSF or blood discovered upon aspiration (> 2 ml) indicates that the catheter is in the intrathecal or intravascular space. The physician should be notified with abnormal aspiration results and catheter use avoided.

7. Small amounts of air in the catheter or infusion line are not harmful.

8. Alcohol, povidone-iodine, and bacteriostatic solutions are not recommended for disinfection at epidural catheter-tubing junctions because they are toxic to the central nervous system.

9. Epidural infusion tubing should not have injection ports. If ports exist, they should be taped to prevent access and a possible entry site for infection.

**11. What monitoring is required during epidural catheter use?**

Respiratory rate should be assessed every hour for 24 hours and then every 4 hours for the duration of the infusion. Assessment of pain is now considered the fifth vital sign. Pain score (using the 0–10 scale) and sedation level should be assessed every 4 hours for the duration of the infusion. If the patient is unable to speak or is asleep, the nurse can assess behavioral cues and physiologic signs (e.g., facial grimace, guarding, tachycardia). Frequency of monitoring other vital signs should be based on the patient's condition. If the patient develops severe itching or nausea or appears unexpectedly somnolent, the administration of naloxone should be considered.

**12. How is the epidural catheter maintained?**

Epidural solution bottles are changed every 48 hours. Infusion tubing is changed every 72 hours. The Luer lock connection between the infusion tubing and catheter can be reinforced with a tongue blade taped under the two connections to help prevent accidental disconnections. It is important not to clamp the catheter because the lumen is small and fluid back-up is negligible.

**13. Are patients with an epidural catheter allowed to walk?**

Yes. However, they must be instructed to ask for assistance when getting up for the first time. Blood pressure (BP) and heart rate (HR) should be assessed for orthostatic changes. A systolic BP < 90 mmHg, HR < 50 or > 120 beats/minute, and associated mental status changes, dizziness, or lightheadedness require further evaluation.

**14. Can epidural analgesia cause respiratory depression?**

Respiratory depression is one of the most serious complications of epidural analgesia. Early respiratory depression occurs within 2 hours of epidural opioid administration and may continue as the drug moves into the epidural veins and systemic circulation. Six to twelve hours after initiation, the drug begins to diffuse into the CSF and bind with opioid receptors in the respiratory center. Respiratory depression may occur up to 24 hours after an epidural bolus. Fortunately the incidence of severe respiratory depression is less than 1%.

**15. What are the early signs of respiratory depression?**

Early signs associated with impending respiratory depression include change in level of consciousness, lethargy, itching, nausea, and decreased respiratory depth with little change in respiratory rate. Patients with abnormal respiratory rates or patterns and altered mental status require close observation. It is important to monitor respiratory status every hour for the first 24 hours. Oxygen saturation, sedation, pain, sensory level, and motor strength should be assessed on a regular basis and recorded according to hospital procedure.

**16. When is naloxone administered for respiratory depression?**

Attempt to arouse the patient, encourage respirations, and apply oxygen if the respiratory rate drops below the prescribed parameter (usually < 8 breaths/min) or respiratory effort is weak. Stop the epidural opioid infusion and administer naloxone as prescribed.

**17. How is naloxone administered?**

Naloxone should be given slowly and in small increments until the patient's respiratory rate increases. It is recommended that 1 ml (0.4 mg) naloxone be mixed with 9 ml of normal saline to make 0.04 mg/ml concentration. The patient should be given approximately 1–3 ml (0.04–0.12 mg) every 2–3 minutes until the respiratory rate is within normal parameters. The goal is to maintain analgesia while reversing the respiratory depression. Additional doses or a continuous naloxone infusion may be required if respiratory depression continues 30–45 minutes after the initial naloxone dose. Respiratory depression can last up to 24 hours, whereas naloxone has a 30-minute duration of action. Therefore, frequent respiratory monitoring is essential for 24 hours after the epidural infusion is discontinued.

**18. How is the rate of a continuous naloxone infusion calculated?**
When the patient's respiratory rate drops, an IV naloxone dose (usually 0.04 mg) is given every 10 minutes until the respiratory rate reaches 8 breaths/minute. The naloxone infusion dose is typically 1–10 μg/kg/hr, tirated to a respiratory rate of 8 breaths/minute. The epidural infusion may or may not be discontinued.

**19. What are the indications for use of naloxone other than respiratory depression?**
Itching that is unrelieved by IV diphenhydramine (Benadryl) is an indication for a continuous naloxone infusion. The hourly dose of naloxone for itching is usually 1–3 μg/kg/hr. Administration of opioids for pain relief should be continued while the patient is receiving the naloxone infusion to relieve itching.

**20. What can be done if pain is not relieved during an epidural infusion?**
1. Assess catheter placement:
   • In the average adult, the catheter is inserted to the 10-cm mark. Epidural catheters are marked with dots and dashes (2 dots indicates 10 cm; 1 dash indicates 12 cm).
   • Some leakage may occur around the catheter. If leaking around the catheter coincides with poor pain relief, notify the appropriate physician, stop the infusion, and administer intravenous or intramuscular opioids to treat the pain.
   • A test dose of local anesthetic plus epinephrine may be administered to rule out potential intravascular or intrathecal catheter placement. The catheter may be replaced or discontinued with a plan for alternative pain therapy (e.g., patient-controlled analgesia).
2. If catheter displacement is ruled out, the patient may require an increase in the infusion dose, supplemental epidural boluses, or bolus administration of IV opioids. Some institutions have protocols that allow nurses to titrate the epidural dose based on the patient's report of pain.

**21. How are other potential side effects treated?**
1. **Nausea and vomiting** result from stimulation of the chemoreceptor trigger zone (vomiting center). Treatment includes antiemetics and insertion of a nasogastric tube, if indicated.
2. **Urinary retention** is related to local anesthetic blockade of sympathetic and sensory pathways that innervate the bladder. Monitor intake and output and insert a urinary catheter, if indicated.
3. **Hypotension** results from effects of the epidural analgesics and anesthetics on the circulatory system. An excessive dose of local anesthetic can cause extensive sympathetic blockade. Hypotension is treated with IV fluid boluses and/or administration of IV ephedrine or phenylephrine boluses.

## BIBLIOGRAPHY

1. DeLeon-Casasola OA, Lema MA: Postperative epidural opioid analgesia: What are the choices? Anesth Analg 83:867–875, 1996.
2. Drain CB. Shipley CS. Recovery Room: A Critical Approach, Philadelphia, W.B. Saunders, 1987.
3. Fetzer-Fowler SJ: Managing sympathetic blockade in the post anesthesia care unit. J Post Anesth Nurs 9:34, 1994.
4. Gruendemann BJ, Fernsbener B: Comprehensive Perioperative Nursing. Boston, Jones & Bartlett, 1995.
5. Hudak C, Gallo BM, Morton PG: Critical Care Nursing: A Holistic Approach. Philadelphia, Lippincott, 1998.
6. Litwack K: Core Curriculum for Peri-Anesthesia Nursing Practice. Philadelphia, W.B. Saunders, 1998.

# VIII. *Drugs and Alcohol*

## 63. DRUG OVERDOSES

*Ted* S. *Rigney*, RN, MS, ACNP

**1. How common are drug overdoses?**

Over the past three decades the incidence of drug overdose (OD) has increased dramatically. Some authorities believe that drug OD and the consequent cost to society constitute a public health crisis. ODs and other drug-related emergencies are responsible for as many as 38% of visits to emergency departments, and OD is the third most common admitting diagnosis after cardiac and pulmonary disorders, accounting for more than 5% of all intensive care unit admissions.

**2. What are the most commonly overdosed drugs?**

Acetaminophen is the most commonly reported drug OD in the United States, followed by antidepressants and stimulants such as cocaine and amphetamine.

**3. What are the priorities in treating any patient after a drug OD?**

Stabilization of airway, breathing, and circulation is always the first priority after a known or suspected OD. Protecting the airway, ensuring adequate oxygenation, and supporting cardiovascular function take precedence over identifying the specific drug ingested. After OD, all patients are at risk for clinical deterioration and require rapid establishment of intravenous access, frequent assessment of vital signs, and continuous cardiac and pulse-oximeter monitoring. Monitoring temperature is essential because either hyper- or hypothermia may complicate treatment. After initial stabilization, treatment should focus on preventing further absorption, enhancing drug elimination, and using drug-specific interventions.

**4. What about patients with altered mental status?**

When a patient presents with altered mental status, an immediate determination should be made about the administration of glucose, thiamine, and naloxone (Narcan). Unless promptly treated, hypoglycemia can cause irreversible brain damage. Alcoholic or malnourished patients may have diminished thiamine stores and should receive parenteral thiamine if glucose is administered. The use of naloxone, a narcotic antagonist, may serve as a diagnostic tool and a therapeutic intervention by reversing narcosis if a narcotic OD has occurred.

**5. What about toxicology screening?**

Routine toxicology screening is of little value in the initial care of patients with drug OD. It is time-consuming, expensive, and frequently erroneous. Blood screening is relatively insensitive for many drugs, including opioids, stimulants, and psychotropics. Serum testing is indicated only if a specific toxin is suspected and treatment will be based on the result. Urine testing is recommended for broad qualitative screening.

**6. What are important nursing considerations in treating any patient after a drug OD?**

Critical care nurses play an essential role in maintaining a safe environment and providing psychological support. Crucial elements of nursing care include assessing suicidal intention, ongoing suicidal risk or risk of harm to the patient or others, and mental state. Patients who have intentionally overdosed are at increased risk for self-destructive behavior. One-on-one nursing care is the most effective preventive method in caring for suicidal patients. Such patients should not be left unattended for any length of time, and all potentially harmful objects, including items that may be on their person, should be removed from the environment. Furthermore, violent behavior, agitation, and aggressiveness place everyone—patient and staff—at risk for injury. Psychological support includes basic emotional support, facilitating psychiatric intervention, referral to substance abuse programs, and information about self-help groups.

**7. What are toxidromes? Why are they helpful in the monitoring and management of patients after an OD?**

Toxidromes are groups of signs and symptoms that often occur consistently with a particular class of drug or toxin. They can be useful in guiding diagnosis and lead to definitive therapies. Many ODs fit into one of the four common toxidromes in the table below.

| TOXIDROME | SIGNS | CAUSES |
|---|---|---|
| Sympathomimetic | Anxiety, agitation, delusions, paranoia, diaphoresis, mydriasis, tachycardia (although with severe hypertension reflex bradycardia may occur), hypertension, hyperpyrexia, hyperreflexia | Cocaine, amphetamine, methamphetamine, and over-the-counter decongestants, such as phenylpropanolamine, ephedrine, and pseudoephedrine |
| Sympatholytic | Lethargy, respiratory depression, coma, miosis, bradycardia, hypotension hypothermia, hyporeflexia, decreased bowel sounds, noncardiac pulmonary edema, seizures (after OD of meperidine or propoxyphene) | Narcotics, barbiturates, benzodiazepines, |
| Anticholinergic | Agitation, delirium, seizures, coma, dry flushed skin, mydriasis, tachycardia, hyperpyrexia, myoclonus, urinary retention | Antihistamines, atropine, scopolamine, antipsychotics, tricyclic antidepressants, antispasmodics, mydriatics, phenothiazines |
| Cholinergic | Anxiety, confusion, agitation, weakness, salivation, lacrimation, diaphoresis, emesis, miosis, bradycardia (or tachycardia), hypertension, muscle fasciculations, hyperperistalsis, incontinence, seizures, pulmonary edema | Physostigmine, nicotine, organophosphates, carbamates |

**8. What methods are used to reduce drug absorption?**

Methods to reduce drug absorption include induced emesis, gastric lavage, and activated charcoal (AC). If more than 60 minutes has passed, however, induced emesis and gastric lavage are relatively ineffective. Exceptions are large ingestions of anticholinergics or salicylates, which often delay gastric emptying, and ingestion of sustained-release or enteric-coated tablets, which may remain intact for several hours. Unfortunately, only a small percentage of the ingested drug is retrieved through gastric lavage; even the largest orogastric tubes are unable to accommodate pill clumps or large pill fragments. Contraindications to induced emesis or lavage include altered mental status and diminished gag reflex, unless the airway is protected by endotracheal intubation. If gastric lavage is begun, there may be some benefit in administering AC before the first bolus of lavage fluid to prevent absorption of highly toxic substances.

**9. How does activated charcoal work?**

AC binds ingested poisons or drugs within the gut, decreasing their absorption and allowing the charcoal-toxin complex to be evacuated with stool. AC effectively adsorbs almost all drugs and poisons. However, ionized chemicals, such as mineral acids, iron, lithium, fluoride, and cyanide, are not well adsorbed by charcoal. The recommended doses are 50–100 gm for adults and 1gm/kg for children. Usually AC is combined with a cathartic such as sorbitol. Contraindications to AC administration are decreased peristalsis, ileus, and ingestion of corrosives. Complications of AC therapy include aspiration and bowel obstruction caused by inspissated charcoal. In addition, AC may prevent the absorption of orally administered therapeutic agents.

**10. What methods are used to enhance elimination of drugs?**
- Cathartics
- Repeat-dose AC
- Whole-bowel irrigation
- Forced diuresis
- Hemodialysis
- Charcoal hemoperfusion
- Surgical removal

**11. How are cathartics used?**
Cathartics, such as sorbitol, magnesium citrate, or magnesium sulfate, enhance elimination by stimulating intestinal motility. Multiple doses of cathartics are to be avoided, however, since the subsequent diarrhea may cause severe electrolyte imbalances. Sodium-based cathartics should be avoided in patients with hypertension, congestive heart failure, and renal failure. Magnesium-based cathartics should be avoided in patients with renal failure.

**12. When are repeat doses of AC used?**
Multiple dosing of AC at regular intervals is an effective method of enhancing the elimination of various drugs, including phenytoin, tricyclic antidepressants, theophylline, phenobarbital, and salicylates. In fact, for drugs such as theophylline and phenobarbital, repeat dosing of AC approaches the efficacy of hemodialysis; hence the term "intestinal dialysis."

**13. When is whole-bowel irrigation used?**
Although whole-bowel irrigation can cause severe electrolyte imbalances, particularly in children, it is effective in removing heavy metals, such as iron, and enteric-coated tablets.

**14. What is forced diuresis? How does it work?**
Diuresis, particularly when coupled with alteration of urinary pH, may prevent the reabsorption of drugs that undergo renal excretion. Acidic drugs, such as salicylates and phenobarbital, are excreted more rapidly with alkaline urine. Although acid diuresis enhances renal elimination of such drugs as cocaine and tricyclic antidepressants, the clinical efficacy of such a method has not been established and its use largely has been abandoned.

**15. What precautions are necessary with the use of forced diuresis?**
Because of its association with significant risks, such as pulmonary edema and electrolyte imbalances, forced diuresis should be used cautiously in patients with renal insufficiency and cardiac disease. In the presence of pulmonary or cerebral edema, which may occur in severe salicylate OD, alkaline diuresis is dangerous and should not be attempted. Bicarbonate is commonly used to alter urinary pH and maintain a pH $\geq 7.5$. Intake and output and urine pH should be monitored hourly with a urinary catheter in place. Serum potassium must be monitored and maintained at normal levels to avoid hypokalemia.

**16. When is hemodialysis or charcoal hemoperfusion indicated?**
Hemodialysis or charcoal hemoperfusion is indicated in patients with ingestion of lethal amounts of a dialyzable drug, clinical deterioration despite conventional therapies, and renal or hepatic failure that impairs clearance of the ingested drug. Dialyzable drugs have a small volume of distribution; that is, they remain largely in the bloodstream as opposed to moving into tissue. Commonly dialyzed drugs include lithium, aspirin, and phenobarbital. Dialysis is also effective at rapidly correcting acid-base and electrolyte imbalances that may accompany OD. Peritoneal dialysis occasionally is used when hemodialysis is not available but is less efficient.

**17. What are the four phases of acetaminophen OD?**
Acetaminophen is a common ingredient in many prescription and over-the-counter products. ODs may be intentional or accidental. Early signs and symptoms may be subtle and can be

overlooked until hepatotoxicity, the major manifestation of OD, develops. Symptoms can be divided into four phases according to time since ingestion:

**Phase I** begins within hours of ingestion. Symptoms include anorexia, vomiting, and diaphoresis, although some patients may be asymptomatic.

**Phase II** begins 24–72 hours after ingestion when liver enzymes begin to rise. Symptoms include right upper quadrant abdominal pain.

**Phase III** begins 3–5 days after ingestion when advanced hepatotoxicity is present, as signaled by marked elevation of liver enzymes, jaundice, hypoglycemia, coagulopathy, encephalopathy, and renal failure due to acute tubular necrosis.

If the patient survives phase III, **phase IV** lasts from 5 days to several weeks and signals the slow resolution of hepatic dysfunction.

### 18. Which patients are at risk for acetaminophen toxicity even at therapeutic doses?

Acetaminophen is metabolized primarily in the liver. An acute ingestion of 140 mg/kg is considered toxic; however, patients with preexisting hepatic dysfunction secondary to alcohol abuse, hepatitis, starvation, or fasting are at risk for acetaminophen toxicity at much lower doses. People who take anticonvulsants are likewise at risk.

### 19. How is an acetaminophen OD managed?

The goal of management is prevention of hepatotoxicity. Limiting absorption through induced emesis or gastric lavage is effective if fewer than 2 hours have passed since ingestion. Otherwise, AC should be administered. The antidote for an acetaminophen OD is N-acetylcysteine (NAC), which reduces the extent of hepatotoxicity by replenishing essential hepatic enzymes and thus allowing continued hepatic clearance of acetaminophen metabolites. Liver transplantation has been attempted when NAC therapy fails.

### 20. How is NAC administered?

The sooner therapy is initiated, the better the prognosis; however, NAC may be effective up to 24 hours after ingestion. Although AC is capable of adsorbing NAC, the overall effect is considered clinically insignificant and AC should be given. If initial acetaminophen levels are in the toxic range (> 200 $\mu$g/ml at 4 hours after ingestion), a loading dose of NAC, 140 mg/kg orally, should be administered, followed by 70 mg/kg every 4 hours for 72 hours. Intravenous NAC is available in Europe and Canada, but there is no approved parenteral formulation in the United States.

### 21. How is the patient with acetaminophen OD monitored?

Serum acetaminophen levels should be obtained 4 hours after ingestion. Levels drawn before then are not accurate because absorption and distribution may not be complete. NAC therapy can be started before the determination of serum acetaminophen levels and then discontinued if levels are not in the toxic range. Hypoglycemia may result from hepatic dysfunction and requires the administration of intravenous glucose. The treatment of nausea and vomiting includes intravenous fluids and antiemetics. Liver function tests and coagulation parameters should be monitored daily.

### 22. How do stimulants such as cocaine and amphetamines work?

Stimulants work by innervating $\alpha$-, $\beta_1$-, and $\beta_2$-adrenergic receptors. This increased stimulation of the sympathetic nervous system results in a sympathomimetic toxidrome. A stimulant OD can have serious cardiovascular effects, such as dysrhythmia, cardiac ischemia, and myocardial infarction.

### 23. How should a stimulant OD be managed and monitored?

Treatment of a stimulant OD is largely symptom management. Orally ingested tablets may be removed by standard measures, but gastric decontamination has no benefit when such drugs are inhaled, snorted, or injected. Continuous cardiac and blood pressure monitoring are essential because hypertension and arrhythmias are common problems. Hypertension can be treated with various vasodilators; however, a pure beta blocker such as propranolol should not be used, because the unopposed $\alpha$-adrenergic effects may paradoxically worsen hypertension. A standard

ECG should be done to assess for myocardial ischemia or evolving myocardial infarction. Temperature should be monitored frequently and measures taken to lower body temperature in patients who are hyperthermic. Seizure precautions and rapid intervention are essential because seizure activity contributes significantly to hyperthermia and rhabdomyolysis. Patients may be agitated, paranoid, or floridly psychotic. Sedation with benzodiazepines or haloperidol is preferred to the use of physical restraints, which can cause extreme agitation.

### 24. How should a patient with respiratory compromise after an opioid OD be treated?

Although opioids have widely varying potencies and durations of action, all act on the central nervous system, producing variable degrees of sedation, respiratory depression, and apnea. Oral ingestion of opioids can be treated with induced emesis, gastric lavage, and AC as long as patients are alert and breathing spontaneously, with intact airway reflexes. A cathartic agent should be administered along with the AC to counteract gut hypomotility. All other narcotic ODs should be treated with naloxone. Naloxone is a specific opioid antagonist that can rapidly reverse narcotic toxicosis. Naloxone has a half-life of 1 hour, which may be considerably less than the half-life of the involved narcotic; thus, narcotic toxicosis may recur. Repeat dosing, continuous naloxone infusion, or administration of nalmefene (Revex), an opioid antagonist with an 8- to 10-hour half-life, may be necessary. Higher naloxone doses may be needed to reverse the effects of semisynthetic oral opiates. Complications after administration of naloxone are rare. They include seizures, arrhythmias, severe agitation, and noncardiogenic pulmonary edema.

### 25. Is naloxone effective after OD of any nonopioid drugs?

Naloxone is useful after clonidine OD. Symptoms of a clonidine OD are similar to those of narcotic toxicosis and respond similarly to the administration of naloxone, although higher doses usually are required.

### 26. Describe the clinical presentation in an acute salicylate OD.

Direct gastric irritation causes nausea, vomiting, and hematemesis. Salicylate effects on the brainstem result in increased respiratory rate and depth, respiratory alkalosis, and lethargy. Decreased production of prothrombin, coupled with salicylate-impaired platelet function, leads to coagulation abnormalities, although overt hemorrhage is rare. Other effects include tinnitus and metabolic acidosis. Salicylates, normally thought of as antipyretics, in toxic doses cause hyperthermia due to cellular derangement. Finally, severe intoxication may result in agitation, confusion, coma, seizures, pulmonary edema, and circulatory collapse.

### 27. What about chronic salicylate toxicity?

Unlike an acute OD, chronic salicylate toxicity is usually accidental and is seen more frequently in older patients with arthritis or some other chronic condition. Chronic toxicity can present with changes in mental status and tachypnea only, without other symptoms associated with acute salicyate OD.

### 28. What is considered a toxic dose of salicylate?

**Acute ingestions**
Mild toxicity: < 140 mg/kg
Moderate toxicity: 140–400 mg/kg
Severe toxicity:> 400 mg/kg
**Chronic toxicity** can occur with use of 120 mg/kg/day over a period of several days.

### 29. What is the Done nomogram? When should it be used?

The Done nomogram was developed to aid in predicting toxicity based on serum salicylate levels. It is useful, however, only with an acute, one-time ingestion, and the initial serum level should be drawn no less than 6 hours after the OD. It should not be used when the time of OD is unknown or for ingestions of sustained-release or enteric-coated salicylates. The Done nomogram also should not be used with chronic ingestions because as salicylates move from blood to tissue, serum levels become progressively less reflective of total body content of salicylate. In addition, if acidemia is present, more salicylate will penetrate the blood-brain barrier, resulting in central nervous system toxicity. Therefore, in a salicylate OD, acidemia is associated with toxicity regardless of the serum level.

### 30. How is salicylate OD managed?

For acute OD (as opposed to chronic use), gastric emptying with lavage or induced emesis limits absorption. Lavage may be useful even several hours after OD because large amounts of aspirin may clump together in the stomach and form concretions, delaying absorption for 24 hours or longer. Elimination can be enhanced with multiple doses of AC. Alkalization of the urine and forced diuresis increase renal excretion of salicylate. Although acetazolamide alkalinizes urine, the associated acidemia increases salicylate toxicity; therefore, use of acetazolamide is not recommended. Short-acting benzodiazepines may be used to treat salicylate-induced seizures. Hemodialysis is indicated for severe metabolic acidosis (pH < 7.10) refractory to treatment, severe central nervous system symptoms (seizures, cerebral edema, coma), salicylate levels > 120 mg/dl, and renal failure.

### 31. How are patients with salicylate OD monitored?

Urine output, urinary pH (target = 7–8), and serum potassium must be monitored closely during alkaline diuresis. Temperature should be monitored and hyperthermia treated with a cooling blanket. Elderly patients and patients with preexisting heart disease should be assessed frequently because the large amounts of fluid required for diuresis can induce pulmonary edema.

### 32. How do patients with OD of sedative-hypnotic drugs typically present?

The sedative-hypnotic drugs include various unrelated tranquilizers, such as barbiturates, benzodiazepines, and chloral hydrate. OD results in a sympatholytic toxidrome; namely, depressed mental status, respiratory depression, and hypotension. Euphoria, slurred speech and ataxia are common with mild intoxication. Fortunately, fatalities are rare.

### 33. How are patients with sedative-hypnotic OD managed and monitored?

The goals of treatment are to reduce absorption and to provide supportive care. Airway, respiratory status, and blood pressure must be monitored continuously. AC should be administered along with a cathartic agent. Gastric lavage and emesis are unlikely to be of benefit if more than 1 hour has passed since ingestion. Alkaline diuresis is effective after phenobarbital OD, and hemodialysis can be used to remove drugs with small volumes of distribution, such as phenobarbital and chloral hydrate. Flumazenil (Romazicon) is a specific treatment for benzodiazepine OD.

### 34. What is flumazenil? How is it used?

Flumazenil is a benzodiazepine antagonist. It has no effect on barbiturates or other sedative-hypnotics. As with naloxone, the duration of action of flumazenil is short, and repeated doses or continuous infusion may be necessary. In contrast to naloxone, empiric administration of flumazenil in the setting of suspected OD is not recommended. Flumazenil can induce withdrawal seizures in chronic benzodiazepine users or breakthrough seizures in patients with an underlying seizure disorder. It also should not be given in the setting of a concomitant tricyclic antidepressant OD because cyclic antidepressants lower the seizure threshold. If seizures occur after flumazenil administration, benzodiazepine anticonvulsants will not be effective. Cardiac monitoring should be instituted whenever flumazenil is administered because dysrhythmias may occur.

### 35. What are the clinical findings in patients with cyclic antidepressant OD?

OD with tricyclic or other cyclic antidepressants (CAs) produces neurotoxicity, cardiotoxicity, and anticholinergic effects. Central nervous system effects range from agitation to lethargy and coma. Additional signs include hallucinations, ataxia, hyperactive reflexes, clonus, and seizures. Cardiovascular toxicity is manifested by supraventricular and ventricular arrhythmias, prolonged QRS and QT intervals, conduction blocks, and hypotension. Anticholinergic effects include mydriasis, ileus, flushed skin, urinary retention, delirium, and psychosis. Hyperthermia may result from seizure activity and anticholinergic-induced impairment of sweating.

**36. Describe the appropriate management of patients with cyclic antidepressant OD.**

Signs of severe intoxication may occur precipitously and without warning. Tricyclic and other CAs are second only to analgesics as the reported cause of death after intentional OD. Stabilization and supportive care, therefore, are critical first steps.

Hypotension can be treated initially with crystalloids, but the addition of vasopressors may be required. Norepinephrine or epinephrine is the vasopressor of choice. Dopamine is less effective because severe CA toxicity causes catecholamine depletion. Physostigmine, a cholinergic agent, can reverse neurotoxic effects rapidly but should not be used routinely because of its serious side effects, including seizures, worsened hypotension, and precipitation of asystole. Seizures can be managed with benzodiazepines and phenobarbital. Phenytoin can exacerbate QT prolongation and should not be used routinely.

Urinary catheterization may be necessary because of the risk for urinary retention. Gastric lavage should be performed regardless of when ingestion occurred because gastric emptying is delayed by CAs. Consideration should be given to endotracheal intubation prior to lavage because of the rapidity with which loss of consciousness can occur. AC with a cathartic can be administered after lavage. Repeat dosing of charcoal is controversial because bowel obstruction may occur in the setting of ileus after CA OD. CAs are highly tissue-bound with a large volume of distribution and therefore are difficult to remove once absorbed. For this reason, forced diuresis and hemodialysis are not effective.

**37. How are patients with cyclic antidepressant OD monitored?**

Continuous cardiac monitoring is essential, and an external pacemaker should be readily available in the event of serious conduction block. Arterial pH should be monitored frequently because cardiac and neurologic toxicity may be enhanced by acidemia. Sodium bicarbonate and hyperventilation (in intubated patients) are used to keep arterial pH at 7.45–7.55. Serum levels of CAs correlate poorly with severity of symptoms and are not useful for clinical management.

**38. What are the clinical findings in a digitalis OD?**

Toxicity may result from a single intentional OD or from accidental chronic ingestion. Hyperkalemia due to acute poisoning can differentiate acute OD from chronic toxicity. Symptoms include nausea and vomiting, cardiac conduction disturbances, and lethargy. The classic description of yellow or green halos around lights is a late symptom and is present only in a minority of cases. Patients predisposed to chronic digitalis toxicosis often have renal insufficiency or underlying hypokalemia or hypomagnesemia due to concurrent diuretic therapy.

**39. How is digitalis OD treated?**

After an acute ingestion, lavage should be performed and AC administered. Induced emesis is not recommended because it may increase vagal tone and precipitate bradycardia or conduction blocks. Signs of severe intoxication (refractory bradycardia, conduction block, or ventricular arrhythmias) or serum levels > 10 ng/ml are indications for treatment with digoxin immune FAB. Hyperkalemia can be treated with sodium bicarbonate, insulin, and glucose. Calcium should not be used to counteract hyperkalemia because it may precipitate arrhythmias.

**40. How is digoxin immune FAB used to treat digitalis OD?**

Hyperkalemia and digitalis toxicity are best treated with the administration of digoxin immune FAB (Digibind). Ideally, the dose of Digibind is based on a steady-state plasma level. Unfortunately, many patients deteriorate before a steady state is reached (6 hours after ingestion); thus, dosing is based on body weight or suspected amount ingested. If treatment is based on serum levels drawn before steady state has been achieved, the Digibind dose will be overestimated, because serum levels are falsely high. In addition, once Digibind has been administered, serum digoxin levels are falsely elevated. Digibind begins to take effect after 30–60 minutes.

## BIBLIOGRAPHY

1. Adams MH, Barnett-Lammon C, Stover LM: Responding to tricyclic antidepressant OD. Dimens Crit Care Nurs 17(2):67–74, 1998.

2. Criddle LM: Toxicologic emergencies. In Newberry L (ed): Sheehy's Emergency Nursing: Principles and Practice, 4th ed. St. Louis, Mosby, 1998, pp 647–663.
3. Derlet RW, Horowitz BZ: Cardiotoxic drugs. Emerg Med Clin North Am 13:771–791, 1995.
4. Heyman EN, LoCastro DE, Gouse LH, et al: Intentional drug OD: Predictors of clinical course in the intensive care unit. Heart Lung 25:246–252, 1996.
5. Kellermann AL, Fihn SD, LoGerto JP, Copass MK: Impact of drug screening in suspected OD. Ann Emerg Med 31:777–781, 1998.
6. Linden CH, Lovejoy. FH Jr: Poisoning and drug overdosage. In Fauci AS, Braunwald E, Isselbacher KJ, et al (eds): Harrison's Principles of Internal Medicine, 14th ed. New York, McGraw-Hill, 1998, pp 2523–2544.
7. Litovitz TL, Klein-Schwartz W, Dyer KS, et al: 1997 Annual Report of the American Association of Poison Control Centers Toxic Exposure Surveillance System. Am J Emerg Med 16:443–497, 1998.
8. Olsen KR: Poisoning. In Tierney LM Jr, McPhee SJ, Papadakis, MA (eds): Current Medical Diagnosis and Treatment, 37th ed. Stamford, CT, Appleton & Lange, 1998, pp 1465–1495.
9. Roberts D, Mackay G: A nursing model of OD assessment. Nurs Times 95(3):58–60, 1999.
10. Seger DL, Murray L: Aspirin, acetaminophen, and nonsteroidal agents. In Ellenhorn MJ, Schonwald S, Ordog G, Wasserberger J (eds): Ellenhorn's Medical Toxicology, 2nd ed. Baltimore, Williams & Wilkins, 1996, pp 1250–1263.

# 64. ALCOHOL WITHDRAWAL

*Laura Greicus*, RN, MSN, ACNP, CCRN

### 1. What is alcohol withdrawal syndrome?

Alcohol withdrawal syndrome (AWS) is a constellation of often life-threatening signs and symptoms that occur when a heavy or prolonged user of alcohol ceases or reduces alcohol intake.

### 2. List the clinical symptoms of AWS.

- Hand tremor
- Insomnia
- Nausea and vomiting
- Tachycardia
- Hypertension
- Pyschomotor agitation
- Anxiety
- Transient visual, tactile, or auditory hallucinations
- Grand mal seizures
- Delirium (in severe cases)

Not all people manifest all of the above symptoms.

### 3. How are symptoms of AWS classified?

1. Early (24–48 hours) or late (more than 48 hours).
2. Major or minor. The level of autonomic hyperactivity and the presence of delirium are the main determinants of progression from minor to major symptoms.

### 4. How long do the symptoms last?

Generally, signs and symptoms of AWS begin within 5–10 hours after decreased use, peak in intensity on days 2 and 3, and are alleviated by day 4–7. However, cases of delirium tremens (DTs) have been reported to last in excess of weeks.

### 5. Define delirium tremens.

Delirium tremens is the most severe manifestation of AWS and occurs in about 5% of cases. If left untreated, it results in a 15% mortality rate; death usually is due to complicating conditions such as pneumonia or cardiac arrhythmia.

### 6. What are the signs and symptoms of delirium tremens?

The **initial signs and symptoms** are mild tachycardia and hypertension, progressive irritability, mild tremor, and low-grade fever. Patients with seizures due to AWS often progress to delirium tremens.

**Full-blown cases** are evidenced by profound confusion; visual, tactile, or auditory hallucinations, and severe signs of autonomic hyperactivity (fever, tachycardia, sweating, and dilated pupils).

### 7. When should delirium tremens be suspected?

Delirium tremens should be suspected in any agitated patient withdrawing from alcohol with blood pressure > 140/90 mmHg, pulse > 100 beats/min, and temperature > 101°F.

### 8. What are alcohol withdrawal-related seizures? When do they occur?

Alcohol withdrawal-related seizures generally occur during the first 48 hours before delirium develops. They usually are generalized (grand mal) and self-limited; they may consist of a single episode or occur in a short series.

### 9. How are alcohol withdrawal-related seizures diagnosed?

Before assuming that the seizures are strictly alcohol-related, other causes should be considered, including head trauma, metabolic disorders, cerebral hemorrhage, infection, fever, drug overdose, cerebral vascular accident, and epilepsy. Imaging of the head and neurologic consultation should be considered, particularly if the seizure occurs after delirium has begun or if the patient has multiple seizures. Lumbar puncture may be necessary in febrile patients with seizures to rule out meningitis.

### 10. How are alcohol withdrawal-related seizures treated?

Intravenous administration of diazepam can be used to stop an acute alcohol-related seizure episode . The use of loading doses of common anticonvulsants (e.g., phenytoin [Dilantin]) is controversial. In general, anticonvulsant therapy should be considered if the patient has recurrent seizures after admission or a history of seizure disorder unrelated to alcohol withdrawal. In Europe, carbamazepine (Tegretol) is often used for short-term therapy in patients with acute withdrawal rather than the benzodiazepines. It has proved effective for both symptom relief and prevention of worsening seizures.

### 11. What is the kindling effect?

It is theorized that past episodes of poorly treated alcohol withdrawal symptoms may lower the threshold for future episodes of severe alcohol withdrawal by sensitizing neural structures. It is important to recognize that this phenomenon, known as the kindling effect, may occur. Adequate doses of medications that suppress kindling (e.g., benzodiazepines or carbamazepine) may have specific efficacy in the prevention of delirium tremens.

### 12. What factors may predict progression to full-blown delirium tremens?

The single best predictor is a previous history of alcohol-related seizures or delirium tremens. Patients with concomitant infections or medical problems and higher quantity and frequency of drinking also are more likely to have severe alcohol withdrawal symptoms.

### 13. Why is it often difficult to differentiate between delirium tremens and other cognitive disorders in the intensive care unit (ICU)?

1. Many ICU patients are tracheally intubated and or require prolonged analgesia and sedation; therefore, cognitive disorders and psychotic symptoms such as hallucinations are difficult to recognize and assess.

2. Most patients in the ICU have comorbidities. Therefore, before AWS can be established in an agitated or otherwise neurologically compromised patient, common complications (e.g., bleeding, metabolic or electrolyte disorders, infection, hypoxia, pain, focal neurologic signs) must be excluded.

Unfortunately because of the complexity in diagnosing acute AWS in many ICU patients, therapy for other medical conditions may be delayed, causing the patient's condition to deteriorate.

### 14. How should the critical care nurse assess alcohol withdrawal in the ICU?

Whenever possible, the critical care nurse should ask the patient about daily alcohol intake and history of previous alcohol withdrawal on admission to the ICU and before intubation. Many sources recommend use of standardized questionnaires (e.g., the CAGE questionnaire) to determine potential alcohol abuse. However if the patient is unable to communicate (emergently intubated or already neurologically compromised), the family should be consulted as soon as possible about the patient's alcohol use and history of alcohol withdrawal signs and symptoms. Other critical care nursing assessments should include monitoring for physiologic signs and symptoms of alcohol withdrawal, abnormal laboratory findings, and alcohol-related complications and disease processes.

### 15. What laboratory findings support a diagnosis of alcohol abuse?
- Increased levels of aspartate transaminase (AST), alanine transaminase (ALT), and gamma glutamyl transpeptidase (GGT)
- Elevated mean corpuscular volume (MCV)
- Abnormal electrolyte concentrations
- Elevated uric acid levels
- Decreased serum albumin
- Elevated triglycerides
- Prolonged prothrombin time
- Positive drug or alcohol screens.

### 16. What complications other than seizures and delirium tremens may be associated with acute alcohol withdrawal?
- Cardiac arrhythmias
- Wernicke-Korsakoff syndrome
- Psychiatric problems (especially agitation and depression)
- Dehydration
- Fluid and electrolyte disturbances
- Infection
- Aspiration
- Alcoholic ketoacidosis

### 17. What disease states should raise suspicion of long-term alcohol abuse that may lead to withdrawal symptoms?
- Cancer of the head and neck, esophagus, or cardia of the stomach
- Cirrhosis
- Unexplained hepatitis
- Pancreatitis
- Bilateral parotid gland swelling
- Peripheral neuropathy

### 18. What is a valid and reliable tool for measuring the severity of alcohol withdrawal?
The Revised Clinical Institute Withdrawal Assessment for Alcohol (CIWA-Ar) has been used in numerous studies and clinical settings to measure the severity of alcohol withdrawal. This 10-item scale is used to monitor severity of symptoms and to guide treatment. It should be used as frequently as every hour in deciding medication doses.

*Revised Clinical Institute Withdrawal Assessment for Alcohol*

| SYMPTOM | RANGE OF SCORES |
| --- | --- |
| Nausea and vomiting | 0–7 |
| Tremor | 0–7 |
| Paroxysmal sweats | 0–7 |
| Anxiety | 1–7 |
| Agitation | 1–7 |
| Tactile disturbances | 0–7 |
| Auditory disturbances | 0–7 |
| Visual disturbances | 0–7 |
| Headache or fullness in head | 0–7 |
| Disorientation and clouding of sensorium | 0–4 |

Adapted from Erstad BL, Cotugno CL; Management of alcohol withdrawal. Am J Health-Syst Pharm 52:697–709, 1995.

### 19. How is the CIWA-Ar scored?

The scores for the 10 items are summed to give a total score (maximal score = 67):

| Total Score | Patient Status |
|---|---|
| < 10 | Stable |
| 10–19 | Mild-to-moderate alcohol withdrawal |
| 20–25 | Moderate alcohol withdrawal |
| > 25 | Severe alcohol withdrawal, with impending delirium tremens |

Results, however, must be intrepreted with caution in patients with comorbid conditions because the symptoms measured by the CIWA-Ar are nonspecific and may be present in other conditions (e.g., sepsis).

### 20. What are the current recommendations for management of mild alcohol withdrawal?

Standard recommendations for managing mild alcohol withdrawal include supportive measures: provision of a quiet environment, reassurance, hydration, nutrition, reality orientation, and administration of thiamine to prevent Wernicke's encephalopathy. Pharmacotherapy may not be indicated initially. If the patient is at a high risk for worsening withdrawal (e.g., history of moderate-to-severe withdrawal or current heavy alcohol use), prophylactic treatment with benzodiazepines should be considered. Finally, safety precautions (e.g., for falls and seizures) should be considered.

### 21. Why are benzodiazepines the first-line therapy for moderate-to-severe symptoms of alcohol withdrawal and delirium tremens?

Benzodiazepines are cross-tolerant with alcohol, reduce agitation, provide sedation and amnestic effects, prevent alcohol withdrawal seizures, and have a wide therapeutic window. Benzodiazepines also produce less respiratory depression than other CNS depressants. Of note, a higher dose of benzodiazepine is generally required for treating the autonomic hyperactivity associated with AWS than for treating anxiety.

### 22. Which benzodiazepine should be used?

The choice among the different benzodiazepines should be guided by duration of action, rapidity of onset, and cost. In the ICU, lorazepam (Ativan) is frequently used because of its moderate duration of action and parenteral availability.

### 23. What adjunctive medications may be used?

Adjunctive medications include beta blockers and clonidine to treat hyperadrenergic symptoms and neuroleptics (haloperidol) to treat alcohol-related psychoses and agitation. However, because these medications reduce the seizure threshold, they should be used only in conjunction with a benzodiazepine.

### 24. Which benzodiazepines should be considered for treating alcohol withdrawal in patients with severe liver disease, evidence of preexisting hepatic encephalopathy, or brain damage?

Oxazepam and lorazepam may be used for patients with severe liver disease because both have short-to-moderate half lives and do not produce active metabolites. Lorazepam has the additional advantage of being available and well absorbed orally, intramuscularly, and intravenously (IV), whereas oxazepam is available only in oral form.

### 25. What three medication regimens are used for treating alcohol withdrawal? How are they implemented?

1. **Gradual tapering:** benzodiazepines are administered at a predetermined dosing schedule for several days and then gradually discontinued.

2. **Loading method:** the rationale is that relatively large doses of the drug can be administered when it is most needed. The half-life of the drug allows gradual pharmacokinetic self-tapering

without the need for additional doses. Chlordiazepoxide commonly is used with this method because of its long half-life.

3. **Symptom-triggered therapy:** the CIWA-Ar is used to assess signs and symptoms. Medication is given only when symptoms are present. For example, lorazepam may be administered orally every 1 hour when the CIWA-Ar score is ≥ 8. The goal is to treat uncomfortable symptoms without oversedation.

### 26. Why should thiamine be administered before or with IV solutions that have a high concentration of glucose in any patient at risk for alcohol withdrawal?

In patients with thiamine deficiency (30–80% of alcohol-dependent people), high glucose solutions can precipitate acute Wernicke-Korsakoff syndrome. This syndrome involves two processes: Wernicke's encephalopathy, which leads to mental confusion, nystagmus, ophthalmoplegia, and gait ataxia, and Korsakoff syndrome, which causes mental confusion and confabulation. The syndrome may become permanent without treatment, but it is partially to completely reversible with thiamine therapy. A good rule of thumb: give all hospitalized alcohol-consuming patients 100 mg/day of thiamine, either before or with (mixed in) IV dextrose solutions.

### 27. How may alcohol withdrawal symptoms differ in elderly ICU patients?

1. Elderly patients often have coexisting conditions and illnesses and are more likely to exhibit more severe symptoms of alcohol withdrawal.

2. Alcohol-related confusion and hallucinations in the elderly may be difficult to distinguish from other causes, such as hypoxia, cognitive changes, drug interactions, reaction to anesthesia, sleep deprivation, malnutrition, ICU psychosis, bladder distention, urinary tract infection, organ system inflammation, or damage due to alcohol abuse (e.g., cirrhosis, hepatitis, pancreatitis, cardiomyopathy, cerebellar degeneration). The critical care nurse needs to have an astute recognition of the cluster of physiologic changes associated with alcohol withdrawal (see question 2) and a thorough knowledge of the patient's history to establish a differential diagnosis.

3. Elderly patients frequently use multiple drugs, both prescription and over-the-counter medications. Drug interactions should be considered with neurologic changes.

4. Elderly people may not metabolize medications as effectively as younger people. Lower dosages of benzodiazepines may be required for withdrawal symptoms to avoid neurologic or respiratory compromise.

### 28. Should IV alcohol be used in hospitalized patients to control withdrawal symptoms?

Although alcohol sometimes is administered intravenously to treat withdrawal symptoms, many sources advise against this approach as routine practice. Reasons include the known toxicities of alcohol (e.g., pancreatitis, hepatitis, bone marrow suppression), its short half-life, and the need for monitoring blood levels. Furthermore, no documented clinical trials show any advantages over benzodiazepines. Finally, administering alcohol may appear to condone drinking behavior in an alcoholic who is considering recovery.

### 29. What are the priorities in treating an ICU patient with severe alcohol withdrawal?

- Airway protection
- Maintenance of hemodynamic stability
- Prevention or control of seizures
- Correction of nutritional and metabolic deficiencies
- Prevention of dehydration
- Relief of signs and symptoms of withdrawal
- Safety precautions (e.g., soft restraints as needed).

## BIBLIOGRAPHY

1. Erstad BL, Cotugno CL: Management of alcohol withdrawal. Am J Health-Syst Pharm 52:697–709, 1995.
2. Erwin WE, Williams DB, Spei, WA: Delirium tremens. South Med J 91:425–432, 1998.
3. Holbrook AM, et al: Diagnosis and management of acute alcohol withdrawal. Can Med Assoc J 160:675–680, 1999.
4. Lohr RH: Concise review for primary-care physicians: Treatment of alcohol withdrawal in hospitalized patients. Mayo Clin Proc 70:777–782, 1995.
5. Morris PR, et al: Alcohol withdrawal syndrome: Current management strategies for the surgery patient. J Oral Maxillofac Surg 55:1452–1455, 1997.
6. Ruppert SD: Alcohol abuse in older persons: Implications for critical care. Crit Care Nurse Q 19:62–70, 1996.
7. Saitz R, O'Malley SS: Pharmacotherapies for alcohol abuse: Withdrawal and treatment. Med Clin North Am 81:881–907, 1997.
8. Schuckit MA: Alcohol and alcoholism. In Fauci AS, et al (ed): Harrison's Principles of Internal Medicine. New York, McGraw-Hill, 1998.
9. Spies CD, Rommelspacher H: Alcohol withdrawal in the surgical patient: Prevention and treatment. Anesth Analg 88:946–954, 1999.
10. Yost DA: Alcohol withdrawal syndrome. Am Fam Physician 54:657–664, 1996.

# IX.  Skin, Wound Care, and Physical Therapy

## 65.  SKIN AND WOUND ASSESSMENT AND MANAGEMENT

*Nancy Stotts, RN, EdD, and Jill Howie, RN, MS, ACNP*

### 1.  How do acute wounds differ from chronic wounds?

**Acute wounds** heal in a predictable timeframe and predictable phases (inflammatory, prolif-
erative, and remodeling). Wounds that close by primary intention (e.g., surgical incision) normally seal within 48–72 hours, although remodeling of scar tissue continues for months to years.
The time it takes to heal by secondary intention (e.g., gunshot wound) depends on the condition
of the wound and its size.

**Chronic wounds** differ from acute wounds in that they do not heal in a timely manner and
do not regain original structure. The affected part of the body may not have full preinjury function. Tissues in various parts of the body heal at different rates; for example, injuries on the face
and head heal faster than those on the feet. Biochemical differences are believed to account for
the delay in healing in chronic wounds. Current research points to higher protease levels in
chronic wounds than in acute wounds. Proteases (e.g., elastase and collagenase) degrade tissue
for wound healing and remodeling.

### 2.  Define partial-thickness and full-thickness wounds.

**Partial-thickness wounds** involve the epidermal layer and may extend to the dermis (e.g.,
skin tear, donor site of a skin graft). **Full-thickness wounds** involve the epidermis and dermis
and may extend to the adipose tissue, muscle, and bone.

### 3.  How do partial-thickness wounds heal?

Partial thickness wounds heal primarily by epithelialization. Epithelial tissue migrates from
the area surrounding the wound, the hair follicles and glands of the skin. Because the skin ap-
pendages are widely dispersed, healing of partial-thickness wounds normally occurs rapidly.

### 4.  How do full-thickness wounds heal?

Full-thickness wounds can heal by primary or secondary intention. Wounds that heal by primary intention have well-approximated edges and are closed with suture, clips, or tape. Wounds
that heal by secondary intention are left open to close by generation of granulation tissue, reep-
ithelialization, and contraction.

### 5.  How do you know if a wound is healing?

The characteristics of a healing wound that was closed by **primary intention** are a well-approximated incision line, inflammation (for approximately 3–5 days), no drainage after 48 hours,
and a healing ridge by day 7–9.

For wounds closing by **secondary intention**, healing is more difficult to characterize. In the
first 3–5 days, an acute inflammatory response is expected and may be seen as warmth, redness,
and induration that extends from outside to inside the wound. During healing, certain characteristics can be observed: beefy red granulation tissue, minimal drainage, an intact epithelial edge
surrounding the wound, and decreasing wound size. Healing wounds have no exudate or
drainage, no slough or eschar, and no unusual odor. Although not a strict measure of healing, the
skin surrounding the wound site should not be warm to touch, erythematous, or indurated.

**6. Summarize the characteristics of healing in partial-thickness and full-thickness wounds.**

| PARTIAL-THICKNESS WOUNDS | FULL-THICKNESS WOUNDS: PRIMARY INTENTION | FULL-THICKNESS WOUNDS: SECONDARY INTENTION |
|---|---|---|
| Wound size is decreasing | Well-approximated incision line | Wound size is decreasing |
| Epithelial tuffs are visible throughout wound at site of hair follicles and glands | Inflammation is present for 3–5 days | Pale pink tissue is replaced with beefy red granulation tissue |
|  | No drainage after 48 hr | Drainage is minimal |
|  | Healing ridge is present by day 7–9 | Intact epithelial edge surrounding wound |

### 7. How do you know if a wound is deteriorating?

A wound is deteriorating when it does not possess the characteristics listed in the table above. An increase in wound size or discharge and decreasing amount or quality of epithelial or granulation tissue, and development of exudate, slough, eschar, and unusual odor (when not previously present) indicate deterioration.

### 8. Distinguish among contamination, colonization, and infection.

**Contamination:** organisms are present on the surface of tissue.

**Colonization:** organisms multiply on the surface of the wound.

**Infection:** organisms invade tissue and provoke a tissue response. Only infection is associated with specific clinical signs and symptoms.

### 9. How do you diagnose wound infection?

Wound infection usually is diagnosed on the basis of clinical signs and symptoms. Most wounds healing by primary intention are **surgical wounds**; infection is called surgical site infection (SSI). SSIs are divided into three categories: superficial, deep, and organ/space. By definition, SSI occurs within 30 days of surgery or, if an implant is in place, within 1 year of surgery. The clinical signs include purulent drainage, positive wound culture, pain, signs of inflammation (tenderness, localized swelling, redness, or heat), abscess formation and dehiscence. Opening of the incision by the surgeon and diagnosis of SSI by physician also are indicative of infection. The following infections are not considered SSIs: stitch abscess, infection of an episiotomy or infection of a newborn circumcision site, and infected burn wound.

Wound infection in **chronic wounds** often is subtle. It may include drainage (excess, change in color, or change in consistency), inflammation around the wound (redness, warmth, pain, induration), poor quality of granulation tissue, change in wound odor (often malodorous), a suddenly high glucose level in a diabetic patient, and pain or a change in sensation in patients with neuropathic extremities.

### 10. What is the role of wound culture?

Wound culture is used to confirm clinical suspicion of infection and to identify the specific antibiotic to which the organism(s) is sensitive. Regardless of the type of culture, it is important to obtain tissue or fluid from the wound. Pus and eschar should not be cultured because the purpose of culture is to determine what, if any, organisms are present *in the wound tissue*.

### 11. What is the best way to culture a wound?

**Biopsy** is the gold standard for wound culture. After the wound is cleansed, a piece of tissue is removed from the wound with a scalpel or punch-biopsy tool. Biopsy has been criticized because it may cause pain; local anesthetic is not used because it may dilute the organisms within the wound. In addition, many labs do not culture wound biopsies because the process is costly or because they lack appropriate facilities.

**Aspiration** of a wound for culture is not commonly done by nurses. It involves cleansing the skin next to the wound and inserting a needle attached to a syringe. Fluid withdrawn from the tissue next to the wound is sent to the lab for culture. This method is painful, requires knowledge of the structures at the site where the aspiration is taken, and often underestimates the number of organisms in a wound.

**Swabbing** a wound involves cleansing the wound and then inserting the tip of a swab to collect fluid from the wound bed. This technique can overestimate the number of organisms, but it is easy to perform and usually not painful. The current recommendation is to obtain fluid from clean tissue by swabbing in a 1-cm$^2$ area.

### 12. What are the goals of treating an infected wound?

Reducing the bioburden (number of microorganisms) and keeping microorganisms from spreading throughout the body

### 13. Describe the usual treatment for infected wounds.

The first line of treatment is to cleanse or debride the wound to reduce the local bioburden. When the organisms have widely invaded the tissues, resulting in cellulitis or sepsis, systemic antibiotics are indicated. Local antiseptics often are used, but their value is questionable. Absorption of topical agents may be limited, and the real concern is the organisms in the tissues, not on the surface.

### 14. What principles guide cleansing of the wound?

Fluid is used to remove loosely adherent debris, exudate, residual topical agents, and metabolic wastes from tissue. Since the advent of the Agency for Health Care Policy and Research Guidelines for Treatment of Pressure Ulcers in 1994, this approach has become the standard of care for all wounds. No data, however, support its use with each dressing change in all types of wounds. The contrary opinion is that such an approach may change the local environment and remove growth factors and agents supportive of healing. Further research will clarify this issue. Until definitive data are available, cleansing is usually done with each dressing change for all types of wounds.

*Principles of Wound Cleansing*

---

- Perform at each dressing change.
- Use sufficient force to be effective (psi 4–15).
- Do not cause trauma; mechanical injury results with psi > 15.
- Consider whirlpool for wounds with heavy exudate; discontinue when no longer needed.
- Use normal saline for most cleansing.
- Use commercial cleansers for adherent material. Select cleansers with low toxicity.
- Do not use antiseptics as cleansers.

---

psi = pounds per square inch.

### 15. What type of wound cleansing fluid should be used?

Often the nurse is responsible for selecting or recommending an appropriate solution. In the hospital setting, sterile normal saline is the standard, whereas in home care tap water is used most frequently. In many ways, this difference makes sense. Hospitalized patients are exposed to a variety of organisms and may be immunosuppressed. At home patients are in their own environment, and immunocompetence is usually less of an issue.

Some cleansers have no antimicrobial action; others do. All cleansers have a toxicity index that refers to the effect on tissue cells. Cleansers with a higher toxicity index are more damaging to the wound than those with a lower index. In general, the antimicrobial cleansers have a higher toxicity index. This information is useful for committees who determine protocols for care of wounds. Skin cleansers should not be confused with wounds cleansers. Skin cleansers contain substances that are cytotoxic to wounds.

*Wound Cleansing Solutions*

| PRODUCT (MANUFACTURER) | TOXICITY INDEX |
|---|---|
| **Non-antimicrobial cleansers** | |
| Dermagran (Derma Sciences, Inc.) | 10 |
| Shur-Clens Wound Cleanser (ConvaTec) | 10 |
| Biolex (CR Bard) | 100 |
| Cara-Klenz Wound & Skin Cleanser (Carrington Labs) | 100 |
| Saf-Clens Chronic Wound Cleanser (ConvaTec) | 100 |
| Constant-Clens Dermal Wound Cleanser (Sherwood Medical–Davis & Geck) | 1,000 |
| Curasol (Healthpoint Medical) | 1,000 |
| **Antimicrobial cleansers** | |
| Clincal Care Dermal Wound Cleanser (Care-Tech Laboratories) | 1,000 |
| Dermal Wound Cleanser (Smith & Nephew United) | 1,000 |

## 16. How should the cleansing solution be delivered?

Delivery devices used for wound-cleansing solutions provide various amounts of force or pressure. Low pressures do not loosen adherent debris, whereas high pressures can cause tissue damage. Pressure delivered at 4–15 pounds per square inch (psi) is optimal for cleansers.

*Delivery Devices for Cleansing Solutions*

| INADEQUATE PRESSURE | OPTIMAL PRESSURE | EXCESSIVE PRESSURE |
|---|---|---|
| Cloth, sponges, or brushes | 35-ml syringe with No. 19 | Water-Pik at medium and high |
| Bulb syringe | Angiocath | settings |
| | Piston syringe | |
| | Water-pik (at lowest setting) | |

## 17. Define debridement and describe the various types.

Debridement is removal of devitalized tissue and debris from the wound.

**Sharp:** removal of devitalized tissue with sterile scissors or scalpel.

**Mechanical:** removal of devitalized tissue with dressings, hydrotherapy, or dextranomers.

**Chemical:** removal of devitalized tissue with topically applied enzymes.

**Autolytic:** removal of devitalized tissue by the use of synthetic dressings that allow the wound to autodigest.

## 18. What are the advantages and disadvantages of each type of debridement?

| TYPE OF DEBRIDEMENT | ADVANTAGES | DISADVANTAGES |
|---|---|---|
| Sharp | Rapid | May remove viable tissue |
| | Indicated when cellulitis or sepsis is present | Requires physician or registered nurse with special training |
| Mechanical | Dressings used as initial form of debridement | Nonselective, potential trauma to new tissue |
| | Hydrotherapy useful for softening eschar | |
| Chemical | Useful for patients who cannot tolerate surgery and in long-term or home care | Slower than sharp |
| | Can be used in conjunction with sharp debridement | May become infected because of rich environment and bioburden |
| | | Requires physician order |
| Autolytic | Easy to use | Slower than chemical |
| | Ideal for superficial areas | Can be used by any provider |
| | Useful for patients who cannot tolerate surgery and in long-term or home care | |

**19. What principles guide the selection and use of dressings in critically ill patients?**

Dressings should provide the optimal environment for healing. The principles that guide wound healing include moisture for the wound, protection of the wound, and prevention of infection. With partial-thickness injuries and wounds healing by primary intention, local care is designed to maintain a physiologic environment and protect the wound from disruption. With wounds healing by secondary intention, local care should minimize contamination and debris in the wound and keep the tissue moist.

**20. Why is a moist environment preferred?**

The development of new dressings was based on research showing that wound healing progresses most rapidly in a moist environment. Moist healing supports rapid epithelialization, angiogenesis, rapid granulation tissue formation, and collagen metabolism. Initially the beneficial effects of moist wound healing were questioned because of the belief that a dry environment inhibited the growth of organisms and helped to prevent infection. Early studies showing that moist healing resulted in increased numbers of organisms in the wound site. Subsequent work showed that although colonization was greater, moist healing was not associated with an increased rate of infection.

**21. What types of dressing are available?**

Until recently, most dressings were made of cotton gauze. Exudate is absorbed in the threads or interstices of the gauze, away from direct contact with the injured tissue, and subsequently removed from the wound with the dressing change. Currently a wide array of dressings is available. Dressings that can be used to heal partial-thickness injuries or full-thickness wounds closed by primary intention include gauze dressings, hydrocolloids, hydrogels, transparent films, absorptive dressings, and foams. Dressings were manufactured to provide different functions for use in wounds. Some provide moisture, others are absorbent, and some provide combinations of both.

**22. Describe the proper use of gauze for wound dressing.**

For a full-thickness injury with a large wound space, gauze is the mainstay of treatment. It is moistened and placed in the wound to keep tissues moist and separated so that healing can progress from the bottom of the wound upward. This approach prevents abscess formation. In the past, gauze dressings often were removed from the wound dry to debride foreign material and exudate. Bleeding of tissue consistently accompanied removal of dry gauze from the wound. Now it is recognized that removal of dry gauze dressing disrupts the new capillary bed and places an added burden on injured tissue. If a wound is excessively exudative or full of debris, other approaches need to be taken, such as more frequent dressing changes or high-pressure irrigation.

**23. What types of dressing are used most often in the intensive care unit (ICU)?**

In the ICU environment, gauze dressings and some hydrocolloid dressings are used most frequently. Gauze dressings require frequent changing. As the patient progresses toward discharge, the type of dressing may change for treatment of the same wound, depending on the needs and abilities of the patient and the progression of wound healing.

**24. What systemic therapies support wound healing?**

Healing wounds need adequate perfusion and oxygenation. Pain and hypothermia cause vasoconstriction that decreases perfusion to the healing wound. Warming and analgesics decrease vasoconstriction, allowing local perfusion, delivery of oxygen and nutrients. Local wound perfusion requires administration of adequate fluid. The febrile patient may require more fluid, whereas the fluid-positive patient may require diuresis. Assessing capillary refill on the forehead is a useful way to monitor fluid status. Refill time should not exceed 1.5 seconds. For patients cooled with surgery, warming should continue until the patient is fully awake and can maintain thermal balance. Hypertension and hypotension impair wound perfusion. Local perfusion is ensured in patients with a normal blood volume and inactivated sympathetic nervous system who are warm and pain-free.

### 25. What other factors affect wound healing?

Other factors that affect wound healing include noise, sleep, and drugs. Providing a restful environment can be challenging in the ICU. Noise can be irritating and stimulate the sympathetic nervous system. Planning for sleep periods when the patient is hemodynamically stable can be helpful, particularly with chronic wounds. Vasoconstrictive drugs should be avoided if possible. Beta blockers and alpha-adrenergic agonists are harmful to tissue healing but may be necessary for critically ill patients.

### 26. Describe the role of nutrition in wound healing.

Wound healing requires adequate nutrition. Increased metabolic rate is related directly to the severity of injury. Caloric and protein needs are increased. These demands generally return to normal in 1–14 days after acute injury.

### 27. What are the newest therapies for the treatment of wounds?

**Growth factors** are polypeptides that control cellular growth, differentiation, and metabolism. Although present in minute amounts, they exert a profound effect on local events in healing by interacting with specific receptors in the cell surface that result in signals to target cells. The effects of growth factors include cell proliferation, chemotaxis, angiogenesis, protein expression, and enzyme production. Initially the growth factors often were named for the tissue of origin (e.g., platelet derived growth factor), the cells on which they act (e.g., epidermal growth factors), or their biologic action (e.g., transforming growth factors beta). Subsequent work demonstrated that growth factors have more than one action and that often the effect is dose-related. The exact dose and timing of their application remains to be determined. Growth factors currently are not used for acute wounds; their application during critical illness is limited.

Although **skin substitutes** have been used in wound healing for many years, the newest types are grown in culture from fetal cells. Because of the low antigenicity of fetal tissue, it is readily incorporated into the wound module, and skin closure occurs rapidly. The cultured cells can be meshed to increase the area that they cover. They are especially useful in patients with burns and patients who have limited donor sites or difficulty with healing.

### BIBLIOGRAPHY

1. Bergstrom N, et al: Treatment of pressure ulcers: Clinical practice guideline. Rockville, MD, U.S. Department of Health and Human Services, Publication number 950652, 1994.
2. Hunt TK, Hopf HW: Wound healing and wound infection: What surgeons and anesthesiologists can do. Surg Clin North Am 77:587–606, 1997.
3. Mangram AJ, Horan TC, Pearson ML, et al: Guideline for prevention of surgical site infection, 1999. Am J Infect Control 27(2):97–132, 1999.
4. Rodeheaver GT: Wound cleansing, wound irrigation, wound disinfection. In Krasner D, Kane D: Chronic Wound Care, 2nd ed. Wayne, PA, Health Management Publications, 1997, pp 97–108.
5. Stadelmann WK, Digenis AG, Tobin GR: Physiology and healing dynamics of chronic cutaneous wounds. Am J Surg 176 (Suppl 2A):26S–38S, 1998.

# 66. IDENTIFICATION AND TREATMENT OF PRESSURE ULCERS

*Nancy A. Stotts, RN, EdD*

**1. How is pressure ulcer risk assessed?**

Pressure ulcer risk is evaluated with clinical judgment or risk assessment tools with established validity and reliability. The instruments most often used are the Braden and the Norton scales. A frequently used British instrument, called the Waterlow scale, is slightly different in that it includes items on age and comorbid conditions; in addition, specific interventions are linked with different levels of risk. Regardless of whether clinical judgment or a risk assessment scale is used, the assessed risk should be documented.

**2. When and how often should pressure ulcer risk be assessed?**

Pressure ulcer risk should be assessed at hospital admission, when a patient's status changes, and at regular intervals. There is no community standard for the frequency at which routine reassessment is needed, but many critical care units assess pressure ulcer risk daily because of the rapid changes in patient status. Identifying patients at-risk has important fiscal implications. Prevention is expensive, but treatment is even more so. Prevention is costly in terms of nursing time, supplies, equipment, and potentially lost opportunity. Therefore, prevention strategies need to address specific areas of risk in specific patients.

**3. What are the major risk factors for pressure ulcers? How are they altered in critical care?**

Pressure, friction, and shear are the major causes of pressure ulcers. They result in tissue damage that is manifest as ischemia and necrosis. In critical care patients, perfusion and oxygenation often are compromised and result in hypoperfusion and hypoxic tissue. Therefore, less pressure or pressure applied for a shorter duration may result in a pressure ulcer. In addition, because critically ill patients often are immobile, their risk of ulcers is increased.

**4. What are the most common sites of pressure ulcer development?**

The sacrum and the heels are the most common sites of pressure ulcer development. Special precautions need to be taken to protect these areas.

**5. What are the basic preventive strategies for critical care patients at risk of pressure ulcers?**

Pressure relief over bony prominences at regular intervals using the "30° rule" probably is the most basic principle. The 30° rule states that patients should be positioned (1) with the head at an angle not greater than 30° or (2) on their side at an angle not greater than 30°. This task seems simple, but critically ill patients often have higher-priority needs (e.g., resuscitation, oxygenation) or cannot tolerate the turning or other activity required to implement simple preventive measures.

The heels are especially vulnerable in immobile patients, largely because they have little subcutaneous tissue. Thus, pressure on the bone readily compresses the vasculature. Often the heels are "floated" using pillows or special protective boots. When protective boots are used, they need to relieve pressure from the heels, not just cushion them.

**6. Compare and contrast the stages of pressure ulcers.**

The four stages of pressure ulcers reflect the depth of tissue injury. In addition, if the ulcer is covered with eschar, it is not stageable and is documented as such.

**Stage I** ulcers are characterized by intact skin with nonblanchable erythema. Discoloration of the skin, warmth, edema, induration, or hardness also may be indicators, especially in patients with dark skin, in whom nonblanchable erythema is difficult to elicit.

**Stage II** ulcers develop with partial-thickness skin loss involving the epidermis, dermis, or both. The ulcer presents clinically as an abrasion, blister, or shallow crater.

**Stage III** ulcers involve full-thickness skin loss and damage of subcutaneous tissue. They may extend down to, but not through, the fascia. Stage III ulcers present as a deep crater that may or may not involve undermining.

**Stage IV** ulcers are the deepest and include full-thickness skin loss with destruction of tissue that extends into the muscle, bone, or supporting structures (tendon, joint capsule). Undermining and sinus tracts may be associated with stage IV ulcers.

### 7. What principles should guide local wound care?

1. **Know the goal of care.** The type of care provided depends on its purpose. For example, when necrotic tissue is present, it is usually debrided. However, if the patient has arterial disease and a heel ulcer with intact skin, the goal of care often is to keep the tissue from becoming infected. In other patients, the goal of care may be to provide comfort (rather than healing); thus, less aggressive wound treatment is used.

2. **Reduce bioburden.** Bioburden is the strain placed on the wound by microorganisms. This strain is reduced at the local level by debriding dead tissue and cleansing the wound (see Chapter 65). Cleansing of the wound is important in reducing bioburden, particularly in undermined wounds. Undermined areas harbor microorganisms, especially gram-negative organisms, which flourish in the warm, dark, moist environment.

3. **Keep the wound moist but not excessively wet.** Moisture supports the formation of granulation tissue and migration of epithelium to close the wound. Excessive moisture results in maceration of the wound bed (and potentially of surrounding tissue), whereas excessive dryness results in dehydration and death of tissue. Dressings that accomplish the goals of care should be selected.

4. **Treat the underlying cause.** The underlying cause of pressure ulcers is pressure that results in ischemia. Treatment is relief of pressure, which may involve use of special support surfaces, adjunctive positioning devices, heel protection, and an aggressive turning schedule.

### 8. What principles guide systemic support for healing of pressure ulcers?

Tissue tolerance for pressure is enhanced with the triad of adequate perfusion, oxygenation, and nutrition. Perfusion is supported with adequate intravascular volume in the setting of normal interstitial fluid. The presence of edema slows the transport of nutrients to tissues and therefore contributes to delayed healing. Normal oxygenation supports cellular integrity. In critical care, fluid and oxygen balance are often precarious and may increase the patient's risk of pressure ulcers and delayed healing. Nutrients are needed to support healing. Adequate calories, high protein, and a multivitamin/mineral supplement normally are provided. Although specific nutrients such as vitamin C and zinc are emphasized because of their role in collagen formation, an adequate and balanced intake—orally or by the enteral or parenteral route—supports healing.

Even if the critically ill patient has adequate intravascular volume, oxygenation, and nutrients, the substrates may not be able to reach the area of injury. Such a situation is seen when the patient is cold, in pain, or receiving vasoconstricting drugs. You should address each of these areas to optimize healing.

### 9. If a patient in the critical care unit develops a pressure ulcer, what should you tell the patient and family?

Patients and families need to understand the patient's risk for pressure ulcers. The basic pathophysiology of ulcer development and the type of treatment should be explained. Sometimes pressure ulcers develop because patients cannot be turned or positioned to relieve pressure. Examples include patients whose blood pressure falls when they are turned from the supine position and patients with respiratory compromise who need to be in semi-Fowler's position. If appropriate, clinical decisions based on the patient's priority needs should be explained. The nurse should document the discussion with the patient and family. You may need to notify the risk management department of your institution.

**10. Should we use newer therapies, such as growth factors, skin substitutes, and electrical stimulation, to assist with healing?**

Such therapies are important and often used with chronic wounds. Most wounds in critical care are acute and will heal without problems. Also, because critically ill patients often are typically unstable, such therapies are not appropriate. They may be used later in the patient's recovery, if healing is delayed.

### BIBLIOGRAPHY

1. Maklebust J, Siegreen M: Pressure Ulcers: Guidelines for Prevention and Nursing Management, 2nd ed. Springhouse, PA, Springhouse Press, 1996.
2. Senecal SJ: Pain management in wound care. Nurs Clin North Am 34:847–860, 1999.
3. Stotts NA, Hunt TK: Pressure ulcers. Managing bacterial colonization and infection. Clin Geriatr Med 13:565–573, 1997.

# 67. PHYSICAL THERAPY

*Kris Ishii*, MS, PT, CCS

**1. Define muscle atrophy and muscle weakness.**

**Muscle atrophy** is a reduction in size of the muscle fibers, but the term often is used to describe a decrease in total muscle size. **Muscle weakness** is a decrease in strength (ability to produce movement or force) compared with the patient's normal status. The reduction in muscle strength is proportional to the degree of atrophy. Muscle weakness may result from pain or reflex muscle guarding of an inflamed joint.

**2. What are the causes of muscle atrophy and weakness? Give clinical examples of each.**

| CAUSE | CLINICAL EXAMPLES |
| --- | --- |
| Cell death and reabsorption | Trauma (laceration, crush or thermal injury), necrosis, gangrene, rhabdomyolysis |
| Pressure | Compartment syndrome, hemorrhage, infection, tight casts or dressings, trauma, neoplasm |
| Neuromuscular disorders | Amyotrophic lateral sclerosis, Eaton-Lambert syndrome, Guillain-Barré syndrome, motor neuron disease, peripheral neuropathies, muscular atrophies or dystrophies, myopathies, myasthenia gravis, collagen vascular disease, glycogen storage disease, porphyria |
| Bacterial toxins | Botulism, tetanus |
| Vascular insufficiency | Peripheral vascular disease, decreased cardiac output |
| Malnutrition | Chronic undernutrition, deficiencies of essential nutrients, alcoholism |
| Decreased activity | Bedrest, inactivity, immobilization (cast, splint, restraint), denervation, spinal cord injury, cerebral vascular accident |
| Hormonal changes | Adrenocortical deficiency, Cushing's disease, Addison's disease, thyroid disease |
| Medications | Neuromuscular blocking agents, corticosteroids, aminoglycosides |

**3. How can the nurse help to prevent or treat skeletal muscle atrophy and weakness?**

After the differential diagnoses listed above have been considered and the appropriate consultations made, primary nursing interventions address physical activity and medications:

1. Muscle weakness is minimized or improved by muscle use. Mobilization of the patient (limb exercises, bed mobility, dangling and standing, transferring) facilitates muscle use. (See questions 20 and 21.)

2. Encourage positions and activities in which patients can use their muscles. For example, ensure that patients have sufficient space to move their limbs, especially against gravity. Many patients develop less upper extremity weakness because they reach and use their hands in bed, whereas the lower extremities become weak from lack of weight bearing and movement.

3. Minimize the use of restraints. If restraints are mandatory, maximize the amount of movement allowed within the range of the restraint.

4. Minimize the use of neuromuscular blocking agents, corticosteroids, and aminoglycosides. Avoid concomitant use of these agents.

5. Minimize muscle weakness related to pain by administering analgesics as needed.

**4. What are the causes joint stiffness? Give clinical examples of each.**

| CAUSE | CLINICAL EXAMPLES |
|---|---|
| Joint effusion/inflammation | Traumatic arthritis, rheumatoid arthritis, infectious arthritis, gout |
| Capsular fibrosis | Prolonged immobilization, restricted mobility, tissue pathology due to trauma, congenital or acquired deformities |
| Connective tissue or neuromuscular diseases | Scleroderma, dermatomyositis, polymyositis, lupus erythematosus, Parkinson's disease, muscular dystrophy |

**5. How can the nurse help to prevent or treat joint stiffness?**

Range-of-motion (ROM) activities help to maintain joint and soft-tissue mobility. Stretches are used to elongate pathologically shortened soft-tissue structures and thereby increase ROM. Stretches are most effective when they are held for at least 30 seconds at the endpoint of the existing range of motion.

**6. What are the three types of ROM exercises?**

| | |
|---|---|
| Passive | Movement produced entirely by external force (another person or mechanical device) |
| Active | Movement produced by active contraction of muscles |
| Active-assistive | Active ROM with some assistance provided (because muscles need assistance to complete the motion) |

**7. How are ROM exercises performed?**

ROM exercises may be performed formally, by moving each limb and trunk segment through various ranges, or incorporated into positioning and functional use. For example, as a patient is moved about for bathing, hips and knees may be extended in the supine but flexed in the side-lying position. The trunk, neck, and limbs are moved to provide access to all areas of skin for cleansing.

**8. What is foot drop?**

Foot drop is defined as plantarflexion of the foot due to weakness or paralysis of the anterior muscles of the lower leg. It is the position of the foot caused by lack of dorsiflexion strength (ability to move the foot up). It causes the toes to drag during ambulation. The term also is used to describe the plantarflexed position of a patient's foot in bed, even when dorsiflexion strength and/or ROM is present, and to identify a plantarflexion contracture.

**9. What is the normal range of dorsiflexion of the foot? How is it assessed?**

The normal range of dorsiflexion is 20°. In other words, from the neutral or 90° foot-to-leg position, the foot should be able to move another 20° upward. When assessing dorsiflexion ROM, be careful to observe movement only at the ankle; do not include movement of the forefoot.

**10. How can the nurse help to prevent or treat foot drop?**
1. To prevent dorsiflexion weakness, the patient should perform active dorsiflexion (e.g., ankle pumps) in bed, in the sitting position, or during normal walking.
2. To prevent a prolonged plantarflexion position, which may lead to calf or ankle tightness and/or contracture, the patient should perform regular dorsiflexion ROM exercises or place the ankles in at least neutral (90°) position.
3. A footboard may be used to position the feet in neutral position. The bottom of the feet are kept in full contact with the board at the foot of the bed. This maneuver may be difficult for short patients whose feet do not reach the end of the bed, mobile patients who do not keep their feet in contact with the footboard, and patients who require lateral positioning with the hips and knees flexed.
4. Pillows may be used to position the ankles in neutral position, with the footboard used to keep the pillows from falling off the end of the bed. This position is temporary at best, because the pillows allow plantarflexion into the soft surface with any movement.
5. While sitting in a chair, the patient may place the feet flat on the floor or on a foot rest to achieve the neutral ankle position. This maneuver may be difficult if the patient is reclining in a position in which the legs do not form a 90° angle with the floor or foot rest.

**11. When is a splint indicated for foot drop?**
A splint is indicated when dorsiflexion positioning is needed; for example, when the patient is not ambulating, standing, or receiving dorsiflexion ROM exercises on a regular basis or cannot perform dorsiflexion exercises or be maintained in positions that support neutral ankle position.

**12. What type of splint is used for dorsiflexion positioning?**
For simple dorsiflexion positioning, any splint that adequately holds the ankles in at least a 90° position will do. Soft, ankle-cradling foam splints are cheapest. They work only if the patient has full dorsiflexion range of motion and no active plantarflexion or plantarflexion tone so that the foot can be easily supported in the correct position. Feet must be monitored carefully for loss of the neutral position due to active ankle movement, position changes, or gravity.

**13. What type of splint is used for dorsiflexion positioning when a soft splint is not adequate?**
A rigid, L-shaped plastic splint with a firm foam liner often is used for foot drop. The splint may be fixed at 90° or hinged to allow varying amounts of plantar- or dorsiflexion. Straps keep the foot in the splint and support or adjust the angle at the ankle. Such splints are best used to maintain or (with the hinged version) increase dorsiflexion by providing prolonged stretch. The splint can handle changes in position, gravitational effects, and intermittent plantarflexion pushing by the patient. However, if persistent, forceful plantarflexion is evident (volitional or due to to increased tone or spasms), the patient may develop skin breakdown at the site where the straps hold the foot into the splint at the anterior ankle. A full-coverage splint or casting may be necessary.

**14. What type of splint is used in patients with fragile skin or circulation problems?**
Splints with lamb's wool liner float the heels and have broader flap coverage (rather than straps) to keep the foot in the splint. Some have at the bottom a kickstand-like peg that can be used to help control rotation in bed (e.g., to keep the foot pointing upward in the supine position).

**15. What should be done for noncompliant patients or patients who persistently plantarflex the feet?**
For patients who are noncompliant with splint-wearing or who persistently plantarflex the feet (e.g., patients with brain injury), casting may be required. Splints that produce a persistent stretching force to the joint and increase ROM also are available.

**16. Describe the typical splint-wearing schedule.**
For maintenance dorsiflexion positioning, a typical schedule begins with 1 hour on, 1 hour off and, if skin integrity and pain allow, increases to 4 hours on, 4 hours off.

If the aim of splinting is to apply stress to increase ROM, the initial amount of stress is set so that the patient can wear the splint without increased pain for at least 20 minutes. A typical starting time in a stretching splint is 1 hour/day (four 15-minute sessions or two 30-minute sessions). The schedule is adjusted as pain is tolerated and ROM progresses.

### 17. Before mobilizing the patient, what should the nurse consider about the physical environment?

As patients move about, they are influenced by the surfaces on which they move. Basic principles include the following:

1. It is easier to move on a firmer surface than on a softer one. Rolling, scooting, and balancing in sitting and standing are easier on harder surfaces. Less energy is absorbed by the surface, and the patient gets more feedback and stability.

2. Stability is the opposite of mobility. More weight, friction, or body contact on a surface increases stability; less increases mobility.

3. It is easier to slide patients in bed if they are lighter, if less of their body is on the bed (e.g., knees bent upward so that only the feet are in contact with the mattress), and if the sheets are slippery (e.g., Goretex instead of regular sheets).

4. It is easier to stand if the patient scoots to the edge of the seat because less buttock area is on the seat and less weight is on the buttocks. In standing from a chair, it is best to get into the "nose over toes" position and shift the weight forward and onto both feet.

5. It is easier to stand from a higher sitting surface. In general, if the hips are higher than the knees in the seated position, it is easier to stand; if you are sitting in a low seat with feet on the floor and knees higher than hips, it is more difficult to stand. However, the surface (e.g., a raised bed) should not be so high that the feet do not reach the floor until the patient is practically standing.

### 18. How should the bed be adjusted before the patient is mobilized?

Flatten the bed if the patient can tolerate it. If the head of the bed is left up, the patient's trunk bends to the side during rolling, causing asymmetric abdominal use and possibly back discomfort. If the knee of the bed is left up, the patient will be sitting on a slope when dangling.

Air mattresses should be deflated. The firmer surface is easier to move on, and the height of the mattress allows both feet to touch the floor in dangling. Transfers are also easier. If the thin amount of padding under the air mattress is uncomfortable for the patient, inflate the mattress to maximal capacity. This technique provides a firm surface for easier movement and balance as well as added height. Because many ICU beds are tall, consider using a stool to assist the patient back to bed after standing.

### 19. How should chairs be adjusted?

Prepare the chair at an appropriate height for the patient to facilitate standing. Use folded blankets rather than pillows to elevate the chair seat. Blankets are firmer and ultimately add more height than squishy pillows; they also facilitate push-off for standing. If a stool is needed to get back to bed, and if the patient is unable to step up onto the stool, the height of the chair seat must be raised accordingly. Place a draw sheet in the chair seat in case the patient needs to be lifted back into bed. Remember that many commodes have adjustable heights.

### 20. What is the best way to position surfaces for patient transfer?

Position the surfaces to be transferred to and from at a 90° angle to each other. This technique usually maximizes the proximity of the two surfaces (e.g., chair and bed), minimizes the distance that the patient must travel, and allows space for the nurse to help. A common mistake is to place the surfaces at a smaller angle because they appear closer. In fact, however, smaller angles leave a smaller working space and create a greater distance for the patient to travel.

### 21. What is the most therapeutic way to move the patient in bed?

In terms of physical rehabilitation, the most therapeutic way maximizes the patient's participation. ROM and strengthening exercises can be incorporated simply by allowing the patient to help. The nurse can cue patients to grab the rails to roll, to push their feet to scoot, or to wiggle their scapulae to adjust back position. This approach also reduces the nurse's effort, although it may take more time.

Consider the mobility precautions (e.g., total hip, spine, sternum) required for each patient as well as the risks for alterations in skin integrity related to shearing. Patients should bend both knees upward. With feet flat on the bed, patients can assist in rolling by letting the knees drop to either side and in scooting by pushing up in bed with both legs. Instruct patients to place both hands on the bed railing to roll or on a trapeze or headboard to scoot upward. Patients should turn their head to the direction in which they are rolling to work on neck mobility and strengthening. Help patients only if they need help. Stand by and let them try before assisting.

**22. What is the most therapeutic way to transfer a patient?**
Again, the most therapeutic way maximizes patient participation and incorporates ROM and strengthening exercises. Consider how the patient can help and how items can be positioned to facilitate participation. For example, a rail, walker, or arms of a chair can be used by patients with strong upper extremities.

During the ideal transfer, the patient works, the nurse assists, and no barriers interfere. A snag in equipment can stop the transfer abruptly or impair safety and body mechanics. The nurse should consider everything that is attached to the patient. Maintain enough slack in various lines and tubes, and determine whether anything needs reinforcement (e.g., nasogastric tube taping), support (e.g., endotracheal tube for prevention of gagging), or removal (e.g., blood pressure cuff). Double check for contraindications to mobility (e.g., femoral line that limits the sitting position).

If the patient must be transferred a significant distance, gather a portable monitor and oxygen tank, or have someone at hand to ventilate the patient, if needed. Check that pumps have a battery source of power and are attached to a portable pole.

**23. How can the nurse prevent falls when the patient attempts to stand?**
When the patient first stands, guard his or her knees. If the patient begins to buckle or fall, block the front of the knees and keep the patient's body balanced over the feet. To demonstrate the efficacy of this technique, try to buckle your own knees while standing with your front against the wall. Your knees cannot buckle because they are blocked.

**24. What is the best way to rehabilitate patients with poor tolerance of the upright position?**
The best strategy is to maximize the time spent in the upright position. Most problems contributing to poor tolerance (e.g., diminished cardiac capacity, reduced plasma and blood volumes, impaired control of blood vessels) result from reduction in hydrostatic pressure in the horizontal position. Thus, minimizing the horizontal position may minimize the adverse effects of bedrest.

Change the patient's position gradually. Slowly elevate the head of the bed, or increase the length of time with the head of the bed elevated. Placing the bed in reverse Trendelenburg position may enhance the patient's upright position. Dangling at the edge of the bed is the next step in the progression to standing and transfers.

Use proactive strategies to promote orthostatic tolerance, including warm-up leg exercises and movements before each position change and support hose. The room temperature should be cool.

**25. When should progression to the upright position be aborted?**
During the transition from supine position to dangling to standing, the patient should be monitored for orthostatic tolerance. Abort the progression if symptoms of intolerance increase, such as nausea, pallor, diaphoresis, lightheadedness, dizziness, visual blurring, impaired consciousness, hyperventilation, yawning, sighing, belching, and vague epigastric distress.

### BIBLIOGRAPHY

1. Bolton C: Neuromuscular function in the ICU. Acta Anaesthesiol Scand 41:109–112, 1997.
2. Brooks GA, Fahey TD: Fundamentals of Human Performance. New York, Macmillan, 1987.

3. D'Ambrosia RD (ed): Musculoskeletal Disorders: Regional Examination and Differential Diagnosis, 2nd ed. Philadelphia, Lippincott, 1986.
4. Gutmann L, Futmann L: Critical illness neuropathy and myopathy. Arch Neurol 56:527–528, 1999.
5. Kessler RM, Hertling D: Management of Common Musculoskeletal Disorders: Physical Therapy Principles and Methods, 3rd ed. Philadelphia, Lippincott-Raven, 1996.
6. Kisner C, Colby LA: Therapeutic Exercise: Foundations and Techniques, 3rd ed. Philadelphia, F.A. Davis, 1996.
7. McClure PW, Blackburn LG, Dusold C: The use of splints in the treatment of joint stiffness: Biologic rationale and an algorithm for making clinical decisions. Phys Ther 75:1101–1107, 1994.
8. Norkin CC, White DJ: Measurement of Joint Motion: A Guide to Goniometry, 2nd ed. Philadelphia, F.A. Davis, 1995.
9. Thomas CL (ed): Tabor's Cyclopedic Medical Dictionary, 18th ed. Philadelphia, F.A. Davis, 1997.
10. Winslow EH, Lane LD, Woods RJ: Dangling: A review of relevant physiology, research, and practice. Heart Lung 24:263–272, 1995.

# X. Family and End-of-Life Issues

## 68. FAMILY CARE

*Daphne Stannard, RN, PhD*

### 1. Who should be considered family?

The legal definition of family, based on blood relations, is purposefully narrow and limiting and is used routinely for informed consents and end-of-life decisions. But its restrictive meaning excludes many types of families; therefore, it is not the best definition to use on a daily basis. When the critically ill patient can communicate, the ideal definition is whomever the patient defines as her or his family. When the patient is unable to communicate, a practical definition of family is anyone who shares a history and a future with the patient. This inclusive definition is helpful for everyday clinical use.

### 2. Why care for a patient's family?

A reciprocal relationship exists between a patient and her or his family. For example, the family is severely affected by the loved one's illness; similarly, a "sick" or dysfunctional family can affect the patient. Nurses who respect this life-long reciprocal relationship understand that caring for a patient's family is simply another way of caring for the patient. By working with patients and their families, critical care nurses can support and strengthen meaningful relationships during times of great stress.

### 3. What are the top ten needs of families in critical care?

*The Ten Most Important Needs of Families of Adult Critically Ill Patients\**

| NEED | FREQUENCY PERCENTAGE |
| --- | --- |
| 1. To have questions answered honestly | 100 |
| 2. To know specific facts about what is wrong with the patient and her or his progress | 100 |
| 3. To know prognosis/outcome/chance for recovery | 90 |
| 4. To be called at home about changes | 90 |
| 5. To receive information once a day | 80 |
| 6. To receive information in understandable language | 80 |
| 7. To believe that hospital personnel care about the patient | 80 |
| 8. To have hope | 70 |
| 9. To know exactly what is being done to the patient and why | 70 |
| 10. To have reassurance that the best possible care is being given to the patient | 70 |

• Based on eight research projects reporting the needs of families of adult critically ill patients.

### 4. Why has assessment of patients and their families become more complex?

Advances in medical knowledge and technology have extended life and cured once incurable diseases. Such advances have complicated patients' medical histories and deepened family members' previous experiences with hospitalization. In addition, delayed marriage, deferred childbirth, dual wage earners, and differing family configurations and lifestyles have altered traditional family forms. As a result, assessing patients and families can be challenging, especially given the rapid-fire pace of most critical care areas.

### 5. What simple approach can facilitate family assessment?

Remembering the three Fs can assist critical care nurses to collect assessment data about even the most complex family units:

1. **Family composition** refers to the individuals composing a particular family. Assessment data may include members of the immediate and extended family, close friends who are considered family, and even pets.

2. **Family experience** points to what the patient and family bring to the situation. Assessment data may include previous hospitalization experiences, employment status, religious and cultural practices, and patient/family strengths and special needs.

3. **Family life** refers to the daily habits, norms, and routines that characterize a particular patient and family's life together. Assessment data may include work schedules, rest and relaxation activities, dietary preferences, and familial roles.

### 6. How should the nurse record family assessment data?

Although assessment data can be challenging to gather for complex family units, it can be even more daunting to record the collected data in a concise manner on already cramped cardexes, flowsheets, and careplans. Yet it is imperative to share assessment data with the entire health care team to ensure that care is tailored to the individual patient and family. One concise way to record family assessment data is the genogram. As information about family composition, family experience, and family life is gathered, the bedside genogram can be modified and further developed.

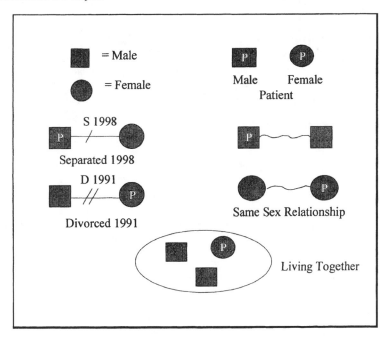

Genogram symbols. (Adapted from Wright LM, Leahey M: Nurses and Families: A Guide to Family Assessment and Intervention, 3rd ed. Philadelphia, F.A. Davis, 2000.)

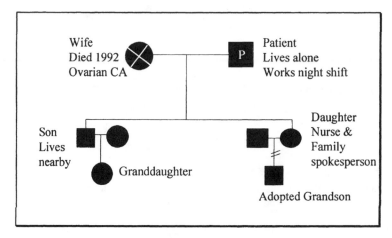

Sample bedside genogram.

### 7. What are common family interventions?

A recent study investigating the everyday interventions of expert critical care nurses in a variety of settings found that common family interventions across the lifespan include:

- Ensuring that the family can be with the patient (to promote family cohesion, connection, and closure; to foster patient well-being; and to provide the family with information)
- Providing the family with additional information and support (caring behaviors and interactions)
- Encouraging family involvement in caregiving activities (to facilitate patient-family bonding and togetherness; to promote patient healing and comfort; to decrease the family's sense of helplessness and anxiety; and to help family members understand the patient's condition).

### 8. Does family visitation have adverse physiologic effects on the patient?

The two main clusters of research examining the physiologic effects of family visitation on critically ill adult patients have focused on cardiopulmonary and neurologic changes:

- No significant cardiovascular changes were found in two recent studies examining blood pressure, heart rate, rate of premature ventricular contractions, ST segment, and oxygen saturation in a total of 72 coronary care patients before, during, and after family visitation. Both studies, however, showed that some patients were physiologically more reactive to visitation than others.
- One study found a clinically significant decrease in intracranial pressure (ICP) in 18 of 24 neurologic patients in the intensive care unit during family visitation; another study found no statistically significant increase in ICP before, during, or after visitation in 15 neurologic patients.

Such studies indicate no overarching physiologic rationale to limit or exclude family visitation. With regard to the cardiovascular reactivity noted in a subgroup of patients, the bedside nurse should monitor the patient's condition carefully during visitation. This practice, however, is commonplace with the advent of central monitoring and alarm systems and thus should not affect family visitation.

### 9. How involved should family members be in the patient's care?

Involvement can range from minor activities (e.g., asking a family member to pass an alcohol wipe) to major activities (e.g., inviting a family member to assist with the patient's bath). Family members speak highly of nurses who involve them in simple ways. It is important, however, to determine the extent to which family participation is desired. Pediatric and neonatal nurses have long involved families in caregiving activities, because participation prepares family members for their caregiving roles once the child returns home. Although the same may be said for adult critical care areas, the societal expectation and ethic of involving parents in their child's care is much stronger than it is for family members of adult patients. Yet familiar grooming and caring rituals by family members can evoke a sense of continuity and comfort for adult patients. On the other hand, in the case of chronically ill adults, hospitalization may provide a much needed respite for family members from their usual caregiving activities. Thus, opening up possibilities for comfort care and direct caregiving activities for adults requires exploration of patient and family preferences.

**10. Should families be allowed to be present during procedures and resuscitation efforts?**
Ensuring family access during procedures and resuscitation efforts is controversial. Many claim that it competes with patient care. Several reports, however, have described successful programs in emergency department settings that offer families the option of staying with their loved ones during resuscitative efforts. Although additional follow-up studies are needed to evaluate the long-term impact on family members, a cornerstone to the success of these programs is the information and support offered to the family before, during, and after resuscitation. The option of letting families stay with loved ones during procedures and resuscitative efforts should be extended to other critical care settings as well, but appropriate resources must be in place. Examples include adequate preparation of the family, presence of support personnel who are not engaged in the immediate lifesaving efforts to help the family through the resuscitation, and debriefing sessions and supportive work with staff.

### BIBLIOGRAPHY

1. Benner P, Hooper-Kyriakidis P, Stannard D: Clinical Wisdom and Interventions in Critical Care: A Thinking-In-Action Approach, Philadelphia, W.B. Saunders, 1999.
2. Emergency Nurses Association: Presenting the Option for Family Presence [educational booklet]. Park Ridge, IL, Emergency Nurses Association, 1995.
3. Hickey M: What are the needs of families of critically ill patients? A review of the literature since 1976. Heart Lung 17:670–676, 1990.
4. Leske JS: Overview of family needs after critical illness: From assessment to intervention. AACN Clin Issues 2:220–226, 1991.
5. Leske JS: Family needs and interventions. In Chulay M, Molter NC (eds): AACN Protocols for Practice. Aliso Viejo, CA, American Association of Critical-Care Nurses, 1997.
6. Titler MG: Family visitation and partnership in the critical care unit. In Chulay M, Molter NC (eds): AACN Protocols for Practice. Aliso Viejo, CA, American Association of Critical-Care Nurses, 1997.
7. Wright LM, Leahey M: Nurses and Families: A Guide to Family Assessment and Intervention, 3rd ed., Philadelphia, F.A. Davis, 2000.

# 69. BRAIN DEATH AND ORGAN PROCUREMENT

*Lisa Day, RN, PhD*

**1. What is brain death?**
Brain death is a medical term used to identify irreversible destruction and/or loss of function of the whole brain, including the brainstem. After brain death, the heart may continue to beat as long as the body is provided ventilatory and vasodynamic support. In the United States, however, brain death is the medical and legal equivalent of death due to cessation of cardiac and respiratory function.

**2. When should a nurse suspect brain death?**
When a severely brain-injured patient with a body temperature ≥ 32°C, who is not under the influence of neuromuscular blocking agents or sedating medications, exhibits the following signs, the nurse should suspect brain death has occurred or is imminent:

- Complete unresponsiveness to any stimuli, noxious or otherwise
- Loss of all brainstem reflexes (pupillary light reflex, oculocephalic or "doll's eye" response; corneal, cough, and gag reflexes; no swallowing or yawning)
- The patient no longer "triggers" the ventilator by initiating a breath, assuming the ventilator is in synchronized mandatory ventilation (SIMV) mode
- Intracranial pressure exceeds mean arterial pressure

**3. What should the nurse do if he or she suspects a patient may be brain dead?**

Continue full support and immediately notify the physician in charge of treatment so that brain death can be confirmed as soon as possible.

**4. What is the nurse's role in the confirmation of brain death?**

In many states, brain death can be confirmed and declared by two licensed physicians at the bedside with use of minimal technology. As recommended by the American Academy of Neurology, the physicians confirming brain death should examine the patient for lack of responsiveness and absence of brainstem reflexes, including response to cold calorics. The apnea test is usually confirmatory. If brain death cannot be confirmed by testing for apnea, a scan or an angiogram of blood flow to the brain may be done. The nurse assists with the physical exam, cold calorics, apnea testing, and, if required, brain blood flow studies.

**5. How is the cold calorics test performed?**

1. Assemble the following equipment: a 50-ml syringe, a butterfly needle attachment with the needle clipped off to leave an open tube, an emesis basin, a towel, and at least 100 ml of ice-water (tap water is fine).

2. At least two people are required to perform the test. Depending on the particular institution, cold calorics may be done by two nurses, two physicians or residents, or any combination.

3. Lay the patient supine with the head elevated 30°, and place the emesis basin and towel under one ear.

4. Draw up 50 ml of ice water, and attach the clipped butterfly to the syringe.

5. Insert the tube as far as possible into the ear, but make sure that the tube does not bend or kink.

6. As one person holds the patient's eyelids open and watches for eye movements, the other injects the ice water into the ear.

7. Do this procedure for both ears.

**6. How is the cold calorics test interpreted?**

Cold calorics measures the vestibuloocular reflex, which involves the eighth cranial nerve. If the vestibooccular reflex is intact, the eyes should deviate toward the affected ear with nystagmus away from the stimulus. Any movement of the eyes, limbs, or face constitutes a positive reflex and the patient cannot be declared dead. The key is to watch the patient carefully while the ice water is injected.

**7. What is the purpose of an apnea test?**

Apnea testing is intended to determine whether the patient demonstrates any effort to breathe and thus to confirm the presence or absence of functional respiratory centers in the brainstem. Once the patient is determined to be unresponsive and to have no brainstem reflexes, an apnea test is usually the only test required to confirm brain death.

**8. How is the patient prepared for the apnea test?**

Make sure that the patient's arterial carbon dioxide tension ($PaCO_2$) is normal or high. For most patients, the drive to breathe is stimulated by rising carbon dioxide levels. If $PaCO_2$ is low, as in many brain-injured patients who are artificially hyperventilated to decrease intracranial pressure, the patient may not make an effort to breathe because the stimulus is lacking. The apnea test requires disconnecting the ventilator, which can interrupt oxygen delivery. Therefore, the patient should be hyperoxygenated before initiating the test. The fractional concentration of oxygen in inspired gas (FiO$_2$) is adjusted to achieve an arterial oxygen tension (PaO$_2$) of 300–400 mmHg. Once the PaCO$_2$ is normal or high and PaO$_2$ is high, the patient is ready for the apnea test.

### 9. How is the apnea performed?

Ideally, an intensive care nurse, physician, and respiratory therapist should be present for the apnea test. Each institution should have a written protocol that indicates required personnel and details the procedure. Essentially, an apnea test involves taking the patient off the ventilator and watching for respiratory effort while monitoring PaCO$_2$ levels.

### 10. How is the apnea test interpreted?

If the patient makes no ventilatory effort by the time that the PaCO2 is 60–70 mmHg, the test is positive, indicating that the patient has no intrinsic drive to breathe. Any patient-initiated ventilatory effort during an apnea test, no matter how minimal and no matter whether it can sustain life, constitutes a negative result.

### 11. What complications may occur during an apnea test?

Patients often become unstable during apnea testing. The oxygen saturation and/or blood pressure may drop, or the patient may have serious cardiac dysrhythmias. Any of these complications necessitates discontinuation of the apnea test.

### 12. What is the nurse's role during apnea testing?

The key nursing responsibilities during apnea testing are to monitor the patient's chest and abdomen for signs of ventilatory effort and to assess tolerance for the procedure. After the apnea test is completed, hyperventilate the patient with a bag-valve-mask device to return PaO$_2$ and PaCO$_2$ levels to normal as quickly as possible.

### 13. What is the best way to offer the family the option of organ and tissue donation?

Research has shown higher consent rates when the decoupled approach is used: the discussion of death is separated in time from the discussion of organ donation. Some studies have shown higher consent rates when a representative of the organ procurement organization (OPO) is involved in the discussion with the family. Although such findings have been put into practice in various forms, the research is flawed. Most studies have been descriptive and/or correlational and have relied on retrospective chart review as the only source of data. Combined with the questionable accuracy of the data, the research, in some cases, has led to unwarranted conclusions. For example, a correlation between higher consent rates and involvement of an OPO representative does not warrant the conclusion that the OPO representative's involvement accounts for the increase in consent rates. The higher rate of consent found with OPO involvement may be attributable to the process of referral to the OPO; perhaps families who are more likely to consent are referred more often than families less likely to consent.

### 14. What is the most significant flaw in research about organ procurement?

The most significant flaw is reliance on consent rates as the main and sometimes only outcome measure. Because organ donation is a choice that the patient and/or family ought to be free to make, the best method for offering the option of donation cannot be measured in terms of consent rates. The best method offers a true choice and allows the family either to consent or to refuse donation.

### 15. What makes a patient a good candidate for organ donation?

Any patient declared brain dead and under the age of 70 years may have the potential to donate solid organs such as the heart, lungs, liver, and/or kidneys. Patients declared dead based on cessation of heart-lung function may have the potential to donate other body tissues, such as corneas, skin, heart valves, or bones. For this reason, all deaths should be reported to the local organ and tissue procurement agency.

## BIBLIOGRAPHY

1. Bernat J: Brain death. In Gilman S, Goldstein GW, Waxman SG (eds): Neurobase CD-ROM, 4th ed. San Diego, Arbor Publishing, 1999.
2. Day LJ: Nursing care of potential organ donors: An articulation of practice, ethics and etiquette. Unpublished doctoral dissertation, University of California, San Francisco, 1999.
3. Garrison RN, Bentley FR, Raque GH, et al: There is an answer to the shortage of organ donors. Surg Gynecol Obstet 173:391–396, 1991.
4. Gortmaker SL, Beasley CL, Sheehy E, et al: Improving the request process to increase family consent for organ donation. J Transplant Coord 8:210–217, 1998.
5. Niles PA, Mattice BJ: The timing factor in the consent process. J Transplant Coord 6:84–87, 1996.
6. Quality Standards Subcommittee of the American Academy of Neurology: Practice parameters for determining brain death in adults (summary statements). Neurology 45:1012–1014, 1995.
7. von Pohle W: Obtaining organ donation: Who should ask? Heart Lung 25:304–309, 1996.

# 70. END-OF-LIFE CARE

*Kathleen A. Puntillo, RN, DNSc, FAAN*

### 1. What is palliative care and how can it be provided at end of life to critically ill patients?

Palliative care is provided to lessen the severity of a symptom or clinical process when cure is not possible. It is comprehensive management of physical, psychological, social, and spiritual needs of patients. Although all critically ill patients should receive aggressive care, the goals of aggressive care at end of life should emphasize the provision of a peaceful death.

### 2. What are the essential roles of communication and goal-setting in the care of dying patients in critical care units?

A primary nursing activity is to be present during team and family discussions of the patient and to facilitate communications with physicians and other health care providers about the dying patient's plan of care. The nurse can encourage a team dialogue that demonstrates respect for others' perspectives about the best plan of care for the individual patient.

Critical care nurses play a major role in setting goals for the patient related to end-of-life comfort care. Nurses are unique in that they are with the patient for up to 12 hours each day or night. Therefore, they can advocate for the patient when they believe, and the patient's condition indicates, that comfort care should be the primary goal.

Goal-setting should be a conscious, deliberate activity performed by the health care team, patient, and patient's family. Incorporating goal-setting into the daily team reports is as important as the review of body systems and diagnostic tests. At this time the team can determine what is best for this patient and family, what can be achieved, and how the team can achieve it.

### 3. What are the most common symptoms faced by dying patients?

Among the most common symptoms experienced by many patients at end of life are pain and anxiety; confusion and agitation; dyspnea; and thirst and dry mouth.

### 4. What is the nurse's role in pain assessment and management?

Pain is one of the most prevalent and distressing symptoms of seriously ill patients dying in large teaching hospitals. Assessment of pain is important in all ICU patients because many patients with pain have conditions that health care providers do not usually associate with pain (e.g., chronic obstructive pulmonary disease, congestive heart failure). For a full discussion of pain management, see chapter 60.

## 5. How can the nurse help to minimize unnecessary procedures?

The many diagnostic and treatment procedures performed in critical care units are sources for pain and anxiety in critically ill patients. Research has shown commonly performed procedures such as central, arterial, peripheral line placements, nasogastric tube placements, chest tube removal, and endotracheal suctioning to be quite painful for patients. Discomfort from invasive and painful procedures may be the primary cause of suffering at the end of life. Other procedures that may be unnecessary, painful, and unpleasant include frequent vital sign assessment, frequent turning, wound debridements, frequent dressing changes, and use of sequential compression devices. Of primary importance is to determine the necessity of any and all procedures after a decision has been made to end life support. Nurses can evaluate the appropriateness of procedures being planned for patients and advocate for the omission of unnecessary ones. The most important procedures for patients to experience at end of life are those which promote comfort.

## 6. What other measures help to decrease anxiety and distress?

Dying patients can also be in a great deal of distress. Providing information, initiating measures to promote relaxation, and/or suggesting the addition of anxiolytics or antidepressants to the pharmacologic regimen are all interventions to be considered to decrease distress.

## 7. What are the causes of confusion and agitation in dying patients?

Dying patients in ICUs frequently have confusion that is evidenced as agitation. Many of the causes are identifiable, such as the effects of certain drugs, metabolic alterations, hypercarbia, hypoxia, environmental problems, and pain. Sometimes, however, causes are not identifiable. Successful detection of confusion requires careful surveillance and screening (see chapter 58). Clinicians can attempt to assess the presence of confusion and, when possible, eliminate the source(s). Even when the causes are unknown, erring on the side of treatment and symptom control may help to reduce that patient's and family's suffering. When indicated, nurses can advocate for the addition of psychotropic medications to the patient's treatment regimen. Neuroleptics such as haloperidol are often the first-line treatment for nonspecific agitation.

## 8. How can the nurse help the family of confused and agitated patients?

The patient's family may become quite concerned about development of confusion in their loved one. They may equate the confusion and agitation with pain, even though pain is not necessarily present during confusion. The nurse can encourage open communication between the patient, when possible, and all family members and encourage them to discuss unresolved issues while the patient is cognitively intact.

## 9. How can dyspnea be managed?

Pharmacologic and nonpharmacologic conditions can be both causes of and treatments for dyspnea. For example, dyspnea can increase when patients are receiving adrenergic agonists (e.g., metaproterenol, albuterol) and theophylline. Morphine can directly improve dyspnea by decreasing cardiac preload, and benzodiazepines can indirectly improve dyspnea through their anxiolytic effects. The nurse can use nonpharmacologic measures to decrease the patient's feeling of shortness of breath. Placing the patient in a position of comfort (e.g., sitting upright) can help to relieve dyspnea, and a bedside fan provides a cool breeze and makes breathing easier. Repeated reassurance is an effective intervention for dyspnea when the patient trusts the professional staff. Alert dyspneic patients can obtain comfort from knowing that they will not be left alone and have some degree of control in their care.

## 10. How are thirst and dry mouth managed?

Thirst and dry mouth can be uncomfortable symptoms at end of life. Dehydration is not a necessary prerequisite to development of thirst and dry mouth; many medications can cause thirst and dry mouth, including opioids, phenothiazines, hyoscine, antihistamines, and antidepressants. In addition, mouth breathing and candidiasis also may cause dry mouth. The patient's mouth should be gently inspected every day with a padded tongue blade and flashlight. Dry mouth and thirst can be helped with meticulous mouth care. When possible, the administration of small amounts of oral fluids and/or ice chips also helps to minimize thirst and dry mouth.

**11. What other comfort care measures can be provided to dying ICU patients?**

The critical care nurse can perform specific hygiene measures that increase patient comfort. Examples include the use of lotion on dry skin and ointment on dry lips. If the patient's eyes are dry and/or do not close completely, use of artificial tears or eye ointments can decrease eye discomfort. Patients should be told that tears or ointments are being used so that they understand why their vision is blurred. The nurse can try to maintain a normothermic body temperature by sponge-bathing the patient with lukewarm water, using fans, and applying just enough linen to maintain the patient's privacy. The nurse can be alert for the development of pressure areas, especially over bony prominences, and use massage and turning as appropriate. Gentle washing and combing of the patient's hair are soothing hygienic measures that help to maintain the patient's dignity. During the provision of these comfort measures, the nurse can talk gently to the patient, informing him or her about what activities are being performed. Part of patient comfort is knowing that their providers care about them and will be with them at all times.

**12. When is it appropriate to withdraw mechanical ventilation?**

Removal from mechanical ventilation is indicated when the informed patient requests its withdrawal; when interventions to save the patient's life are deemed to be futile; and when withdrawal reduces a terminally ill patient's pain and suffering.

**13. What methods are used to withdraw patients from mechanical ventilation?**

Two primary methods are used. The first, described as terminal weaning, is gradual withdrawal of ventilator assistance, which is done by decreasing the amount of inspired oxygen, decreasing the ventilator rate and mode, removing positive end-expiratory pressure (PEEP), or using a combination of these maneuvers. The second method is a more abrupt removal of the patient from ventilator assistance by extubation. Recommendations for specific procedures for withdrawal are available.

**14. What role does the nurse play in withdrawal of mechanical ventilation?**

Regardless of the method used, the critical care nurse plays a major role during the decision and implementation of withdrawal from mechanical ventilation. Specifically, the nurse can ensure that a rationale for, and all elements of, the plan have been adequately discussed among the team, patient, and family. The nurse can ensure that adequate time is given to families and their support persons, such as clergy, to reach as positive a resolution as possible. The family needs reassurance that the patient and they will not be left alone and that the patient will be kept comfortable with the use of medications and other measures. Opioids alone or in combination with benzodiazepines can be used during withdrawal to ensure optimal comfort.

**15. What is the role of paralytic agents during ventilator withdrawal?**

Paralytic agents should not be used during ventilator withdrawal. Their use makes it almost impossible to assess patient comfort. Although appearing comfortable, the patient may be experiencing pain, respiratory distress, or severe anxiety. The primary goal during the process of withdrawal should be to ensure that patient and family members are as comfortable as possible, both psychologically and physically.

**16. What interventions can be provided to the dying patient's family?**

Comprehensive care of the dying patient includes care of the patient's family. Caring for families encompasses three major aspects: (1) access; (2) information and support; and (3) involvement in caregiving activities. Nurses can offer family members the opportunity to spend as much time as possible with their loved one by appreciating the fact that their remaining time together is limited. Nurses can also share information in a timely manner by using clear and understandable language and by explaining all procedures in lay terms. They can help the family to understand the implications of prognostic information and assist them to participate in the transition from aggressive care-saving goals to palliative care goals. Nurses can help families prepare for the patient's death; this may include having family members participate in various aspects of care (e.g., bathing, hair combing, making the patient as comfortable as possible). A primary focus of the nurse should be care of the family so that their experience of the loss of a loved one in the ICU is as positive and painless as possible.

**17. What interventions can help critical care nurses to cope with caring for dying patients and their families?**

Although many nurses receive much satisfaction from providing good care to patients at end of life and even volunteer for such care, many nurses experience stress. Our culture does not prepare health professionals adequately for dealing with the discomfort associated with death and dying. Ensuring and promoting care for the caregiver cannot be overemphasized. Staff meetings can be set aside to review stresses that nurses experience in providing end-of-life care. These meetings can provide a setting for involved health professionals to process their own feelings about death and their inability to prevent it. Developing a unit philosophy and practice protocols related to care of dying patients can be a concrete method of recognizing the value of such important nursing work.

**18. How can critical care nurses assist in comforting families after the patient's death?**

When a patient in critical care dies, family members continue to need the support of health professionals. This support can come in the form of written materials about coping with grief and lists of available community resources. Some nurses attend the funeral or memorial services of patients for whom they cared, especially if they developed a close relationship with the family. Many family members appreciate follow-up contact by the nurses who cared for their loved one. This contact can be through telephone calls and/or sympathy cards at certain times (e.g., every three months) during the first year after the patient's death. The use of volunteers in the implementation of a unit bereavement program can be helpful to a busy critical care staff. A bereavement program that includes some or all of these actions can be an important component of care. Providing this type of follow-up care to families also can be a helpful intervention for the critical care nurse. It provides a mechanism for coping with the deaths of patients and can provide acknowledgment of the importance of their extraordinary work.

### BIBLIOGRAPHY

1. Campbell ML: Forgoing Life-sustaining Therapy. Aliso Viejo, CA, AACN Critical Care Publication, 1998.
2. Campbell ML, Carlson RW: Terminal weaning from mechanical ventilation: Ethical and practical considerations for patient management. Am J Crit Care 1(3):52–56, 1992.
3. Coolican MB, Pearce T: After care bereavement program. Crit Care Clin North America 7:519–527, 1995.
4. Daly BJ, Newlon B, Montenegro HD, Langdon T: Withdrawal of mechanical ventilation: Ethical principles and guidelines from terminal weaning. Am J Crit Care 2:217–223, 1993.
5. Ellershaw JE, Sutcliffe JM, Saunders CM: Dehydration and the dying patient. J Pain Symptom Manage 10:192–197, 1995.
6. Kaye P: Symptom Control in Hospice and Palliative Care. Essex, CT, Hospice Education Institute, 1990.
7. Levetown M: Palliative care in the intensive care unit. New Horizons. 1998;6(4):383-397.
8. Lynn J, Teno JM, Phillips RS, et al: Perceptions by family members of the dying experience of older and seriously ill patients. Ann Intern Med 126:97–106, 1997.
9. Morrison RS, Ahronheim JC, Morrison GR, et al: Pain and discomfort associated with common hospital procedures and experiences. J Pain Symptom Manage 15:91–101, 1998.
10. Puntillo K: Dimensions of procedural pain and its analgesic management in critically ill surgical patients. Am J Crit Care 3:116–122, 1994.
11. Puntillo KA: The role of critical care nurses in providing and managing end-of-life care. In Curtis R, Rubenfeld GD (eds): The Transition from Cure to Comfort: Managing Death in the Intensive Care Unit. (In press).
12. Puntillo KA, Stannard D: Palliative care in intensive care units. In Ferrell B, Coyle N (eds): Palliative Nursing. (In press).
13. Shuster JL: Delirium, confusion, and agitation at the end of life. J Palliat Med 1:177–186, 1998.
14. Storey P: Symptom control in advanced cancer. Semin Oncol 21:748–753, 1994.
15. Stannard D: Reclaiming the house: An interpretive study of nurse-family interactions and activities in critical care [unpublished doctoral dissertation]. University of California at San Francisco, San Francisco, 1997.
16. Taskforce on Palliative Care: Precepts of palliative care. J Palliat Care 1:109–112, 1998.

# 71. CRITICALLY ILL OBSTETRIC PATIENTS

*Maribeth Inturrisi, RN, MS, and Debra Busta-Moore, RN, MS*

**1. How do normal physiologic changes of pregnancy affect the cardiovascular presentation of critically ill obstetric patients?**
- Cardiac output (CO) increases by 40–50% (6–7 L/min)
- Plasma volume and stroke volume (SV) increase by 50%
- A grade I systolic ejection murmur, associated with increased SV, is present in 95% of pregnant women
- Heart rate increases by 15–20 beats/minute
- Systemic and pulmonary vascular resistance are decreased
- Tissue edema related to low intravascular oncotic pressure may be present

**2. How does pregnancy affect the respiratory presentation of critically ill patients?**
Oxygen consumption increases up to 25%. To meet this increased demand, the respiratory rate, tidal volume, and minute ventilation are increased. The increased minute ventilation produces hyperventilation and compensated respiratory alkalosis. The partial pressure of carbon dioxide in arterial blood ($PaCO_2$) is 27–32 mmHg. The kidneys compensate for the alkalosis by increasing bicarbonate excretion. The functional residual capacity of the lungs is reduced as pregnancy progresses.

**3. How does pregnancy affect the renal and hematologic presentation of critically ill patients?**
**Renal.** Renal blood flow is increased by 50%. Creatinine clearance and medication clearance are enhanced. Glucosuria is present in up to 20% of pregnant women.
**Hematologic.** Pregnancy is a risk factor for thromboembolic disorders. Platelet counts are normal. Fibrinogen levels increase by 30–50%, and many of the coagulation factor levels increase. At the same time fibrinolytic activity is diminished.

**4. What are the effects of maternal position on cardiac output?**
Position-related compromise of maternal CO is due to decreased venous return caused by mechanical obstruction of the inferior vena cava by the uterus. CO can be significantly compromised in the supine position. This compromise may manifest as hypotension, which can be readily treated by repositioning the mother on her left side with a right knee-chest angle.

| Position | Cardiac Output (L/min) |
| --- | --- |
| Knee-chest | 6.9 (± 2.1) |
| Right side | 6.8 (± 1.3) |
| Left side | 6.2 (± 2.0) |
| Supine | 6.0 (± 1.4) |
| Standing | 5.4 (± 2.0) |

**5. What conditions commonly bring pregnant women to the intensive care unit (ICU)?**
- Sepsis
- Trauma
- Severe cardiac lesions
- Pulmonary hypertension
- Malignancies
- Pulmonary embolism
- Status asthmaticus or severe asthma exacerbation
- Diabetic ketoacidosis
- Complications of systemic lupus erythematosus
- Neurologic lesions

**6. What complications of pregnancy may require critical care?**
- Severe preeclampsia/eclampsia
- HELLP syndrome (see question 24)
- Acute fatty liver of pregnancy
- Complications of tocolytic therapy
- Amniotic fluid embolism
- Postpartum hemorrhage

#### 7. What factors influence fetal oxygenation?

Oxygen delivery to the placenta and fetus depends on both maternal arterial oxygen content and uterine blood flow. The uterine vasculature is normally dilated. A decrease in maternal CO can adversely affect fetal oxygenation. Maternal hypotension as well as endogenous or exogenous catecholamines may constrict the uterine artery. Maternal alkalosis causes decreased uteroplacental perfusion and decreases oxygen transfer related to a left shift in the oxygen dissociation curve. Umbilical venous blood returning to the fetus has a lower oxygen tension than uterine blood. Fetal hemoglobin (Hgb) is 80–90% saturated at a partial pressure of oxygen ($PO_2$) of 30–35 mmHg because of the marked left shift of the oxygen dissociation curve. Fetal Hgb concentrate is ~150 mg/L.

#### 8. What are the normal results of fetal blood gas analysis?

The umbilical vein delivers oxygenated blood to the fetus from the placenta. Normal umbilical venous blood gas has a $PO_2$ of 35 mmHg and $PCO_2$ of 55 mmHg. The umbilical artery delivers deoxygenated blood from the fetus to the placenta. Normal umbilical artery blood gas has a $PO_2$ of 20–25 mmHg and $PCO_2$ of 30–35 mmHg,

#### 9. How long can a fetus sustain oxygen debt without irreversible brain damage?

The 50% decrease in fetal arterial oxygen does not usually cause fetal acidosis. The fetus compensates by redirecting cardiac output to the brain, heart, and adrenal glands. Irreversible brain damage does not usually occur until oxygen supply has been absent for approximately 10 minutes.

#### 10. How can fetal oxygen supply be optimized?

The oxygen-carrying capacity can be increased by (1) increasing maternal oxygen saturation with administration of supplemental oxygen at high flow (> 10 L) and high oxygen concentration (100% nonrebreather mask); (2) avoiding red cell loss and transfusion when maternal Hgb is < 28 gm/dl; and (3) increasing maternal circulation (CO). Hypovolemia and hypotension should be avoided and mean arterial pressure (MAP) maintained at > 60 mmHg. CO is optimized by positioning head of the bed at 45° and avoiding venacaval compression by lateral positioning.

#### 11. How are changes in fetal oxygenation detected?

- Fetal movement: the deoxygenated fetus avoids movement to conserve oxygen.
- Fetal heart-rate monitoring (FHRM): prolonged deceleration (< 100 beats/min for > 10 min) and late decelerations indicate poor oxygenation.
- Biophysical profile (BPP): nonstress test (NST), amniotic fluid index (AFI), fetal movement (FM), fetal breathing (FB), and fetal tone.
- Cordocentesis
- Scalp sampling
- Cord blood at delivery

#### 12. How do maternal acid-base abnormalities influence fetal pH?

Maternal alkalosis can mask fetal acidosis. Maternal acidosis can result in a low fetal pH without fetal compromise.

#### 13. How do radiologic procedures affect the fetus?

Potential adverse effects of uterine exposure to radiation include oncogenicity and teratogenicity, but the risks are minimal (< 1%) in exposures < 5 rads. Higher levels of fetal absorbed radiation doses have been calculated for abdominal radiographic and pelvic computed tomography (CT) scans.

#### 14. What drugs are known to have adverse effects on the fetus during pregnancy?

Angiotensin-converting enzyme inhibitors, tetracycline, warfarin, nitroprusside (prolonged use), and drugs that diminish uterine blood flow (e.g., epinephrine). Ephedrine is a systemic vasoconstrictor that actually increases uterine blood flow. Morphine and fentanyl do not lead to fetal opioid dependence and are safe to use in pregnancy as needed.

**15. What should be kept in mind when the pregnant patient is mechanically ventilated?**

Normal $PaCO_2$ during pregnancy is 30 mmHg. Avoid respiratory alkalosis ($PaCO_2 < 17$), which adversely affects uterine blood flow and fetal oxygenation. Upper airway edema and nasal obstruction are often present during normal pregnancy.

**16. How does cardiopulmonary resuscitation (CPR) differ in pregnant patients?**

It is technically more difficult to perform adequate CPR because of the enlarged uterus and breasts. The uterus must be tilted to the left to relieve compression of the major vessels. A perimortem cesarean section may be life-saving for both mother and infant if done within 4 minutes of the arrest and should be considered if there is no response to initial resuscitative efforts.

**17. Why are pregnant women more susceptible to pulmonary edema?**

During pregnancy, serum albumin levels are decreased because of the dilution of plasma protein with the increase in plasma volume. The result is a decrease in plasma colloid oncotic pressure (COP), which is associated with a marked increase in interstitial fluid. In states of reduced COP, the critical pulmonary capillary pressure at which pulmonary edema forms is less than normal.

**18. Is maternal fever harmful to the fetus?**

Hyperthermia (temperature > 39° C) during the first trimester may be teratogenic, causing an increased incidence of neural tube defects.

**19. What are the effects on the fetus when the mother must avoid oral ingestion (NPO status)?**

Initially the fetus is provided nutrients from maternal stores, but when these stores are depleted, the fetus is not protected. Therefore, total parenteral nutrition and lipids should be considered if NPO status is to continue for more than 3–4 days.

**20. What is severe preeclampsia?**

Preeclampsia, also called toxemia, is an unpredictable disease that occurs only when a placenta is present. The cause is unknown but is thought to be an immune-mediated event in which a substance or substances released into maternal circulation cause an abnormality in the maternal vascular endothelium. The vascular changes are unlike those seen in other types of hypertension. They result in arterial vasoconstriction accompanied by reduction in plasma volume. Microthrombi and vasospasm develop, leading to decreased organ perfusion and multiple organ dysfunction.

**21. What are the signs of preeclampsia?**
- Hypertension: systolic blood pressure (BP) > 160 mmHg, diastolic BP > 110 mmHg
- Oliguria: < 30 ml/hr
- Proteinuria: > 5 gm/24 hr
- Platelet count: < 100,000
- Epigastric pain
- Headache
- Blurred vision
- Pulmonary edema
- Increased liver function tests (LFTs)
- Intrauterine growth retardation (IUGR)

**22. What is eclampsia?**

Eclampsia is the presence of seizures in a patient with symptomatic preeclampsia.

**23. What other complications can result from severe preeclampsia?**

Other potential sequelae of preeclampsia include pulmonary edema, hepatic rupture, renal failure, stroke, disseminated intravascular coagulation (DIC), placental abruption, and fetal demise.

**24. What is HELLP?**

HELLP is a severe form of preeclampsia that requires immediate delivery. It accounts for 12–17% of all maternal deaths in the U.S. HELLP is characterized by **h**emolysis (red blood cell smear with histocytes), **e**levated **l**iver enzymes (aspartate aminotransferase, alanine aminotransferase), and **l**ow **p**latelets (< 100,000).

### 25. How is severe preeclampsia managed?

Severe preeclampsia, with or without HELLP syndrome, is treated with steroids (betamethasone) and antihypertensive agents if the fetus is younger than 35 weeks. The fetus and mother are monitored continually for increasing severity of symptoms. The only definitive treatment is delivery of the fetus and placenta, preferably by the vaginal route. Magnesium sulfate is administered to prevent eclampsia and usually is continued 24 hours after delivery. It is given intravenously to obtain a plasma level around 5 mg/dl.

### 26. What is an amniotic fluid embolus?

This catastrophic complication is uncommon (1 in 80,000 births) and has a high mortality rate (~ 86%). It accounts for 10% of all maternal deaths. Most cases occur during labor and delivery. The clinical presentation includes sudden onset of severe dyspnea, hypoxemia, cardiovascular collapse, and possible seizures. It is less common, but the initial presentation can be hemorrhage from DIC. The respiratory symptoms can progress quickly to acute respiratory distress syndrome (ARDS). Prognosis is poor; 25–50% of patients die within the first hour of the initial event. Diagnosis is usually presumptive, and treatment is supportive.

### 27. How is postpartum hemorrhage (PPH) managed differently from hemorrhage in non-pregnant patients?

PPH is often the result of uterine atony. The uterine musculature fails to contract around uterine arteries at the placental site at delivery. Other possible causes of PPH are vaginal and/or cervical lacerations or an inverted uterus. Beside the usual resuscitative measures, such as IV access, crystalloid, and blood replacement, measures should be taken to treat uterine atony. These include manual uterine massage and administration of oxytocin, misoprostil, hemabate, and/or methergine.

If the above interventions are ineffective, consider (1) dilatation and curettage to remove retained placental fragments, (2) embolization of the internal iliac or uterine arteries in interventional radiology, or (3) hysterectomy. Expect a dilutional coagulopathy and/or DIC after resuscitation. Rule out posthemorrhage anterior pituitary necrosis (Shehan's syndrome). An early sign of Shehan's syndrome is the mother's inability to produce breast milk. Treatment includes pituitary hormone replacement.

### 28. What is acute fatty liver of pregnancy (AFLP)? How is it managed?

AFLP is acute fulminant hepatic failure during the third trimester of pregnancy. It affects 1 in 15,000 pregnancies. Maternal mortality rates range from 0–18%; fetal demise occurs in 23– 60% of cases. AFLP may be associated with the spectrum of severe preeclampsia. It is characterized by a prodrome of malaise, vomiting, and epigastric pain after 30 weeks' gestation. Other signs include jaundice, profound hypoglycemia, increased LFTs, coagulopathy, and increased ammonia levels contributing to metabolic encephalopathy. AFLP is managed with supportive therapy and delivery.

### 29. Why are tocolytic medications used in pregnancy?

During pregnancy the onset of uterine activity that either dilates or effaces the cervix after 20 weeks' and before 37 weeks' gestation is called preterm labor (PTL). To prevent PTL from resulting in preterm birth, tocolytic medications (e.g., terbutaline, nifedipine, magnesium sulfate, indomethacin) are administered soon after onset of PTL.

### 30. What are the adverse effects of tocolytic medications? How are they managed?

Terbutaline and magnesium have been associated with an increased incidence of pulmonary edema, primarily when given intravenously and in conjunction with large amounts of IV fluids. Exact mechanisms of action are unknown. Other side effects of terbutaline include hyperglycemia, hypokalemia, sodium and water retention, tachycardia, arrhythmias, and myocardial ischemia. Betamethasone often is given to enhance fetal lung maturation and can contribute to fluid retention.

Fluid restriction to 3000 ml in 24 hours and avoidance of fluid boluses help to prevent pulmonary edema. If it occurs, the tocolytic should be discontinued and the usual measures taken. If the edema does not resolve within 24 hours after cessation of the drug, rule out other potential causes.

**31. How is diabetes managed during pregnancy?**

Hyperglycemia is teratogenic in the first trimester and can lead to abnormal fetal growth and have life-long effects on the offspring (obesity, hypertension, type 2 diabetes). Glucose control must be tight to avoid these complications. Fasting blood glucose levels should be < 95 mg/dl and postprandial levels < 130 mg/dl. Levels also should be greater than 70 mg/dl. Overzealous treatment of hypoglycemia should be avoided. Maintaining glucose at ~ 100mg/dl is optimal. Both type 1 and type 2 diabetes require insulin for optimal management. Gestational diabetes mellitus (GDM) is generally diagnosed by universal screen between 18 and 24 weeks' gestation. The same parameters of control are indicated, regardless of the source of hyperglycemia, although GDM often does not require insulin management.

**32. What preparations should be made for delivery in the ICU?**

An interdisciplinary conference, including the ICU team, obstetric team, neonatologist, and anesthesiologist, should be held as soon as possible to establish a plan for emergency delivery, both vaginal and cesarean. If a vaginal delivery is planned to take place in the ICU, review the following critical points:

1. Birth is a normal process and can occur safely without medical intervention.

2. If the mother is intubated, an early sign of labor may be increasing oxygen needs, grimacing at intervals, or uncooperativeness.

3. A cervical exam can establish that labor is occurring.

4. Contractions decrease blood flow through the placenta, disrupting the diffusion of oxygen to the fetus. Maximize oxygen delivery to both mother and fetus.

5. Pain can increase oxygen consumption and catecholamine release, which can decrease uterine blood flow. Pain management with IV opioids or regional anesthesia usually is indicated.

**33. What supplies are essential for delivery in the ICU?**

- Pads for under the patient's buttocks (to absorb blood and amniotic fluid)
- Two clamps (to clamp the umbilical cord)
- Scissors (to cut the cord)
- Bulb syringe (to clear the newborn's airway)
- Warm blankets (to dry and wrap the newborn, especially the head)
- Warm ambient temperature (because a cold, wet newborn uses glucose to maintain heat, profound hypoglycemia may result)
- Oxytocin (Pitocin) for IV administration to keep the fundus firm immediately after delivery of the placenta

**34. What hemodynamic changes occur immediately after delivery?**

Immediately after the delivery of the placenta, dramatic hemodynamic changes begin. CO increases by 60% and stroke volume by 80% within 10 minutes after delivery. The high CO most likely results from increased venous return to the heart as the blood shifts from the uterine vessels to the central circulation. CO returns to prepregnancy values by 2 weeks after delivery.

**35. What are the essentials of postpartum care?**

1. Monitoring of vital signs and observation for bleeding are important.

2. The fundus should be firm. This natural occurrence may be assisted by fundal massage or IV oxytocin. Check for firmness at least every 15 minutes for 1 hour, then every 30 minutes for 1 hour, and then then every hour for 2 hours. If findings are stable, checks can decrease to every 4–6 hours.

3. While checking the fundus, observe the perineum for vaginal bleeding (approximately 1 pad per hour is normal). Small clots (< 3 cm) are normal. Large clots may contain retained pieces of placenta and should be examined by the obstetric team.

4. Breasts should be soft. Engorgement usually does not occur for several days. If the mother does not plan to breastfeed, use an Ace bandage to hold ice packs under the axilla for 1–2 days to stop the milk from coming in. There are no safe drugs to suppress lactation.

5. A risk of deep venous thrombosis (DVT) is associated with increased coagulability during the postpartum period. Assess lower extremities for signs and symptoms of DVT.

**36. Can postpartum critically ill patients breastfeed their newborns?**
Most women who are critically ill after delivery have the potential to breastfeed. Although breast pumping is a low priority in the critical care unit, the mother who places a high value on breastfeeding will be extremely grateful for adequate milk supply once she recovers and is re-united with her infant. Breast stimulation, through either infant suckling or mechanical pumping, is necessary to establish lactogenesis. As soon as possible, pumping or infant breast-feeding should be initiated, with a schedule of 8 times/day, 10–15 minutes per breast. A piston-style, hospital-quality pump with a double kit is preferable for effectiveness and efficiency. Little or no milk flow is not unusual for the first few days. Regular, frequent pumping should continue. If the mother remains critically ill, her milk supply will take longer to become established.

**37. How can breast milk be collected in bottles?**
To collect breast milk in bottles, the mother should sit upright or lie on her side. If she is unable to assume either of these positions, it is difficult to collect the milk. Continue pumping to sustain milk production. Place towels around the breasts to absorb the milk, and begin collecting as soon as possible.

**38. Is transfer of medications through breast milk a major concern?**
A common concern for critically ill, breastfeeding mothers is the transfer of medications through breast milk. Although all drugs penetrate milk to some degree, in most cases the concentrations are exceedingly low, and subclinical doses are delivered to the infant. The amount of drug excreted into milk depends on several factors. The Physicians' Desk Reference is not the best source for information about breastfeeding and medications. An excellent resource is Thomas Hale's *Medications and Mothers' Milk.*

BIBLIOGRAPHY

1. Dildy GA, Clark DL: Cardiac arrest during pregnancy. Obstet Gynecol Clin North Am 22:30–314, 1995.
2. Hale TW: Medications and Mothers' Milk. Amarillo, TX, Pharmasoft Medical Publishing, 1999. www.perinatalpub.com
3. Harvey M: Critical care for the maternity patient. Matern Child Nurs 17:296–309, 1992.
4. Harvey CJ: Critical Care Obstetrical Nursing. Gaithersburg, MD, Aspen, 1991.
5. Lapinsky SE, Kruczynski K, Slutsky AS: Critical care in the pregnant patient. Am J Respir Crit Care Med 152:427–455, 1995.
6. Mullaly LM, Belgrave L, Wentzel M: Collaborative planning for critically ill obstetrical patients. Matern Child Nurs 19:202–206, 1994.
7. Shailer TL, Harvey CJ: Management of the intrapartum patient in the intensive care unit. Crit Care Nurs Clin North Am 4:675–685, 1992.
8. Simpson KR: A collaborative approach to fetal assessment in the adult intensive care unit. AACN Clin Issues 8:558–563, 1997.

# 72. ETHICS

*Anna Omery, RN, DNSc*

**1. Define ethics.**
Ethics may be defined as a discipline or body of abstract knowledge that is practiced by philosophers who deliberate on and clarify ethical theories and language. Ethics also can be de-fined as a set of standards or criteria that a group uses to determine appropriate action. When

ethicists refer to normative ethics, they are referring to this definition. Examples of concrete expressions of normative ethics include do not resuscitate (DNR) or withdrawal of life-sustaining therapy policies and protocols. The most common expression of ethics is as a set of values that frame the way in which an individual views or makes choices in interpersonal situations.

## 2. How does ethics function in the critical care setting?

One may think of ethics as one thinks of monitors in critical care. Generally, monitors function to give structure to data such as heart rate and rhythm as well as various pressures. Critical care nurses think of the monitors only when something on the screen or read-out is inconsistent with what is expected—when it identifies a problem. The same can be said of ethics. Ethical values give structure to every clinical decision, but until there is an ethical conflict or dilemma (i.e., a moral problem), the presence of ethics and ethical values goes unrecognized.

## 3. Is there such a thing as nursing ethics?

A few philosophers contend that nurses do not have the authority and autonomy that are required for an ethical system. They believe that nurses depend on physicians and hospital administrators for ethical decisions. As a result, they are moral agents of physicians and administrators.

Other philosophers do not deny that nurses face ethical dilemmas and make moral decisions. But they do not believe that ethics should be affiliated with any specific professional groups. In their view, the only issue is bioethics.

The largest groups of professionals support the reality of nursing ethics as applied ethics; that is, application of ethical reflection to the decision-making process to resolve the conflict between the ideal (optimal outcome) and the real (possible outcome) in a rational and responsible way.

## 4. Name 10 ethical issues that critical care nurses have identified as significant in their clinical practice?

Between 1984 and 1993, critical care nurses in several hospitals were surveyed to identify the ethical issues that most nurses face. They are listed below from most to least frequent:

1. Do-not-resuscitate decisions
2. Quality-of-life decisions
3. Organ transplantation
4. Dealing with difficult patients
5. Issues of beneficence
6. Conflict of interest
7. Cost of care to the patient
8. Pain relief/management
9. Patient-physician-nurse relationship
10. Dying with dignity

## 5. How can a nurse distinguish the ethical from the clinical or administrative dimensions of any given professional situation?

**Clinical questions ask:** What can I do? For example, what is the amount of pain medication generally required on day 0 after cardiac surgery? Answers to clinical questions come from research and practice.

**Administrative questions ask:** What do the organization's policies or procedures tell me to do? For example, guidelines may indicate the amount of pain medication when a patient has been diagnosed as terminally ill. Answers to administrative questions come from research and the organizational leadership.

**Ethical questions ask:** What should I do? For example, a nurse is taking care of a terminally ill patient. The policy states that more medication than the patient has currently received is acceptable. The nurse is concerned, however, that additional medication may depress the rate of respiration sufficiently for death to occur. Should the nurse still give the medicine? Answers to ethical questions come from or are given language by ethical knowledge.

## 6. What kinds of ethical knowledge can help a critical care nurse analyze an ethical dilemma?

Ethical knowledge can be organized as four different types that provide particular, specific arguments for distinct ethical positions: (1) consequential ethics (teleologic theory), (2) principle-based ethics (deontologic theory), (3) care theory, and (4) virtue theory.

### 7. What is consequential theory?

Consequential theory bases or justifies an ethical decision on the belief that consequence alone (i.e., outcomes) determine the rightness of an act. From this perspective, the first question to be answered is: What is the good (outcome) desired? The second question becomes: What should be done? That is, what action or behaviors need to be undertaken to achieve the good outcome? A common axiom associated with consequential theory is that the ends justify the means.

Consequential theory has received increasing emphasis in terms of health care outcomes. Although there are good reasons for focusing on optimizing outcomes, there are also dangers. A frequently asked question is: What will be done to a particular patient to achieve an end that is good for many patients?

### 8. What are the most common principles of principle-based theory?

Ethical principles are generalizations or concepts that are used as prescriptions for action. They identify particular ethical duties or obligations. The most frequently identified ethical principles in bioethics are autonomy, beneficence and maleficence, and justice.

### 9. Define autonomy.

Autonomy is a form of personal liberty in which the individual determines his or her own course of action in accordance with a plan made by him- or herself. The autonomous person is one who not only deliberates about and chooses such plans, but who also is capable of acting on the basis of such deliberation. The principle is different from the principle of respect for persons in that it entails respect for self-determined choice of action. Autonomy is the principle that legitimizes durable power of attorney documents and living wills and underlies the policy of informed consent.

### 10. What problems are involved in using autonomy as a guide to ethical decisions?

Autonomy is a fundamental principle in Western culture, based on the rights and duties of the individual. Persons raised in other cultures or groups that give priority to obligations to the community have difficulty in accepting autonomy as a guiding ethical principle.

### 11. Explain beneficence and nonmaleficence.

**Beneficence** is the duty to help others further their own important and legitimate interests when we can do so with minimal risk to ourselves. Much of what we do as professional health care providers is based on this principle. But this principle is binding only when risk to the nurse is minimal. Nurses are also bound by the ANA Code of Ethics not to abandon patients. Clarifying the boundary between unacceptable risk and abandonment in any given situation can be extremely difficult. The converse of beneficence is **nonmaleficence**. Nonmaleficence is the duty not to inflict harm on others. It includes both intentional harm and risk of harm.

### 12. Define justice.

Justice is the duty to act with impartiality and equality and to be fair and evenhanded. Justice can be individual, distributive, and social. Individual justice obligates the individual to treat others fairly and without bias. Distributive justice supports equitable distribution of goods. Social justice is the obligation of a society to develop laws and policies that treat each member fairly and impartially.

### 13. Are these the only principles that nurses can use to address an ethical dilemma?

No. In fact, they are not necessarily the most important principles for nurses. Other principles described as important for nursing practice are fidelity, veracity, and those found in American Nurses Association's Code of Ethics. **Fidelity** is the duty to be faithful to one's patients; promise-keeping is one aspect. It is the moral covenant between people in a relationship to work together to achieve some goal. In health care the goal is usually to work toward health or well-being. **Veracity** is the duty to tell the truth and not to lie or deceive. The **ANA Code of Ethics** is a list of principles to guide moral nursing practice.

## 14. What problems are inherent in principle-based ethics?

Part of the difficulty is determining which principle should take priority in any given situation. When is autonomy more important than beneficence? If autonomy is a more binding obligation, whose autonomy should be maximized, the patient's or the health care provider's? Philosophers also remind us that beneficence run amok becomes paternalism.

## 15. Where does care theory fit into the ethical picture?

Care theory is the newest of the ethical theories. It is different from the other theories in that it has a group or community rather than an individual locus. The greatest ethical obligation is rooted in being receptive and responsive to others in order to maintain relationships. This view does not deny rationality. However, the affective response is fundamental to being an ethical person. The right thing to do in any given situation is not based on rational consideration of consequence or application of principles; it is what can be negotiated to result in minimal harm to all involved persons.

## 16. What is virtue theory?

Virtue theory, like care theory, holds that every ethical decision requires an appreciation of the situation. Right or wrong decisions do not depend on applying rules, considering consequences, or maintaining relationships. Instead, the appropriate decision depends on the development or socialization of character traits, such as kindness, courage, and compassion.

The priority of any specific virtue changes over time, reflecting societal changes. For example, in the early part of this century obedience was a desired virtue for nurses as illustrated in the following excerpt from Dock in 1917:

> In my estimation, obedience is the first law and very cornerstone of nursing. The first and most helpful criticism that I ever received from a doctor was when he told me that I was supposed to be simply an intelligent machine for the purpose of carrying out his orders.

Currently obedience has a lower priority as a virtue to guide decision making. More modern nursing virtues include independence, caring, and advocacy.

## 17. How does a nurse apply these theories in practice?

Faced with a moral dilemma, nurses often find information about ethical theories useless, ineffectual, and frustrating. For ethical knowledge to be functional, it has to be integrated into a decision-making model. Such models include steps that assist the nurse with making ethical decisions. Although many models have been proposed, the basic phases of the nursing process are an adequate guide. The nurse simply needs to know where to integrate the ethical content.

## 18. How does each phase of the nursing process guide ethical decision-making?

**Assessment phase.** Nurses gather data about clinical parameters. When faced with an ethical dilemma, the only addition to the assessment phase is identification of the persons involved in the dilemma and the ethical issues and values in play. Many people may be interested in the dilemma. The nurse taking care of the patient in the next bed and the peripheral family member may want to know what is going on and give an opinion. However, if the dilemma is to be resolved effectively and efficiently, the nurse needs to identify the critical players. Often it is only the patient, one or two close family members, the attending physician, and the nurse. Then the nurse needs to listen to each player's desired solution and determine the types of ethical knowledge that are being expressed: consequences, principles, caring, or virtue.

**Diagnosis phase.** First, the nurse identifies the clinical diagnosis and treatment options. For example, if the patient has arrested several times and is nonresponsive, the nurse determines the physical status of the patient, arrives at traditional nursing diagnoses, and reviews polices to determine what administrative direction there might be. Finally, the nurse assesses the ethical knowledge at play and determines the ethical diagnosis. One such diagnosis may be the potential for DNR status with conflict between physician and family because of opposing consequential and caring values. From there, the nurse determines the goal that may be most appropriate for the patient. For example, the goal may be to maximize the patient's autonomy. Appropriate interventions include a family conference to determine (1) whether the patient has a durable attorney for health care and (2) whether the patient has had any conversations with family members in which they expressed their wishes.

**Evaluation phase.** Questions to be asked include the following: What was the outcome of the family conference? Was the goal of maximizing the patient's autonomy achieved? Was a surrogate decision-maker identified to speak for the patient? If so, were mechanisms set in place so that the patient's perceived desires could be implemented? Are further steps required?

### 19. What kinds of resources are available to help address ethical issues?

Ethical dilemmas can be psychologically intensive. Just as in health care, it is more effective to prevent dilemmas than to deal with one. Not all dilemmas can be prevented. In such cases, preparation is still the best course of action. There are significant resources for both preventing and addressing the dilemmas. The kinds of resources available can be organized in the following categories:(1) societal, (2) professional, (3) institutional, (4) unit-based, and (5) personal.

### 20. What societal resources can the nurse access?

Laws are the reflection of a society's ethics. They are the values that either the group or the group's leaders believe are so important that they give authority to some body (such as courts or police) to enforce them. Although nurses should use available lawyers and risk managers to clarify the finer points, they also should have a basic knowledge of the laws that apply to their practice. At the federal level, the Patient Self-Determination Act of 1990 mandated health care organizations receiving Medicare funds to develop mechanisms by which the organization could identify advance directives and to educate staff about such mechanisms. States also have laws and regulations. Two areas relevant to nurses concern advance directives and the scope of nursing practice (i.e., Nurse Practice Acts). Because laws vary from state to state, nurses should educate themselves after any geographical move. As nursing practice integrates new technologies, the nurse also needs to understand the legal implications; for example, how a telephone practice that goes across state lines may be regulated.

Advancing technologies also are a resource for nurses. Several different types of websites are available. General bioethics resources are available at bioethic.net. The American Nurses Association website at ana.org has ethics resources, as does the National Library of Medicine's medline at igm.nlm.nih.gov. Search engines such as Yahoo and Excite can be used to locate other resources.

### 21. What do professional organizations provide to assist critical care nurses?

Probably the most important contribution from any professional organization is the ANA Code of Ethics with Interpretative Statements. One of the first codes of ethics, it is a list of eleven principles to guide ethical decisions in nursing practice. These principles range from duties to retain competencies to obligations to advocate and increase nursing knowledge. The ANA Code makes plain the nature of nursing's contract with society. It identifies for each nurse the duties and obligations that are fundamental to the profession of nursing.

In addition to the ANA Code, professional organizations are frequently sources of position statements about common ethical dilemmas. The ANA currently has thirteen position statements, ranging from assisted suicide to risk vs. responsibility in providing nursing care. The American Association of Critical Care Nurses (AACN) has a position statement on ethics in research.

### 22. What institutional resources are common in health care?

Since 1991, the Joint Commission on Accreditation of Healthcare Organizations (JCAHO) has required that all hospitals desiring accreditation must have in place policies, procedures, and resources for dealing with ethical dilemmas arising out of health care. This information is to be readily available to any employee. In the mid 1990s, JCAHO also required that organizations have in place policies and procedures relating to organizational ethics—that is, policies for ensuring ethical conduct of the business of health care in that organization.

Health care organizations that did not already have an ethics committee formed or affiliated with one. Ethics committees have as their mission the education of members of the organization about ethical issues; review of cases (dilemmas) with recommendations for action; and development of policies and procedures. Common policies developed by ethics committees of interest to critical care nurses are DNR policies, policies for the use of opioids in terminally ill patients, and policies for signing and implementing durable power of attorney for health care.

### 23. What are the arguments for and against Nursing Ethics Committees?

Most organizations have one committee, usually called the Bioethics or Medical Ethics Committee, to address the ethical education and issues for that organization. Other organizations have developed Nursing Ethics Committee or Subcommittees. Opponents of Nursing Ethics Committees are concerned that discussions that should include many different disciplines will not occur if discipline-specific committees are allowed. Proponents argue that certain ethical issues are of major concern to nursing and would not get the attention that they deserve in a multi-disciplinary committee.

### 24. What type of action can the nurse initiate at the unit level?

When faced with an ethical issue in practice, societal and institutional resources can seem far away. Nurses can develop unit-based activities that assist in preparing for and dealing with ethical issues. A common strategy is to develop unit-based discussions of issues such as pain management or daily unit rounds to assess the potential for ethical dilemmas in the care of specific patients. Nurse managers can add ethical issues as discussion items on the staff meeting agenda, allowing enough time for education and discussion. Finally, standards of care or guidelines should be developed for patients who frequently present with ethical concerns, such as patients with DNR orders.

### 25. What can the nurse do for herself or himself?

In some settings, experts called ethicists are available for consultation. They may have the professional background of a philosopher, lawyer, physician, or nurse with special education in ethics and ethics consultation. They can help the nurse to explore dilemmas and identify the ethical knowledge that best supports the nurse's sense of moral integrity.

Even when unit-based resources or professional consultants are not available, the nurse still has options. Frequently the most important resources are nursing peers in the same critical care unit. What has been their experience? What decision have they made and why? Through such discussions, nurses can explore their own ethical perspectives and knowledge for actual or potential use.

Finally, the nurse can use the literature. Case studies can provide direction or clarification If the dilemma happens once in the nurse's practice, it probably will happen again. Ethical analysis of issues such as allocation of resources, DNR orders, and pain management also can be helpful.

### 26. What does all of this mean to me as a critical care nurse?

Making an ethical decision is rarely easy. Differences in professional power relations, feelings of inarticulateness, and struggling with the right thing to do are common to the process. Knowledge of ethics, ethical decision-making, and available resources offer a meaningful start for the critical care nurse who is seeking to maintain moral integrity in times of change.

### BIBLIOGRAPHY

1. American Nurses Association: Code of Ethics with Interpretive Statements. Washington, DC: American Nurses Association, 1985.
2. Caswell D, Omery A: The dying patient in the critical care setting: Making the critical difference. AACN Clin Issues Crit Care Nurs 1:179–186, 1990.
3. Dock S: The relationship of the nurse to the doctor and the doctor to the nurse. Am J Nurs 17:392–395, 1917.
4. Omery A: Values, moral reasoning, and ethics. Nurs Clin North Am 24:499–508, 1989.
5. Omery A., Henneman E., Billet B, et al: Ethical issues in hospital-based nursing practice. J Cardiovasc Nurs 9(3): 43–53, 1995.
6. Viens DC: A history of nursing's code of ethics. Nurs Outlook 37:45–49, 1989.

# INDEX

Page numbers in **boldface type** indicate complete chapters.